Skin
Moisturization

Compliments of Dove®

Dove, a trusted source for
advanced skincare for over 45 years

COSMETIC SCIENCE AND TECHNOLOGY

Series Editor

ERIC JUNGERMANN

Jungermann Associates, Inc.
Phoenix, Arizona

ADDITIONAL VOLUMES IN PREPARATION

Skin
Moisturization

edited by

James J. Leyden

University of Pennsylvania School of Medicine
Philadelphia, Pennsylvania

Anthony V. Rawlings

Unilever Research
Bebington, Wirral, United Kingdom

MARCEL DEKKER, INC.   NEW YORK · BASEL

ISBN: 0-8247-0643-9

This book is printed on acid-free paper.

Headquarters
Marcel Dekker, Inc.
270 Madison Avenue, New York, NY 10016
tel: 212-696-9000; fax: 212-685-4540

Eastern Hemisphere Distribution
Marcel Dekker AG
Hutgasse 4, Postfach 812, CH-4001 Basel, Switzerland
tel: 41-61-261-8482; fax: 41-61-261-8896

World Wide Web
http://www.dekker.com

The publisher offers discounts on this book when ordered in bulk quantities. For more information, write to Special Sales/Professional Marketing at the headquarters address above.

Current printing (last digit):
10 9 8 7 6 5 4 3 2 1

PRINTED IN THE UNITED STATES OF AMERICA

Series Introduction

The Cosmetic Science and Technology series was conceived to permit discussion of a broad range of current knowledge and theories in the field. The series is composed of books either written by one or more authors or edited with multiple contributors. Authorities from industry, academia, and the government are participating in writing these books. The purpose of this series is to cover the many facets of cosmetic science and technology. Topics are drawn from a wide spectrum of disciplines ranging from chemistry, to physics, to biochemistry, and include analytical and consumer evaluations, safety, efficacy, toxicity, and regulatory questions. Organic, inorganic, physical, and polymer chemistry, emulsion and lipid technology, microbiology, dermatology, and toxicology all play important roles in cosmetic science.

There is little commonality in the scientific methods, processes, and formulations required for the wide variety of cosmetics and toiletries in the market. Products range from preparations for hair care, oral care, and skin care to lipsticks, nail polishes and extenders, deodorants, and body powders and aerosols, to quasi-pharmaceutical over-the-counter products such as antiperspirants, dandruff shampoos, antimicrobial soaps, and acne and sunscreen products.

Cosmetics and toiletries represent a highly diversified field involving many subsections of science and "art." Even in these days of high technology, art and intuition continue to play an important part in the development of formulations, their evaluation, the selection of raw materials, and, perhaps most importantly, the successful marketing of new products. The move toward the application of more sophisticated scientific methodologies that gained momentum in the 1980s has grown in such areas as claim substantiation, safety testing, product testing, and chemical analysis and has led to a better understanding of the properties of skin and hair. Molecular modeling techniques are beginning to be applied to data obtained in skin sensory studies.

Emphasis in the Cosmetic Science and Technology series is placed on reporting the current status of cosmetic technology and science, changing regulatory climates, and historical reviews. The series has grown to over 20 books dealing with the constantly changing technologies and trends in the cosmetic industry, including globalization. Several of the books have been translated into Japanese and Chinese. Contributions range from highly sophisticated and scientific treatises to primers, practical applications, and pragmatic presentations. Authors are encouraged to present their own concepts, as well as established theories. Contributors have been asked not to shy away from fields that are in a state of transition, nor to hesitate to present detailed discussions of their own work. Our intention is to develop the series into a collection of critical surveys and ideas covering diverse phases of the cosmetic industry.

Skin Moisturizers, the twenty-fifth book published in the series, represents a truly global effort. The 28 chapters cover the following areas: the stratum corneum and epidermal biology, xerotic skin conditions, efficacy of moisturizers and moisturizing ingredients, evaluation methodologies, formulation, and safety and regulatory considerations. Ten chapters have been contributed by authors from the United States, nine from the United Kingdom, four from Japan, and the remainder from France, Germany, Italy, and Belgium.

Skin moisturization and moisturizers represent the dominant growth area in cosmetics and toiletries, reflecting the consumer's perpetual interest in looking young. Youthful, healthy skin is perceived as soft, moisturized, and free of wrinkles. Moisturizing products have become the proverbial "hope in a bottle" resulting in the creation of thousands of products and moisturizing claims. This interest in youthful skin becomes even more important as the population ages and concerns over dry skin conditions increase. Practical formulation chemists have long realized that there are two basic mechanisms perceived as moisturization: hydration with water-miscible agents (glycerine is the classical example) and occlusion (classically, petrolatum). The concept of moisturization is, of course, far more complicated. The stratum corneum is recognized as a heterogeneous system of protein-enriched cells embedded in lipid-laden intercellular domains. It is an epidermal barrier governing water penetration and loss, cohesion, and desquamation. The dependence of skin conditioning on the lipids in these systems is due to the fact that essential fatty acids play an important role, together with the natural moisturizing factor, a mixture of hydroscopic water-soluble substances, such as lactic acid and PCA. In addition, collagen, hyaluronic acid, and elastin play a role in these systems. This book identifies these new concepts, increases our understanding of the skin and skin moisturization, and provides the scientific basis of skin moisturization.

I would like to thank the contributors for participating in this project and particularly the editors, Drs. James Leyden and Anthony Rawlings for conceiving, organizing, and coordinating this book. Special thanks are extended to Sandra Beberman and the editorial and production staff at Marcel Dekker, Inc. Finally, I thank my wife, Eva, without whose constant support and editorial help I would not have undertaken this project.

Eric Jungermann, Ph.D.

Preface

The focus of this book is the scientific basis of skin moisturization. The contents range from biological aspects of the skin through active ingredients and their formulation, evaluation methodology, and the regulatory and safety aspects of skin moisturizers. This book will be an invaluable resource for dermatologists, cosmetic scientists, and clinical scientists interested in treatment of xerotic skin conditions. Each chapter reviews the relevant literature in the particular area and gives an up-to-date account of recent research findings. The biology of the epidermis and stratum corneum is the subject of intense review, as well as changes in structure and function in a variety of xerotic skin conditions. Overviews of clinical and consumer testing approaches together with ex vivo evaluation procedures are presented in the evaluation section. The action efficacy and formulation of various moisturizing ingredients are also covered, including emollients, humectants, ceramides and other barrier lipids, alphahydroxyacids, and enzymes. The final section discusses safety and regulatory guidelines in the industry.

This book is a result of contributions by experts in their own areas and is the work of an international team. The authors represent a cross-section of the scientific community in academia as well as industrial research. Cosmetic scientists, dermatologists, and researchers will find this book a valuable, in-depth account of skin moisturization.

James J. Leyden
Anthony V. Rawlings

Contents

FORMULATION

SAFETY AND REGULATORY

Contributors

Kavssery P. Ananthapadmanabhan, Ph.D. Principal Research Scientist, Skin Care and Cleansing Department, Unilever Research, Edgewater Laboratory, Edgewater, New Jersey

Steve Barton, M.Sc., C.Biol. Skincare Scientific Adviser, Strategic Marketing Unit, The Boots Company, Nottingham, United Kingdom

Enzo Berardesca, M.D. Department of Clinical Dermatology, University of Pavia, San Matteo, Pavia, Italy

Lynn Blaikie, Ph.D. Unilever Research, Colworth Laboratory, Sharnbrook, Bedford, United Kingdom

Steven S. Braddon, Ph.D. Senior Research Consumer Test Coordinator, Department of Consumer Science, Unilever Home and Personal Care North America, Trumbull, Connecticut

Prem Chandar, Ph.D. Research Scientist, Skin Care and Cleansing Department, Unilever Research, Edgewater Laboratory, Edgewater, New Jersey

Mitsuhiro Denda, Ph.D. Research Scientist, Skin Biology Research Laboratories, Shiseido Life Science Research Center, Yokohama, Japan

Anna Di Nardo, Ph.D., M.D. Department of Dermatology, University of Modena, Modena, Italy

Christopher Flower, M.Sc., Ph.D., C.Biol. M.I.Biol. Head of Safety and Toxicology, The Cosmetic, Toiletry, and Perfumery Association, London, United Kingdom

Joachim Fluhr, Ph.D. University of Pavia, San Matteo, Pavia, Italy, and University of California, San Francisco, California

Ruby Ghadially, MB, Ch.B., F.R.C.P.(C) Veterans Administration Medical Center and University of California School of Medicine, San Francisco, California

Miklos Ghyczy, Ph.D. Director, Applications Research, Nattermann Phospholipid GmbH, Cologne, Germany

Paolo U. Giacomoni, Ph.D. Executive Director, Research and Development, Clinique Laboratories, Inc., Melville, New York

Veroniqué Goffin, M.D., Ph.D. Department of Dermatology, University Medical Center Sart Tilman, Liège, Belgium

Gary L. Grove, Ph.D. KGL Skin Study Center, Broomall, Pennsylvania

Clive R. Harding, M.Sc. Research Biochemist, Department of Cell and Molecular Biology and Biorecognition, Unilever Research, Colworth Laboratory, Sharnbrook, Bedford, United Kingdom

Walter M. Holleran, Ph.D. Associate Adjunct Professor, Department of Dermatology and Pharmaceutical Chemistry, University of California, San Francisco, San Francisco, California

Genji Imokawa, Ph.D. Kao Biological Science Laboratories, Haga, Tochigi, Japan

Gwendolyn S. Jarrett, B.S. Manager, Consumer Science, Department of Research and Development, Unilever Home and Personal Care North America, Trumbull, Connecticut

Anthony W. Johnson, Ph.D. Manager, Skin/Bioscience, Global Technology Center, Unilever Home and Personal Care North America, Trumbull, Connecticut

Robert Lavker, Ph.D. Department of Dermatology, University of Pennsylvania School of Medicine, Philadelphia, Pennsylvania

Jean Luc Lévêque, Ph.D. L'Oréal, Clichy, France

James J. Leyden, Ph.D. Department of Dermatology, University of Pennsylvania School of Medicine, Philadelphia, Pennsylvania

Daniel Maes, Ph.D. Vice President, Department of Biological Research, Estee Lauder, Melville, New York

Thomas Mammone, Ph.D. Director, Department of Skin Biology, Estee Lauder, Melville, New York

Kenneth Marenus, Ph.D. Estee Lauder, Melville, New York

Takuji Masunaga, Ph.D. Manager, Fundamental Research Laboratory, Kosé Corporation, Tokyo, Japan

Gopinathan K. Menon, Ph.D. Senior Research Fellow and Head, Skin Biology Research, Global Research and Development, Avon Products, Inc., Suffern, New York

Neelam Muizzuddin, Ph.D. Director, Biological Research Department, Estee Lauder, Melville, New York

Alejandra M. Muñoz, M.Sc. President, International Resources for Insights and Solutions, Mountainside, New Jersey

Gregory Nole, B.Sc. Manager, Biophysical Evaluation Department, Unilever Home and Personal Care North America, Trumbull, Connecticut

Lars Norlén, Ph.D. Department of Physics, University of Geneva, Geneva, Switzerland

Marc Paye, Ph.D. Colgate-Palmolive, Milmort, Belgium

Edward Pelle, B.S., M.S. Principal Scientist, Research and Development, Estee Lauder, Melville, New York

Gérald E. Piérard, M.D., Ph.D.   Professor, Department of Dermatology, University Medical Center Sart Tilman, Liège, Belgium

Claudine Piérard-Franchimont, M.D., Ph.D.   Department of Dermatology, University Medical Center Sart Tilman, Liège, Belgium

Elizabeth Pierce, B.A.   Clinical Research Specialist, KGL Skin Study Center, Broomall, Pennsylvania

David J. Pocalyko, Ph.D.   Category Platform Manager, Department of Skin Bioscience, Unilever Research, Edgewater Laboratory, Edgewater, New Jersey

Gail B. Rattinger, Ph.D.   Category Platform Manager, Skin Care and Cleansing Department, Unilever Research, Edgewater Laboratory, Edgewater, New Jersey

Anthony V. Rawlings, Ph.D.   Science Area Leader, Biosciences Department, Unilever Research, Port Sunlight Laboratory, Bebington, Wirral, United Kingdom

Didier Saint-Leger, Ph.D.   Staff Prospective, Research and Development, L'Oréal, Clichy, France

Junko Sato, Ph.D.   Shiseido Research Center, Yokohama, Japan

Ian R. Scott, Ph.D.   Chief Scientist, Unilever Research, Edgewater Laboratory, Edgewater, New Jersey

Frederick Anthony Simion, Ph.D.   Research Principal, Product Development, The Andrew Jergens Company, Cincinnati, Ohio

Rose Marie Sparacio   Director, Clinical Research, Biological Research Division, Estee Lauder, Melville, New York

David C. Story, B.S., M.S., R.Ph.   Associate Director, Product Development, The Andrew Jergens Company, Cincinnati, Ohio

Kumar Subramanyan, Ph.D.   Research Scientist, Skin Care and Cleansing Department, Unilever Research, Edgewater Laboratory, Edgewater, New Jersey

Vladimir Vacata, Ph.D.   Biophysicist, Institute for Hygiene and Public Health, University of Bonn, Bonn, Germany

Allan Watkinson, Ph.D., D.I.C.   Research Scientist, Department of Skin and Hair Biology, Unilever Research, Colworth Laboratory, Sharnbrook, Bedford, United Kingdom

Philip W. Wertz, Ph.D.   Professor, Dows Institute for Dental Research, University of Iowa, Iowa City, Iowa

Simon Young   Head of Regulatory Affairs, Unilever Research, Port Sunlight Laboratory, Bebington, Wirral, United Kingdom

Charles Zerweck, Ph.D.   KGL Skin Study Center, Broomall, Pennsylvania

1

The Skin Moisturizer Marketplace

Anthony W. Johnson
Unilever Home and Personal Care North America
Trumbull, Connecticut

1 INTRODUCTION

Nearly everyone has used a skin moisturizer product. In fact many people use a moisturizer every day of their life. Moisturizers are so familiar we seldom think to ask "what is a moisturizer?" A visit to the local supermarket, convenience store, or pharmacy should surely provide the answer. And, yes, the products on the moisturizer shelves do appear to be much the same, a variety of creams and lotions. But why are there so many different creams and lotions? And what are all these other moisturizers? There are sprays and foams, gels and serums, oils and jelly, balms and lipsticks, foundations and mascara, and even sunscreens, all labeled as moisturizing. And there are more. Back in the cleansing aisle we find bar soaps and shower liquids described as moisturizers. Moisturizing baby wipes and moisturizing tissues are on display in the paper and disposable products section. In hair care we encounter moisturizing shampoos and conditioners and some moisturizing hair colorants. There are even some moisturizing antiperspirants! It seems that nearly everything on the personal care shelves is moisturizing, so what is a moisturizer?

Each of the products mentioned has a label (pack copy) that describes the product, lists the ingredients, provides instructions for use, and describes the benefits to be expected. With all this information it should be easy to discover what a

1

moisturizer is. However, the mass of pack label information is often confusing for the average consumer. The concept of a product to keep skin moisturized is simple enough, but why are there so many different products to do this? How can a consumer decide which product to buy? Some moisturizers appear to contain one or more special moisturizing ingredients, whereas other products that claim to be highly effective skin moisturizers do not. Some moisturizers are described as natural in a way that suggests that naturalness is important. But many moisturizers seem not to be natural and yet are apparently excellent moisturizing products. Then there are moisturizers described for different types of skin, for different parts of the body, for different times of the day, for younger or older consumers, and for different ethnic groups. New products keep appearing and old favorites seem to disappear for no particular reason. With such a vast array of products, so many different ingredients in these products, and so much information about products—in advertising, in women's magazines, and now everywhere on the internet—the marketplace for moisturizers can seem bewildering.

In fact there is structure to the moisturizer market and there are reasons for all the different products, although not very obvious ones. The purpose of this chapter is to explain the moisturizer market and why there are so many different moisturizing products. Explaining consumer needs and the structure, dynamics, and driving forces of the moisturizer marketplace will do this, providing a backcloth to the detailed scientific and technical chapters of the book.

2 THE MARKETPLACE

Products for the care of skin are part of a larger category of consumer products for personal care and hygiene. Personal care embraces skin care as well as hair and oral care products, with skin care the largest of the three categories. Skin care is big business. The global skincare industry was valued at $20 billion in 1997, with facial care products accounting for $10.6 billion, over 50% [1]. There was enormous growth of the personal care market in the last two decades of the 20th century, building on the continuous evolution of skin care over 50 years or more [2]. That growth continues, fueled by intense global competition to satisfy ever-increasing consumer expectations. As we shall see, consumer expectations are driven by the claims and promises of skin product manufacturers and encouraged by health and beauty writers in a plethora of specialist magazines. Since 1999, more and more of this communication has reached consumers via the internet, where the quality of information is widely variable. The difficulty for consumers seeking information on the world wide web is to distinguish accurate information from misinformation and fantasy.

The personal care market is segmented according to classes of trade. There are several segmentation schemes but the main practical divisions of the marketplace are (1) mass market, (2) prestige, and (3) direct sale. There are subdivisions of these segments that vary around the world, particularly between regions with "mature" markets and those with so-called developing and emerging (D&E) markets. Nevertheless, the main segments can be found in all countries.

2.1 Mass Market Products

Mass market is usually divided into *food* (the major supermarket chains), *drug* (the major pharmacy chains), and *mass* (all other retail outlets). Historically mass market outlets were the local store selling a full range of domestic goods at a price the working consumer could afford. Skin care products like other products were always branded products from manufacturers. Each store stocked a limited range of products and the marketplace was supplied by a relatively small number of manufacturers. During the 1960s to 1980s there was an expansion in the number of manufacturers followed by contraction and consolidation of the big players in the 1990s. By 1999, a handful of multibillion dollar major international companies dominated the global skin care market [3,4].

With the advent of supermarkets it was not long before the emergence of a new category of product, the store brand, or distributor own brands (DOBs). Supermarket chains recognized that their national sales networks gave them the opportunity to sell their own products alongside the branded products of manufacturers at a discounted price. Supermarkets usually obtain their own brand products from custom manufacturers. Some manufacturers have developed lines of products at budget prices specifically to compete with the store brands as low cost products. Store brands are typically good basic products, but manufacturer branded products usually have a little extra in performance or esthetic qualities. However, the branded products cost a little more. The consumer has a choice.

2.2 Prestige Products

Prestige products are the specialist skin care products sold in department stores at individual counter areas for each manufacturer. The counters are staffed by "cosmetic consultants" who provide one-on-one skin care advice and product recommendations to consumers. Prestige manufacturers sell mostly face care products, color cosmetics, and fragrances. Most prestige moisturizers are face care products. Unlike the mass market, there are relatively few hand and body moisturizers in prestige, a reflection that face care is the overwhelming priority for most women. Similarly, prestige manufactures sell facial cleansers but relatively few body and hand cleansing products. Most specialist skin care products are good moisturizing formulations containing additional ingredients intended to promote a particular skin benefit. Many specialist moisturizers are intended to help reduce the visible signs of skin aging—lines, wrinkles, laxity, uneven pigmentation. Another term for prestige products is upscale, implying something better than regular mass market products. Prestige products certainly cost a great deal more than mass market products, but there is no simple measure to assess relative value. However, prestige products are typically more complex than mass market products and are sold in more elaborate containers and packaging with the promise of a wider range of skin benefits. Many women see prestige products as special and likely to do more for their skin than the less expensive mass brands. There is an emotional element in the consumer assessment of prestige products. Using a special moisturizer can make a difference to self-image and confidence.

2.3 Upper Mass

At one time there was a very clear separation between mass market skin care products and the specialist products in prestige. However, during the 1990s manufacturers of mass market products developed ranges of products including moisturizers that offered a promise and performance that was previously the exclusive domain of the prestige sector. These products are more expensive than the basic mass market products and offer a broader range of skin care benefits. This sector of mass market skin care is sometimes referred to as upper mass. Examples of upper mass products in the year 2000 were L'Oreal's Plenitude range, Ponds's Age Defying range, and Oil of Olay.

2.4 Direct Sale

The direct sale segment of the market includes those manufacturers who sell direct to consumers rather than through a retail store. Avon is the archetypal direct sale organization, with a long-standing international direct sale business. The traditional direct sale operation is based on a network of representatives who interact directly with consumers. Mail order from catalogs is another method of direct sale that has operated for many years. In advanced markets, with the United States leading the way, catalog sales are being progressively replaced by direct order from TV. Special programs, known as infomercials, have evolved that are part advertising and part information, intended to induce the consumer to place a telephone order from home. The best infomercials are valuable sources of skin care information and education for the consumer, but there are others that peddle unsubstantiated claims, folklore, and other misinformation. As is often the case in the skin care marketplace, it is difficult for the average consumer to distinguish good information from bad. This is a major issue with the latest channel for direct sale of skin care products, the internet. However, web sites of major manufacturers are usually reliable because these manufacturers have the resources to get it right and also the business imperative to protect their image and reputation.

2.5 The Breakdown of Market Segmentation

As the marketplace evolves rapidly in the internet world of 2001 and beyond, the boundaries between skin care categories become less clear. Mass marketers are selling via the internet, direct sale companies are entering the retail arena, and prestige marketers are setting up specialist stores outside of department stores [5].

3 REGIONAL VARIATION OF SKIN CARE MARKETS

Dynamics underlying the continuing development of skin care markets around the world are economic prosperity and scientific progress. Mature markets like the United States, Japan, and Western Europe are highly developed with a wide range of products available to consumers through multiple levels of trade. Nevertheless, growth of these markets continues, driven by innovation, prosperity, and ever-increasing longevity. As people live longer they give greater priority to maintaining a youthful appearance. At one time it was assumed that skin aging was inevitable, that lines and wrinkles, sags and bags, were unavoidable. We now realize that a great deal of skin aging change is due to environmental factors, particularly ultraviolet radiation, and is therefore avoidable [6,7]. Even if not avoided, we now have the capability to eliminate many of the unwanted signs of skin aging using laser resurfacing of skin [8]. The improvement in skin appearance from laser surgery can be very dramatic [9]. Now that the laser has shown us that old skin can be rejuvenated to look and function as it was decades earlier, consumer expectations have been raised. Many consumers believe that it will not be long before topical skin care products will achieve the impressive results obtained with lasers. Belief is strong that there is a fountain of youth after all, just waiting to be discovered. This belief is a key driving force in the skin care market place. It is the reason why so many consumers are prepared to keep on trying each new technology in skin care. This strong consumer pull provides an incentive for manufacturers and stimulates intensive innovation of skin care products [10].

In D&E markets such as China, Eastern Europe, parts of Africa, and South America, the skin care marketplace includes all of the classes of trade described but with a different balance between sectors compared to developed markets. Mass market outlets predominate with a concentration on low price/discount products. Prestige is limited to a few department stores in major cities. In the 1990s the D&E markets were where the developed markets had been 30–40 years earlier, but catching up very fast, propelled by modern communications and advances in technology.

The development of mass communications was a critical factor in the explosive growth of the skin care and moisturizer market in the last half of the 20th century. The 50 years that spanned the discovery of DNA in 1953 to the mapping of the entire human genome by the year 2000 saw the skin care market progress from bars of soap, basic moisturizers, and make-up to a sophisticated, complex, highly structured, multibillion dollar segment of the consumer product marketplace. In 1950 there was one product for everyone; by year 2000 there were thousands of products to chose from. The competitive advantage of providing consumer choice led to highly customized products. The multiplication and diversity of product types and compositions have been linked to accelerating scientific progress and increased understanding of consumer needs and motivations. As described later, each variation of need creates an opportunity for a new or different product.

The wide choice now available to consumers is bewildering to many, and regrettably the information available to help them make their choices is not always reliable. To understand the moisturizer marketplace we need to understand the consumer need for moisturizers and the ways in which moisturizer products satisfy these needs.

4 THE CARE OF NORMAL SKIN

The skin is without doubt the most complex organ of the human body and the one with most need for everyday care and attention. The approximately two square meters of skin covering the average adult body provides a remarkable protective interface with the outside world, both physical and immunological. But skin does much more than protect. It is our means for adjusting to variations in environmental temperatures through elegant controls that regulate the microcirculation. The skin provides us with our ability to feel and sense ourselves, and others, and our environment, though touch, pain, temperature, and pressure receptors. The appearance and feel of skin are central to human interpersonal perception and attraction, while pheromones released on the skin are drivers of sexual attraction and activity. Our skin plays a vital role in maintaining our physical and mental health [11]. Keeping this most important tissue in best condition has many advantages for the individual, and therefore the care of skin has always been a priority of human behavior in all races and all cultures throughout history.

Cleansing and moisturizing are the two basic processes for keeping skin in good condition [12]. Cleansing is necessary to remove environmental dirt, skin secretions, and microorganisms that would otherwise produce odors and disease. Cleansing is more than keeping skin clean, it is a contribution to keeping skin healthy. Important as cleansers are for keeping skin clean and healthy, they are potentially damaging to the skin's outer protective layer, the stratum corneum. Cleansers deplete the stratum corneum of water by disturbing the skin's normal mechanisms for maintaining optimum water content [13]. Cleansing is therefore a major factor creating the need for moisturizing products. However, it is not only cleansers that rob the skin of moisture: UV damage, environmental factors (water, detergents), age, and skin diseases can all come into play (see Sec. 7). Moisturizers are definitely needed once the stratum corneum thickens and becomes flaky and rough, otherwise there can be rapid deterioration with cracking, inflammation, exudation, and bleeding.

5 NATURAL MECHANISMS OF SKIN MOISTURIZATION

As detailed in several reviews [14,15] and explained in more detail in other chapters of this book, the structure of the stratum corneum is often likened to the bricks and mortar of a wall. The bricks are the dead skin cells of the stratum corneum (corneocytes), and these are embedded in a matrix of intracellular lipid bilayers (the mortar). Corneocytes are flat pancakelike protein structures approximately 1 µm thick and 50–80 µm in diameter. The protein matrix of corneocytes contains a specific mix of hygroscopic low molecular weight compounds that keep the corneocytes hydrated. The main components of this mix, collectively known as skin's natural moisturizing factor (NMF), are lactic acid, urea, various salts, and amino acids derived from degradation of the protein filaggrin in the lower regions of the stratum corneum. There are three types of lipid that combine to form the intercellular lipid matrix of the stratum corneum. These are fatty acids, ceramides, and cholesterol. Each lipid type is bipolar with a hydrophilic (water loving) head group/region and a hydrophobic (water hating) side chain/region. When thrown together these lipids spontaneously form alternating layers of hydrophilic and hydrophobic regions. It is these alternating lipid bilayers that form the water barrier of the stratum corneum. The layers control the movement of water through the stratum corneum, measured as trans-epidermal water loss (TEWL) and also form a seal around each of the corneocytes, locking in the NMF, which being water soluble would otherwise diffuse away.

Distilling this to the essential components, skin has two mechanisms for retaining moisture:

1. Natural moisturizing factor within the protein matrix of corneocytes
2. Triple lipid bilayers around and between corneocytes

Moisture is required in the stratum corneum, particularly in the superficial layers

1. To keep the stratum corneum soft, supple, and flexible
2. To activate desquamation (exfoliation)

Desquamation, the shedding of corneocytes from the skin surface, is an enzymic process (degradation of desmosomes) which requires an optimum water activity. If desquamation is impaired, superficial corneocytes remain attached to those below and pile up as visible flakes on the skin surface and are responsible for the characteristic dullness, white scaly appearance, roughness, and flaking of dry skin.

6   CLEANSING CREATES NEED FOR MOISTURIZERS

Cleansers are of two types, surfactant based or oil/solvent based. Surfactant types are most common and are used for general cleansing. Oil- and solvent-based cleansers have specific applications such as removal of make-up, engine grime, oil-based paints, and other oily soils. Surfactant- and oil-based cleansers damage the skin in two ways. By somewhat different mechanisms, both can disturb, dissolve, and remove the intercellular lipid bilayers of the stratum corneum and both can interact with and damage the protein composition of corneocytes, the "dead" cells of the stratum corneum [16]. Damage to corneocytes releases and washes away the NMF dispersed throughout the protein matrix of the cells. In this way the cleansing process tends to remove the two skin components essential to keep the outer stratum corneum hydrated, the lipids and NMF. Not all cleansers and cleansing routines are bad for skin. The extent to which cleansers cause dry skin depends upon the formulation of the cleanser and the duration and frequency of skin contact. Repetitive and excessive contact with cleansers and water, as can be the case for nurses, mothers with a number of infants, etc., can be very drying and irritating to skin. On the other hand, limited contact with mild cleansers can help to maintain skin in good condition.

The biological and physicochemical mechanisms by which optimum hydration of the stratum corneum facilitates desquamation and maintains skin flexibility will be described in other chapters. Likewise the mechanisms of surfactant skin interaction are described elsewhere [17]. But it is the understanding of these mechanisms that spawned the wide range of "moisturizing cleansers" available in the skin marketplace by the year 2000.

Manufacturers have used two strategies to address the issue that cleansing damages and dries the skin:

1.   To formulate less damaging cleansing products
2.   To add moisturizing ingredients to cleansers to compensate for damage

The first branded cleansers to become widely available were bars of soap in the late 1800s. Soap is the sodium salt of fatty acids, made by adding caustic soda to triglycerides of plant or animal origin [18]. The triglycerides are hydrolyzed forming soap molecules and releasing glycerol. The early products were crude blocks of unrefined soap, promoted more for washing clothing than for cleansing the body. Soap is a very effective cleanser but also very effective at stripping lipids and NMF from the skin [19]. The effectiveness, lathering action, and drying effects of soap are all related to chain length. C12 chain lengths are best for lathering but also the most irritating [20]. Longer chain lengths are less soluble, making them less irritating, less drying, and more resistant to mushing in the soap bowl. Bars of soap usually contain a range of chain lengths, often in proportions of 80/20 or 70/30 longer chain (C16/18 and above)–to–shorter chain (C12/14) soap molecules.

Before considering how the search for less drying and more moisturizing cleansers led to the diversity of cleanser products in the current marketplace it is appropriate to switch attention to skin moisturizers. Moisturizers arose from a consumer need to treat and prevent dry skin, but over the years the term moisturizer and the technology of moisturizers has evolved to address all aspects of skin care required to keep normal skin in healthy youthful condition. However, dry skin remains the most common problem of normal skin and if left unchecked opens the door to irritation, impaired function, and accelerated skin aging. In the consumer products marketplace "skin aging" is not a statement of chronology but an expression of premature decline of function and appearance.

7   SKIN MOISTURIZERS

In simplest terms a moisturizer is a product designed to restore and maintain optimum hydration of the stratum corneum. Notwithstanding the thousands of moisturizer products available to consumers there are only two cosmetic ways to do this:

1. The first way is to increase water-holding capacity of the stratum corneum by external application of hygroscopic ingredients, collectively known as humectants. These ingredients serve to replace skin NMF that has been washed away or otherwise depleted. Humectants act in the same way as NMF, and indeed some of the humectants commonly used in moisturizers are components of the skin NMF, e.g., lactic acid and urea.

2. The second way is to trap water in the stratum corneum by depositing an impermeable layer of water-insoluble oily material on the skin surface. Oily materials mimic the effect of the natural lipid bilayers of the skin to restrict evaporation from the surface and to seal NMF/humectants in corneocytes. These oily emollient materials also help to restore impaired water barrier function in regions where natural skin lipids have been lost.

Oily materials that form stable continuous films on the skin surface, e.g., petrolatum, are known as occlusives; they occlude the skin surface. There are other oils and lipids used in moisturizers that are less sticky and greasy than petrolatum, but also less effective at sealing the stratum corneum. These other fatty materials are often referred to as emollients, reflecting their ability to render skin soft, supple, and flexible by lubricating and moisturizing. The term emollient is also used to describe fully formulated products containing oils and lipids. Fats and lipids are terms used interchangeably by cosmetic scientists. "Oil" and "emollient" are the descriptors used most commonly on product packaging because "fat" and "lipid" have negative connotations for many consumers.

Emulsions are the most effective way to combine oils and water-soluble ingredients in a single product suitable for application to skin. Stable emulsions are formed using ingredients called emulsifiers. Simple emulsions are moisturizing, but adding a humectant ingredient to an emulsion greatly enhances moisturizing effectiveness.

Already we see that there is scope for a wide range of moisturizer formulations based on combinations of many oils, many humectants, and different types of emulsion. It could be imagined that there would be little reason to choose between one emulsion moisturizer over the next and therefore no need for multiple variations in composition of products in the marketplace. In fact the ability to adapt and tweak compositions to achieve an almost endless variety of product formulations has enabled manufacturers to customize moisturizers to meet the many variations of consumer need and consumer preference. These variations relate to the following main factors:

1. *Esthetic preference.* Consumers vary greatly in their appreciation of product attributes, particularly product in-use properties like product texture, speed of absorption, rub-in, and after-use feel. Given that many products are similar in delivery of actual skin benefit it is often esthetic factors which ultimately determine purchase intent. Some consumers like heavy products and some like light products, while some are greatly influenced by fragrance. Because fragrance preference is very personal and very important to consumers it is often the attribute that drives consumer selection of personal care products. Many moisturizers are only lightly perfumed so that they appeal to the widest possible range of consumers. Given that skin benefit technology in the marketplace is usually at par between major manufacturers over any extended period of time, it is often esthetics and claims that determine the consumer's choice of skin moisturizer product.

2. *Perceptions of product performance.* Consumers will chose what they think works. Perception of performance is complex, related to actual performance (perceived benefit) and the impact of concept and communication (how compelling is the product proposition, how appealing and convincing are the product claims). For example, many women who believe that dry skin leads to wrinkles perceive moisturizers as essential for maintaining youthful skin condition. Note that using moisturizing products does not prevent wrinkling except for

those products that contain sunscreens. In the consumer product marketplace it is what the consumer thinks/believes about performance that drives preference and purchase. Therefore perception of performance is ultimately paramount, notwithstanding all the clinical evaluations that may be conducted by the manufacturers [21]. Perception of skin problems and of product performance is influenced by external factors. For example, perception of skin oiliness is increased with increased temperature and humidity. Some individuals who have dry skin in winter may feel that their skin is oily in the summer.

3. *Skin type.* Facial skin is usually categorized as *normal, oily, dry,* or *combination.* Superimposed on these skin types is skin sensitivity—with approximately 40–50% of female consumers classifying their facial skin as sensitive [22,23]. Body skin is less variable. The main subdivisions are *dry* and *dry/sensitive.* Individuals with an atopic trait (i.e., have suffered with atopic dermatitis or have it in their family and therefore in their genes) have a tendency toward dry, itchy, and easily irritated skin [24]. Many women experience changes in their skin related to menopause, particularly increased dryness [25,26].

4. *Environment/climate.* As described in the next section, environmental conditions are key drivers of dry skin conditions; heavy duty products are required in very harsh conditions, whereas much lighter products are suitable for milder climates.

5. *Ethnic skin.* The variations of consumer needs for moisturizers related to ethnic origins are less than might be imagined. Although there are several differences in skin physiology between different races [27,28], other than the obvious differences in pigmentation, the mechanisms of dry skin formation are essentially the same in all skin types. However, dry skin once formed impacts dark skin appearance more than lighter skin. Slight dryness that is hardly perceptible on white skin imparts a distinctive gray ashy appearance to black skin. Apart from this and the obvious variations of need for sun protection, it seems that cultural difference more than different skin needs explains the variation of basic product types and attributes seen in different regions of the world [29,30].

6. *Emotional factors.* The fact that perception can play a critical role in consumer perception of product benefits introduces a new element for considering the moisturizer marketplace—there is an emotional component to consumer assessment of product performance and benefits. Therefore, moisturizers like other skin care products are developed to satisfy a mix of functional and emotional needs. The prestige sector in particular seeks to address the emotional component of consumer skin care needs.

7. *Body parts.* Consumer concerns and needs for skin care start with the face and may or may not move to the body. This distinction between face and body is mirrored in the marketplace where there is a clear distinction between face and body (including hands) products. Within the two main categories of face care and body care there are further subdivisions. For face care there are general moisturizing products, eye area moisturizers, and products intended for the neck. For the body there are all-purpose products and then products specific for hand care, foot care, heels and elbows, thigh area, and breasts and chest areas.

8. *Occupation.* Some occupations are more challenging and damaging to skin condition than others. Deep sea fishing and nursing are examples of outdoor and indoor occupations which subject the hands in particular to very drying activities, long periods of soaking in near freezing water for North Atlantic fishermen and multiple hand washes in the case of nurses. These are two somewhat extreme examples but there are many more. Heavy barrier creams are often available in the workplace but also need to be available for general sale. Severe dry skin doesn't observe an eight hour day. Indoor environments can also adversely affect the skin, particularly the drying effects of air conditioning. The work environment is a significant factor determining skin condition for many people [31].

9. *Travel.* While not a major factor in determining product types in the marketplace, it is of interest that air travel moves people from one environment to another more quickly than the ability of their skin to adapt. Skin adjusts its level of NMF to match what is needed in the prevailing environment. In a hot humid environment production of NMF is less than in a cold dry environment. It takes several days for a new level to be established whereas a person flies from a humid to a drying environment in a matter of hours. The drying out starts with the low humidity on the plane, which explains the moisturizing lotion included in the comfort pack provided to first and business class passengers!

10. *Age.* The moisturizer market shows an age segmentation that relates to the changing needs of skin through life. Specific consumer needs for moisturizers have developed within the age spectrum. Youngsters, particularly females, are becoming appearance aware at younger and younger ages. At the other end of the spectrum, we have a new generation of appearance conscious seniors determined to look as young for their age as modern technology will allow [32]. In between, there is a growing appreciation that relationship between skin condition and age is influenced greatly by environmental exposure to skin-dam-

aging forces such as UV from sunlight [33] and, in the case of females, some significant negative changes in skin condition that occur during menopause [34]. These extensions of consumer interest, active involvement, and associated needs provide additional areas of opportunity for skin care manufacturers.

We now start to see why there are so many different moisturizer products in the marketplace even though there are basically only two methods to moisturize skin. The large number of products arises when we factor in all the variables. There are many different types of humectant, occlusive, emollient, and sensory ingredients that impact the skin, as well as emulsifiers and other ingredients of the product base (excipients).

The CTFA *Cosmetic Ingredient Handbook* lists the many thousands of ingredients used in skin care products [35]. There are over 3000 ingredients listed as emollient, humectant, occlusive, or miscellaneous skin conditioning agents. Some of the more widely used of these ingredients are detailed in Table 1. Emollients are defined as cosmetic ingredients which help maintain the soft, smooth, and pliable appearance of skin. Emollients function by their ability to remain on the skin surface or in the stratum corneum to act as lubricants, to reduce flaking, and to improve the skin's appearance. Humectants are cosmetic ingredients intended to increase the water content of the top layers of skin. This group of ingredients includes primary hygroscopic agents employed for this specific purpose. Occlusives are cosmetic ingredients which retard the evaporation of water from the skin surface. By blocking the evaporative loss of water, occlusive materials increase the water content of skin. The miscellaneous group is defined as cosmetic ingredients used to create special effects on skin. This group includes substances believed to enhance the appearance of dry or damaged skin and substantive materials which adhere to the skin to reduce flaking and restore suppleness.

These long lists of ingredients are used in countless combinations and levels to produce the myriad skin care products now available to consumers everywhere. The variations in formula are designed to account for different skin types, different ethnic needs, and different environmental conditions. Further variations are made to achieve differentiated formulations and compelling claims, some functional and some designed to provide empathy with consumer emotional needs. And there are still more variations to tailor products to a particular market segment and for either face care or body care. Leaving aside the detailed arithmetic, it is clear that the number of legitimate product variations is very large. It is an impossible task for the consumer to try more than a small proportion of all these products to decide which might be best suited. Instead, most consumers are guided to the products they purchase by advertising, promotions, and the recommendations of specialist magazines and skin care professionals. These are key drivers of the skin care/moisturizer marketplace and will be reviewed later.

TABLE 1 Widely Used Skin Care Moisturizing and Conditioning Ingredients

Emollients	Humectants	Occlusives	Miscellaneous
Acetylated lanolin	Acetamide MEA	Acetylated castor oil	**Allantoin**
Acetyl trihexyl citrate	Agarose	Acetylated lanolin alcohol	Aloe barbadensis
Avocado sterols	Ammonium lactate	Behenyl isostearate	Arachidonic acid
Butyl myristate	Arginine PCA	C12-18 acid triglyceride	Ascorbic acid
C 14-15 alcohols	Betaine	C20-40 alcohols	Azulene
C 12-13 alkyl ethylhexanoate	Copper PCA	C20-40 alkyl dimethicone	Beta-carotene
Caprylyl glycol	Corn glycerides	C16-36 alkyl stearate	Betaglucan
Cetyl acetate	Diglycereth-7 Malate	Canola oil	Bioflavonoids
Cetyl oleate	Diglycerin	Caprylic/capric triglyceride	Bisabolol
C 14-16 glycol palmitate	Dimethyl imidazolidinone	Cetearyl methicone	Butylene glycol
C 12-20 isoparaffin	Erythritol	Cetyl ricinoleate	Caproyl sphingosine
Diethylhexyl adipate	Glucose	Cholesteryl oleate	Capsaicin
Diethylhexyl malate	Glucuronic acid	C18-70 isoparaffin	Carnitine
Diisodecyl adipate	Glucuronolactone	C20-24 olefin	Carnosine
Dimethicone copolyol	Glutamic acid	C10-18 triglycerides	Ceramides 1/2/3/4/5/1A/6II
Dipropyl adipate	Glycereth-12	Decyl myristate	Cholesterol
Ethylhexyl palmitate	**Glycerin**	**Dimethicone**	Coco-betaine
Ethyl linoleate	Honey extract	Distearyl ether	Collagen
Glyceryl dioleate	Hydrolyzed wheat starch	Glycol dioleate	Dimethicone copolyol acetate
Glyceryl ricinoleate	Hydroxyethyl sorbitol	Hexyldecyl isostearate	Gelatin
Glyceryl stearates	Lactamide	Hydrogenated castor oil	Glucose
Glycol palmitate	Lactic acid	Hydrogenated lanolin	Glycosphingolipids
Glycol stearate	Maltitol	Isocetyl myristate	Hyaluronic acid

Hexyl laurate	Melibiose	Lanolin linoleate	Hydrolyzed keratin
Isocetyl alcohol	Pantolactone	Lauryl cocoate	Hydrolyzed soy starch
Isodecyl stearate	PCA	**Mineral Oil**	Isodecyl salicylate
Isohexyl palmitate	PEG-10 propylene glycol	Myristyl myristate	Lactic acid
Isopropyl myristate	Polyglucuronic acid	Neatsfool oil	Linoleic acid
Lanolin	Polyglycerin-10	Octyldodecyl stearate	Maltodextrin
Methyl palmitate	Potassium lactate	Oleyl linoleate	Methyl nicotinate
Myristyl propionate	Propylene glycol	Palm kernel wax	Milk protein
PEG-4 lanolate	Saccharide hydrolysate	Paraffin	Mineral salts
PEG-5 tristearyl citrate	Sea salt	Pentaerythrityl tetracocoate	Niacin
Polyglyceryl-6 oleate	Seasame amino acids	**Petrolatum**	Papain
Polyglyceryl-2 triisostearate	Sodium aspartate	Propylene glycol dioleate	PEG-5 tall oil sterol
PPG-20 cetyl ether	Sodium malate	Shark liver oil	Phospholipids
PPG-4 laureth-2	Sodium PCA	Soybean lipid	Retinol
Propylene glycol linoleate	Sodium polyaspartate	Squalane	Salicylic acid
Squalene	Sorbitol	Tall oil	Skin lipids
Sucrose oleate	TEA-lactate	Tocopherol	Superoxide dismutase
Sunflower seed oil glycerides	Triglycereth-7 citrate	Trihexyldecyl citrate	Theophylline
Tall oil glycerides	Urea	Triisostearin	Tocopheryl acetate
Tridecyl stearate	Xylose	Vegetable oil	Tyrosine
Wheat germ glycerides			Ubiquinone
			Undecylenyl alcohol
			Zinc gluconate
928[a]	117[a]	507[a]	1489[a]

[a]Total number of this type of ingredient listed in CTFA Cosmetic Ingredients Directory.

Note: Bold indicates ingredients listed as skin protectants in proposed rule published by U.S. Food & Drug Administration [54].

Effective moisturizers must do more than simply restore water to the stratum corneum. They must also facilitate the recovery of dry damaged skin and provide protection against future damage and further water loss [36]. Modern moisturizer products perform these functions and often a great deal more. Moisturizers have become the vehicle for providing a wider range of skin care benefits intended to maintain and improve overall skin condition. Before considering the more broadly based benefits of moisturizer products we will review the factors which influence the consumer need for moisturization.

7.1 Factors Influencing the Need for and Types of Moisturizers

Environmental factors other than cleansers induce and exacerbate dry skin [37]. Some of the drying factors actually remove water from the skin, while others disturb or damage the skin processes for holding water, namely, the lipid bilayers and NMF. Product variations designed to address the impact of environmental influences on skin condition add further to the diversity of moisturizer products in the marketplace.

Anything that removes water from the skin surface faster than it can be replaced by normal trans-epidermal water movement will disturb desquamation and cause the signs of skin dryness described. It must be remembered that dry skin is only dry (lacking water) in the superficial layers of the stratum corneum. These layers become dry because they lose the ability to hold water even though water is available from the lower regions of the stratum corneum.

Cleansers and water are the main factors damaging the water-holding mechanisms of the superficial stratum corneum. Wind and low humidity are the main environmental factors removing water from damaged regions of the superficial stratum corneum. In the same way that wind dries clothes on the washing line by increasing evaporation it dries out corneocytes at the skin surface. How effectively the wind removes water depends on humidity and the amount of NMF in the stratum corneum. Relative humidity is the percentage of water in air compared with saturated water content at that same temperature. When the relative humidity is high the skin's NMF has little difficulty in holding water in the protein matrix of corneocytes. At low humidity the NMF is unable to hold water against the pull of low partial pressure at the skin surface. If the NMF is depleted, there is nothing to hold water at low relative humidity (RH) and the skin surface becomes very dry.

Temperature can also play a role in determining dry skin condition. Cold temperature has two effects. The colder the air, the less water it can hold, so skin in equilibrium with 60% RH cold air has much less moisture than skin in equilibrium with 60% RH warm air. Also, cold temperature greatly reduces the mobility and flexibility of stratum corneum lipids and predisposes it to physical cracks in regions like knuckles where skin is subject to stretching forces. Normal hot weather temperatures are not drying unless the relative humidity is low. However, the UVB in strong sunlight can interfere with the skin's normal mechanisms for generating NMF, resulting in a deficiency of NMF that predisposes to dry, flaky skin.

Having considered factors which actually remove water from skin, the next group of skin drying agents are those that disturb the skin processes for water retention. Cleansers, we have seen, are potentially very damaging to the skin's water-holding mechanisms. Perhaps surprisingly, water itself can also be very drying by washing away NMF. Overexposure to solar UVB radiation can reduce the NMF content of skin by interfering with filaggrin degradation in the mid-lower regions of the stratum corneum. Ultraviolet radiation also interacts with stratum corneum lipids to generate lipid peroxides, and these are a further contribution to dry skin by disturbing the regularity and efficiency of the lipid bilayers.

Each of the different circumstances leading to dry skin conditions creates the opportunity for a customized product [38]. In 1950, a few basic moisturizers were available, but by 2000 there was not only a separate product for each eventuality but often multiple product offerings, each trying to be a little different from the next. To argue that not all these products are necessary is to invite the response that choice is good for the consumer. And so it is, provided the consumer is able to make an informed choice with comfort and confidence. It appears that the marketplace has reached such a degree of complexity that many consumers simply find a zone of comfort and disregard the rest. This encourages manufactures to intensify their efforts to attract consumers to their products. Notwithstanding these efforts, it is consumers who ultimately determine products that last in the market place. There may be thousands of moisturizer products on sale at any one time, but only a few of these products have real staying power. The rest disappear in a continuous cycle of withdrawal and replacement. Products that are not successful are discontinued and replaced by new products containing new ingredients and making new claims.

8 THE PRODUCT CYCLE

Because moisturizers fullfil such a fundamental consumer need they are a huge category of the consumer products market. Moisturizers are big business all around the world, and the moisturizer market is intensively competitive. Each manufacturer is vying with all others to gain the largest possible share of market. Manufacturers do this by supporting their existing products with advertising (TV, print, radio, and others) and promotions (discounts, bonus offerings, product tie-in competitions, etc.) and by launching new products. Advertising support for existing products is very expensive and launching a new product is even more expensive, particularly for large manufacturers. In developed markets like the

United States the failure rate for new product launches is about 95%. Approximately 19 of every 20 newly launched products are not successful and disappear within a year or so. Most of these failures are from smaller manufacturers who can afford to be entrepreneurial. They are able to try products and recycle quickly when not successful. The cost of investment for large manufacturers is so high—millions of dollars in both development costs and advertising support for new product launches—that they have to be sure that a new product has high potential for success before they enter the marketplace. They do this using sophisticated consumer testing, test marketing, and ancillary techniques that enable an estimate of approximate market share for a new product. Only product developments that show a high probability of success proceed to launch.

9 FACE AND BODY SEGMENTS OF THE MOISTURIZER MARKETPLACE

As indicated, the skin care and moisturizer market is divided between face care and hand and body care products. The dynamics of each of these two market categories are very different. There are thousands of moisturizer products for the face and relatively few for the body. This reflects the different consumer needs for the face and body.

9.1 Facial Moisturizers

The face is our interface with the outside world. The face is also the part of the body that most shows the signs of aging. The face is constantly exposed to the environment, whereas clothing may protect other parts of the body. Lines and wrinkles appear on the face but not much on the body. The recognition of the first permanent wrinkle is a pivotal moment for most people and perhaps surprisingly is often experienced in the early 30s. At one time facial moisturizers were simply moisturizing products. They were used to balance the drying effects of cleansing and to protect the skin against the elements—moisturized skin is better able to resist a drying environment. Moisturized skin also looks healthier and more radiant than dry skin. Facial moisturizers have always contained emollients, with or without humectants, typically in esthetically pleasing formulations. More recently, moisturizers have become the vehicle to address other problems of facial skin, particularly those age-related changes which are perceived as the visible signs of aging. Products designed to address the signs of aging are known as anti-aging products [39,40].

Historically, anti-aging was the province of the prestige marketplace with a variety of ingredients added to moisturizers to create anti-aging products. For example, in the 1970s a number of products contained placental extract as a skin rejuvenating ingredient. At that time, mass market products mostly continued to offer moisturizing benefits as the way to maintain skin in healthy condition and looking younger for longer. This changed in 1992 with the introduction of alpha-hydroxy acids (AHAs) in mass market moisturizers, the first really effective anti-aging technology introduced in mass market skin care products [41]. As explained in chapter 16 dedicated to AHAs, these ingredients produce clinically demonstrated and consumer perceivable improvements in the visible signs of facial aging. The use of AHAs was so successful that it created a new category of moisturizing product, initially in the United States and then extending around the world. Interestingly, an AHA (lactic acid) had been used as a moisturizing ingredient in mass market moisturizers since the early 1970s [42], but it turned out that a low pH is necessary for the anti-aging benefits beyond simple moisturizing (pH 3.8 is used in mass market AHA moisturizers).

AHAs transformed the moisturizer marketplace, not only by creating a new sector, but by enhancing the credibility of anti-aging claims and creating a new expectation in mass market consumers. The success of AHAs and associated change in consumer need stimulated manufacturers to search for even more effective ingredients for anti-aging moisturizers. The result has been intensified research by both skin care manufacturers and the ingredient supply industry [43]. In the period between 1992 and 2000, several ingredients were promoted as the next generation of cosmetic anti-aging technology. The main contenders were retinol and retinol esters, vitamin C and stable derivatives of vitamin C, other anti-oxidant vitamins, and a variety of botanical and marine extracts. The efficacy of these ingredients is discussed in other chapters of this volume, but each has been the platform for a new range of products in the marketplace. Impressive and compelling claims of anti-aging benefits have been made for each technology, but so far nothing has made a step change in consumer perceived efficacy comparable with that seen when AHAs were introduced in 1992.

9.2 Hand and Body Moisturizers

The main consumer skin care need for the body is universal, an all-family need to treat and prevent dry skin. There are many products that do this very effectively. In fact, the treatment and prevention of dry skin is such a well-satisfied need that it has become difficult for manufacturers to find a competitive edge. With all leading dry skin products similarly very effective for everyday dry skin we see manufacturers broadening the benefits of hand and body moisturizers as a way to achieve novelty and competitive edge [44,45]. A recent significant development is the addition of sunscreens to regular hand and body moisturizers [46].

Other body care needs exist but have a narrower focus. For example, women with photodamaged hand and arm skin seek moisturizers to address the associated signs of aging, particularly age spots and coarse/crepey texture (crinkled appearance). In older women, thinning, sagging, and laxity are additional problems of skin that are unmet needs. A specific problem for a surprisingly high proportion of women is cellulite [47], creating a need for products to eliminate or reduce the cellulite appearance of thighs and buttocks. There are moisturizer products with additional specific ingredients aimed at each of these consumer needs.

Products to treat and prevent dry skin are the main products in the hand and body moisturizer market worldwide, but there are some regional differences. Moisturizers to maintain a fair skin color are a large segment of the moisturizer market in India and Southeast Asia, a reflection that uneven skin tone is the number one skin care concern of some consumers [48].

Cleansing and the environment induce dry skin, but there are also personal factors that come into play. There are some people, particularly atopics, who have no overt skin disease but who are more prone to develop dry skin than the rest of the population [49]. The atopic condition is explained later in chapter 9. Atopics tend to have dry skin all year round regardless of weather, and they often develop severe dry skin in winter or in drying environments [50]. It is now recognized that many cases of occupational hand dermatitis occur in atopics and reflect their decreased ability to resist conditions that dry out the skin, leaving them more susceptible to environmental irritants. The number of atopics in the population has been rising steadily around the world since the 1970s [51]. Because many individuals with an atopic tendency are unaware of their condition they often continue the patterns of product use and environmental contacts that promote and propagate their dry skin condition.

Dry skin is without doubt the most common skin problem for consumers around the world, but for many it is not a serious skin problem. Some consumers are content to live with some level of dry skin and regard this simply as their normal skin condition. Use of body moisturizers tends to parallel cleansing routines. In the United States and increasingly around the world, daily showering has become a common practice. This represents a considerable challenge to the natural moisturizing processes of the skin, and in drying weather it is not long before consumers experience distinctly dry and itchy skin after each and every shower. Use of a body moisturizer becomes a necessity. As we will see later, the need for moisturizing to combat the drying effects of showering led to the development of an entirely new product category in the skin care market place, the moisturizing body wash [52].

The market for hand and body moisturizers shows a clear segmentation based on price and positioning. The main categories are value/low price brands, everyday products, therapeutic, and cosmetic. Within each category there are two main product forms, creams and lotions, with lotions the most common. There is also petroleum jelly that is unique as a treatment for dry skin and as a skin protectant.

Value brands are low price products, usually store brands or "unknown" products that sell at a discount to the rest of the market. Everyday products include the main branded products that offer performance at a competitive price. Therapeutic is a smaller category with products that sell at a significant premium over everyday brands based on a positioning of superior efficacy. Products in all these categories are effective for treating and preventing dry skin. Relative effectiveness, as measured by controlled clinical trials, varies (but not greatly) and depends on the particular moisturizing ingredients and their concentration in the formulation. Although there are differences in effectiveness for most consumers, most of the time there is little practical difference for dealing with everyday dry skin needs. The consumers who could be expected to most notice small differences in efficacy are those with the greatest problems and needs. This would be the groups exposed to particularly harsh conditions or individuals with a personal increased susceptibility to developing dry skin, particularly the 20–30% of the population who have an atopic tendency.

Product effectiveness and product esthetic properties pull in different directions; in general, the greater the content of oils and humectants, the greater the efficacy but also the heavier the product for rubbing into the skin.

The cosmetic category of the hand and body moisturizer market includes products that are light, elegant, and esthetically pleasing. These formulations contain lower levels of humectants and emollient oils than mainline dry skin products to achieve faster rub-in and better skin feel. Cosmetic moisturizers usually have a feminine positioning, often centered around fragrance, botanicals, and other emotive ingredients. Nevertheless, many cosmetic category products contain sufficient moisturizing ingredients to be effective for their main use as daily maintenance products to keep skin moisturized and in good condition, rather than to treat dry skin.

9.3 Other Subdivisions of the Body Category

By now the reader has a good appreciation that nearly every subdivision of consumer activity, both physical and emotional, represents a consumer need that immediately becomes a stimulus for moisturizer products customized to that need. The main hand and body lotions described are good for general use, but within the broad category it is possible to find moisturizers targeted at rather specific needs, such as care of the finger nails and for foot care.

10 SKIN MOISTURIZERS AND DERMATOLOGY

Dermatologists dealing with skin diseases that predispose toward development of dry skin need their patients to use skin care products that help rather than worsen their underlying skin condition. They need their patients to use a mild cleanser and moisturizing cream or lotion. The nonprescription products recommended by dermatologists are the same as those available to the general consumer. Although the dry skin experienced by skin disease patients and by consumers generally may have different origins, the solution is much the same—a well-formulated emollient cream or moisturizing lotion [53]. However, patients often have more intractable dry skin than the average consumer and therefore need the heavier more effective moisturizing formulations.

11 REGULATORY CATEGORIES OF SKIN MOISTURIZERS

Moisturizers generally are not specifically regulated in the United States. There is no requirement for premarketing approval or registration. However, in the United States there is an over-the-counter (OTC) drug category for many everyday skin care products, including acne, first aid, and antibacterial treatments as well as sunscreen and skin protectants [54]. Some hand and body moisturizers fall within the aegis of the OTC skin protectant monograph and are therefore subject to controls including labeling requirements and allowed claims. Monograph products typically must contain particular "active" ingredients (see Table 1). In the case of the OTC skin protectant monograph, two specified active ingredients are petrolatum and dimethicone, at specified minimum levels—30% or higher for petrolatum and 1% or higher for dimethicone. If the difference between these concentrations is surprising it is a reflection that limit values built into regulations often reflect the actual compositions of products in the marketplace at the time that regulations were formulated. There is no scientific rationale for the large differences in the monograph minimum levels of these two ingredients. The OTC monograph products are required to list active ingredients on the pack above and separate from the list of other ingredients. Most U.S. consumers are not aware of the OTC monograph system and therefore may wonder why some moisturizers have active ingredients and other similar products do not. This regulatory overlay is a further complication for consumers trying to understand the skin moisturizer market.

As described in later chapters on regulations, the European and Japanese regulation of skin moisturizers is different from the United States. European regulations tend to control the ingredients used in products and therefore, unlike the United States, do not lead to separate regulated and unregulated products in the marketplace. Japan is somewhat like Europe in the sense that the main regulation impacting skin and moisturizers is a quasi drug regulation that directs what ingredients can be used in cosmetics, including moisturizers.

12 COSMECEUTICAL

Readers will find the term *cosmeceutical* used frequently in cosmetic and skin care journals, magazines, and other publications [55]. If you visit a prestige counter in the department store, the consultant may offer you the latest cosmeceutical treatment to combat aging skin. The term is widely used to describe moisturizing products that go beyond moisturizing to offer some additional skin benefit [56]. There have been international conferences to present and review the role and future trends for cosmeceuticals [57]. Many people have come to believe that "cosmeceutical" is a regulatory category of consumer products. Nothing could be further from the truth [58]. The term has no regulatory status anywhere around the world, although the Japanese quasi drug category is close in concept to the now accepted use of the term cosmeceutical.

There now is a generation who believe that the term cosmeceutical was introduced in the early 1990s with the emergence of alpha-hydroxy acid anti-aging products as the first moisturizers to do more than moisturize the skin. In fact the term cosmeceutical originated in 1962 [59] and was expanded upon years later by Dr. Albert Kligman [60]. In the early 1980s, at a symposium organized by the Society of Cosmetic Chemists, Dr. Kligman pointed out that simple moisturizers had a profound effect on the stratum corneum. They clearly had a beneficial effect on the stuctural elements and proper functioning of the stratum corneum. They were cosmetics having a therapeutic action; they were "cosmeceuticals." Ten years later, Vermeer put forward proposals to define and regulate cosmeceuticals [61], but the cosmetics industry in the United States remains bound by legislation developed in 1937 that defined any material having an effect on the structure or function of skin as a drug and subject to drug regulations.

13 MOISTURIZING CLEANSERS

13.1 Cleansing Bars

The skin care industry understood many years ago that bar soap caused dry skin, creating a need for products to restore moisture. Clearly there would be a consumer benefit by reducing the drying action of soaps. There are two types of soap bars, the regular opaque colored bars everyone is familiar with and clear glycerin bars which are made by a completely different manufacturing process. Regular soap is made by hydrolyzing natural fats and oils (glycerides) to yields fatty acid and glycerol, separating out the glycerol, and converting the fatty acid to soap (soap is the sodium salt of fatty acid). Glycerin bars are made by leaving in the glycerin to produce a different form of regular soap that develops transparency when aged under controlled conditions for 2 months.

Back in the 1960s there were two approaches to reduce the drying action of soaps:

1. To balance the chain length distribution toward the milder longer chain lengths
2. To add fatty acid to the soap mix to produce so-called superfatted soap

While these variations were a little milder than regular soap, it was not until the early 1960s that there was a real advance in reducing the drying effects of cleansing. This was the introduction of a cleansing bar based on nonsoap synthetic detergent, fatty acid isethionate, and addition of a large proportion of fatty acid to the bar (>20%). This product, called Dove, was dramatically milder than soap [62] and was unequaled in the marketplace until its patents expired in 1992, at which time other manufacturers copied the technology to make their own version of the mild synthetic detergent (syndet) bar. The Dove bar was not only less drying than soap but deposited some fatty acid on skin during the washing process. As discussed, fatty acids are one of the three lipid types that make up the intercellular lipid bilayers of the stratum corneum. The deposition of fatty acid by Dove largely compensated for the natural fatty acid lost during the wash process. Because the milder syndet bars induce less dryness than soap bars, regular use of a mild syndet bar, particularly in cold drying weather, helps keep skin relatively more moisturized than regular use of soap. In addition to regular soap bars there are translucent/transparent bars, often referred to as glycerin bars, that are intermediate between regular soap and syndet bars for skin drying [63]. By year 2000, the cleansing bar market was still predominantly soap bars (60%), syndet bars (25%), and combination bars, mixtures of soap and syndet (15%). However, the bar market had evolved from simple cleansing to offering a wider range of benefits [64].

13.2 Moisturizing Cleansing Liquids

Liquid detergent products are an alternative to bar soap for hand cleansing and general body cleansing, particularly in the shower. The first shower products were simple formulations based on combinations of relatively mild surfactants. These products were generally less drying than soap but also less effective for cleansing. However, during the 1990s, frequent showering, often daily, was the norm, and this was more for refreshment and removal of body odors than for washing away dirt and grime. The cleansing power of soap was not needed. Liquid products, although usually milder than soap, were still inclined to leave the user feeling tight and dry after showering. This problem created a product opportunity, and skin care manufacturers responded with a new category of shower products called moisturizing body washes. These product were very different from the previously available shower liquids, most particularly by containing a high level of emollient oil and a deposition system, often polymer based, to promote deposition of emollients and resistance to rinsing away. The moisturizing benefits of these products, particularly when skin is a little dry before showering, is readily perceived and many women report that they have less need to use a moisturizing lotion after showering. The skin moisturizing effect can also be demonstrated clinically using instruments to reveal an increase in hydration and visual grading to demonstrate a reduction of visual dryness [65].

13.3 Moisturizing Cleansing Wipes

The disposable wipes segment of the cleansing market has been growing steadily since the late 1980s. The common products are everyday wipes and baby wipes, but toward the end of the 1990s a number of new disposable wipe type products appeared. There were make-up removal wipes, antibacterial cleansing wipes, foaming cloths for facial cleansing, and skin moisturizing wipes. While most wet wipes provide a transient hydration of skin, wipes designed to be moisturizing usually contain a humectant such as glycerol.

14 SKIN MOISTURIZERS AND SUN PROTECTION

Sunscreens containing specific moisturizing ingredients were introduced in the United States in the 1980s. These products contained the usual sunscreen ingredients to give a full range of sun protection factors (SPF) as well as humectants for moisturizing benefit. Over the years many manufacturers have added moisturizing ingredients to their sunscreen product range. Notwithstanding this extension of benefits, products in the sunscreen segment of the marketplace are seasonal products intended primarily to protect against sunburn.

In addition to sunscreen products containing moisturizing ingredients there are face and body moisturizing products which contain sunscreen ingredients. For many years facial moisturizing creams and lotions have contained sunscreens for protection against lines, wrinkles, and other long-term effects of solar UV. In this context sunscreens are used as anti-aging ingredients. Facial products are segmented into day and night products. Not surprisingly, it is the day creams that contain sunscreens. Most manufacturers also offer day creams without sunscreens, as these are lighter formulations and preferred by some consumers.

Prior to 1998, sunscreens were not added to body moisturizers, but now several leading manufacturers of hand and body products have at least one variant containing sunscreen in their dry skin product range. These products are intended to provide protection from everyday UV exposure in addition to treating and preventing dry skin. It is interesting to note that one manufacturer introduced a dry skin product containing sunscreens in the 1980s but the product failed. Consumers did not perceive a need for such a product at that time and did not buy it. Now, over 20 years later and with intensive medical and media focus on escalating skin cancer rates, protection from everyday UV exposure makes sense for consumers and the new generation of sunscreen moisturizers seem assured of success.

15   THE MEDIA AND THE MESSAGE

With so many different moisturizers available it is not surprising that many consumers earnestly seek information to guide their choice of skin care products.
One thing is certain: no consumer could ever try all the available skin products to
determine in practice the ones most appropriate for one's individual needs. Fortunately, or maybe not, information on skin care and skin care products is everywhere: magazine and newspaper articles and advertisements; radio and television
programs and advertisements; products labels; promotional pamphlets and junk
mail; friends, acquaintances, relatives, coworkers, beauty consultants, and dermatologists; and now on the internet.

　　Some of the information from these sources is excellent; regrettably some
is little more than piffle. Most of the information on skin care products and technologies falls between these two extremes. One common source of misinformation is the expectation that an activity demonstrated for an ingredient in a test tube
system will apply when the ingredient is incorporated in a moisturizer and applied to skin. Unfortunately, a lot of misinformation cycles between the different
sources and acquires familiarity and credibility in the process. How much of what
you know about skin care products is what you have heard or read in sources other than peer reviewed scientific journals?

　　The internet has become a major source of information for skin care products with numerous sites offering both products and advice [66]. All of the major
manufacturers have web sites to promote their products and to provide relevant
technical information. Because the internet is open to all and not regulated for
content, it may seem that anything goes. However, the web sites of the major
manufacturers can be regarded as reasonably reliable because the posted information will have been subject to internal legal review and approval.

　　Prior to the internet, and probably still true for a majority of consumers,
specialist magazines were the primary source for information and advice about
moisturizers and skin care generally. Magazines come and go but all have the
same categories of contents. Most women's magazines have a selected target audience such as teenagers, young mothers, sophisticated women, executives, older
women, active seniors, or other groups. All the magazines have many pages de-
voted to advertisements for skin care, beauty, and fashion items. Unlike advertisements on television, which must package the product message into a few
memorable sound bites, full-page print advertisements can contain a great deal of
information, although usually in headline form and with no reference to source or
explanation. All magazines have a number of feature articles and regular sections
that typically include reviews of new products, market trends, and skin health issues and treatments. Each article in a magazine is selectively tailored to the particular readership of that magazine.

　　The reliable sources of information on skin care issues and effective treatments are the peer reviewed journals. There is the *International Journal of Cosmetic Science,* several peer reviewed journals in dermatology, such as the *Journal of Investigative Dermatology,* and several more broadly based medical journals, such as the *New England Journal of Medicine.* These journals are not the normal reading for most of the individuals who write or contribute to skin care articles.

16 THE FUTURE

The trend in the skin care market at this time is ever increasing specialization and customization of products [67,68]. Accompanying this trend is an explosion of information that serves to direct consumers toward products most relevant to individual needs and also creates an expectation that these needs can be satisfied. Hope has always been ahead of technology in skin care. Expectations, based on what is communicated from the marketplace, are also moving ahead of technology. The challenge for the marketplace is to provide good information as well as better products. The consumer needs both.

There is a book to be written about the sources and communication of skin care information. While information about skin care products and technologies seems almost endless there is an issue of reliability, but not because of any malicious intent to deceive. There is an element of truth in almost everything that is reported. Much of the misinformation that could be identified as unsound by an expert is very plausible and can often seem reasonable to the informed nonexpert. In this situation how does the consumer figure out what to believe and what to reject? One answer is to ensure the widest possible readership of books such as this. Another answer is the consumer answer: what matters is not what is said or written but only how a product performs. If a product works, the consumer will find it. If the consumer is led to expect performance but it is not delivered, the consumer will be disappointed, move on to something else, and the product will die.

The mass market for moisturizers started over 100 years ago with products such as Vaseline Petroleum Jelly and Pond's Cold Cream as single products to meet most every need for body and face care. From this humble beginning the marketplace has evolved to the sophistication and customization of the 21st century. Moisturizers certainly work. Regular use will keep the skin in good condition and help to maintain that good condition over time. Addition of a select number of ingredients, as described elsewhere in the book, has enhanced the benefits of moisturizers beyond simple hydration of the stratum corneum, but these advanced products fall well short of satisfying unmet consumer skin care needs. The skin moisturizer marketplace is highly fragmented and very complex. There seems little reason to expect this will change unless and until there are some big breakthroughs in the science and technology of skin care—not just another ingredient or product form adding incremental benefit, but something fundamental. The science fiction writers have envisioned wands to diagnose and treat the skin.

The medical profession is making gene therapy a reality for select disease conditions. A wand or a gene product that worked for skin would certainly change the face of the moisturizer market. In the meantime, what you read in this book is likely to remain the current position for a long time to come.

REFERENCES

1. Global Skin Care. Datamonitor. 1998. www.datamonitor.com.
2. Nacht S. 50 years of advances in skin care. Cosmet Toil 1995; 110(12):69–82.
3. Bitz K. The international top 30. Happi 2000; 37(8):74–75.
4. Branna T. The top 50. Happi 2000; 37(7):67–68.
5. Hartfield E. Is it the end of the mass market? Cosmet Int 2000; 23(538):8.
6. Benedetto AV. The environment and skin aging. Clin Dermatol 1998; 16:129–139.
7. Fisher GJ, Wang AQ, Datta SC, Varani J, Kang S, Voorhees JJ. Pathophysiology of premature skin aging induced by ultraviolet light. N Engl J Med 1997; 337(20):1419–1428.
8. Ratner D, Tse Y, Marchell N, Goldman MP, Fitzpatrick RE, Fader DJ. Cutaneous laser resurfacing. J Am Acad Dermatol 1999; 41:365–389.
9. Guttman C. Branching into cosmetic procedures no stretch. Dermatol Times 1999; 20(2):1,23.
10. Tenerelli MJ. The State of the skincare industry revealed. Global Cosmet Ind 1999; 164(6):42–48.
11. O'Sullivan RL, Lipper G, Lerner EA. The Neuro-immuno-cutaneous-endocrine network: relationship of mind and skin. Arch Dermatol 1998; 134:1431–1433.
12. Johnson AW, Nettesheim S. The care of normal skin. In: Arndt KA, Leboit PE, Robinson JK, Wintroub BU, eds. Cutaneous Medicine and Surgery. Vol. 1: Philadelphia: WB Saunders 1995:75–83.
13. Polefka TG. Surfactant interactions with skin. In: Zoller U, Broze G, eds. Handbook of Detergents. Part A: Properties. New York: Marcel Dekker, 1999:433–468.
14. Rawlings AV, Scott IR, Harding CR, Bowser PA. Stratum corneum moisturization at the molecular level. J Invest Dermatol 1994; 103:731–740.
15. Johnson AW. Dry skin. Recent advances in research and therapy: a continuing education program for pharmacists. Drug Store News for the Pharmacist 1994; 4:51–58.
16. Dykes P. Surfactants and the skin. Int J Cosmet Sci 1998; 20:53–61.
17. Misra M, Ananthapadmanabhan KP, Hoyberg K, Gursky RP, Prowell S, Aronson M. Correlation between surfactant-induced ultrastructural changes in epidermis and transepidermal water loss. J Soc Cosmet Chem 1997; 48:219–234.
18. Whalley GR. Solid soap phases. Happi 1998; 35(7):72–74.
19. Rawlings AV, Watkinson A, Rogers J, Mayo A, Hope J, Scott IR. Abnormalities in stratum corneum structure, lipid composition, and desmosome degradation in soap-induced winter xerosis. J Soc Cosmet Chem 1994; 45:203–220.
20. Prottey C, Ferguson T. Factors which determine the skin irritation potential of soaps and detergents. J Soc Cosmet Chem 1975; 26:29–46.
21. Wiechers JW, Wortel VAL. Bridging the language gap between cosmetic formulators and consumers. Cosmet Toil 2000; 115(5):33–41.

22. Morizot F, Guinot C, Lopez S, Le Fur I, Tschachler E. Sensitive skin: analysis of symptoms, perceived causes and possible mechanisms. Cosmet Toil 2000; 115(11):83–89.
23. Bogensberger G, Baumann L. What you should know about "sensitive skin." Skin & Aging 1999; 7(9):75–78.
24. Nassif A, Chan SC, Storrs FJ, Hanifin JM. Abnormal skin irritancy in atopic dermatitis and in atopy without dermatitis. Arch Dermatol 1994; 130:1402–1407.
25. Bolognia JL, Braverman IM, Rousseau ME, Sarrel PM. Skin changes in menopause. Maturitas 1989; 11:295–304.
26. McKinlay SM. The normal menopause transition: an overview. Maturitas 1996; 23:137–145.
27. Robinson MK. Population differences in skin structure and physiology and the susceptibility to irritant and allergic contact dermatitis: implications for skin safety testing and risk assessment. Contact Dermatitis 1999; 41:65–79.
28. Berardesca E, Maibach H. Racial differences in skin pathophysiology. J Am Acad Dermatol 1996; 34:667–672.
29. MacDonald V. Ethnic skin care. Happi 2000; 37(10):65–81.
30. Cosgrove J. Emerging trends in multicultural skin care needs. Soap & Cosmetics 2000; 76(12):58–60.
31. Funke U, Fartasch M, Diepgen TL. Incidence of work-related hand eczema during apprenticeship: first results of a prospective cohort study in the car industry. Contact Dermatitis 2001, 44.166–172.
32. Billek DE. Cosmetics for elderly people. Cosmet Toil 1996; 111(July):31–37.
33. Yaar M, Gilchrest BS. Aging versus photoaging: postulated mechanisms and effectors. J Invest Dermatol 1998; 3:47–51.
34. Callens A, Vallans L, Leconte P, Berson M, Gull Y, Lorelle G. Does hormonal skin aging exist? A study of the influence of different hormone therapy regimens on the skin of postmenopausal women using non-invasive measurement techniques. Dermatology 1996; 193:289–294.
35. Wenninger JA, Canterbery RC, McEwen GN Jr, eds. International Cosmetic Ingredient Dictionary and Handbook. Vol. 2. 8th ed. Washington, D.C.: The Cosmetic, Toiletry, and Fragrance Association, 2000:1767–1785.
36. Halkier-Sorensen L. Understanding skin barrier dysfunction in dry skin patients. Skin & Aging 1999; 7(5):60–64.
37. Parish WE. Chemical irritation and predisposing environmental stress (cold wind and hard water). In: Marks R, Plewig G, eds. The Environmental Threat to the Skin. London: Martin Dunitz, 1992:185–193.
38. Idson B. Dry skin moisturizing and emolliency. Cosmet Toil 1992; 107(7):69–68.
39. Owen DR. Anti-aging technology for skincare 1999. Global Cosmet Ind 1999; 164(2):38–43.
40. Owen DR. Anti-aging technology for skincare. Part II 1999. Global Cosmet Ind 1999; 164(3):40–43.
41. Hermitte R. Aged skin, retinoids, and alpha hydroxy acids. Cosmet Toil 1992; 107(7):63–64.
42. Middleton JD. Development of a skin cream designed to reduce dry and flaky skin, J Soc Cosmet Chem 1974; 25:519–534.

43. Radd BL. Antiwrinkle ingredients. Skin Inc 1997; 9(1):89–99.
44. Hand/body lotions solid performers. Chain Drug Rev 1999; November:21–24.
45. Hand, body creams incorporate traits of facial care items. Chain Drug Rev 1999; January:51.
46. Nole GE, Johnson AW, Cheney MC, Znaiden A. Cumulative lifetime UVR exposure in the United States and the effect of various levels of sunscreen protection. Cosmet Dermatol 1999; July:23–26.
47. Kligman AM. Cellulite: facts and fiction. J Geriatr Dermatol 1997; 5(4):136–139.
48. Tenerelli MJ. Ethnic skin-care: special products for a special sector. Global Cosmet Ind 2000; 167(4):32–37.
49. Loffler H, Effendy I. Skin susceptibility of atopic individuals. Contact Dermatitis 1999; 40:239–242.
50. Leung DYM, Soter NA. Cellular and immunologic mechanisms in atopic dermatitis. J Am Acad Dermatol 2001; 44(Suppl 1):1–12.
51. Taieb A. Hypothesis: from epidermal barrier dysfunction to atopic disorders. Contact Dermatitis 1999; 41:177–180.
52. Marchie MK. Liquids move up in the soap market. Happi 2000; 37(12):72–84.
53. Emollients: current uses and future trends. Skin & Aging 1999; 7(Suppl 6):5–15.
54. US FDA Skin protectant drug products for over-the-counter human use. 48 Fed. Reg. 6820, February 15, 1983; amended 58 Fed. Reg. 54458, October 21, 1993; amended 59 Fed. Reg. 28767, June 3, 1994.
55. Labous J. Mother nature shows. Cosmet Int 2000; 24(547):8–9.
56. Levine N, Draelos ZD. Rising tide of cosmeceuticals provokes physician questions. Dermatol Times 2001; 22(1):59–60.
57. Steinberg DC. Cosmeceuticals: an advanced forum for manufacturers. Cosmet Toil 1996; 111(6):43–49.
58. Branna T. Is the industry really ready for cosmeceuticals? Happi 1996; 33(8):60–66.
59. Reed RE. The definition of "cosmeceutical." J Soc Cosmet Chem 1962; 13:103–106.
60. Vermeer BJ. Cosmeceuticals, a proposal for rational definition, evaluation, and regulation. Arch Dermatol 1996; 132:337–340.
61. Kligman AM. Why cosmeceuticals. Cosmet Toil 1993; 108(8):37–38.
62. Frosch PJ, Kligman AM. The soap chamber test. A new method for assessing the irritancy of soaps. J Am Acad Dermatol 1979; 1:35.
63. Whalley GR. Better formulations for today's bar soaps. Happi 2000; 37(12):86–88.
64. Kintish L. Soap: it's not just for cleansing anymore. Soap/Cosmet/Chem Specialties 1998; 74(10):50–54.
65. Patrick E, Tallman DM. Studies exploring moisturization potential of personal washing products. American Academy of Dermatology Academy, Chicago, IL, July 31–August 4, 1998.
66. The growing beauty of the internet. Cosmet Int 2000; 24(543):4.
67. Skin care in the 21st century. Soap/Cosmet/Chem Specialties 1996; 72(4):68–73.
68. MacDonald V. The skin care market. Happi 2000; 37(5):114–124.

2

Stratum Corneum Ceramides and Their Role in Skin Barrier Function

Gopinathan K. Menon
Avon Products, Inc., Suffern, New York

Lars Norlén
University of Geneva, Geneva, Switzerland

1 INTRODUCTION

Although encompassing a multitude of attributes, in its most widely appreciated context the skin barrier function refers to the epidermal barrier to water permeability. Indeed, this is one of the most crucial of integumentary functions that make terrestrial life possible. Large-scale damage to this barrier, as in third-degree burns, results in death by dehydration (due to unchecked water loss). An intact impermeable barrier allows the organism to soak in water without flooding its internal organs and keeps out many xenobiotics. The stratum corneum (SC), a tough, paper-thin superficial layer of skin, has evolved to meet this primary requirement. Compared to the rest of the skin, which weighs around 16% of the total body weight, the mass of SC is rather insignificant. However, its average surface area (1.6 to 1.9 m^2 in an adult person) is a clear indication of its functional significance to the integumentary system. The skin serves as a primary defense, a sensory and an excretory organ, a key to temperature regulation, and a visual signal for intraspecific communication. Its barrier function extends to UV, oxidants, and immune barriers, as well as barriers in interracial relations that have shaped human destiny. Functions and dysfunctions of skin affect not only the physical health, but also the self-esteem of the person. The latter aspect, once trivialized as vanity, is being increasingly recognized as important to emotional well being. This scientific attitude also has made the cosmetic and personal care industries focus on truly functional ingredients and products that perform, with an objective means of measuring the functional efficacy. As a result, research in skin biology has taken a truly interdisciplinary approach to encompass polymer sciences, measurement sciences (analytical), bio- and tissue-engineering and instrumentation, controlled-release and transdermal delivery of actives, in addition to the classic dermatological sciences, which have added molecular biology and genome sciences to its armamentarium of diagnosis and treatment.

Many of these advances have paralleled the developments in understanding the structural organization and functional properties of the stratum corneum. As the interface between the body and the environment, the SC has to perform a myriad of functions. Its own functional status depends on being in a plasticized state, i.e., having adequate water-holding ability, while its waterproofing function is crucial for the survival of the organism. Both these are achieved by utilizing lipids, nature's most ubiquitous waterproofing molecules [1]. Indeed, the primary function of the keratinocytes appears to be generation of this protective sheath by their terminal differentiation into corneocytes. In mammalian SC, these lipids consist of intercellular sheets of ceramides, cholesterol, and fatty acids, but in the deeper layers of epidermis, phospholipids are predominant [2]. We will briefly review the histologic organization of the skin and the cellular events leading to terminal differentiation of keratinocytes before describing the organization of the SC, the crucial role of ceramides, the physical properties of key barrier lipids, and a model for their organization.

2   HISTOLOGY OF THE MAMMALIAN SKIN

The skin consists of two distinct layers. The dermis (making up the bulk of skin) is made up of connective tissue elements. The overlying, avascular epidermis is composed primarily of keratinocytes (Fig. 1). Dermis is made up of collagen, elastin, glycosaminoglycans, as well as fibroblasts that elaborate these substances. Dermis is highly vascular and also includes the pilosebaceous units, sweat glands, dermal adipose cells, mast cells, and infiltrating leucocytes. About 95% of the epidermis layer is composed of keratinocytes, of which the lowermost are anchored to the basement membrane via hemidesmosomes. Other cell types seen in the epidermis are melanocytes, Langerhans cells, and Merkel Cells (mechanoreceptors). This stratified layer is approximately 100 to 150 μm thick and has keratinocytes in various stages of differentiation—reflected in the expression pattern of keratins and consequently in histological appearance. Based on histologic criteria, the epidermis is divisible into four strata: the stratum basale

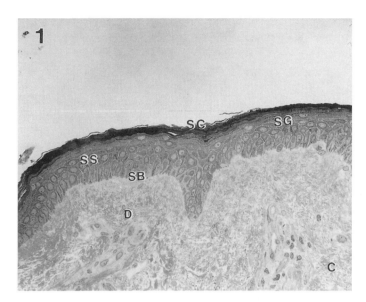

FIGURE 1 Histology of human skin showing the dermis and epidermis. C = collagen, D – stratum basale, SG – stratum granulosum, SC = stratum corneum, and SS = stratum spinosum.

(SB), stratum spinosum (SS), stratum granulosum (SG), and stratum corneum (SC).

The *stratum basale* consists of one layer of columnar basal cells which are composed of epidermal stem cells and transiently amplifying cells derived from the stem cells. They remain attached to the basement membrane via the hemi-desmosomes. Morphologically, they have a high nucleo/cytoplasmic ratio, cell organelles such as mitochondria, and keratin filaments that are inserted into the hemidesmosomes. They also have desmosomes connecting adjacent and overlying cells. Biochemically, keratins K14 and K5 are expressed in the basal cells.

The *stratum spinosum,* or "spinous layer," is so designated due to the spine-like appearance of the cells in histological preparations that result from the large numbers of desmosomes (Fig. 2). In addition to the typical cell organelles seen in the basal layer, the SS also shows the presence of lipid-enriched lamellar bodies (Odland bodies, keratinosomes, membrane-coating granules) that first appear in this layer. These organelles play a crucial role in the formation of the permeability barrier.

Morphologically, they are round or ovoid bodies 0.2 to 0.5 μm in diameter and contain parallel stacks of lipid-enriched disks enclosed by a trilaminar membrane. In near perfect cross-sections, each lamella shows a major electron dense

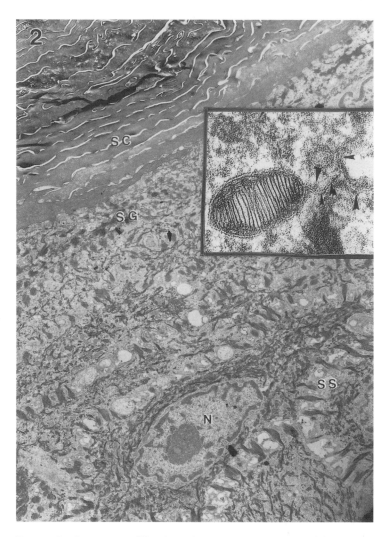

FIGURE 2 Low magnification electron micrograph of human epidermis and part of SC. Note progressive flattening of cells from the upper SS layers. Inset: lamellar body from murine epidermis showing its internal organization as well as connection with cytosolic tubular membrane system (arrowheads). (OSO4 fixation.)

band that is shared by electron lucent material divided centrally by a minor electron dense band (Fig. 2 inset). Their appearance marks the dual aspects of epidermal differentiation, viz., protein and lipid synthesis. Proteins that are expressed in the SS are keratins 1 and 10. An increase in cellular keratin filaments is noticeable compared to the basal cells. In the upper layers of the SS, the cells begin to flatten and elongate. Above this layer is the stratum granulosum.

The *stratum granulosum* layer is characterized by the presence of distinct, darkly staining keratohyalin granules (KHGs), composed of profilaggrin, loricrin, and a cysteine-rich protein as well as keratins 1 and 10. Keratohyalin granules become progressively larger in the upper granulocytes (Fig. 3) due to a quantitative increase in keratin synthesis. The filaggrin subunits of profilaggrin play the role of matrix molecule to aggregate and align the keratin filaments. Keratin filaments in upper granular layers are highly phosphorylated and have extensive disulfide bonds, compared to the cell layers below. The increase in protein synthesis is accompanied by an upregulation in lipogenesis as well, reflected in the boost in numbers of lamellar bodies reaching their highest density in the uppermost granulocytes, where they occupy about 20% of the cell cytosol. The uppermost cells in the SG display a unique structural and functional organization of the lamellar bodies (LBs), consistent with their readiness to terminally differentiate into a corneocyte, during which the lamellar bodies are secreted to the extracellular domains. As seen in electron micrographs of oblique sections, they are highly polarized in the apical cytosol of upper granulocytes. A battery of techniques, such as confocal scanning and electron microscopy, together with enzyme cytochemistry [3] show that in these secretory cells, lamellar bodies are interconnected and appear to bud off a transgolgi-like network. Biochemical characterization of the LBs by preparing an enriched fraction [4] as well as by cytochemical studies [2] show that they are enriched in glucosyl ceramides, phospholipids, and cholesterol, as well as hydrolytic enzymes like lipases, sphingomyelinase, β-glucosylcerebrosidase, and phosphodiesterases. Once secreted, their lipid contents are processed by the co-secreted enzymes, transforming the short stacks of probarrier lipids into the ceramide-enriched final barrier lipid structures.

Some rare electron microscopic images (Fig. 4 upper inset) also suggest that the disk structures within individual lamellar bodies are already continuous, having an accordionlike folded pattern, and that these contents unfurl on secretion. However, whatever form the disks are within the LBs, further fusion of the secreted contents mediated by co-secreted enzymes and/or fusogenic lipids formed due to enzyme activity (lysophospholipids) are involved in formation of the SC extracellular bilayers. A recently described, unique arrangement of the lamellar body secretory system within the secretory granular cell explains the ability for rapid LB secretion to support the homeostasis and/or rapid repair of the permeability barrier [3]. Confocal microscopic images first suggested that

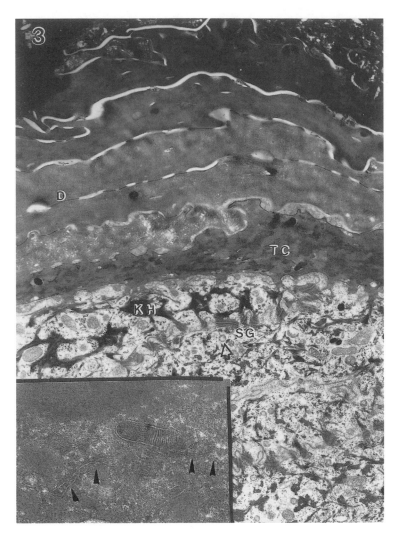

FIGURE 3 Higher magnification view of SG and part of SC. Note keratohyalin granules (KH) and mitochondria in SG and features of transitional cell, as well as prominent corneodesmosomes in the stratum compactum (arrows). (OSO4 fixation.) Inset: RUO4 postfixation reveals tubular profile of a lamellar body, connected (arrowheads) to a transgolgi-like network (arrows) in the cytosol.

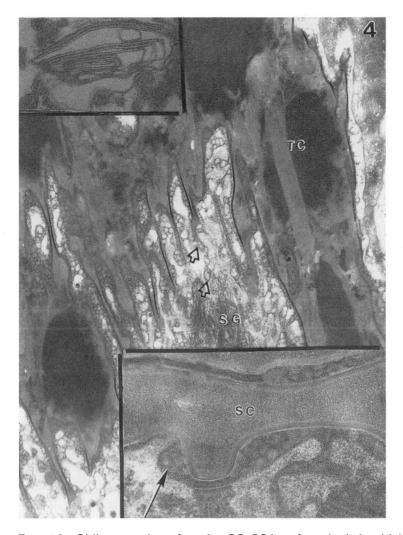

FIGURE 4 Oblique section of murine SG–SC interface depicting highly tortuous intercellular junction, abundance of secreted LBs, and deep invaginations that are portals of LB secretion. Lower inset: in a near-perfect cross-section of SG–SC interface, the tortuosity is not evident. Secreted contents of
LBs fill the expanded intercellular domains (arrows). (Modified from Ref. 85
with permission from Blackwell Sciences, LTD.) Upper inset: unfurling LBs
showing the continuity of LB disks within. (OSO4 fixation.)

LBs are organized into a previously unrecognized cytosolic, tubuloreticular network. Electron microscopic observations of RUO4 postfixed, obliquely sectioned murine epidermis further confirmed that LBs appear not as discrete organelles, but are arranged in an end-to-end/side-by-side orientation. An extensive intracellular cisternal system that is spatially associated with LBs frequently appears to be in direct contact with the envelope of adjacent LBs. Most significantly, continuities between the extracellular domains of SG–SC interface with deep, interdigitating invaginations form an extensive honeycomb-like latticework within the apical cytosol of the uppermost SG cell. To sum up, these ultrastructural data correlated well with the confocal images of fluorescent lipid staining of epidermis and demonstrate (1) deep invaginations of the extracellular domains, (2) a trans-golgi-like tubuloreticular network, and (3) arrays of contiguous LBs in the apical cytosol of the outermost SG cell. This organization provides for portals of LB secretion as the granulocyte elaborates a thickened envelope, the cornified envelope, in preparation for its final transition to a corneocyte. The cornified envelope is a thickened, electron dense band (as seen in electron micrographs) underlying the apical plasma membrane. The thickening represents the sequential deposition of proteins, cross-linked by (glutamyl) lysine isopeptide linkages, bis(glutamyl) polyamine linkage, and disulfide bonds [4]. The cross-linking is catalyzed by transglutaminases, whose major substrate is involucrin. Loricrin, the major structural protein of the envelope, is incorporated at a relatively late stage. Other putative constituents of the envelope are cornifin, keratolinin, and a cystein-rich protein related to cystatin A. Coincident with cornification, the plasma membrane of the outermost SG cell is replaced by a solvent-resistant envelope. This structure is enriched in ω-hydroxyceramides covalently bound to peptides in the outer cornified envelope (primarily glutamine/glutamic acid residues in involucrin). The origin of this structure is now believed to be the lamellar body contents (see Figs. 5 and 7), more precisely, ω-hydroxyceramides transesterified in situ to the cornified envelope peptides by transglutaminase 1, the calcium-dependent enzyme. Although the corneocyte lipid envelope (CLE) itself may not possess intrinsic water barrier function, it is thought to be crucial for normal deposition of the lipid lamellae (scaffold function), corneocyte cohesion, and/or regulation of access/egress of molecules from the corneocyte cytosol. The initiation of the formation of cornified envelope, the large-scale secretion of lamellar bodies, the dissolution of the cellular organelles, the condensation of keratin filaments, etc., that lead to the irreversible process of cornification depend on many signals, the nature of which is still being elucidated. One such signal that triggers the process is ionic calcium. In vitro studies have shown that keratinocyte differentiation can be induced by elevating the calcium concentration of their culture media [5]. Cytochemical techniques [6] as well as particle beam analysis [7] have demonstrated an extracellular calcium gradient in mammalian epidermis in vivo, with low Ca^{2+} content in the basal proliferating layers and progressively higher concentrations as the epi-

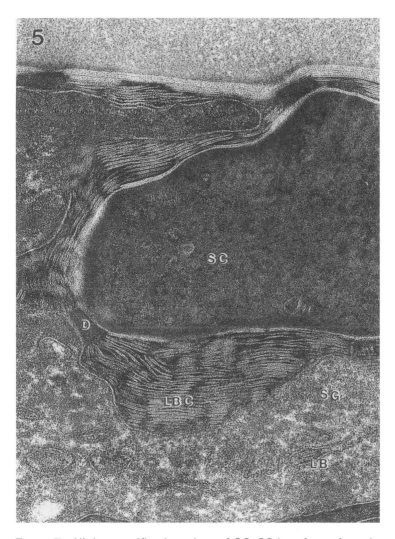

Figure 5 High magnification view of SG–SC interface of murine epidermis following RUO4 postfixation. Note superior visualization of lipid-enriched LB contents. Postsecretory processing of LB derived lipid disks such as end-to-end fusion and their transformation into broad, compact bilayers at the distal portions of the intercellular (extracellular) domain. The RUO4 technique illuminates details of the relation between desmosomes (D) and the lipid disks that seem to be anchoring onto the desmosomes. While cytosolic LBs are stained, keratohyalin granules and other cytosolic structures are obliterated by RUO4. (Modified from Ref. 22.)

dermis stratifies and differentiates. An influx of Ca^{2+} into the cytosol of upper granulocytes is believed to trigger the rapid transformation of granulocyte into a corneocyte. Via an intermediate stage, the transitional cell which is characterized by remnants of nuclei and other cytosolic components, unidentifiable vacuoles; dense, keratin-filled cytosol, and cornified cell envelope. This process of transition from granular to first cornified cell is rapid (5 to 6 hr) and the mechanism of cytoplasmic degradation involving activation of several proteases, despite no morphological evidence of autolysosomes, is poorly understood [8] and has been termed *difpoptosis* [9] to distinguish it from the classic apoptotic pathway.

3   CORNEOCYTES AND THEIR EXTRACELLULAR DOMAINS

The stratum corneum is a composite of the corneocytes (terminally differentiated keratinocytes) and the secreted contents of the lamellar bodies (elaborated by the keratinocytes), which give it a brick-and-mortar organization and unique functional properties. These properties are based on the nature of sequestration of proteins to the cytosol of corneocytes (stacked one upon another and spot-welded at several points by corneodesmosomes) and lipids to the extracellular space, where they form a continuous phase (Fig. 6). This arrangement creates a tortuous path through which substances have to traverse in order to cross the SC. In the human skin, the stratum corneum typically has about 18 to 21 cell layers. Individual corneocytes are 20 to 40 µm in diameter (as opposed to 6 or 8 µm for the basal cell). They may differ in their thickness, packing of keratin filaments, number of desmosomes (corneodesmosomes), etc., depending on the body site and their location within the SC (inner stratum compactum versus outer stratum disjunctum). These features also may influence their degree of hydration, which varies from 10 to 30% bound water. Water-holding properties of corneocytes are influenced by the rate of proteolysis (filaggrin breakdown) that leads to formation of amino acids collectively known as natural moisturizing factors [10]. Corneocytes have ridges and undulations which aid the overlapping cells to interdigitate, enhancing the stability of the layer. In addition, corneodesmosomes ensure the cohesiveness of the layer, especially in the stratum compactum, where they appear intact (Fig. 3). In contrast, slow degradation of these structures in the stratum disjunctum allow the normal process of corneocyte desquamation.

   The SG–SC interface shows (1) invaginations of the apical cell membrane of uppermost granulocytes serving as portals of LB secretion and (2) greatly expanded intercellular space filled with secreted contents of lamellar bodies. As shown in Fig. 5 the lamellar body contents fuse end to end on secretion, forming elongated bilayer structures that go through chemical and structural modulations mediated by a battery of lipid metabolizing enzymes such as acid and neutral lipases, phospholipases, sphingomyelinase, β-glucocerebrosidase, etc. [2]. At the

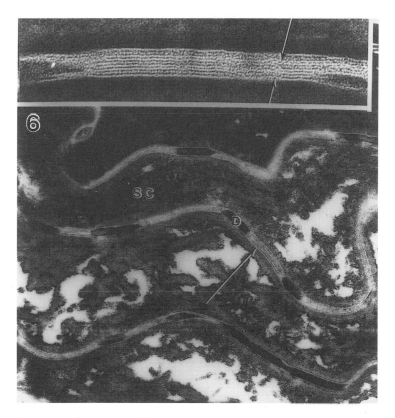

FIGURE 6 Low magnification electron micrograph of human SC as a composite structure showing the tortuous extracellular domains filled with lipid bilayers (arrows) and desmosomes (D) that rivet the corneocytes. The large "holes" within some of the corneocytes are artifacts (due to keratin digestion by the reactive RUO4). (Reprinted from Ref. 86, with permission from Springer Verlag, GMBH & Co. KG.) Inset: a high magnification view of intercellular bilayer structures with repeat pattern of lucent and dense bands (arrows) in normal human SC.

SG–SC interface, a string of fused LB disks can still be identified, but closer to the membrane of the first layer of corneocytes the individual disk outlines have already disappeared, and long continuous bilayer structures are already formed. This offers morphological evidence for the postsecretory processing of LB contents in the extracellular domains and lends support for earlier biochemical data that suggested ongoing lipid modulations that characterize epidermal differentiation and stratification [11]. One of the most crucial events in the processing of LB contents is glucosyl ceramide-to-ceramide metabolism by the enzyme β-glucosyl cerebrosidase. Investigations by Holleran et al. [12,13] have shown that the pro-barrier lipids originating from lamellar bodies have a predominance of glucosy-lated lipids, and that the enzyme β-glucocerebrosidase is crucial in removing the glucose moiety and giving rise to the ceramides of stratum corneum. Inhibitors of the enzyme, as well as genetic deficiency of β-glucocerebrosidase, lead to well-characterized lipid processing defects, structurally immature lipid bilayers in the SC, and consequent barrier abnormalities and defective desquamation. The desmosomes initially appear to provide anchorage to the disk contents of LBs. But toward the outer SC, they begin to appear surrounded by lipid lamellae. Lamellar body–derived proteases are involved in degradation of desmosomes leading to the normal process of desquamation, from the outer SC (stratum disjunctum). However, the lipid bilayers may protect the stratum compactum from proteolytic degradation, ensuring integrity of this stratum that is crucial to the barrier function. An interesting observation that sugars protect desmosomes [14] may have implications in the specific sequence of lipid processing during barrier formation. Other aspects of extracellular lipid processing include phospholipid to free fatty acids by phospholipases, and cholesterol sulfate to cholesterol by steroid sulfatases. Several observations linking enzyme deficiencies and abnormal lipid structural morphology in the SC correlate well with the functional significance of the three major lipid species and their critical ratios to the barrier. The sequestration of lipids as membrane bilayers within the SC extracellular domains can be appreciated from the ultrastructural appearance of RUO4-stained SC. Static images in electron micrographs provide a glimpse, albeit a frozen moment, of the dynamic postsecretory modulations in the probarrier lipids (Fig. 5). Whereas the proximal parts of the SG–SC interface contain separate disks or those in the process of fusing with each other, close to the membrane of the first corneocyte the fused LB disks have already formed continuous lipid bilayers. The basic unit pattern of the bilayers consists of a series of six electron lucent lamallae alternating with five electron dense lamellae (Fig. 6, inset). Double and triple basic units occur frequently. The basic unit structures persist all the way to the outermost layer of SC (Fig. 6), although contamination with sebum results in loss of the tight arrays of bilayers. Additionally, the structural relation of the bilayers to the corneodesmosomes shows gradual changes associated with the progressive degradation of desmosomal structures. Ultrastructurally, the process of desmosomal breakdown involves (1) the formation of electron lucent areas in their core and (2) eventual expansion or ballooning of the cores to form the lacunar domains which are gradually engulfed by the extracellular bilayers. The near total segregation of lipids to intercellular domains of SC was also confirmed by isolating SC membrane sandwiches containing trapped intercellular lipids [15]. These preparations comprised about 50% lipids by weight, accounting to over 80% of SC lipids, and had the same lipid profile of whole SC. Additionally, it had the same freeze fracture and x-ray diffraction pattern of whole SC [16]. These lipids are composed of ceramides, cholesterol, and fatty acids [17] present in roughly equimolar ratios, in addition to small amounts of triglycerides, glycosphin-golipids, and cholesterol sulfate that are detected in the SC [18]. Ceramides amount to approximately 50% of the total lipid mass and 40% of the total number of lipids, and are crucial to the lipid organization of the SC barrier [19]. Based on chromatographic separation, six classes of ceramides were indentified in porcine epidermis. However, chromatographic profile of human stratum corneum some-what differs from that of porcine stratum corneum due to differences in amide-linked fatty acids. Hence a new system of nomenclature based on structure, rather than chromatographic mobility, was proposed by Motta et al. [32]. This system, named CER FB (F indicates the type of amide-linked fatty acids; B indicates the base), the details of which are given by DiNardo and Wertz elsewhere in this vol-ume, is adopted here (Table 1). Of these, ceramide 1 is believed to be uniquely significant in the formation of the covalently bound lipid envelope of corneocytes [20]. Ceramide 1 consists of sphingosine and long chain unsaturated, mono- and di-unsaturated ω-hydroxy acids in the amide linkage. Cholesterol is the second most abundant lipid in the SC and amounts to approximately 25% by weight or 30 mol% of SC [21] and is crucial for promoting the intermixing of different lipid species. Free fatty acids account for about 10% of SC lipids or 15 mol%, and con-sist predominantly of long chain saturated fatty acids having more than 20 carbon atoms. Oleic (6%) and linoleic (2%) are the only unsaturated fatty acids detected as free in the SC [17].

Deficiencies in any one of these three lipid species result in barrier abnor-malities characterized by increased trans-epidermal water loss (TEWL) as well as observable alterations in the ultrastructural features of the SC extracellular do-mains [22]. These abnormalities could arise from experimental inhibition of key epidermal enzymes involved in synthesis of cholesterol (HMG Co A reductase), glycolipid synthesis (serine palmitoyl transferase), fatty acid synthesis (fatty acyl co carboxylase), or in extracellular processing of glycolipids that are secreted as probarrier lipids via the lamellar body secretory system (β-glucocerebrosidase). These barrier defects also lead to epidermal hyperproliferation, as well as dry, flaky skin conditions. Epidermal sterologenesis has been shown to be indepen-dent of circulating levels of cholesterol [23], and hence systemic cholesterol-low-ering drugs do not usually impact the epidermal barrier. However, a few cases where hypocholesteremic drugs have resulted in skin barrier defects and scaly skin have been reported [24]. Much of the research in this area has centered around ceramide deficiency and will be discussed. Other dermatological condi-tions that arise due to deficiency of enzymes/activators include the Netherton syn-drome.

4 SPECIAL ROLE OF CERAMIDES

In the past two decades, the special role of ceramides in skin barrier has attracted considerable research efforts, broadly divided in the following categories: (1)

TABLE 1 Mean Number of Carbons and Double Bonds per Alkyl Chain of Stratum Corneum Lipids from Epidermal Cysts

Lipid species	Description	Mean carbons per alkyl chain	Mean double bonds per alkyl chain	>95 mol%	Notes
CER-EOS (Ceramide 1) (3 wt% of total)	Long chain base (sphingosine)	18.7	0.8	C17–22	33 mol% C18:1
	Amide linked fatty acid (ω-OH)	29.9	0.0	C26–32	59 mol% C30:0
	Ester linked fatty acid (non-OH)	18.4	0.8	C14–24	24 mol% C18:2
CER-NS (Ceramide 2) (9 wt% of total)	Long chain base (sphingosine)	18.7	0.8	C17–22	37 mol% C18:1
	Amide linked fatty acid (non-OH)	23.5	0.0	C16–30	54 mol% C24–26
CERs-EOH+NP (Ceramide 3) (5 wt% of total)	Long chain base (phytosphingosine)	20.2	0.0	C16–25	61 mol% C19–22
	Amide linked fatty acid (non-OH)	23.4	0.0	C16–28	51 mol% C24–26
CERs-AS+NP (Ceramide 4/5) (12 wt% of total)	Long chain base (sphingosine)	18.4	0.7	C16–22	32 mol% C18:1
	Amide linked fatty acid (α-OH)	23.3	0.0	C16–26	70 mol% C24–26

Component				
CER-AH (Ceramide 6I) (2 wt% of total)				
Long chain base (phytosphingosine)	19.5	0.0	C16–25	61 mol% C18–20
Amide linked fatty acid (α-OH)	23.1	0.0	C18–28	69 mol% C24–26
Ester linked fatty acid (α-OH)	20.4	0.0	C16–26	70 mol% C16,24,26
CER-AP (Ceramide 6II) (11 wt% of total)				
Long chain base (phytosphingosine)	20.2	0.0	C16–24	48 mol% C20–22
Amide linked fatty acid (α-OH)	23.9	0.0	C16–26	81 mol% C24–26
Free fatty acids (9 wt% of total)	21.3	0.1	C16–26	45 mol% C22–24
Cholesteryl esters (10 wt% of total)	17.9	0.7	C16–18	69 mol% C18:1
Cholesterol (27 wt% of total)				

Source: Calculated from Ref. 17.

Physical chemical investigations on lipid mixtures that mimic SC lipid composition and the impact of different types and ratios of lipids on these parameters, [19,25]; (2) in vitro studies on keratinocytes, with emphasis on ceramide synthesis and transport into lamellar bodies [26]; (3) in vivo studies of barrier repair in animal models, experimental conditions of altered ceramide synthesis and metabolism, as well as transgenic animals with enzyme deficiencies [27–29]; and (4) quantification of ceramide levels and types in human skin disorders such as atopic dermatitis [30,31] and psoriasis [32]. All of these approaches have provided valuable information on the multiple roles of this crucial lipid species, not only in barrier formation, but also in regulating epidermal homeostasis (via cell proliferation, apoptosis) and skin microbial population [33].

Although the details of the molecular organization of lipids in the SC has not been clearly elucidated, studies using mixtures of lipids that mimic SC composition (or are extracted from SC) with a diverse range of physical techniques such as x-ray, TEM, DSC, AFM, NMR, and FTIR show that they are organized in lamellar bilayer structures in which the lipid chains are highly ordered [34–40]. Bouwstra et al. [35] indicated that at an equimolar CHOL/CER molar ratio, the lamellar organization is least sensitive to a variation in CER composition, while at a reduced CHOL/CER molar ratio, the CER composition plays a more prominent role in the lamellar phases.

Studies on keratinocyte cultures by Madison et al. [26] have shown that ceramide glucosyltransferase (CGT), the golgi enzyme responsible for lamellar body glucosylceramides, is upregulated on inducing keratinocyte differentiation, and parallels the appearance of lamellar bodies. They also found that ceramides are converted to glucosylceramides within the golgi, which points to a transgolgi origin of lamellar bodies. Besides, electron microscopic images of LBs showed shapes consistent with cross-sections of tubules or buds from tubules, in addition to vesicles, similar to what was described in vivo (Fig. 3 inset) [3].

Several in vivo studies by Holleran and colleagues [13,27,28] have firmly established the crucial role of ceramide synthesis in barrier repair process and β-glucocerebrosidase enzyme in converting the probarrier lipids (β Gluc Cer) to ceramides, i.e., processing of the secreted LB contents during barrier repair. Additionally, inhibition of the enzyme by topically applied inhibitors (in normal skin) as well as the deficiency of the enzyme in transgenic animals, lead to defective processing of LB contents, resulting in morphologically abnormal lipid bilayers and increased TEWL. Similar defects occur in patients of Gaucher's disease. The role of ceramides in formation of the corneocyte lipid envelope was mentioned earlier in this chapter. A very recent study by Behne et al. [40] provided the first direct evidence for the crucial role of ω-hydroxy ceramides in CLE as well as barrier function. They found that aminobenzotriazole (ABT), an inhibitor of ω-hydroxylation, significantly inhibited the ω-hydroxylation of very long chain fatty acids in cultured human keratinocytes, but did not alter the synthesis of other ceramides and fatty acid species. Topical application of ABT to murine epidermis following barrier disruption (tape stripping) led to a significant delay in barrier recovery. The barrier abnormality resulting from ABT treatment (but not from its inactive chemical analog used as a control) correlated with (1) significantly decreased ω-hydroxyceramides in both the unbound and covalently bound pools of ceramides; (2) pronounced alterations in LB internal structure; (3) abnormal SC extracellular lamellar membranes; and (4) ultrastructural evidence of numerous foci with absent CLE. These observations provided firm support to earlier contentions that the CLE is a significant component of the epidermal permeability barrier. Figure 7 provides a schematic representation of the CLE formation and the steps affected by ABT treatment.

Compromised barrier functions that correlate with alterations in SC ceramide levels have been documented in seasonal changes [41], aging [42], psoriasis [33], and in atopic dermatitis [30], which have been addressed in other chapters of this volume.

It is also worth mentioning here that a wealth of literature exists on the roles of ions, cytokines, and various ligands for the superfamily of nuclear receptors, in barrier development as well as maintaining the barrier homeostasis. For these aspects, the reader is referred to two of the recent reviews [43,44].

5 PHYSICAL PROPERTIES OF SKIN BARRIER LIPIDS

5.1 Ceramides

Ceramides are sphingolipids that consist of a long chain amino alcohol (sphingosine or one of its derivatives) to which a long chain fatty acid is linked via an amide bond (Fig. 8) [45]. The sphingosine molecule behaves like a surfactant in its free form since it is charged at physiological pH [46]. In addition, it contains a couple of hydroxyl groups along the chain.

Sphingolipids may undergo a plethora of lyotropic and thermotropic phase transitions, which in part may be due to different packing arrangements of their two hydrocarbon chains. This is probably because there is typically a considerable length difference between the carbon chain of the amino alcohol (usually an 18-carbon sphingosine or phytosphingosine base) and a saturated very long (usually 24-carbon) amide-linked fatty acid [47].

Pascher [48] determined the crystal structure of the ceramide group of sphingolipids. Crystal space groups of membrane ceramides have not yet been reported. However, the crystal forms of N-tetracosanoylphytosphingosine (i.e., C18 phytosphingosine with an amide-linked C24 fatty acid) pack in a *splayed chain* conformation where the phytosphingosine and fatty acid chains form separate matrices. However, packing with folded molecules, like in liquid crystalline biological membranes, can be obtained by crystallization from solvent. A detailed

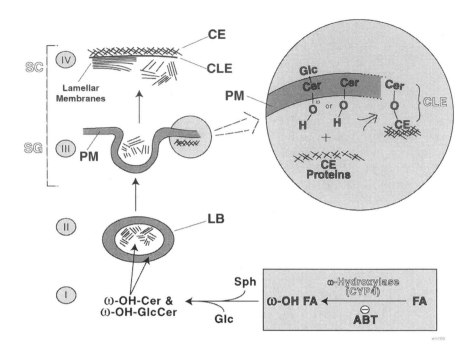

Figure 7 Stepwise formation, packaging, and organization of epidermal ω-hydroxyceramides (ω-OH-Cer). Step I (in both lower and upper epidermal layers): Omega-hydroxylation of very long chain fatty acids (FA) precedes condensation with sphingoid base (Sph) to form ω-OH-Cer species, including glucosylated and ω-acylated forms. The process is interrupted by ABT. Step II (primarily in the mid- to outer epidermal layers): The ω-OH-Cer species are then packaged, along with other barrier lipids, into both the limiting membranes and the central core of lamellar bodies (LB) Step III: (Subsequent fusion of the LB-limiting membrane with the apical plasma membrane (PM) of the outermost stratum granulosum (SG) cell delivers LB contents into the interstices between SG and cornified cells. This process also putatively enriches the apical plasma membrane with ω-OH–containing ceramide species (i.e., from the LB-limiting membrane), with subsequent covalent attachment of ω-OH-Cer to cornified envelope (CE) proteins to form the corneocyte lipid envelope (CLE) (inset). Step IV: Finally, mature lamellar membrane unit structures form in the extracellular domains of the SC, the organization of which appears to depend upon the presence of an intact CLE. (From Ref. 40 with permission from Blackwell Science, Inc.)

FREE CERAMIDES

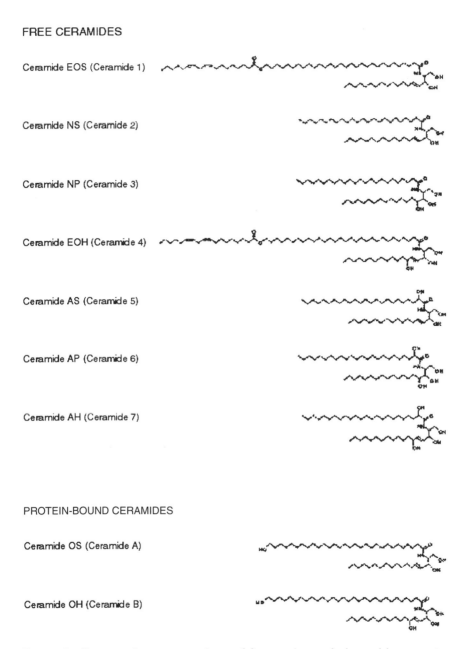

Ceramide EOS (Ceramide 1)

Ceramide NS (Ceramide 2)

Ceramide NP (Ceramide 3)

Ceramide EOH (Ceramide 4)

Ceramide AS (Ceramide 5)

Ceramide AP (Ceramide 6)

Ceramide AH (Ceramide 7)

PROTEIN-BOUND CERAMIDES

Ceramide OS (Ceramide A)

Ceramide OH (Ceramide B)

FIGURE 8 Structural representations of free and protein-bound human stratum corneum ceramides. (Modified from Ref. 84.)

structural analysis of this crystalline phase is still lacking, but it is assumed that the fatty acid tails interdigitate deeply with the opposite half of the bilayer. The hexagonal packing (α form, or plastic-crystal) exists from 106°C down to 21°C. However, the diffraction pattern undergoes a continuous, and reversible, change from a hexagonal to a more orthorhombic packing, where the hexagonal or orthorhombic subcell a_s axis remains constant (~5 Å), while the b_s axis continuously decreases from approximately 8.8 Å in the hexagonal matrix to 7.5 Å in the orthorhombic matrix. According to Dahlén and Pascher [47], the transformation of the fatty acid chain matrix proceeds continuously over a large temperature range until at 21°C the short phytosphingosine chains also change their packing state [47].

The structure of a plasma membrane cerebroside has been shown to form a bilayer structure with tilted chains [49]. Above 70°C, cerebrosides from bovine brain give an L α phase (i.e., a lamellar liquid crystalline phase) where the hydrocarbon chains are melted and consequently there is solely a crystalline periodicity in the direction corresponding to the bilayer thickness [50]. No other liquid crystalline phases have been observed [46]. Electron paramagnetic resonance studies of cerebrosides and phosphatidylcholine in liposomes show a similar mobility for the fatty acid chains of the two lipids.

At physiological skin temperatures (28 to 32°C), the ceramides of SC have been claimed to be necessary for the existence of an L β structure (i.e., a lamellar gel structure) with alkyl chains pointing in a direction perpendicular to the bilayer plane [51] that is free of both crystalline cholesterol and liquid crystalline H_{II} character [52].

5.2 Cholesterol

Cholesterol is the next most abundant lipid species among the skin barrier lipids in the SC extracellular domains, at approximately 30 mol% [53,54]. The physical properties of cholesterol are much less known than its biochemistry. Cholesterol monohydrate, the biological crystalline form of cholesterol [55], forms a bilayer with hydroxyl groups and water forming a hydrogen bonded sheet [56]. It is clear that the phase behavior of cholesterol in biological membranes is exceedingly complicated. In general, cholesterol decreases the chain mobility and reduces the mean molecular polar head group area of lipids in the liquid crystalline state, while it increases the chain mobility of lipids in the gel state [57]. It also decreases transition enthalpies of biological membranes and broadens transition regions from gel to liquid crystalline state in model membranes [57,58]. At high concentrations (>30 mol%) cholesterol prevents alterations of the bilayer structure in biological membranes (dielaidoyl phosphatidylethanolamine, DEPE). However, at low concentrations (<20 mol%), cholesterol stabilizes reversed structures [58]. Cholesterol incorporation into phosphatidylcholine (PC) bilayers increases the phase transition temperatures for lamellar phases having hydrocarbon chains of 16 or fewer carbons. It also decreases the phase transition temperature for lamellar phases having hydrocarbon chains of 18 or more carbons. At 50 mol% cholesterol, a separate cholesterol phase forms and a cooperative lipid transition is no longer observable by differential scanning calorimetry (DSC) [59].

For cholesterol dipalmitoyl phosphatidylcholine (DPPC) mixtures with high cholesterol concentration (>25 mol%) at low temperature, the bilayer behaves as a liquid with much reduced area compressibility (i.e., a viscous liquid). At these high concentrations, the cholesterol strongly favors the liquid phase over the solid phase, since the liquid phase is stable down to temperatures far below the transition temperature (Tm). In the liquid phase, cholesterol increases the conformational order of the alkyl chains but does not induce a concomitant decrease of molecular mobility. At low concentrations, cholesterol is almost as soluble in ordered solid as in disordered liquid phase [60].

It has been suggested that cholesterol can operate as a line-active substance (cf. two-dimensional surfactant, or "lineactant") situated at the interzone between crystalline and liquid crystalline structures [61]. Thus cholesterol is likely to promote intermixing of different lipid species. However, two-dimensional, elongated microcrystals have been observed in binary monolayers of synthetic ceramides and cholesterol [62]. Recently, detergent-resistant membrane domains (DRMs) have been isolated from a variety of eukaryotic cells. These are composed of a mixture of saturated long acyl chain sphingolipids and cholesterol and exist as a liquid ordered structure (i.e., properties intermediate between those of the gel and liquid crystalline states) [63–65].

In mixtures of fatty acids and their soaps (30 wt% water), more than 20 mol% cholesterol is needed for crystalline cholesterol to appear [52,66]. In SC lipid model membranes [cholesterol/bovine brain type III ceramides/medium chain fatty acids (C14–C18) (35 mol% unsaturated), 26.2:27.4:46.6 (30 wt% water)] the ceramides were required for solubilization of the cholesterol [52]. Also, no separate crystalline cholesterol phase was observed in a skin lipid model mixture containing human ceramide 3/cholesterol/palmitic acid/oleic acid (neutralized to 53 mol%), 1:1:0.5:0.5 (32 wt% water) [74].

5.3 Free Fatty Acids

The third or fourth most abundant lipid species among SC barrier lipids is saturated long chain free fatty acids (approximately 10–15 mol%) (Table 1) [53,54,67]. In an aqueous milieu, free fatty acids are partly or fully ionized, acid-soaps (AS) or soaps (S), and their physical properties greatly differ from fully protonated fatty acids. The nomenclature of fatty acid crystal structures is based on X-ray long spacings (i.e., angle of tilt of the hydrocarbon chains toward the bilayer plane). Saturated even- and odd-chained fatty acid crystals are either organized in parallel *triclinic* or perpendicular orthorhombic packing. Unsaturated fatty acids form bilayers with tilted hydrocarbon chains where there is a change in the direction of tilt at the cis double bond [46].

Condensed phase diagrams of dry free fatty acid-soap mixtures show complex phase behavior. Unique crystal unit cells of both the acid and the soap are formed below the chain melting temperature. The palmitic acid-sodium palmitate phase diagram of McBain and Field [45] shows that, except for an acid and soap crystal, both an acid-soap crystal (AS, S = 0.50) and an acid-soap 2 crystal (AS2, S = 0.67) are formed in the dry state. The effect on phase behavior by neutralization is well exemplified by the oleic acid-sodium oleate–water system above the chain melting temperature. Here a decreased salt concentration or increased pH favors the formation of normal phases due to an increased interfacial charge density (and consequently larger effective lipid headgroup areas) [68]. At lipid–water interfaces, fatty acids are more difficult to ionize the higher the negative surface charge density. It is evident that segregation of fatty acids in lipid mixtures can lead to increased surface charge densities locally.

5.4 Cholesteryl Esters

These are the fourth most abundant lipid species in SC barrier lipids (approximately 10–15 mol%) (Table 1) [52,53]. In cholesteryl oleate (constituting about 70% of SC cholesteryl esters), the crystal space group is monoclinic with the molecules packed antiparallelly and with long axes tilted about 30° with respect to the layer planes [69]. Generally, the interlocking of cholesteryl stacks determines the tilt of molecular long axes. The ester chain part may exhibit disorder as well as considerable thermal motion and the hydrocarbon chains are therefore not packed according to a repeating subcell pattern [45]. In contrast to the boomerang shape of crystal structures of oleic acid, cholesteryl oleate exhibits an almost straight chain. In the cholesteryl oleate the kink section is larger [the cis double bond is situated in the middle of the chain, C(36) = C(37)], but the overall perturbation of the chain is smaller than for oleic acid [45].

Liquid crystals of cholesteryl esters show exceedingly complex phase behavior. They can form smetic (i.e., having long-range order in the direction of the long axis of the molecules), cholesteric, and blue phases depending on the chain length of the fatty acid [46,69]. For the cholesteryl esters the smetic phase is similar to the L α phase [46]. The cholesteric phase is a twisted type of nematic phase (i.e., the lipid molecules are aligned side by side, but not in specific layers), where each molecule is slightly displaced in relation to the next giving rise to a helical arrangement of the molecules. Because it was first described for cholesteryl esters, it was termed cholesteric liquid crystalline phase [45]. The blue phases are cubic and the blue color is due to the long periodicity of the phases.

5.5 Cholesterol Sulfate

Cholesterol sulfate, the fifth most abundant lipid species of SC lipids (approximately 1–5 mol%), is almost exclusively found in the interzone between the SG and SC. Further up in the SC, the relative amount of cholesterol sulfate decreases rapidly [70,71]. Cholesterol sulfate crystalizes as its sodium salt with two molecules of water. The predominant aqueous phase is a gel phase (α form). Water is needed for a certain degree of ionization, which is in turn required for the electyrostatic repulsion and swelling [46,71].

In model membranes of equimolar quantities of ceramide and cholesterol sulfate, it has been shown that one molecule of ceramide and one molecule of cholesterol sulfate together bind about 11 molecules of water, as compared to pure cholesterol sulfate membranes where each molecule of cholesterol sulfate binds about 12 molecules of water [72]. This indicates that cholesterol sulfate is a much stronger surfactant than ceramide, and that cholesterol sulfate therefore has a very different role in the stratum corneum as compared to ceramides and other nonpolar lipids. The accumulation of cholesterol sulfate at the SG–SC interzone, and the fact that cholesterol sulfate accumulation in the SC as a whole may be responsible for barrier abnormality in recessive X-linked ichthyosis [71], also supports this notion. It is therefore proposed here that cholesterol sulfate under normal conditions takes active part in the *formation* of the skin barrier, but *is not* part of the SC intercellular, stacked, lamellar lipid matrix constituting the barrier.

6 THE PLASTIC-CRYSTAL, OR SINGLE GEL PHASE, MODEL FOR THE STRUCTURE AND FUNCTION OF THE PERMEABILITY BARRIER

The principal objective of the permeability barrier is to be as tight as possible, except for a minute "leakage" of water needed for the hydration of the keratin in the corneocytes (for plasticizing the SC). The integument must also ensure that the barrier capacity is optimal, even under widely and abruptly changing ambient conditions (e.g., temperature, pH, salt concentrations, relative humidity, etc.). Consequently, (1) sudden transitions of the physical state of the intercellular lipid matrix of SC, with possibly different permeabilities between the two phases, on either side of the transition temperature and (2) phase separation between lipids, where permeabilities could be locally enhanced at the interface between different domains [73], will therefore be avoided as much as possible. Thus from a functional point of view, the skin barrier should be as homogeneous as possible (i.e., ideal physical state, no abrupt transitions, no large differences in permeability between different morphologies, and as little phase separation as possible). This can, however, only be achieved by heterogeneity in the lipid composition, which broadens phase transition zones, stabilizes an ideal lipid morphology, and ensures that the lamellar structures remain intact and that no pores or nonlamellar structures are induced. It has therefore been proposed that the mammalian SC barrier is composed of lipids in a lamellar arrangement that are in a plastic-crystalline state (i.e., α form or "gel" state) stabilized by cholesterol and heterogeneities in hydrocarbon chain length distributions (i.e., broad chain length distributions) with or without water present between the lamallae [74].

Cholesterol is proposed to be the key component for the structure and function of the skin barrier while the ceramides are regarded as constituting the bulk lipid matrix [74]. This is mainly because cholesterol stabilizes "gel" phases [58,59] and probably promotes intermixing of different lipid species [61]. In fact, a depressant effect on the water permeability has been observed on addition of cholesterol to ceramide containing sphingomyelin and phosphatidylcholine membranes [4,52,75,76]. Further, a high cholesterol/ceramide ratio has been shown to render the lamellar lipid organization of mixtures of SC lipids less sensitive to variations in skin ceramide composition [19]. Since the most salient features of skin barrier lipid composition are (1) widespread heterogeneity and (2) an almost complete dominance of saturated very long chain lipid acyl chains with broad, very stable, chain length distributions [53,54] (cf. Table 1), it is logical to suggest that the extracellular lipid matrix of the SC is a plastic-crystal (i.e., "gel" phase) stabilized by cholesterol and heterogeneities in hydrocarbon chain length distributions with or without water present between the lamallae [74]. The stable alkyl chain distributions of ceramides and free fatty acids (mainly C24:0–C26:0, Table 1) [53,54] and the large relative amounts of cholesterol may aid intermixing of different lipid species. Consequently, the combination of (1) a lamellar plastic-crystalline structure (i.e., with low permeability as well as relatively low viscosity and great tendency to remain in a lamellar conformation due to the presence of cholesterol) and (2) relatively impermeable corneocytes would present a barrier of maximum resistance irrespective of environmental conditions, i.e., ideal in a biological context [74].

The proposed structural morphology of the epidermal permeability barrier of terrestrial mammals is a lamellar plastic-crystalline lipid structure, *either*

1. Without water, with ceramides in the "hairpin" conformation (i.e., the two alkyl chains pointing in the same direction) and/or splayed chain conformation (i.e., the two alkyl chains pointing in opposite directions) [77], which is supported by the absence of swelling of the intercellular lipid matrix upon hydration of the SC [19]
   or
2. With water, which is supported by the finding that hydration of the SC decreases lipid transition temperatures [78] and increases lipid disor-

dering [79]. The presence of water will necessitate a hairpin ceramide conformation or mixed splayed chain *and* hairpin ceramides [74].

The notion of a *single and coherent* lamellar "gel" phase in the stratum corneum is not inconsistent with the WAXD findings of Bouwstra et al. [81] and the electron diffraction studies of Pilgram et al. [82], who reported coexistence of orthorhombic (β form) and hexagonal (α form) chain packing lattices in isolated stratum corneum. This is because for ceramides the phase transition from hexagonal to a more orthorhombic chain packing is thought to be reversible and *continuous* (cf. previous discussion and Ref. 47). This implies that the same amide-linked fatty acid chain may have an orthorhombic packing in the upper part (i.e., closest to the polar headgroup) and a looser, more hexagonal packing in the lower part (i.e., the end of the hydrocarbon chain) at the same time in cholestrol-deficient regions. However, the "impurity," or compositional heterogeneity (i.e., many different chain lengths), of the crystal remains unperturbed (i.e., no lateral diffusion of molecules takes place during the continuous phase transition). This implies in turn that even in the case of almost complete "orthorhomicization" of the molecular chain packing in cholestrol-deficient regions, the single and coherent "gel" crystal remains intact, i.e., *no phase separation occurs.*

In conclusion, it is proposed that the extraordinary barrier capacity of terrestrial mammalian skin is due to the presence of a single and coherent plastic-crystalline lipid structure (i.e., "gel" phase) in the SC extracellular space. The proposed model could fully account for the extraordinary barrier capacity of mammalian skin and differs in a most significant way from earlier models, in that it predicts that no phase separation [e.g., between liquid crystalline and "gel" phases or between hexagonal ("gel" phases) and orthorhombic phases] is present in the intact barrier structure.

ACKNOWLEDGMENTS

The present work was made possible by the generous support from the Wenner-Gren Foundations (L.N.), the Swedish Council for Work Life Research (96-0486; 98-0552) (L.N.), and the Edward Welander Foundation (L.N.). We acknowledge the excellent editorial help from Sheri Vanderzee, Avon Products, Inc., Global R&D, Suffern, NY, and Dr. W. Holleran (UCSF), who kindly provided Figure 7.

REFERENCES

1. Hadley NF. Lipid water barriers in biological systems. Prog Lipid Res 1989; 28:1–34.

2. Elias PM, Menon GK. Structural and biochemical correlates of the epidermal permeability barrier. In: Elias PM, ed. Advances in Lipid Research. Vol. 24. Skin Lipids. New York: Academic Press, 1991:1–26.

3. Elias PM, Cullander C, Mauro T, Rassner U, Komuves L, Brown B, Menon GK. The secretory granular cell: the outermost granular cell as a specialized secretory cell. J Invest Dermatol Symp Oroc 1998; 3:87–100.

4. Schaefer H, Redelmeier TE. The Skin Barrier—Principles of Percutaneous Absorption. Basel:Karger, 1996.

5. Hennings H, Michael D, Cheng C, Steinert P, Holbrook K, Yuspa SH. Calcium regulation of growth and differentiation of mouse epidermal cells in culture. Cell 1980; 19:245–254.

6. Menon GK, Elias PM, Grayson S. Ionic calcium reservoirs in mammalian epidermis: ultrastructural localization with ion capture cytochemistry. J Invest Dermatol 1985; 84:508–512.

7. Warner RR. The distribution and functions of physiological elements in skin. In: Loden M, Maiback HI, eds. Dry Skin and Moisturizers: Chemistry and Function. Boca Raton: CRC Press, 2000:71–88.

8. Holbrook K. Ultrastructure of the epidermis. In: Leigh IM, Lane BE, Watt FM, eds. The Keratinocyte Handbook. Oxford: Cambridge University Press, 1994:3–39.

9. Whitfield JF. Calcium: cell cycle driver, differentiator and killer. New York: Chapman and Hall, 1997.

10. Rawlings AV, Scott IR, Harding CR, Bowser PA. Stratum corneum moisturization at the molecular level. J Invest Dermatol 1994; 103:731–740.

11. Lampe MA, Burlingame AL, Whitney J, Williams ML, Brown B, Roitman BE, Elias PM. Human stratum corneum lipids: characterization and regional variations. J Lipid Res 1983; 24:120–130.

12. Holleran WM, Takagi Y, Menon GK, Jackson SM, Lee JM, Feingold KR, Elias PM. Permeability barrier requirements regulate epidermal β-glucosylceramidase. J Lipid Res 1994; 35:903–911.

13. Holleran WM, Takagi Y, Menon GK, Legler G, Feingold KR, Elias PM. Processing of epidermal glucosylceramides is required for optimal mammalian cutaneous permeability barrier function. J Clin Invest 1993; 91:1656–1664.

14. Chapman SJ, Walsh A. Desmosomes, corneosomes and desquamation: an ultrastructural study of pig epidermis. Arch Dermatol Res 1990; 262:304–310.

15. Grayson S, Elias PM. Isolation and lipid biochemical characterization of stratum corneum membrane complexes: implications for the cutaneous permeability barrier. J Invest Dermatol 1982; 78:128–135.

16. Elias PM, Feingold KR. Lipid-related barriers and gradients in the epidermis. Ann NY Acad Sci 1988; 548:4–13.

17. Wertz PN, Downing DL. Epidermal lipids. In: Goldsmith LA, ed. Physiology, Biochemistry and Molecular Biology of the Skin. New York: Oxford University Press, 1991:205–236.

18. Schurer N, Elias PM. The biochemistry and functions of stratum corneum lipids. In: Elias PM, ed. Advances in Lipid Research. Vol. 24. New York: Academic Press, 1991:27–56.

19. Bouwstra JA, Dubbelaar FER, Gooris GS, Weerheim AM, Ponec M. The role of ceramide composition in the lipid organization of the skin barrier. Biochim Biophys Acta 1999; 1419:127–136.
20. Wertz PN, Downing DL. Ceramides of pig epidermis: structure determination. J Lipid Res 1983; 24:759–765.
21. Norlén L, Nicander I, Lundh-Rozell B, Ollmar S, Forslind B. Inter and intra individual differences in stratum corneum lipid content related to physical parameters of skin barrier function in-vivo. J Invest Dermatol 1999; 112:72–77.
22. Menon GK, Ghadially R. Morphology of lipid alterations in the epidermis: a review. Micros Res Technique 1997; 37:180–192.
23. Menon GK, Feingold KR, Moser AH, Brown B, Elias PM. De novo sterologenesis in the skin. II. Regulation by cutaneous barrier requirements. J Lipid Res 1985; 26:418–427.
24. Feldman R, Mainetti C, Saurat J-M. Skin lesions due to treatment with simvastatin (Zocor). Dermatology 1993; 186:272.
25. Bouwstra JA, Thewalt J, Gooris GS, Kitson NA. Model membrane approach to the epidermal permeability barrier: an x-ray diffraction study. Biochemistry 1998; 36:7717–7725.
26. Madison KC, Sando GN, Howard EJ, True CA, Gilbert D, Swartzendruber DC, Wertz PN. Lamellar granule biogenesis: a role for ceramide glucosyltransferase, lysosomal enzyme transport and the Golgi. J Invest Dermatol Symp Proc 1998; 3:80–86.
27. Holleran WM, Man M-Q, Gao WN, Menon GK, Elias PM, Feingold KR. Sphingolipids are required for mammalian barrier function. II. Inhibition of sphingolipid synthesis delays barrier recovery after acute perturbation. J Clin Invest 1991; 88:1338–1345.
28. Holleran WM, Sidransky E, Menon GK, Fartasch M, Grundman J-U, Ginns EI, Elias PM. Consequences of (β-)glucocerebrosidase deficiency in epidermis: ultrastructure and permeability barrier alterations in Gaucher's disease. J Clin Invest 1994; 93:1756–1764.
29. Doering T, Holleran WM, Potraz A, Vielhaber G, Elias PM, Suzuki K, Sandhoff K. Sphingolipid activator proteins are required for epidermal permeability barrier formation. J Biol Chem 1999; 274:11038–11045.
30. Di Nardo A, Wertz P, Giannetti A, Seidenari S. Ceramide and cholesterol composition of the skin of patients with atopic dermatitis. Acta Derm Venereol 1998; 78:27–30.
31. Hara J, Higuchi K, Okamoto R, Kawashima M, Imokawa G. High-expression of sphingomyelin deacylase is an important determinant of ceramide deficiency leading to barrier disruption in atopic dermatitis. J Invest Dermatol 2000; 115:406–413.
32. Motta S, Monti MS, Mellesi L, Caputo R, Carelli S, Ghidoni R. Ceramide composition of the psoriatic scale. Biochim Biophys Acta 1993; 1182:147–151.
33. Geilen CC, Wieder T, Orfanos CE. Ceramide signaling: regulatory role in cell proliferation, differentiation, and apoptosis in human epidermis. Arch Dermatol Res 1997; 289:559–566.
34. White SH, Mirejovsky D, King GI. Structure of lamellar lipid domains and corneo-

cyte envelopes of murine stratum corneum: an x-ray diffraction study. Biochemistry 1988; 27:3725–3732.
35. Bouwstra JA, Dubbelaar FER, Gooris GS, Ponec M. The lipid organization in the skin barrier. Acta Derm Venereol 2000; 208(Suppl):23–30.
36. Kitson N, Thewalt J, Lafleur M, Bloom M. A model membrane approach to the epidermal permeability barrier. Biochemistry 1994; 33:6707–6715.
37. Gay CL, Guy RH, Golden GM, Mak VHW, Francoeur ML. Characterization of low temperature (i.e., <65°C) lipid transitions in human stratum corneum. J Invest Dermatol 1994; 103:233–239.
38. Moore DJ, Rerek ME. Insights into the molecular organization of lipids in the skin barrier from infrared spectroscopy studies of stratum corneum lipid models. Acta Derm Venereol 2000; 208(Suppl):16–22.
39. Pilgram GSK. A Close Look at the Stratum Corneum Lipid Organization by Cryo-electron Diffraction: Significance for the Barrier Function of Human Skin. Ph.D. thesis, Leiden University, Amsterdam. 2000.
40. Behne M, Uchida Y, Seki T, de Montellano PO, Elias PM, Holleran WM. Omega-Hydroxyceramides are required for corneocyte envelope (CLE) formation and normal epidermal permeability barrier function. J Invest Dermatol 2000; 114:185–192.
41. Yoshikawa N, Imokawa G, Akimoto K, Jin K, Higuchi Y, Kawashima M. Regional analysis of ceramides within the stratum corneum in relation to seasonal changes. Dermatology 1994; 188:207–214.
42. Denda M, Koyama J, Hori J, Hori I, Takahashi M, Hara M, Tagami H. Age- and sex-dependent changes in stratum corneum sphingolipids. Arch Dermatol Res 1993; 285:415–417.
43. Feingold KR. Permeability barrier homeostasis: its biochemical basis and regulation. Cosmet Toil 1997; 112:49–59.
44. Williams ML, Elias PM, Feingold KR. Regulation and differentiation in newborn human keratinocytes by endogenous ligands of nuclear hormone receptors. J Skin Barr Res 2000; 2:3–26.
45. Small DM. The physical chemistry of lipids. Handbook of Lipid Research. New York: Plenum Press, 1986.
46. Larsson K. Lipids: Molecular Organization, Physical Functions and Technical Applications. Dundee, Scotland: The Oily Press, 1994.
47. Dahlén B, Pascher I. Molecular arrangements in sphingolipids. Thermotropic phase behavior or tetracosanoylphytosphingosine. Chem Phys Lipids 1979; 24:119–133.
48. Pascher I. Molecular arrangements in sphingolipids. Conformation and hydrogen bonding of ceramide and their implication on membrane stability and permeability. Biochim Biophys Acta 1976; 455:433–451.
49. Pascher I, Sundell S. Molecular arrangements of sphingolipids: the crystal structure of cerebrosides. Chem Phys Lipids 1977; 20:175–191.
50. Friedel MG. Les estats mesomorphes de la matiere. Annals de Physique 1922; 273 (November–December):474.
51. Evans FD, Wennerstrom H. The Colloidal Domain: Where Physics, Chemistry, Biology and Technology Meet. New York: VCH Publishers, 1994.
52. Lieckfeldt R, Villalain J, Gomez-Fernandez JC, Lee G. Diffusivity and structural

polymorphism in some model stratum corneum membrane systems. Biochim Biophys Acta 1993; 1151:182–188.

53. Wertz PW, Downing DT. Covalently bound hydroxyacylsphingosine in the stratum corneum. Biochim Biophys Acta 1987; 917:108–111.

54. Norlén L, Nicander I, Lundsjo A, Cronholm T, Forslind B. A new HPLC-based method for quantitative analysis of inner stratum corneum lipids with special reference to the free fatty acid fraction. Arch Dermatol Res 1998; 290:508–516.

55. Bogren H, Larsson K. An X-ray diffraction study of crystalline cholesterol in some pathological deposits in man. Biochim Biophys Acta 1963; 75:65–69.

56. Craven BM. Crystal structure of cholesterol monohydrate. Nature 1976; 260:727–729.

57. de Kruyff B, van Dijck PWM, Demel RA, Scjuijff A, Brants F, van Deenen LLM. Non-random distribution of cholesterol in phosphatidylcholine bilayers. Biochim Biophys Acta 1974; 356:1–7.

58. Takahashi H, Sinoda K, Hatta I. Effects of cholesterol on the lamellar and the inverted hexagonal phases of dielaidoyl phosphatidylethanolamine. Biochim Biophys Acta 1996; 1289:209–216.

59. McMullen TPW, McElhaney RN. New aspects of interaction of cholesterol with dipalmitoyl phosphatidylcholine bilayers as revealed by high-sensitivity differential scanning calorimetry. Biochim Biophys Acta 1995; 1234:90–98.

60. Ipsen JH, Karlström G, Mouritsen OG, Wennerström H, Zuckermann MJ. Phase equilibria in the phospphatidylcholine-cholesterol system. Biochim Biophys Acta 1987; 905:162–172.

61. Sparr E, Ekelund K, Engblom J, Engstrom S, Wennerstrom H. An AFM study of lipid monolayers. II. The effect of cholesterol on fatty acids. Langmuir 1999; 15:6950–6955.

62. Ekelund K, Eriksson L, Sparr E. Rectangular solid domains in ceramide–cholesterol monolayers—2D crystals. Biochim Biophys Acta 2000; 1464:1–6.

63. Ahmed SN, Brown DA, London E. On the origin of sphingolipid/cholesterol-rich detergent-insoluble membranes: physiological concentrations of cholesterol and sphingolipid induce formation of a detergent-insoluble, liquid ordered lipid phase in model membranes. Biochemistry 1977; 36:10944–10953.

64. Brown DA, London E. Structure of detergent-resistant membrane domains: does phase separation occur in biological membranes? Biochem Biophys Res Commun 1997; 240:1–7.

65. Brown RE. Sphingolipid organizationn in biomembranes: what physical studies of model membranes reveal. J Cell Sci 1998; 111:1–9.

66. Engblom J, Engström S, Jonsson B. Phase coexistence of cholestyerol-fatty acid mixtures and the effects of the penetration enhancer Azone. J Control Rel 1998; 52:271–280.

67. Norlén L, Engblom J, Anderson M, Forslind B. A new computer based evaporimeter system for rapid and precise measurements of water diffusion through stratum corneum in-vitro. J Invest Dermatol 1999; 113:533–540.

68. Engblom J, Engström S, Fontell K. The effect of skin penetration enhancer Azone on fatty acid-sodium soap-water mixtures. J Control Rel 1995; 33:299–305.

69. Craven BM, Guerina NG. The crystal structure of cholesterol oleate. Chem Phys Lipids 1979; 24:91–98.
70. Long SA, Wertz PW, Strauss JS, Downing DT. Human stratum corneum polar lipids and desquamation. Arch Dermatol Res 1985; 277:284–287.
71. Zettersten E, Man M-Q, Sato J, Denda M, Farell A, Ghadially R, Williams ML, Feingold KR, Elias PM. Recessive X-linked ichthyosis: role of cholesterol sulfate accumulation in the barrier abnormality. J Invest Dermatol 1998; 111:784–790.
72. Abrahamson J, Abrahamson S, Hellquist B, Larsson K, Pascher I, Sundell S. Cholesteryl sulfate and phosphate in the solid state and in aqueous solutions. Chem Phys Lipids 1977; 19:213–222.
73. Faure C, Tranchant J-F, Duforc EJ. Interfacial hydration of ceramide in stratum corneum model membrane measured by H NMR of D2O. J Chim Phys 1998; 95:480–486.
74. Clerc SG, Thompson TE. Permeability of dimyristoyl phosphatidylcholine/dipalmitoyl phosphatidylcholine bilayer membranes with coexisting gel and liquid crystalline phases. Biophys J 1995; 68:2333–2341.
75. Norlén L. The plastic-crystal model: a new theory for structure, function and formation of the mammalian skin barrier. J Invest Dermatol. Submitted.
76. Finkelstein A, Cass A. Effect of cholesterol on the water permeability of thin lipid membranes. Nature 1967; 216:717–718.
77. Fettiplace R. The influence of lipid on the water permeability of artificial membranes. Biochim Biophys Acta 1978; 513:1–10.
78. Corkery RW, Hyde ST. On the swelling of amphiphiles in water. Langmuir 1996; 12:5528–5529.
79. Golden GM, Guzek DB, Harris RR, McKie JE, Potts RO. Lipid thermotropic transitions in human stratum corneum. J Invest Dermatol 1986; 86:255–259.
80. Alonso A, Meirelles NC, Tabak M. Effects of hydration upon the fluidity of intercellular membranes of stratum corneum: an EPR study. Biochim Biophys Acta 1995; 1237:6–15.
81. Bouwstra JA, Gooris GS, Salmon-de Vries MA, Van der Spek JA, Bras W. Structure of human stratum corneum as a function of temperature and hydration: a wide-angle x-ray diffraction study. Int J Pharmaceut 1992; 84:205–216.
82. Pilgram GSK, Engelsma-van Pelt AM, Bouwstra JA, Koerten HK. Electron diffraction provides new information on human stratum corneum lipid organization studied in relation to depth and temperature. J Invest Dermatol 1999; 113(3):101–107.
83. Forslind B. A domain mosaic model of the skin barrier. Acta Derm Venereol (Stockh.) 1994; 74:1–6.
84. Robson KJ, Stewart ME, Michelsen S, Lazo ND, Downing DT. 6-hydroxy-4-sphingenine in human epidermal ceramides. J Lipid Res 1994; 35:2060–2068.
85. Halkier-Sorensen L, Menon GK, Elias PM, Thestrup-Pederson K, Ferngold K. Cutaneous barrier function after cold exposure in hairless mice: A model to demonstrate how cold interferes with barrier homeostasis among workers in the fish processing industry. Br J Dermatol 1995; 132:391–401.
86. Menon GK, Elias PM. In: Hengge UR, Volc-Platzer B, eds. The Skin and Gene Therapy. Berlin: Springer-Verlag, 2001:3–26.

3

Stratum Corneum Moisturizing Factors

Clive R. Harding

Unilever Research, Colworth Laboratory, Sharnbrook,
Bedford, United Kingdom

Ian R. Scott

Unilever Research, Edgewater Laboratory, Edgewater, New Jersey

1 INTRODUCTION

The skin is a complex structure that affords protection from the ravages of the external environment. The outermost layer, the stratum corneum (SC) represents the true interface with the environment and is a magnificent example of the successful adaptation of a tissue. Its efficient function is a prerequisite for terrestrial life itself, and it has become highly specialized to protect against the invasion of microorganisms and toxic agents and, perhaps most critically, to limit loss of water. The SC is heterogeneous in structure and at the simplest level has been likened to a brick wall in which the noncontinuous, essentially proteinaceous, terminally differentiated keratinocytes or corneocytes (bricks) are embedded in the continuous matrix of specialized lipids (mortar) [1]. The SC consists typically of 12–16 layers of flattened corneocytes [2]. Corneocytes have a mean thickness of around 1μm and a mean surface area of approximately 1000 μm^2, but ultimately the surface area is dependent upon age, anatomical location and conditions that influence epidermal proliferation such as UV irradiation [3].

  The corneocyte itself is devoid of intracellular organelles and cytoplasm and consists almost entirely of a keratin macrofibrillar matrix stabilized through inter- and intrakeratin chain disulfide bonds encapsulated within a protein shell called the cornified cell envelope [4]. This latter structure is composed of a number of specialized proteins that are extensively cross-linked through the action of at least two members of the transglutaminase family [5]. The cornified envelope is 15–20 nm thick [6], consisting of two components: a 15-nm-thick layer composed of defined structural proteins [7] and a 5-nm-thick layer of ceramide lipids [8] that are covalently attached to the protein envelope on the extracellular surface. The overall integrity of the SC itself is achieved primarily through specialized intercellular protein structures called corneodesmosomes [9,10], which effectively rivet the corneocytes together but which ultimately must be degraded to facilitate desquamation.

Within this complex structure, water plays a vital function, influencing elasticity, tensile strength, barrier characteristics, electrical resistance, and of course the overall appearance of the skin. In the absence of water the SC is an intrinsically rigid and brittle structure prone to cracking. Quite simply the SC must remain hydrated to maintain its integrity, and in healthy skin the tissue contains greater than 10% water [11]. Ultimately the state of hydration of the SC is governed by three factors: first, the water that reaches it from the underlying epidermis, second, water lost from the surface by evaporation, and, third, the intrinsic ability of this layer to hold water.

The maintenance of water balance in the SC is preserved through two major biophysical mechanisms. The first of these is the intercellular lamellar lipids that provide a very effective barrier to the passage of water through the tissue [12,13]. The second mechanism is provided by the natural moisturizing factor (NMF), a term first coined by Jacobi in 1959 [14] to describe the complex mixture of low molecular weight, water-soluble compounds present within the corneocytes [15]. Collectively, the NMF components have the ability to bind water against the desiccating action of the environment and thereby maintain tissue hydration. The highly structured intercellular lipid lamellae as well as the restricting of water movement through the SC also effectively prevent the highly water-soluble NMF from leaching out of the surface layers of the skin.

In this chapter we will concentrate on the second of these two complementary mechanisms and consider the origin, nature, and role of the NMF. We will describe in detail our understanding of the complex yet elegant biochemical pathway leading to its production and consider how this process has shaped our thinking of the SC as a dynamic tissue responding to the external environment.

2 NATURAL MOISTURIZING FACTOR

The NMF consists of a mixture of amino acids, organic acids, urea, and inorganic ions (see Ref. 16). These compounds are collectively present at high concentrations within the cell and may represent 10% dry weight of the SC [17]. The major constituents apart from amino acids are sodium lactate, urea, and pyrrolidone carboxylic acid (PCA).

The importance of the NMF lies in the fact that its constituent chemicals, in particular, sodium lactate and PCA salts, are intensely hygroscopic. Essentially they absorb atmospheric water and dissolve in their own water of hydration thereby acting as very efficient humectants. Biologically, this property allows the outermost layers of the SC to maintain liquid water against the desiccating action of the environment. Traditionally it was felt that this liquid water plasticized the SC, keeping it resilient by preventing cracking and flaking that might occur due to mechanical stresses.

In this chapter, with one exception, we will not discuss the properties of the individual components of the NMF in any detail. The exception is urocanic acid. Although historically considered as a component of the NMF, urocanic acid has unique properties which influence not only the SC but also the body as a whole.

2.1 Urocanic Acid

Urocanic acid (UCA) is formed by the action of the enzyme histidase [18] on free histidine present within the SC. As this enzyme is only found in one other organ in the body, the liver, its presence in the SC is significant. Urocanic acid absorbs ultraviolet light in the most damaging part of the solar spectrum and upon UV exposure is induced to isomerize from the naturally occurring trans isomer to the cis isomer. For many years UCA was considered to be an important part of the skin defense against UV-induced damage [19,20]. However, the in vivo efficacy of UCA as a natural photoprotective agent is debatable. In a clinical study [21] a 5% *trans*-UCA–containing formulation provided a minimal SPF of 1.58 (despite containing 20–200 times the level of UCA naturally present in the SC). The lack of correlation between naturally occurring levels of UCA in the SC and the UV sensitivity of each subject determined by the minimal erythemal dose further supports the lack of a truly significant photoprotective effect of UCA [21,22].

cis-UCA has been demonstrated to initiate suppression of selected immune responses and mimics the effects of UVB irradiation in suppressing delayed hypersensitivity responses in herpes simplex virus infection [23]. The precise mechanism by which *cis*-UCA alters the immune system remains to be clarified, but there is both supporting [24,25] and contradicting [26] evidence that histamine-like receptors are involved. Recent evidence suggests that UCA isomers may also serve as natural scavengers of hydroxyl radicals generated through UV exposure [27]. The levels of *cis*-UCA present in the SC are, not surprisingly, prone to seasonal variation. Norval and coworkers [28] have found that in Western Europeans the levels of *cis*-UCA on exposed body sites peak in July/August at close to 50–60% of total UCA. During the winter months the percentage of *cis*-UCA fell below 7% for all body sites.

3 MECHANISM OF ACTION

The view of NMF as humectants is simplistic; and the precise mechanism by which these molecules collectively influence SC functionality, the role of other molecules (lipids) in water retention, and indeed the precise locations of water within the SC remain points of considerable discussion. Three species of water are identifiable in the SC: tightly bound primary water of hydration bound to polar sites on SC proteins; less tightly bound secondary water, hydrogen-bonded to primary water of hydration, which increases in an amount up to around 40% total water content, and, finally, bulk liquid water which does not appear until about 40% total water is reached. It is the secondary water that is most dependent on the presence of NMF [29]. Nuclear magnetic resonance (NMR) studies by Vavasour et al. [30] indicated that there is a single major pool of water which resides within a relatively homogeneous and large compartment of the SC that they concluded must be within the corneocyte itself, which as we will see later is consistent with the initial localization of NMF. Based on T2 NMR relaxation times these authors also concluded that the water within the corneocyte interacts strongly with macromolecules, namely keratins. Imokawa and coworkers has demonstrated that the depletion of water-extractable materials from acetone/ether-treated SC causes a marked increase in molecular interaction between the individual filaments of keratin fibers as measured by C13 NMR [31]. This increased interaction between keratin filaments could be reversed by the application of water-extractable material back to the SC, specifically the neutral and basic free amino acids. These observations led Imokawa to conclude that the NMF plays the critical role in reducing the intermolecular forces between the nonhelical regions of the keratin filaments through interaction with water molecules, and is therefore vital in providing keratin fiber assembly with enhanced molecular mobility.

Imokawa also concludes from these and many studies [32] that the structural lipids play a considerable role in the water-holding potential of the SC. Application of acetone/ether (1:1) to human skin induces a lasting chapped and scaly skin, with a significant decrease in water content, despite the fact that such treatment could not induce a substantial release of NMF. The defect in water-holding properties in such solvent-damaged skin appears directly related to the depletion of intercellular lipids, especially the ceramides, which comprise up to 50% of the total SC lipids.

4 THE ORIGIN OF THE SKIN'S NMF

Until the early 1980s the source of the NMF and what controlled the levels to which these compounds accumulated in the SC were essentially unknown. Dowling and Naylor [33] disproved suggestions that NMF was formed by the concentration of sweat, and it became generally accepted that the majority of NMF elements were formed by the general degradation of nonessential, nonkeratinous protein during the process of terminal differentiation: "The dustbin hypothesis." Studies conducted in our own laboratory indicated strongly that this was not the case, and that there was a single unique protein responsible for the generation of free amino acids in the SC. This protein was a high molecular weight, histidine-rich protein (Mr >350,000), intrinsically very basic and with an unusual amino acid composition [34]. The extensive phosphorylation of serine residues within the protein rendered it extremely insoluble, and upon dialysis from urea containing buffers the purified protein formed dense aggregates essentially indistinguishable under microscopic examination from intact keratohyalin granules (KHG). In light of the earlier pioneering studies of Ugel [35], and the elegant autoradiographic studies conducted by Fukuyama and Epstein, which localized tritiated histidine-labeled proteins to the granular layer [36], we concluded that this protein was a major component of the KHG.

The most significant evidence supporting the theory that this protein was the source of the amino acid–derived components of the NMF was deduced from the remarkable similarity between the amino acid profile of the protein and that of the NMF itself (Fig. 1) [37]. This similarity became even more striking with the discovery that several of the free amino acids produced from the protein degradation were subsequently and specifically modified by reactions taking place within the SC to produce functional molecules. Glutamine was converted to PCA itself [38], and, as already discussed, histidine was converted to urocanic acid [22]. When these and other enzymatic pathways active within the SC were taken into account the conclusion was that the histidine-rich protein represented the *only source* of the free amino acids [37,39].

Further studies indicated that this protein was rapidly dephosphorylated during the transition of the mature granular cell into the corneocyte and then underwent selective proteolytic processing to form lower molecular weight, and soluble, basic species within the SC [40]. Based upon their ability to aggregate keratin fibers in vitro into macrostructures reminiscent of the keratin pattern seen in the SC vivo [41], Dale and coworkers named this class of basic proteins filaggrins [42]. The phosphorylated, high molecular weight precursor protein subsequently became known as profilaggrin. However, regardless of this putative structural role, and consistent with the biochemical evidence outlined herein, filaggrin was shown to be a transient component of the SC. Radiolabel pulse chase [37], immunohistochemical, and biochemical studies [43] revealed that filaggrin did not persist beyond the deepest two to three layers of the SC. Once formed it became extensively deiminated through the activity of the enzyme peptidylarginine deiminase, which served to reduce the affinity of the filaggrin/keratin complex [40,77], and, second, it was rapidly and completely degraded through small peptides to free amino acids. This fate of filaggrin within the SC mirrors electrical conductance measurements undertaken on isolated SC [44] which indicate that water-

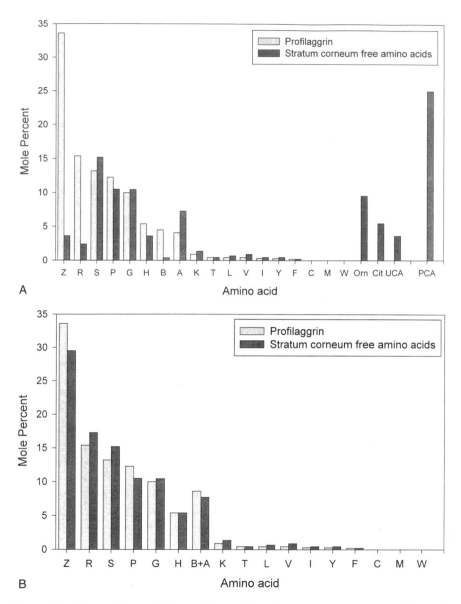

Figure 1 Comparison of the amino acid mole percentage composition of profilaggrin and stratum corneum free amino acids. (A) Actual analysis including amino acid derivatives found in the stratum corneum. (B) Comparative profile showing the marked similarity when these compounds are added to the total for the amino acid from which they are derived through enzymic and nonenzymic pathways. Cit, citrulline; Orn; Ornithine.

holding capacity is high in the superficial layers, maximal in the mid-portion (where filaggrin breakdown is initiated), and very low in the newly formed, immature SC (where filaggrin awaits hydrolysis).

In Caucasian skin the ratio of free amino acids to PCA in the SC varies from 7- to 12-fold (w/w). A remarkable correlation is evident between free amino acid levels and PCA content in the upper layers of the SC, which serves to emphasize that filaggrin hydrolysis is complete well before the corneocytes reach the surface (Fig. 2). This correlation also provides circumstantial evidence to support the studies that indicate that the majority of the PCA is formed spontaneously by nonenzymatic cyclization of glutamine [38].

This tortuous pathway of filaggrin synthesis, phosphorylation, subsequent dephosphorylation, selected proteolysis, followed inevitably by complete hydrolysis has both confused and intrigued scientists over the past 20 years, and while

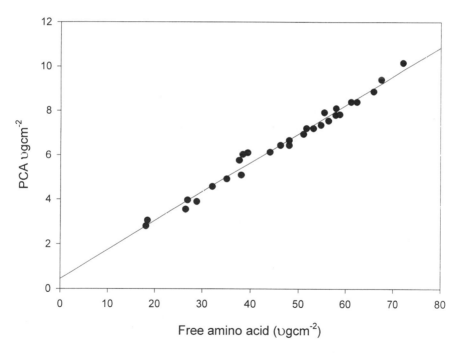

FIGURE 2 Correlation between the free amino acid levels (estimated as glutamic acid) and PCA levels in superficial stratum corneum. Eight consecutive tape strips of stratum corneum were taken from four adjacent sites on the volar forearm. Following extraction PCA was determined by reverse phase HPLC and free amino acids concentration determined using a modified colorimetric assay.

many questions remain unresolved, researchers have begun to unravel some of the mysteries associated with this unique protein.

In the following sections we will seek to explain how some of the apparent complexity of profilaggrin/filaggrin processing merely reflects nature's logical route to generate NMF effectively within the SC. We will also consider evidence that suggests further functions for this enigmatic class of proteins in terminal differentiation await clarification.

5 PROFILAGGRIN: SYNTHESIS, STRUCTURE, AND PROCESSING

Profilaggrin is first expressed in the granular layer and many studies have now confirmed the localization of profilaggrin to the KHG, and specifically to the so-called F-granules [45]. The profilaggrin molecule itself consists of multiple repeats of filaggrin joined by short hydrophobic linker peptides and flanked by N- and C-terminal domains. Ten to twelve filaggrin repeats are observed in the human protein and the repeat number is inherited in classical Mendelian fashion [46]. The filaggrin repeats show marked heterogeneity occurring in nearly 40% of the amino acid residues, whereas the linker peptides sequences are highly conserved. The N-terminal domain is subdivided into an A domain, which contains S100-like Ca^{2+} binding domains, and a B domain of unknown function [47]. Expression of filaggrin constructs in cell systems has indicated that both the filaggrin unit and the linker peptide are required for granule formation [48]. The disappearance of KHG (and hence the processing of profilaggrin), concomitant with the conversion of the granular cell into a corneocyte, argues strongly that this molecule plays an important role in the terminal differentiation process. Calcium binding in the N-terminal region of profilaggrin is likely to be pivotal in this process, just as it is to the terminal differentiation process itself. Although the nature of the critical initiating step in profilaggrin processing remains conjectural, several of the enzymatic processes occurring are now understood. Both the amino terminus and the C terminus beyond the last filaggrin repeat are cleaved [49,50]. The unique amino terminus with the distinct Ca^{2+} binding domains undergoes specific proteolysis [51], as do the linker regions. Extensive dephosphorylation by one or more phosphatases including PP2A [52], or possibly an acid phosphoprotein phosphatase [53], also occurs. Somewhat surprisingly the in vitro studies conducted do not support a critical role for dephosphorylation in changing the solubility of the protein, although the behavior of the macroprotein is likely to be significantly different from the low molecular weight filaggrin constructs prepared to study protein processing. The presence of glycosaminoglycan-like material associated with the keratohyalin granule and first alluded to by Fukuyama [54] may yet prove to play a critical role in influencing profilaggrin/filaggrin insolubility.

Collectively these studies indicate that profilaggrin processing is extremely complex. This complexity may represent the mechanism by which the cell maintains control of this critical process and thereby prevents premature collapsing of the cytoskeleton by inappropriate and untimely release of active filaggrin, which would have drastic consequences for the keratinocyte [55].

6 KERATIN/FILAGGRIN INTERACTION AND FILAGGRIN PROTEOLYSIS

Although the association of filaggrin with keratin intermediate filaments to form macrofibrils is a proven property in vitro [40,42], the in vivo relevance of this function remains controversial. Named for this property before the realization of its other perhaps more significant role, there is convincing and often overlooked evidence that casts doubt upon the need for a specific keratin aggregating protein for the SC. Significantly, close-packed keratin structures can be produced in vitro simply by adding inorganic salts to purified keratin preparations [56]. The species specificity of most antifilaggrin antibodies, the marked heterogeneity in the size of the mature filaggrin protein, and the diversification of amino acid sequence indicate that size and sequence of the protein are not critical for keratin aggregating ability. Indeed recent studies [48] indicate that filaggrin sequences as short as 16 residues (against a mature filaggrin repeat size of 324 residues) can effectively bind intermediate filaments.

Significantly, the ability of other, unrelated but importantly intrinsically basic proteins such as histones to effectively aggregate keratin (I. R. Scott, unpublished observations) indicates that this particular property is more dependent on overall charge distribution than on a precise sequence. Detailed studies led Mack [57] and coworkers to propose the "ionic zipper model" to explain filaggrin's aggregating potential. This model stipulates that filaggrin binds to filaments through simple ionic or H-bonding interactions between positionally conserved positive and negative charges (evident in the secondary structure of the B-turns of filaggrin) and the conserved distribution of positive and negative regions on the rod domains in keratin filaments.

The importance of filaggrin ionic charge for effective keratin interaction in vivo is emphasized by the loss of keratin binding affinity of filaggrin as the positively charged arginine residues within the protein are progressively converted to neutral citrulline residues by the action of peptidylarginine deiminase [40]. This deimination is not restricted to filaggrin, and keratin is also deiminated during SC maturation [77]. Further studies suggest that the ureido group on the citrulline functions to unfold proteins through a combination of a decrease in net charge, loss of potential ionic bonds, and interference with H-bonds [58]. As we shall discuss later dissociation of the filaggrin/keratin complex is a prerequisite for effective filaggrin proteolysis.

On close consideration of species differences the more highly conserved nature of the linker regions and phosphorylation sites inevitably leads one to the tentative conclusion that the constraints in the evolution of profilaggrin/filaggrin are more strongly linked to the processing events than to protein function itself. The in vivo evidence arguing against a critical keratin-aggregating role for filaggrin is even more compelling. In certain pathological conditions [59,60,61] the poor expression of filaggrin has no apparent effect on the keratin pattern observed in the affected SC. The same is true for the hard palate lining the oral cavity. This tissue is highly keratinized with a well-ordered keratin pattern [62], but no immunologically detectable filaggrin in the SC (Fig. 3a) [63].

7 FILAGGRIN IN ORAL EPITHELIA

The varied epithelia lining the oral cavity provide a unique opportunity to study further the fate and functions of filaggrin. In the hard palate, profilaggrin is readily detectable, but the apparent complete absence of processing to filaggrin infers an intrinsic, unknown function for profilaggrin itself. Likewise, if one accepts that the primary role of filaggrin is as a source of NMF, then whilst the presence of these molecules are undoubtedly critical for the exposed skin surface, one would argue that NMF (and hence filaggrin) should be absent, or reduced, in the wet-surfaced keratinized epithelia of the oral cavity, since these tissues have no requirement for hygroscopic material. Some keratinized tissues do lack filaggrin, but in others it is clearly present, for example, in the junctional region between the hard and soft palate (Fig. 3c). Logically, therefore, one must seek further functions for this complex family of proteins or their breakdown products. The possibility that filaggrin breakdown products play a role in controlling keratinocyte differentiation (i.e., proteolyzed elements act as chalones), although attractive, has not been substantiated [64], and no known filaggrin sequence matches that of the putative pentapeptide reported by Elgjo et al. to inhibit epidermal proliferation [65]. A third function for filaggrin—as a component of the cornified cell envelope—has been proposed [6,66], and human cornified cell envelopes contain around 10% filaggrin. If this cross-linked filaggrin retains an ability to interact with keratin, it may function to promote subsequent cross-linking of elements of the internal keratin macrofibrillar network into the cornified cell envelope.

However, it is an understanding of the subtleties of profilaggrin functionality itself that may prove pivotal in describing the control of, and sequence of events leading to, terminal differentiation. Recent evidence points to a role of the cleaved N-terminal peptide of profilaggrin having a potential role in inducing an apoptotic process in transitional cells just below the SC [67], and similarly filaggrin itself is also hypothesized to aid in the terminal differentiation process by potentiating apoptotic machinery [68].

Against a background of continued debate over whether filaggrin is a true structural protein, one fact is irrefutable, filaggrin is only present within the in-

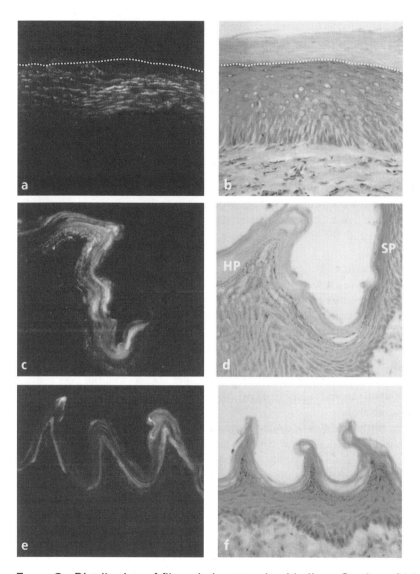

FIGURE 3 Distribution of filaggrin in rat oral epithelium. Section of (a) hard palate, (c) junctional epithelium, and (e) soft palate, stained with an antibody against filaggrin. Plates b, d, and f show comparable hematoxylin and eosin staining for the same sections. Filaggrin staining is noticeably present in the stratum corneum of junctional epithelium (c) between regions of hard (HP) and soft palate (SP), variably present in the soft palate (e), but completely absent from the hard palate (a), despite the presence of immunoreactive protein (profilaggrin) in the underlying granular layer.

nermost layers of the SC, and hence any structural role within the SC is transient. Nevertheless, within the newly formed layers of the SC, filaggrin may serve a specific short-lived function as a "scaffold" protein helping in the overall stabilization of the keratins macrofibrils. This proposal is based on the observation that when this protein is added in small amounts to keratin microfilaments, it catalyzes interchain disulfide bonds in keratin leading to macrofibril formation and subsequent insolubility [69].

8 ACTIVATION OF FILAGGRIN PROTEOLYSIS

As emphasized by immunolocalization studies, the degradation of filaggrin within the SC is abrupt and dramatic. Many proteases with the potential to degrade filaggrin in vitro have been characterized in the SC [70,71], but unequivocal demonstration that these proteases serve a comparable role in vivo remains elusive.

In contrast, the "trigger" which initiates filaggrin proteolysis at a precise stage of SC maturation was first identified in our laboratory in 1986 [43] following careful observation on patterns of filaggrin distribution in the SC after UV irradiation. In these studies it was observed that the effective filaggrin half-life within the SC was reduced dramatically to maintain the same overall distribution within the deepest layers, despite the greatly accelerated rate of cell turnover during the hyperplastic response to the UV stimulus. This indicated that filaggrin hydrolysis was not dictated by the age of a particular corneocyte, but was instead dependent upon the cell reaching a critical point during its transit through the SC to the skin surface.

From further studies in developing tissue we concluded that the signal initiating filaggrin breakdown was, in fact, the gradient of water activity existing across the SC [72].

In developing tissue (and as we have seen in certain oral epithelia) there is no indication of any proteolytic breakdown of filaggrin in the outer regions of the SC. However, within a few hours of birth, the breakdown of filaggrin is initiated in these regions. This triggering could be prevented in a very humid environment. Subsequent studies on filaggrin breakdown in isolated SC revealed that hydrolysis only occurred if the SC was maintained within a certain range of humidity (70–95%). These studies indicated that it is the very process of SC dehydration that initiates filaggrin hydrolysis.

Similarly, if the skin is occluded for a long period [73], filaggrin hydrolysis is blocked, the corneocytes remain filled with the protein, and the filaggrin-derived NMF components of the SC fall close to zero (Fig. 4). Under these conditions of occlusion, although filaggrin is not degraded, the process of deimination continues unabated and, in the absence of proteolysis, eventually produces a form of filaggrin that is incapable of interacting with keratin. These and more recent

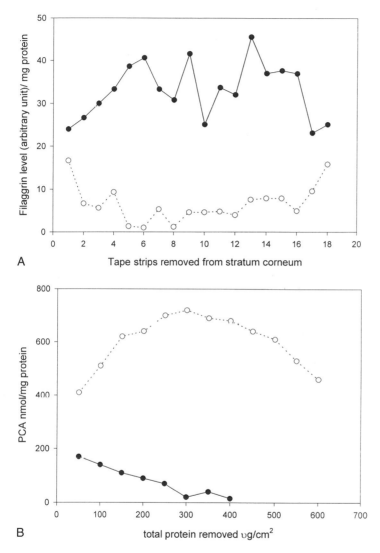

FIGURE 4 Influence of occlusion on the distribution of filaggrin, PCA, and urocanic acid (UCA) in superficial human stratum corneum. Skin surface was occluded for 10 days with a vapor-impermeable membrane. An adjacent un-occluded site served as a control. After 10 days occlusive patch was removed and both sites were repeatedly tape-stripped. (A) Filaggrin immunoreactive material in consecutive tape strips (1, skin surface). (B and C) Depth distribution profiles for PCA and UCA, respectively. Closed circles, occluded site; open circles, nonoccluded (control) site.

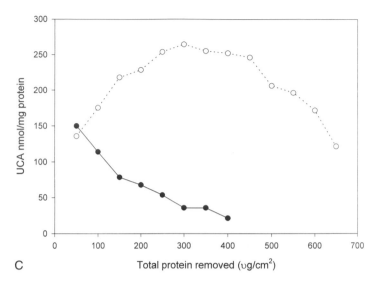

C

FIGURE 4   Continued

studies [74] suggest strongly that peptidylarginine deiminase activity is not the fi-laggrin-processing step regulated by changes in water activity within the SC. Traces of this deiminated form of filaggrin are also observed in the superficial layers of normal, nonoccluded skin, suggesting that deimination, in modifying the protease-labile arginine residues within filaggrin, eventually renders the protein resistant to the proteases otherwise responsible for its degradation.

9   THE COMPLEX NATURE OF NMF GENERATION

At first sight the process by which the skin generates the NMF within the SC seems unnecessarily complicated. However, the rationale of nature's complexity becomes apparent once it is appreciated that the epidermis cannot afford to generate NMF either within the viable layers or within the newly formed immature corneocyte itself, due to the risk of osmotic damage. It is essential that the activation of the filaggrin protease systems is controlled and delayed until the corneocytes containing it have flattened and the cornified cell envelopes have strengthened [75] and moved far enough out into the dryer areas of the SC. Only then is the structure likely to be able to withstand the osmotic effects generated by the sudden release of a concentrated NMF pool. The underlying epidermis prevents the potentially disastrous effects of osmotic pressure and the risk of cytoskeletal collapse through two strategies. First, profilaggrin once synthesized is precipitated within the keratohyalin granule where it acts as an insoluble, inert filaggrin precursor (profilaggrin cannot aggregate keratin). Most importantly, within the keratohyalin granule, profilaggrin exists as an osmotically inactive repository of the NMF. Second, the interaction between keratin and filaggrin forms a proteolytically resistant complex [69] that prevents premature proteolysis of the filaggrin (an intrinsically labile protein containing 10–15 mol% arginine residues) during the intensely hydrolytic processes that accompany SC formation. The value of this property of the filaggrin/keratin complex should not be underestimated. It is essential that filaggrin is exquisitely sensitive to proteolysis so that it can be completely and rapidly degraded to NMF when required, but first it must survive the massive and general cellular proteolysis that accompanies SC formation. This represents an enormous challenge for such a labile protein. Forming a complex with keratin provides the mechanism by which filaggrin can escape untimely hydrolysis. Indeed this may be the raison d'être of the affinity of filaggrin for keratin. As we have indicated, keratin does not need filaggrin to aggregate properly, but filaggrin may need keratin to elude the massive hydrolytic processes associated with SC formation. The importance of peptidylarginine deiminase is now evident. Deimination of filaggrin is essential to enable its subsequent dissociation, and ultimate hydrolysis.

In summary, these mechanisms are part of a subtle process which ensures that it is only as filaggrin-containing corneocytes migrate upward from the deepest layers and begin to dry out that proteases, by a poorly understood mechanism (but one intimately related to decreased water activity), are activated and the NMF is produced. The point at which this hydrolysis is initiated is independent of the age of the corneocyte [72] and is dictated ultimately by the environmental humidity. When the weather is humid, the proteolysis occurs almost at the outer surface; in conditions of extreme low humidity, the proteolysis is initiated deep within the tissue so that all but the deepest layers contain the NMF required to prevent desiccation. The SC has thus developed an elegant self-adjusting moisturization mechanism to respond to the different climatic conditions to which it is exposed.

The various processes leading from profilaggrin synthesis to conversion to filaggrin and then to NMF are under tight control. However, as we shall consider in Chapter 6 of this volume, these mechanisms are readily perturbed in different ways by a range of external factors including UV light, exposure to surfactants, and of course changes in the environmental humidity. These very different factors can, in isolation or in concert, contribute to the complex phenomenon recognized as dry skin.

10 CONCLUSIONS

Natural moisturizing factor is essential for the correct functioning of the SC. Working together with the interlamellar lipids it assists in the retention of water within the corneocytes vital for the barrier and mechanical properties of the SC. Our understanding of the terminal differentiation and SC maturation processes has increased enormously over the last two decades, and it has now become clear that by maintaining hydration of the SC, the NMF also facilitates key biochemical events. The coordinated activity of specific proteases is essential for optimum SC function, and these hydrolytic processes can only function in the presence of water, which is effectively maintained by NMF. Perhaps the most striking example of this is the regulation of the proteases ("filaggrinases") within the corneocyte which are responsible ultimately for the generation of the NMF itself. Insights into the process of NMF generation dismiss the notion that the SC is simply a passive barrier and emphasize the dynamic, responsive nature of this unique tissue.

REFERENCES

1. Elias PM. Epidermal lipids, barrier function and desquamation. J Invest Dermatol 1983; 80(Suppl 1):44–49.
2. Zhen YX, Suetake T, Tagami H. Number of cell layers of the stratum corneum in normal skin—relationship to the anatomical location on the body, age, sex and physical parameters. Arch Dermatol Res 1999; 291:555–559.
3. Marks R, Barton SP. The significance of the size and shape of corneocytes. In: Marks R, Plewig G, eds. Stratum Corneum. Berlin: Springer-Verlag, 1983:161–170.
4. Ricé RH, Green L. Cornified envelope of terminally differentiated human epidermal keratinocytes consists of cross-linked proteins. Cell 1977; 11:417–422.
5. Reichert U, Michel S, Scmidt R. The cornified envelope: a key structure of terminally differentiated keratinocytes. In: Darmon M, Blumberg M, eds. Molecular Biology of the Skin: The Keratinocyte. New York: Academic Press, 1994:107–150.
6. Jarnik M, Simon MN, Steven AC. Cornified cell envelope assembly: a model based on electron microscopic determinations of thickness and projected density. Cell Biol 1998; 111:1051–1061.
7. Steinert PM, Marekov LN. The proteins elafin, filaggrin, keratin intermediate filaments, loricrin, and small proline-rich proteins are isodipeptide cross-linked components of the human cornified cell-envelope. J Biol Chem 1995; 270:17702–17711.
8. Wertz PW, Madison KC, Downing DT. Covalently bound lipids of human SC. J Invest Dermatol 1989; 92:109–111.
9. Chapman S, Walsh A. Desmosomes, corneosomes and desquamation, an ultrastructural study of adult pig epidermis. Arch Dermatol Res 1990; 282:304–310.
10. Skerrow CJ, Clelland DG, Skerrow D. Changes to desmosomal antigens and lectin-binding sires during differentiation in normal epidermis: a quantitative ultrastructural study. J Cell Sci 1989; 92:667–677.
11. Blank IH. Factors which influence the water content of the SC. J Invest Dermatol 1952; 18:433–430.
12. Wertz PW, Miethke MC, Long SA, Strauss JS, Downing DT. Composition of ceramides from human SC and comedones. J Invest Dermatol 1985; 8:410–412.
13. Elias PM, Menon GK. Structural and lipid biochemical correlates of the epidermal permeability barrier. In: Elias, PM, ed. Advances in lipid research. Vol. 240 New York: Academic Press, 1991:1–26.

14. Jacobi O. About the mechanism of moisture regulation in the horny layer of the skin. Proc Scient Sect Toil Goods Assoc 1959; 31:22–26.

15. Tabachnick J, Labadie JH. Studies on the biochemistry of epidermis. IV. The free amino acids, ammonia, urea and pyrrolidone carboxylic acid content of conventional and germ free albino guinea pig epidermis. J Invest Dermatol 1970; 54:24–31.

16. Cler EJ, Fourtanier A. L'acide pyrrolidone carboxylique (PCA) et la peau. Int J Cosmet Sci 1981; 3:101.

17. Trianse SJ. The search for the ideal moisturizer. Cosmetics and Perfumery 1974; 89:57.

18. Scott IR. Factors controlling the expressed activity of histidine ammonia lyase in the epidermis and the resulting accumulation of urocanic acid. Biochem J 1981; 194:829–838.

19. Angelin JH. Urocanic acid a natural sunscreen. Cosmet Toil 1976; 91:47–49.

20. Baden HP, Pathak MA. The metabolism and function of urocanic acid in the skin. J Invest Dermatol 1967; 48:11–17.

21. Olivarius FD, Wulf HC, Crosby J, Norval M. The sunscreening effect of urocanic acid. Photodermatol Photoimmunol Photomedicine 1996; 12:95–99.

22. Olivarius FD, Wulf HC, Therkilsden P, Poulson T, Crosby J, Norval M. Urocanic acid isomers: relation to body site, pigmentation, SC thickness and photosensitivity. Arch Dermatol Res 1997; 289:501–505.

23. de Fabo EC, Noonan FP. Mechanism of immune suppression by ultraviolet irradiation in vivo. J Exp Med 1983; 157:84–98.

24. Gilmour JW, Norval M, Simpson TJ, Neuvoken K, Pasenen P. The role of histamine-like receptors in immunosuppression of delayed-hypersensitivity induced by cis-urocanic acid. Photodermatol Photoimmunol Photomedicine 1993; 9:250–254.

25. Koizumi H, Shimizu T, Nishino H, Ohkawara A. cis-Urocanic acid attenuates histamine-receptor mediated activation of adenylate cyclase and increase in intracellular Ca^{2+}. Arch Dermatol Res 1998; 290:264–269.

26. Laihia JK, Attila M, Neuvonen K, Pasenen P, Tuomisto L, Jansen CT. Urocanic acid binds to GABA but not to histamine (H-1, H-2, or H-3) receptors. J Invest Dermatol 1998; 111:705–706.

27. Kammeyer A, Eggelte TA, Bos JD, Teunissen MBM. Urocanic acid isomers are good hydroxyl radical scavengers: a comparative study with structural analogues and with uric acid. Biochim Biophys Acta 1999; 1428:117–120.

28. Olivarius FD, Wulf HC, Crosby J, Norval M. Seasonal variations in urocanic acid isomers in human skin. Photochemistry and Photobiology 1997; 66:119–123.

29. Takahashi M, Kawasaki K, Tanaka M, Ohra S, Tsuda Y. The mechanism of SC plasticisation with water. In: Marks R, Pine PA, eds. Bioengineering and the Skin. Lancaster: MTP Press, 1981:161–170.

30. Vavasour I, Kitson N, MacKay A. What's water got to do with it? A nuclear magnetic resonance study of molecular motion in pig SC. J Invest Dermatol Symp Proc 1998; 3:101–104.

31. Jokura Y, Ishikawa S, Tokuda H, Imokawa G. Molecular analysis of elastic properties of the SC by solid-state C-13 nuclear magnetic resonance spectroscopy. J Invest Dermatol 1995; 104:806–812.

32. Imokawa G. Skin moisturizers: development and clinical use of ceramides. In: Lo-

den M, Maibach H, eds. Dry Skin and Moisturizers. London: CRC Press, 2000:269–298.

33. Dowling GB, Naylor PFD. The source of free amino acids in keratin scrapings. Br J Dermatol 1960; 72:59–63.

34. Scott IR, Harding CR. Studies on the synthesis and degradation of a histidine rich phosphoprotein from mammalian epidermis. Biochim Biophys Acta 1981; 669:65–78.

35. Ugel AR. Bovine keratohyalin: anatomical, histochemical, ultrastructural and biochemical studies. J Invest Dermatol 1975; 65:118–126.

36. Fukuyama K, Epstein WL. A comparative autoradiographic study of keratohyalin granules containing histidine and cysteine. J Ultrastruct Res 1975; 51:314–325.

37. Scott IR, Harding CR, Barrett JG. Histidine rich proteins of the keratohyalin granules: source of the free amino acids, urocanic acid and pyrrolidone carboxylic acid in the SC. Biochim Biophys Acta 1982; 719:110–117.

38. Barrett JG, Scott IR. Pyrrolidone carboxylic acid synthesis in guinea pig epidermis. J Invest Dermatol 1983; 81:122–124.

39. Horii I, Kawasaki K, Hoyama J, Nakajima Y, Ohazaki K, Seiji M. Histidine-rich proteins as a possible source of free amino acids of stratum corneum. J Dermatol (Tokyo) 1983; 10:25–33.

40. Harding CR, Scott IR. Histidine-rich proteins (filaggrins). Structural and functional heterogeneity during epidermal differentiation. J Mol Biol 1983; 170:651–673.

41. Brody I. The keratinization of epidermal cells of newborn guinea pig skin as revealed by electron microscopy. J Ultrastruct Res 1959; 2:482–511.

42. Steinert PM, Cantieri JS, Teller JD, Lonsdale-Eccles JD, Dale BA. Characterization of a class of cationic proteins that specifically interact with intermediate filaments. Proc Natl Acad Sci USA 1981; 78:4097–4101.

43. Scott IR. Alterations in the metabolism of filaggrin in the skin after chemical and ultraviolet induced erythema. J Invest Dermatol 1986; 87:460–465.

44. Hashimotokumasaka K, Horii H, Tagami H. In vitro comparison of water holding capacity of the superficial and deeper layers of the stratum corneum. Arch Dermatol Res 1991; 283:342–346.

45. Steven AC, Bisher ME, Roop DR, Steinert PM. Biosynthetic pathways of filaggrin and loricrin—two major proteins expressed in terminally differentiated epidermal keratinocytes. J Struct Biol 1990; 104:150–162.

46. Gan SQ, McBride O, Idler WW, Markova N, Steinert PM. Organisation, structure and polymorphisms of the human profilaggrin gene. Biochemistry 1990; 29:9432–9440.

47. Presland RB, Bassuk JA, Kimball JR, Dale BA. Characterization of two distinct calcium binding sites in the amino terminus of profilaggrin. J Invest Dermatol 1995; 104:218–223.

48. Kuechle M, Thulin CD, Presland RB, Dale BA. Profilaggrin requires both linker and filaggrin peptide sequences to form granules: implications for profilaggrin processing in vivo. J Invest Dermatol 1999; 112:843–852.

49. Yamazaki M, Ishidoh K, Suga Y, Saido TC, Kawashima S, Suzuki K, Kominami E, Ogawa H. Cytoplasmic processing of human profilaggrin by active μ-calpain. Biochem Biophys Res Comm 1997; 235:652–656.

50. Resing KA, Thulin C, Whiting K, Al-Alawa N, Mostad S. Characterization of profilaggrin endoproteinase. 1. A regulated cytoplasmic endoproteinase of epidermis. J Biol Chem 1995; 270:28193–28298.
51. Presland RB, Kimball JR, Kautsky MB, Lewis SP, Lo CY, Dale BA. Evidence of specific proteolytic cleavage of the N-terminal domain of human profilaggrin during epidermal differentiation. J Invest Dermatol 1997; 108:170–178.
52. Kam E, Resing KA, Lin SK, Dale BA. Identification of rat epidermal profilaggrin phosphatase as a member of the protein phosphatase 2A family. J Cell Sci 1993; 106:219–226.
53. Ohno J, Fukuyama K, Hara A, Epstein WL. Immuno-histochemical and enzyme-histochemical detection of phosphoprotein phosphatase in rat epidermis. J Histochem Cytochem 1989; 37:629–634.
54. Kimura H, Fukuyama K, Epstein WL. Effects of hyaluronidase and neuriminidase on immunoreactivity of histidine-rich protein in new born rat epidermis. J Invest Dermatol 1981; 76:452–458.
55. Dale BA, Presland RB, Lewis SP, Underwood RA, Fleckman P. Transient expression of epidermal filaggrin in cultured cells causes collapse of intermediate filament networks with alteration of cell shape and nuclear integrity. J Invest Dermatol 1997; 108:179–187.
56. Fukuyama K, Murozuka T, Caldwell R, Epstein WL. Divalent cation stimulation of in vitro fibre assembly from epidermal keratin protein. J Cell Sci 1978; 33:255–263.
57. Mack JW, Steven AC, Steinert PM. The mechanism of interaction of filaggrin with intermediate filaments. J Mol Biol 1993; 232:50–66.
58. Tarcsa E, Marekov LN, Mei G, Melino G, Lee SC, Steinert PM. Protein unfolding by peptidylarginine deiminase—substrate specificity and structural relationships of the natural substrates trichohyalin and filaggrin. J Biol Chem 1996; 271:30709–30716.
59. Sybert VP, Dale BA, Holbrook KA. Ichthyosis vulgaris: identification of a defect in the synthesis of filaggrin correlated with an absence of keratohyalin granules. J Invest Dermatol 1985; 84:191–194.
60. Manabe M, Sanchez M, Sun TT, Dale BA. Interaction of filaggrin with keratin filaments during advanced stages of normal human epidermal differentiation and in Ichthyosis vulgaris. Differentiation 1991; 48:43–50.
61. Weidenthaler K, Hauber I, Anton-Lamprecht I. Is filaggrin really a filament-aggregating protein in vivo? Arch Dermatol Res 1993; 285:111–120.
62. Schroeder HE. Differentiation of human oral stratified epithelium. London: S Karger, 1981:35–67.
63. Scott IR, Harding CR. Profilaggrin phosphatase: a key step in the pathway of epithelial differentiation. J Invest Dermatol (abstr) 1991; 96:1006.
64. Mansbridge J, Knapp M. Effects of filaggrin breakdown on the growth and maturation of keratinocytes. Arch Dermatol Res 1987; 279:465–469.
65. Jensen PKA, Elgjo K, Laerum OD. Synthetic epidermal pentapeptide and related growth regulatory peptides inhibit proliferation and enhance differentiation in primary and regenerating cultures of human epidermal-keratinocytes. Cell Sci 1990; 97:51–58.
66. Richards S, Scott IR, Harding CR, Liddell E, Curtis GC. Evidence for filaggrin as a component of the cell envelope of the newborn rat. Biochem J 1988; 253:153–160.

67. Ishida-Yamamoto A, Tanaka H, Nakane H, Takahashi H, Hashimoto Y, Iizuka H. Programmed cell death in normal epidermis and loricrin keratoderma. Multiple functions of profilaggrin in keratinisation. J Invest Dermatol Symp Proc 1999; 4:145–149.
68. Kuechle MK, Presland RB, Lewis SP, Fleckman P, Dale BA. Inducible expression of filaggrin increases keratinocyte susceptibility to apoptotic cell death. Cell Death and Differentiation 2000; 7:566–573.
69. Steinert PM. Epidermal keratin: filaments and matrix In: Marks R, Plewig G, eds. Stratum Corneum. Berlin: Springer-Verlag, 1983:25–38.
70. Kawada A, Hara K, Morimoto K, Hiruma M, Ishibashi A. Rat epidermal cathepsin B: purification and characterization of proteolytic properties towards filaggrin and synthetic substrates. Int J Biochem, Cell Biol 1995; 27:175–183.
71. Kawada A, Hara K, Hiruma M, Noguchi H, Ishibashi A. Rat epidermal cathepsin L-proteinase: purification and some hydrolytic properties towards filaggrin and synthetic substrates. J Biochem (Tokyo) 1995; 118:332–337.
72. Scott IR, Harding CR. Filaggrin breakdown to water binding components during development of the rat SC is controlled by the water activity of the environment. Dev Biol 1986; 115:84–92.
73. Scott IR, Harding CR. Physiological effects of occlusion-filaggrin retention (abstr). Proc Dermatol 1993; 2000:773.
74. Akiyama K, Senshu T. Dynamic aspects of protein deimination in developing mouse epidermis. Exp Dermatol 1999; 8:177–186.
75. Harding CR, Long S, Rogers J, Banks J, Zhang Z, Bush A. The cornified cell envelope: an important marker of stratum corneum maturation in healthy and dry skin (abstr). J Invest Dermatol 1999; 112:306.
76. Nirunsuksiri W, Presland RB, Brumbaugh SG, Dale BA, Fleckman P. Decreased profilaggrin expression in Ichthyosis vulgaris is a result of selectively impaired post-translational control. J Biol Chem 1995; 270:871–876.
77. Senshu T, Kan SH, Ogawa H, Manabe M, Asaga H. Preferential deimination of keratin K1 and filaggrin during the terminal differentiation of human epidermis. Biochem Biophys Res Comm. 1996; 225:712–719.

4

Desquamation and the Role of Stratum Corneum Enzymes

Junko Sato
Shiseido Research Center, Yokohama, Japan

In the surface area of the skin, layers of corneocytes are tightly and stably bound to each other to form the stratum corneum (SC), the thin but tough barrier at the outermost area of the skin directly facing the external world. Each corneocyte originates from a keratinocyte which is actively proliferating in the epidermis under the SC, i.e., new layers of the corneocyte are supplied continuously from below the SC (Fig. 1). Concurrently, corneocytes serially detach and smoothly drop off from the skin surface for replacement to maintain the integrity and thickness of the SC, keeping it healthy. This shedding process of the corneocyte from the SC, *desquamation,* has strongly attracted the interest of many skin researchers because this is the process which regulates the condition of the skin.

The data obtained from the earlier "SC disaggregation tests," in which an SC sheet was incubated in a buffer solution and dissociation of corneocytes was measured, suggested that desquamation is controlled by an enzyme (or a set of enzymes) since heat treatment of the SC sheet irreversibly blocked the disaggregation [1]. The adhesive substance(s) connecting corneocytes in the SC has remained unidentified for a long time since the corneocytes are embedded in a lipid-enriched intercellular matrix. Bissett et al. proposed a charming hypothesis in 1987 that calcium ion–dependent proteinous linker molecules on the surface of corneocytes should connect the cells in the SC, as they observed promoted disso-

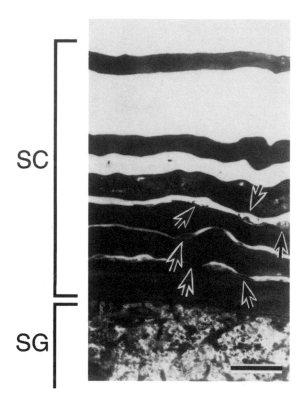

Figure 1 Ultrastructure of SC of mouse skin. Keratinocytes, which are actively dividing in the basal layer, differentiate into extremely flattened corneocytes to form the stratum corneum (SC) over stratum granulosum (SG). Between lower layers of corneocytes, desmosomes (arrows) are visible. (From Ref. 36.)

ciation of corneocytes by supplementation of proteases such as subtilisin and trypsin, divalent metal ion chelators like EDTA, and a surfactant 6-octadecyl-dimethyl ammoniohexanoate to the incubation buffer [2]. In the following year, Lundström and Egelrud suggested that desmosomes are involved in the cohesion of corneocytes because the plantar SC has desmoglein I, a transmembrane protein characteristic of desmosomes [3–5]. Later, Haftek et al. discovered another SC desmosomal protein, corneodesmosin, which is synthesized at the late stage of the epidermal differentiation in the stratum granulosum and is transported via keratinosomes to the cell periphery [6–8]. Both corneodesmosin and desmoglein I persist before desquamation in the SC, but disappear together after desquamation [6,7]. These findings and the fact that several protease inhibitors block both desquamation in vivo and the disaggregation of the SC in vitro suggest that breakdown of desmosomal proteins by proteolytic digestion catalyzed by the protease is the principal event of desquamation.

So far, several different protease activities have been detected in the SC [1,9–11]. Some of them have been purified and further characterized [12,13]. The results of these analyses suggested that it is not one particular enzyme but a combination of enzymes that is required for the shedding process of corneocytes. In addition, some factors of the SC such as the water content, cholesterol sulfate, calcium ion, and pH may also play substantial roles in desquamation, although how these factors regulate desquamation still remains mostly unknown. Inhibition of SC protease activities by endogenous inhibitors or oxidation of substrate molecules potentially connecting corneocytes may regulate the cell shedding in the SC as well. In this chapter, I review the SC proteases implied to be involved in desquamation mainly from the biochemical and molecular view points, as well as other SC factors which may be critical for regulation of desquamation.

1 PROTEASES

The inhibition profile obtained from SC disaggregation tests suggested that proteolytic digestion of adhesive molecules on the corneocytes leading to desquamation is mainly catalyzed by serine proteases because aprotinin, a specific inhibitor of serine proteases, inhibited disaggregation severely, but those protease inhibitors that block other types of proteases exhibited no effect [14]. Topical application of serine protease inhibitors induced scales on the skin [15] indicating that function of this type of protease is indeed required in vivo. Two different serine proteases, the chymotrypsin-like protease and the trypsin-like protease, have been isolated from the SC and characterized already. Recently, two other types of proteases, a cathepsin D type aspartic protease and a cysteine protease, were found in the SC and these proteases seem to be secondary proteases for desquamation and may be involved in the fine adjustment of the shedding process.

1.1 Chymotrypsin-Like Serine Protease

The first SC protease whose activity was detected by the disaggregation test was the chymotrypsin-like serine protease in the plantar SC [5,17]. Later this enzyme was shown immunohistochemically to be distributed in all types of SC on the whole body [18]. The active form of this enzyme, with an apparent molecular weight of 25 kD but molecular weight of 28 kD after reduction and full denaturation, was purified from the plantar SC [12]. Hansson et al. cloned of the cDNA of this enzyme [19]. There are two mRNA species of this enzyme, one is 1.2 and the other 2.0 kilo bases in size. Both of them are highly expressed only in skin; however, very low expression was detected in the brain and kidney, or undetectable in other tissues. A full-length cDNA of 968 nucleotides was cloned from the keratinocyte cDNA library by immunoscreening with the rabbit antisera raised against the purified enzyme, and it was confirmed that this enzyme has most of the highly conserved residues among various serine proteases, such as the active triad histidine–aspartate–serine residues. On the other hand, the overall identity in the amino acid sequence to other chymotryptic proteases (pancreatic chymotrypsin, cathepsin G, mast cell chymase) was less than 40%. Moreover, one position in the primary specificity pocket [20] is occupied by a bulky asparagine residue where a rather smaller serine or alanine residue is normally found in other chymotryptic enzymes. These structural differences from other chymotryptic enzymes may cause the peculiar substrate specificity and inhibitor profile exclusively exhibited by this enzyme [12].

The SC chymotrypsin-like protease is primarily synthesized as an inactive precursor protein of 253 amino acid residues. From the N terminus of the precursor, a signal peptide of 22 amino acid residues is cleaved off, and the resulting intermediate protein, still inactive because of the seven–amino acid propeptide at the N terminus, is stored in lamellar bodies harbored in the keratinocyte [18]. When a keratinocyte differentiates into a corneocyte, an intermediate is released into the extracellular spaces, and there the intermediate is processed by a tryptic enzyme to be the fully active protease.

The chymotrypsin-like protease may be the principal protease which digests the adhesive molecules connecting corneocytes. Nevertheless, the fact that the SC of an aged individual is thicker than that of a youth despite the absence of large differences in the activity of the chymotrypsin-like protease between the two SC [21] suggests that some factor(s) other than this enzyme itself is essential for regulation of desquamation.

1.2 Trypsin-Like Protease

The SC in the human skin contains another serine protease activity other than the chymotrypsin-like protease [1,5,12,14]. In a zymography experiment, the two bands of about 30 kD that developed on the SDS-polyacrylamide gel containing 1% casein disappeared when tryptic proteolysis was specifically inhibited by leupeptin, while two other bands of about 25 kD, which were attributed to the chymotrypsin-like protease, were not affected by the inhibitor (Fig. 2). This suggests that the human SC contains a trypsin-like enzyme [1]. Brattsand and Egelrud purified the enzyme and determined its primary structure by cDNA cloning [13]. The amino acid sequence of this enzyme is similar to those of the other serine proteases which have trypsin-like substrate specificity: the porcine enamel matrix protease exhibited the highest score (55% similarity) in the homology search in the available amino acid sequences in the database, followed by the human and mouse neuropsin. However, expression of the mRNA of this enzyme is high in

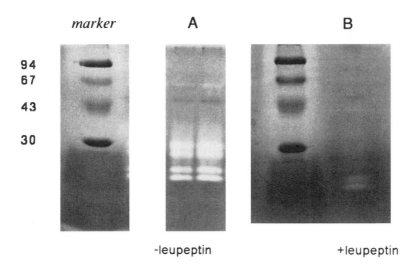

-leupeptin   +leupeptin

Figure 2 Stratum corneum contains proteolytic activity which is inhibited by leupeptin. Extract of SC was applied to SDS-polyacrylamide gel containing 1% casein with (B) or without (A) leupeptin. After electrophoresis, the gels were incubated in buffer with (B) or without (A) leupeptin. The bands around 30 kD which are visible in (B) are absent in (A). (From Ref. 1.)

the epidermis but low or undetectable in other tissues, suggesting that this enzyme is localized specifically in the skin. The SC trypsin-like protease, which consists of 227 amino acid residues, is synthesized initially as a preproprotein of 293 amino acid residues, and serially processed to be an active enzyme like the SC chymotryptic enzyme, but in contrast to the case of the other, the final step of maturation of the trypsin-like enzyme may be independent of other proteolytic activity, i.e., autocatalytic. Ekholm et al. studied maturation and localization of this enzyme in the SC immunochemically with the polyclonal antibodies raised against the overexpressed proteins in *E. coli* and compared the localization of this enzyme and the chymotrypsin-like enzyme [22]. They showed that the SC contains both the inactive proprotein, which still has the 37 amino acid long propeptide at the N terminus, and the active form of this enzyme. The apparant molecular mass of these two isoforms is about 37 and 33 kD, respectively, on the SDS-PAGE under the reduced condition. Interestingly, localization of this enzyme is almost completely the same in the skin as that of the chymotripsin-like SC protease, from the top region of the stratum granulosum to the surface of the skin. As both of these two serine proteases—the SC chymotrypsin-like and trypsin-like enzymes—are capable of exhibiting activity alone even at pH 5.5, the physiological pH of the surface of the skin, co-localization of these two SC serine proteases suggests that the chymotrypsin-like enzyme can be activated throughout the depth of the SC.

1.3 Other Proteases Found in SC

As ordinary serine proteases prefer a neutral to alkaline condition, they are unlikely to be fully active in an acidic environment like the skin surface, even if they can exhibit limited activities. Indeed, the fact that PMSF, a specific inhibitor against the serine protease, inhibits the SC disaggregation at pH 5.0 no more than 30% suggested that there should be other types of proteases which can promote dissociation of the SC at such a low pH [11]. Horikoshi et al. searched for a protease which can function at an acidic pH and discovered a new SC protease other than the serine protease, the cathepsin D type aspartic protease [23]. This enzyme is active between pH 2 to 6 with the optimum pH for activity being 3. Immunochemical data suggested that this enzyme is primarily synthesized in the keratinocyte as the inactive precursor of 52 kD and processed to the 48-kD intermediate probably in the lysozomes, and is finally activated to the functional 33-kD form at the boundary between the stratum granulosum and SC. As an in vitro experiment using liver cathepsin D as the substitute for the SC enzyme sufficiently suggested that this type of protease can have a function in desquamation [11], further characterization of the SC enzyme itself is awaited in order to clarify whether this enzyme is indeed involved in desquamation.

It has been reported that the epidermis contains cystein protease activity [10,24,25]. Watkinson reported that the cystein protease, which can be detected in all types of SC except for the palmoplantar SC, is active between pH 3 and 7, exhibits its highest activity at pH 6, and a partially purified extract exhibiting the cystein protease activity can degrade desmocollin in vitro [10]. However, the fact that E-64, the cysteine protease inhibitor, has no inhibitory effect in the SC disaggregation test [11,14,16] suggests that involvement of this enzyme in desquamation is probably negligible compared to that of other proteases.

2 OTHER SC FACTORS REGULATING DESQUAMATION

2.1 Cholesterol Sulfate

The content of cholesterol sulfate in the epidermis increases gradually along with the differentiation of the keratinocyte and reaches its maximum (about 5% of the total lipid) in the stratum granulosum, then drops at the boundary between the stratum granulosum and SC [26]. Within the normal SC, a difference in the content of cholesterol sulfate is also observed: it is higher in deeper layers of the SC and lower close to the surface of the skin where few desmosomes are observed [27]. On the other hand, the abnormally thickened SC of the patient suffering from recessive X-linked ichthyosis (RXLI), a disease which is caused by a deficiency of steroid sulfatase, accumulates fivefold more cholesterol sulfate than the normal SC, and the desmosome which is normally absent from the outer SC is observed even in the outermost layers of the SC [28]. As the transit time of nucleated cell layers of epidermis is normal, this symptom—retention hyperkeratosis—found in the SC of the RXLI patient is thought to be caused by delay of turnover of the SC [26]. These facts suggested that cholesterol sulfate in the SC is involved in the regulation of desquamation [29].

Topical application of cholesterol sulfate to the normal skin induced abnormal scaliness and an increase in thickness of the SC [30,31] and prolonged persistence of desmoglein I [15] without affecting the labeling index. However, phosphatidylcholine did not exhibit these effects [15]. In addition, cholesterol sulfate inhibited dissociation of the cells in the SC disaggregation test, but other amphopathic lipids—phosphatidylcholine, palmitic acid, and taurocholic acid—exhibited no inhibitory effect [15]. These results suggest that cholesterol sulfate can directly regulate the cell shedding in the SC and it is not simply because this substance has a detergent effect. Indeed cholesterol sulfate can inhibit activities of the serine protease: porcine pancreatic chymotrypsin and bovine pancreatic trypsin are inhibited competitively by cholesterol sulfate with Ki values of 2.1 micromolar and 5.5 micromolar, respectively, but cholesterol, phosphatidylcholine, palmitic acid, and taurocholic acid did not show any inhibitory activity in the same enzyme assay [15] In addition, the physicochemical properties of cholesterol sulfate may also lead to inhibition of desquamation in vivo. The study of behavior of lamellar phase suggested that cholesterol sulfate is one of the key factors which stabilize dissolution of cholesterol in the lamellar phases, i.e., cholesterol sulfate should stabilize the whole SC lamellar phase [32]. Therefore cholesterol sulfate in the SC may regulate the action of the SC protease in two ways: inhibiting its activity directly and obstructing the accessibility of the enzymes to the substrate with the stabilized lamellar phases of the intercellular lipids.

2.2 Water Content

Rawlings et al. showed that desmosomal degradation is inhibited under a dry condition as compared to a moist condition [33]. As environmental humidity influences the water content of SC [34,35], the water content of the SC has been suggested to be one of the important factors regulating desquamation.

Does the humidity of the environment alone alter the water content of SC and affect desquamation in vivo? To answer this question, we examined the change of the skin condition of mice kept under controlled humidity conditions [36]. The water content of the SC of mice kept under a dry condition (relative humidity of 10%) showed a decrease on and after day 1. Scales were induced on the skin surface and the thickness of SC increased without inducing epidermal hyperplasia on day 3. The tryptic activity assayed in vitro was the same in the dry SC and the control, suggesting that the dry SC contains the same amount of the trypsin-like protease as the control at that time point, but more undegraded desmosomal protein was observed in the dry SC. This suggests that scarcity of water in the SC may suppress desquamation through inhibition of the activity of SC protease. On the other hand, the number of scales on the surface of the skin of mice reared under the moist condition (relative humidity above 80%) decreased promptly and the water content of SC increased on and after day 1. However, the thickness of the SC was unchanged and the amount of intact desmoglein I was constant as well. These results suggested that desquamation was locally accelerated under this condition exclusively at the surface of the SC by excess water in the SC and, as a result, visible scales disappeared quickly, but promotion of desquamation was not observed as a whole.

Our experimental data imply the substantial involvement of the water in the SC in desquamation as a physiological regulatory factor, especially at the surface of the SC. However, change in the water content does not always affect the condition of the skin critically, as the thickness of the SC was stable in the SC of the moist skin. It can be explained by the following hypothesis: as illustrated in Figure 3, the efficiency of desquamation may depend on the relative humidity in the atmosphere and reaches a plateau at a critical point (a in Fig. 3). Therefore, as long as the relative humidity is higher than the critical point, no change in either desquamation or thickness of CS is observed, but when the relative humidity

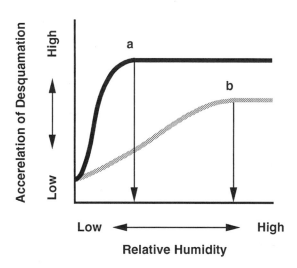

FIGURE 3 Hypothesis on the dependence of desquamation on relative humidity. The efficiency of desquamation may depend on the relative humidity in the atmosphere (black line) and reach a plateau at a critical point (a). The skin with reduced water-holding capacity (gray line) has a critical point at a higher humidity (b), resulting in its higher sensitivity to the dry condition than normal.

drops to below the critical point, inhibition of desquamation would be observed. The skin of an aged individual may have lower capacity to hold water in it, and possibly has a critical point at a higher relative humidity (b in Fig. 3) than that of a youth. So it is more sensitive to the dry condition and shows more severe scaliness in the dry season [37].

2.3 Other Factors

Öhman and Vahlquist observed an abnormal pH gradient in the SC in two different types of hyperkeratosis diseases, autosomal dominant ichthyosis (IV) and recessive X-linked ichthyosis [38]. These abnormalities of the skin pH may affect the desquamation and result in the abnormally thickened SC observed in these diseases. On the contrary, the altered pH gradient may be caused by the abnormality of the SC in these skin diseases. To clarify whether the pH in the SC is actually the cause and desquamation is the result, an experiment in which the pH in the skin surface is controlled for at least a few days in required, though such an experiment is technically difficult.

Oxidation of proteins is known to be correlated to aging, oxidative stress, and a number of diseases [39], and in general, proteases degrade oxidized proteins more rapidly than unoxidized forms [40,41]. In the healthy SC, the amount of the oxidized form of keratin 10 is high in the outer layers but low in the lower layers, suggesting that there is a gradient in the general protein oxidation through the SC which may concern the regulation of desquamation [42]. At the same time, oxidation of SC proteases may occur in the SC and decelerate desquamation.

From the view of regulation of desquamation, existence of physiological protease inhibitors is not surprising. Two different serine protease inhibitors, antileukopeptidase [43] and elafin [44], have been found in the psoriatic epidermis. As Franzke et al. showed that both of these inhibitors efficiently inhibit the SC chymotrypsin-like protease and block the cell shedding in the cell disaggregation test [16], these endogenous protease inhibitors may be involved in the regulation of desquamation even in the healthy skin, though the antileukopeptidase has not been detected in the normal skin yet [43].

Alpha-hydroxy acids such as glycolic acid promote desmosomal degradation [45]. Dicarboxylic acids with a small number of carbon atoms between the two carboxyl groups such as oxalic acid and malonic acid exhibit the same effect, while those with a large number of spacing carbon atoms, e.g., pimelic acid and suberic acid, do not [21]. Wang hypothesized that α-hydroxy acids may chelate calcium ions by their hydroxyl and carboxyl group and reduce intercellular concentration of the calcium ion [46]. Desmosomes may be stabilized by the calcium ion [47]. α-Hydroxy acids do not damage the barrier structures of the SC itself [45], and cosmetic and dermatological formulas containing these substances improve hyperkeratotic skin conditions [48,49]. These facts support that calcium ion affects desquamation by regulating desmosomal degradation.

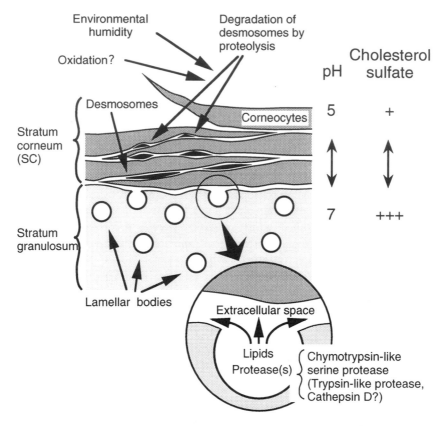

Figure 4 Scheme of desquamation and regulatory factors in the stratum corneum.

3 PROSPECTS

Despite the rapid advance in the past 20 years (summarized in Fig. 4), there remains many mysteries in the process and regulation of desquamation. Several regulatory factors have been proposed; some of them may actually regulate desquamation, but others may be the products which merely reflect the change occurring in the SC. Further studies will enable their discrimination.

As the SC exhibits many critical functions of the skin, such as barrier function, it must be able to respond to the environmental changes dynamically and steadily. Scaliness and thickening of the SC began within 3 days after shift to a low environmental humidity [36]. Following these alterations of the condition of the SC, hyperproliferation in the nucleated cell layer under the SC began in the second week accompanied with changes in barrier homeostasis and number of keratohyalin granules [50], although these changes were still not obvious at this stage [36]. An environmental signal which triggers these secondary changes involving the whole epidermis may be transferred to the nucleated cell layer possibly via the SC water flux, which becomes obvious within 12 h after the event [51]. Therefore, the SC can counteract the environmental change both in short and long time ranges with its autonomous function (desquamation) and those secondary alterations which require the aid of the downward epidermis.

Some moisturizers work quite well, but their action mechanisms in the skin are not so simple and are largely unknown. As the skin has the ability to adapt to the environment, it is desirable to encourage the ability to improve the condition of the damaged skin. Elucidation of the whole mechanism of desquamation will lead to new insight into skin care methodology, new substances, and new application techniques.

REFERENCES

1. Suzuki Y, Nomura J, Hori J, Koyama J, Takahashi M, Horii I. Detection and characterization of endogenous protease associated with desquamation of stratum corneum. Arch Dermatol Res 1993; 285:372–377.
2. Bissett DL, McBride JF, Patrick LF. Role of protein and calcium in stratum corneum cell cohesion. Arch Dermatol Res 1987; 279:184–189.
3. Egelrud T, Lundström A. Immunochemical analyses of the distribution of the desmosomal protein desmoglein I in different layers of plantar epidermis. Acta Derm Venereol (Stockh) 1989; 69:470–476.
4. Lundström A, Egelrud T. Cell shedding from plantar stratum corneum in vitro involves endogenous proteolysis of the desmosomal protein desmoglein I. J Invest Dermatol 1990; 94:216–220.
5. Lundström A, Egelrud T. Stratum corneum chymotryptic enzyme: a proteinase which may be generally present in the stratum corneum and with a possible involvement in desquamation. Acta Derm Venereol (Stockh) 1991; 71:471–474.
6. Serre G, Mils V, Haftek M. Identification of late differentiation antigens of human cornified epithelia, expressed in re-organized desmosomes and bound to cross-linked envelope. J Invest Dermatol 1991; 97:1061–1072.
7. Haftek M, Serre G, Mils V, Thivolet J. Immunocytochemical evidence of the possible role of keratinocyte cross-linked envelopes in stratum corneum cohesion. J Histochem Cytochem 1991; 39:153–158.
8. Montézin M, Simon M, Guerrin M, Serre G. Corneodesmosin, a corneodesmosome-specific basic protein, is expressed in the cornified epithelia of the pig, guinea pig, rat and mouse. Exp Cell Res 1997; 231:132–140.
9. Lundström A, Egelrud T. Cell shedding from human plantar skin in vitro: evidence of its dependence on endogenous proteolysis. J Invest Dermatol 1988; 91:340–343.
10. Watkinson A. Stratum corneum thiol protease (SCTP): a novel cysteine protease of late epidermal differentiation. Arch Dermatol Res 1999; 291:260–268.

11. Horikoshi T, Igarashi S, Uchida H, Brysk H, Brysk MM. Role of endogenous cathepsin D–like and chymotrypsin-like proteolysis in human epidermal desquamation. Br J Dermatol 1999; 141:453–459.

12. Egelrud T. Purification and preliminary characterization of stratum corneum chymotryptic enzyme: a proteinase which may be involved in desquamation. J Invest Dermatol 1993; 101:200–204.

13. Brattsand M, Egelrud T. Purification, molecular cloning, and expression of a human stratum corneum trypsin-like serine protease with possible function in desquamation. J Biol Chem 1999; 274:30033–30040.

14. Suzuki Y, Nomura J, Koyama J, Horii I. The role of protease in stratum corneum: involvement in stratum corneum desquamation. Arch Dermatol Res 1994; 286:3249–253.

15. Sato J, Denda M, Nakanishi J, Nomura J, Koyama J. Cholesterol sulfate inhibits proteases which are involved in desquamation of stratum corneum. J Invest Dermatol 1998; 111:189–193.

16. Franzke C-W, Baici A, Bartels J, Christophers E, Wiedow O. Antileukoprotease inhibits stratum corneum chymotryptic enzyme. J Biol Chem 1996; 271:21886–21890.

17. Egelrud T, Lundström A. A chymotrypsin-like proteinase that may be involved in desquamation in plantar stratum corneum. Arch Dermatol Res 1991; 283:108–112.

18. Sondell B, Thornell L-E, Egelrud T. Evidence that stratum corneum chymotryptic enzyme is transported to the stratum corneum extracellular space via lamellar bodies. J Invest Dermatol 1995; 104:819–823.

19. Hansson L, Strömqvist M, Bäckman A, Wallbrandt P, Carlstein A, Egelrud T. Cloning, expression, and characterization of stratum corneum chymotryptic enzyme. J Biol Chem 1994; 269:19420–19426.

20. Polgár L. In hydrolytic enzymes. In: Chaplin MF, Kennedy JF, eds. New Comprehensive Biochemistry. Vol. 16. Amsterdam: Elsevier Science, 1987:159–200.

21. Koyama J, Nakanishi J, Masuda Y, Sato J, Nomura J, Suzuki Y, Nakayama Y. The mechanism of desquamation in the stratum corneum and its relevance to skin care. In: Tagami H, Parrish JA, Ozawa T, eds. Skin: Interface of a Living System. The Netherlands: Elsevier Science, 1998:73–86.

22. Ekholm IE, Brattsand M, Egelrud T. Stratum corneum tryptic enzyme in normal epidermis: a missing link in the desquamation process? J Invest Dermatol 2000; 114:56–63.

23. Horikoshi T, Arany I, Rajaraman S, Chen S-H, Brysk H, Lei G, Tyring SK, Brysk MM. Isoforms of cathepsin D and human epidermal differentiation. Biochimie 1998; 80:605–612.

24. Ito Y, Fukuyama K, Yabe K, Epstein WL. Purification and properties of aminoendopeptidase from rat epidermis. J Invest Dermatol 1984; 83:265–269.

25. Fukuyama K, Ito Y, Yabe K, Epstein WL. Immunological detection if a cystein protease in the skin and other tissues. Cell Tissue Res 1985; 240:417–423.

26. Williams ML. Epidermal lipids and scaling diseases of the skin. Seminars in Dermatology 1992; 11:169–175.

27. Cox P, Squier CA. Variations in lipids in different layers of porcine epidermis. J Invest Dermatol 1986; 87:741–744.

28. Mesquita-Guimaraes J. X-Linked ichthyosis. Dermatolgica 1981; 162:157–166.

29. Williams ML. Lipids in normal and pathological desquamation. In: PM Elias, ed. Advances in Lipid Research. Vol. 24. San Diego: Academic Press, 1991:211–262.
30. Maloney ME, Williams ML, Epstein EH, Michael Y, Law L, Fritsch PO, Elias PM. Lipids in the pathogenesis of ichthyosis: topical cholesterol sulfate–induced scaling in hairless mice. J Invest Dermatol 1984; 83:252–256.
31. Elias PM, Williams ML, Maloney ME, Bonifas JA, Brawn BE, Grayson S, Epstein EH. Stratum corneum lipids in disorders of cornification. J Clin Invest 1984; 74:1414–1421.
32. Bouwstra JA, Gooris GS, Dubbelaar EFR, Ponec M. Cholesterol sulfate and calcium affect stratum corneum lipid organization over a wide temperature range. J Lipid Res 1999; 40:2303–2312.
33. Rawlings AV, Harding C, Watkinson A, Banks J, Ackerman C, Sabin R. The effect of glycerol and humidity on desmosome degradation in stratum corneum. Arch Dermatol Res 1995; 287:457–464.
34. Blank IH. Factors which influence the water content of the stratum corneum. J Invest Dermatol 1952; 18:433–440.
35. Hashimoto-Kumasaka K, Takahashi K, Tagami H. Electrical measurement of the water content of the stratum corneum in vivo and in vitro under various conditions: comparison between skin surface hygrometer and corneometer in evaluation of the skin surface hydration state. Acta Derm Venereol 1993; 73:335–339.
36. Sato J, Denda M, Nakanishi J, Koyama J. Dry condition affects desquamation of stratum corneum in vivo. J Derm Sci 1998; 18:163–169.
37. Horii I, Nakayama Y, Obata M, Tagami H. Stratum corneum hydration and amino acid content in xerotic skin. Br J Dermatol 1989; 121:587–592.
38. Öhman H, Vahlquist A. The pH gradient over the stratum corneum differs in X-linked recessive and autosomal dominant ichthyosis: a clue to the molecular origin of the "acid skin mantle"? J Invest Dermatol 1998; 111:674–677.
39. Oliver CN, Ahn B-W, Moerman EJ, Goldstein S, Stadtman ER. Age-related changes in oxidized proteins. J Biol Chem 1987; 262:5488.
40. Davies KJA, Lin SW, Pacifici RE. Protein damage and degradation by oxygen radicals: degradation of denatured protein. J Biol Chem 1987; 262:9914–9920.
41. Stadtman ER. Protein oxidation and aging. Science 1992; 257:1220–1224.
42. Thiele JJ, Hsieh SN, Briviba K, Sies H. Protein oxidation in human stratum corneum: susceptibility of keratins to oxidation in vitro and presence of a keratin oxidation gradient in vivo. J Invest Dermatol 1999; 113:335–339.
43. Molhuizen HOF, Alkemade HAC, Zeeuwen PLJM, de Jongh GJ, Wieringa B, Schalkwijk J. SKALP/elafin: an elastase in inhibitor from cultured human keratinocytes. J Biol Chem 1993; 268:12028–12032.
44. Wiedow O, Schröder J, Gregory H, Young JA, Chrisophers E. Elafin: an elastase-specific inhibitor of human skin. J Biol Chem 1990; 265:14791–14795.
45. Fartasch M, Teal J, Menon GK. Mode of action of glycolic acid on human stratum corneum: ultrastructural and functional evaluation of the epidermal barrier. Arch Dermatol Res 1997; 289:404–409.
46. Wang X. A theory for the mechanism of action of the α-hydroxy acids applied to the skin. Med Hypotheses 1999; 53:380–382.
47. Skerrow CJ. Desmosomal proteins. In: Bereiter-Hahn J, Matoltsy AG, Richards KS,

eds. Biology of the Integument. Vol. 2. Vertebrates. Berlin: Springer-Verlag, 1986:762–787.

48. Van Scott EJ, Yu RJ. Hyperkeratinization, corneocyte cohesion and alpha hydroxy acids. J Am Acad Dermatol 1974; 11:867–879.

49. Van Scott EJ, Yu RJ. Alpha hydroxy acids: therapeutic potential. Can J Dermatol 1989; 1:108–112.

50. Denda M, Sato J, Masuda Y, Tsuchiya T, Kuramoto M, Koyama J, Elias PM, Feingold KE. Exposure to a dry environment enhances epidermal permeability barrier function. J Invest Dermatol 1998; 111:858–863.

51. Sato J, Denda M, Ashida Y, Koyama J. Loss of water from the stratum corneum induces epidermal DNA synthesis in hairless mice. Arch Dermatol Res 1998; 290:634–637.

5

The Cornified Envelope: Its Role in Stratum Corneum Structure and Maturation

Allan Watkinson and Clive R. Harding
Unilever Research, Colworth Laboratory, Sharnbrook, Bedford,
United Kingdom

Anthony V. Rawlings
Unilever Research, Port Sunlight Laboratory, Bebington, Wirral,
United Kingdom

1 INTRODUCTION

The stratum corneum is the outermost layer of the skin and is the principal barrier tissue preventing water loss from the body and providing mechanical protection. It is produced as the end product of epidermal terminal differentiation, a process which involves several coordinated biochemical processes. The final result is a tissue that prevents water loss by the formation of a continuous matrix of highly organized lipid lamellae, into which is embedded an extensive network of "dead" cells called corneocytes [1,2].

Corneocyte morphology is crucial to the role of the stratum corneum as a mechanically resistant barrier tissue. The cells themselves are platelike with dimensions of approximately 50 μm across and 1 μm thin, stacked in layers, the number of which varying throughout the body [3–5]. As a remnant of the differentiating keratinocytes, corneocytes retain structural characteristics of the parent cell; they are packed with keratin intermediate filaments that provide the structural integrity and also an elasticity to resist stretching and compressional forces. Furthermore, as with the keratinocytes, they are linked together by rivetlike desmosomes to provide stratum corneum cohesion and integrity, although in the stratum corneum the desmosomes are modified structures and termed corneodesmosomes [6,7]. The most marked difference between corneocytes and their parent keratinocytes is that the former are largely devoid of cellular organelles, which degrade during corneocyte formation. As a result the corneocytes are only capable of catabolic reactions [8].

Since the corneocyte is localized within the hydrophobic lipid lamellae and requires a mechanically stable structure, the standard phospholipid-based plasma membrane used by cells in an aqueous environment is not a suitable cellular envelope. Instead the corneocyte replaces the phospholipid membrane with a highly cross-linked structure made up of specialized structural proteins. Hence a "protein cage" called the cornified envelope (CE) encapsulates the corneocyte. Morphologically, this structure can be detected by electron microscopy as an electron-dense layer of approximately 15 nm thick, adjacent to the intercellular spaces [9–12]. The CE has a more electron-lucent outer coating of approximately 5 nm thick which represents the covalently bound envelope [13,14].

The purpose of this chapter is to review the role of the CE in stratum corneum structure and function. However, it must be realized that all the structural elements of the corneocyte, the CE, the intermediate filaments, and the corneodesmosomes, are interlinked, making these cells, and indeed the stratum corneum itself, a giant macromolecule. Hence alterations in any one of these structures will drastically affect the others.

2 CORNIFIED ENVELOPE BIOCHEMISTRY

The CE has been likened to a protein cage. It is comprised of specialized structural proteins linked by specific γ-glutamyl-ε-lysine and γ-glutamyl-polyamine isopeptide bonds, and to a lesser extent disulfide linkages [15–18]. This results in each corneocyte being enclosed by a protein shell that in essence is a single macromolecule. In addition the specialized nature of the γ-glutamyl-ε-lysine confers a resistance to general proteolytic action. Moreover, a characteristic of the CE is that it is insoluble in SDS/reducing agent conditions, which are used in the isolation of these structures from stratum corneum tissue [19].

The biochemical composition of the CE is not homogeneous. The outermost region of the CE, adjacent to the intercellular space, is rich in the protein involucrin [20–22]. This is a rodlike protein rich in glutamine/glutamate and therefore suited as major structural protein in the CE; although only a specified fraction of the glutamate residues are cross-linked in vivo. Deeper within the CE structure, involucrin gives way to be replaced by the protein loricrin. Loricrin is an insoluble protein rich in glycine, serine, and cysteine and comprises the major component of the CE [23–26]. Probably the third most important component of the CE are the small proline-rich proteins (SPRs). The SPRs comprise a family of small proteins which are characterized into three groups; SPR 1 through 3, of which SPR 1 and 2 have been identified as epidermal CE components [21,26,27]. It is believed that these proteins function as cross-linking agents strengthening the CE against mechanical forces, supported by the correlation of CE SPR content with mechanical stress [28–30]. Additional minor CE components include cystatin-α (keratolinin) [31–33], elafin (SKALP) [26], envoplakin [34], periplakin [35], cystine-rich envelope protein (CREP) [36], S100 proteins, annexins, plasminogen activator inhibitor 2 [21] and filaggrin [37,38]. In addition, since the CE interacts with corneocyte structures such as the keratin intermediate filaments and the corneodesmosomes, keratins and desmoplakins have also been detected cross-linked to CE proteins [12,21,26].

2.1 Cornified Envelope Formation

The major function of the cornified envelope is to produce a mechanically robust alternative to the phospholipid-based plasma membranes of viable keratinocytes. Instantly replacing the keratinocyte plasma membrane is not feasible; hence one of the processes of epidermal terminal differentiation is to construct the CE while the plasma membrane is intact, prior to cornification.

The enzymes responsible for catalyzing γ-glutamyl-ε-lysine isopeptide bond formation are the transglutaminases (TGases) [15,39], Transglutaminases are Ca^{2+}-dependent enzymes and form a bond between the γ-glutamyl amino group and a primary amino group, the latter being normal provided by the side chain of lysine or by the polyamines putrescine and spermidine (Fig. 1)[16,17].

The epidermis produces three types of TGase. TGase 1 (TGase K) is expressed suprabasally, arising in the mid-spinous layer [40–42]. It is produced as a 106-KDa protein and due to N- and S-linked fatty acyl groups at its N-terminal region is membrane bound [43]. Following synthesis the protein is proteolytically processed to give soluble components of 10, 33, and 67 KDa, the complex of which is membrane bound and has enhanced activity [44]. TGase 3 (TGase E) is produced later in terminal differentiation in the granular layer [45–47]. It is produced as a soluble 77-KDa inactive pro-enzyme but subsequently cleaved to give the 50-KDa active form. TGase 2 (TGase C) is ubiquitous and has no role in CE formation but may play a role in apoptosis [48].

TGase 1 is accredited with initiating CE formation due to its earlier appearance in epidermal differentiation [42]. The first steps in CE construction appear to be the production of a scaffold using soluble involucrin as the major component [22]. Cornified envelope construction occurs immediately adjacent to the inner face of the keratinocyte plasma membrane. Precisely how this complex structure assembles is not fully understood. Studies using cultured keratinocytes suggest that involucrin, cross-linked in a head–tail and head–head orientation, spreads out from interdesmosomal regions to link with the desmosomal complexes, anchor-

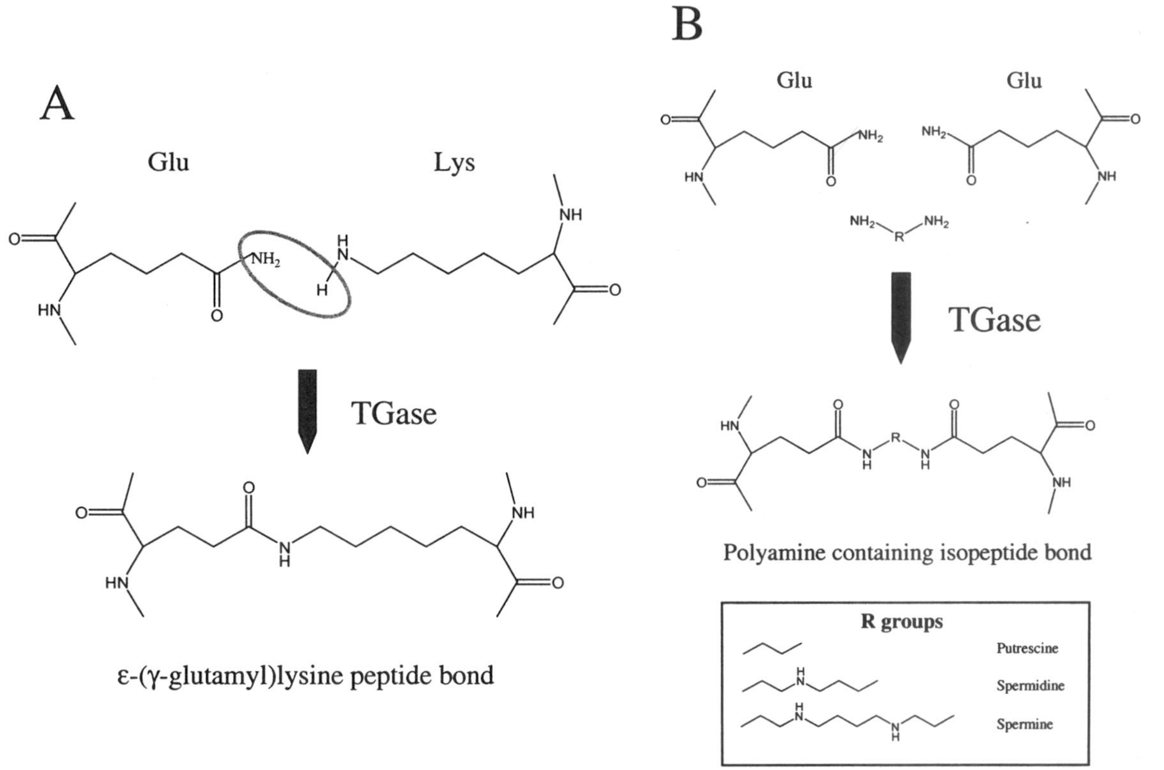

FIGURE 1   Schematic representation of TGase action to produce (A) ε-(γ-glutamyl))lysine peptide bond and (B) polyamine pseudo-isopeptide bond.

ing the forming CE into the keratinocyte cytoskeleton and tissue matrix [49]. Involucrin molecules may self-assemble on the keratinocyte plasma membrane by interacting with phosphatidylserine residues in a calcium-dependent manner and subsequently be linked by the action of membrane-bound TGase 1 [50]. Additional elements linked with this scaffold assembly process are envoplakin and possibly periplakin [49]. Envoplakin co-localizes with involucrin in the early steps of this process and similarly spreads from interdesmosomal regions to link with the desmosomes to produce a continuous layer adjacent to the plasma membrane. Once the involucrin envoplakin scaffold is produced, the structure is strengthened by the addition of loricrin, SPRs, and other CE components. Interestingly, it has been shown that loricrin associates initially with the desmosomal plaque in the granular layer keratinocytes and subsequently becomes incorporated in the CE during or after the cornification process [51]. This suggests that the desmosome may be a focal point for the accumulation and subsequent attachment of CE precursor proteins to the scaffold, possibly by the action of the annexins [21,51,52].

The synthesis of TGase 3 in the granular layer, subsequent to that of TGase 1, provides a supplementary soluble pool of TGase enzyme to facilitate CE completion. As the CE forms, membrane-bound TGase 1 is likely to become, at least partially, entrapped. TGase 3 has a higher affinity for loricrin than other CE components [53] and since this protein comprises about 70% of the CE, this suggests that it is the main enzyme involved in the completion of CE construction. However, both TGase 1 and 3 are required for the strengthening phase since SPR incorporation appears to require both enzymes, each acting at a different site on the molecule. For these same reasons, TGase 3 may also be the major enzyme of CE maturation within the stratum corneum, but currently there is little evidence to support this concept.

Isopeptide bonds are not the sole covalent bond involved in CE structure. Disulfide bonds also link CE components, being produced by the enzyme sulfydryl oxidase [54,55]. Little is known about their contribution to CE structure, especially since they are normally lost in CE isolation due to the use of reducing agents. Cysteine-containing CE components that could be involved in disulfide bond formation include CREP and loricrin [24,25,36]. The major function of disulfide bonds within the CE may be between loricrin and the keratins of the intermediate filaments, providing an additional link into the keratinocyte/corneocyte cytoskeleton [25].

2.2 Covalently-Bound Lipid

Whereas the polar head groups of the phospholipids in the plasma membrane allow interaction with the aqueous environment, in the SC the CE must interact with the hydrophobic lipid lamellae in the intercellular spaces. Since the outer regions of the CE comprise the involucrin scaffold and involucrin is a glutamine/glutamate-rich hydrophilic protein, additional modifications are required. Increasing the hydrophobicity of the outer layer of the CE is achieved by coating the protein with lipid molecules to produce a layer approximately 5 nm thick [13,14,56–58]. This layer is termed the covalently bound lipid and, it not only allows interaction with the intercellular space lipid, but also is believed to help stabilize the lamellar structure and may contribute to corneocyte cohesion [59,12].

The covalently bound lipid envelope is formed during cornification. The lamellar bodies extrude their lipid and enzyme contents, from the rapidly transforming granular layer keratinocytes into the intercellular space [8]. Among the extruded lipid are ω-hydroxy lipids that become covalently linked to the scaffold proteins. The covalently bound lipid is predominantly comprised of ceramide, composed of long-chain 28–34 carbon ω-hydroxyacids, amide-linked to the sphingosine moiety. Alkaline hydrolysis followed by high performance thin layer chromatography (HPTLC) fractionation reveals two variants of ceramide: ceramide A and B. The component fatty acids of both these ceramides are predominantly saturated or mono-unsaturated. Additional covalently bound lipid components are fatty acids and ω-hydroxyacids and again these are mainly saturated or mono-unsaturated [14,56–58].

These lipid components are linked to the involucrin scaffold by ester bonds to glutamate/glutamine residues on the protein [60]. For the ω-hydroxyceramides there are three potential ways of linking to the involucrin protein; these are through the ω-hydroxyl group of the fatty acid or through either hydroxyl group of the sphingosine residue. Certainly in pig stratum corneum, ω-hydroxyl (40%) and the sphingosine 1-hydroxyl groups (60%) make up the ester linkages, whereas the 3-hydroxy-sphingosine residue is not utilized (Fig. 2) [61]. Moreover, the spacial arrangements of the glutamate/glutamine residues on the involucrin molecule are orientated such as to provide regular spacing of the covalently bound lipids [62].

The enzyme responsible for linking the lipid moieties to the involucrin scaffold is currently unknown. It has recently been proposed that TGase 1 may be bifunctional, cross-linking the precursor proteins and esterifying the ω-hydroxyceramides to the glutamine/glutamate residues of this scaffold protein [63]. Incubation of TGase 1 with involucrin and ω-hydroxyceramide in a synthetic lipid vesicular system resulted in the esterification of the ceramide moiety to the involucrin protein. Moreover, the ω-hydroxy group was preferentially linked to the protein. However, whether TGase 1 functions in vivo to esterify lipids to the CE remains to be determined. If so, it is unlikely to be the only enzyme involved due to its specificity for the ω-hydroxyl over the 1-sphinogsine-hydroxyl. Furthermore, analysis of stratum corneum from patients with lamellar ichthyosis, a genetic condition in which TGase 1 activity is deficient or absent (see subsequent

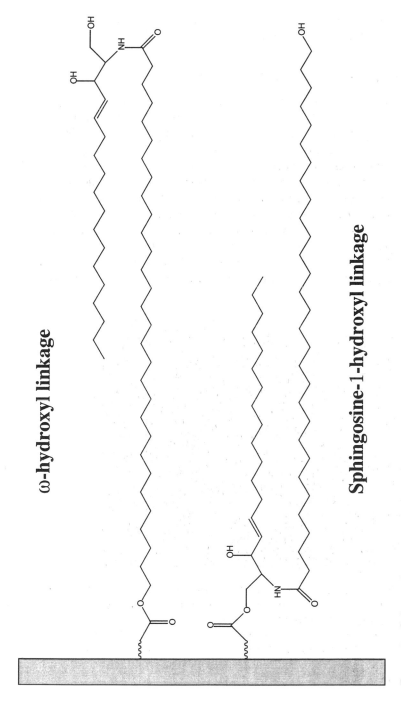

FIGURE 2 Schematic representation of covalently bound lipid ω-hydroxyl and sphingosine-1-hydroxyl ester linkages to involucrin.

discussion) revealed an apparently normal covalently bound lipid layer despite the presence of an abnormal CE [64].

3 CORNIFIED ENVELOPE MATURATION

During epidermal terminal differentiation, the formation of the CE occurs prior to conversion of granular layer keratinocytes to inert corneocytes. Hence during the cornification process, where the keratinocyte plasma membrane is degraded, the preformed CE leaves the corneocyte with a robust, encapsulating protein cage. However, this is only the "beginning of the end" for the CE. Although technically a dead tissue, the stratum corneum undergoes a series of biochemical changes until the corneocytes are ultimately lost, desquamated at the surface of the skin. As part of this maturation process the CE undergoes biochemical changes as it migrates through the layers of the stratum corneum, recognizable as morphological changes when isolated CEs are viewed using Nomarski contrast microscopy (Fig. 3). Cornified envelopes from the deeper, less mature layers of the stratum tend to have an irregularly shaped, ruffled appearance and are referred to as "frag-

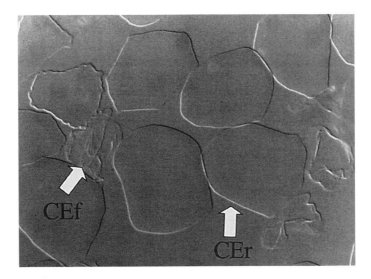

FIGURE 3 Normarski phase contrast microscopy of cornified envelopes demonstrating CEr and CEf maturation types. Corneocytes harvested by tape-stripping were exhaustively extracted with SDS/β-mercaptoethanol and the resultant cornified envelopes were then visualized using Normarski phase contrast microscopy. Immature CEf have an irregularly shaped, ruffled appearance; in contrast, the more mature CEr were polygonal in shape with a smoother surface.

ile" envelopes (CEf). In contrast, CE from the more mature, peripheral layers of the stratum corneum tend to be more polygonal in shape with a smoother surface and are called "rigid" cornified envelopes (CEr) [65]. The reasons for these morphological differences between mature and immature CE are unknown. Cyanogen bromide cleavage of CE to produce peptide maps did not reveal any significant difference between the two variants [66]. However, as well as being discernible under the microscope, the two CE variants can be differentiated by their interaction with the fluorescent label tetramethylrhodamine isothiocyanate (TRITC). CEr stain with an intense yellow-orange fluorescence whilst CEf stain weakly under the same conditions [18,66] (Fig. 4). This staining pattern can be used to follow the CE maturation process by determining the bulk fluorescence of tape-stripped CE which have been treated with TRITC. In the deeper SC, lower levels of fluorescence are detected, consistent with there being predominantly immature CEf; as the CE approach the surface of the SC, there is a marked increase in fluorescence (tape strips 9–12) consistent with a rapid, rather than gradual, maturation event to produce CEr (Fig. 5).

Interestingly, this maturation-associated change in fluorescence occurs after filaggrin has largely been hydrolyzed and therefore appears to be closely associ-

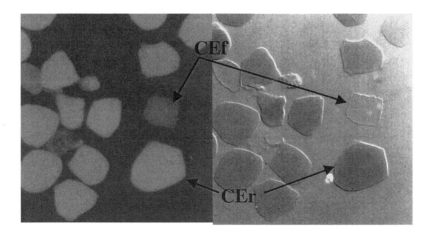

TRITC   **Normarski**

Figure 4 Fluorescence and Normarski phase contrast microscopy of TRITC stained cornified envelopes demonstrating increased fluorescence labeling of CEr compared to CEf. Exhaustively extracted corneocytes were treated with TRITC (200 µl/mL) for 2 hr, then washed and visualized by fluorescence microscopy followed by Normarski phase contrast microscopy. The mature CEr show increased fluorescence labeling compared to the immature CEf.

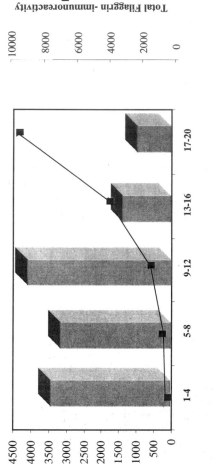

FIGURE 5 Depth distribution of TRITC labeling of CE in human stratum corneum. Corneocytes were harvested from the volar forearm by sequential tape-stripping, pooled in groups of four tapes and converted to CE by exhaustive extraction with SDS/β-mercaptoethanol containing protease inhibitors. After TRITC labeling, fluorescence (ex, 530 nm; em, 590 nm) was determined and normalized to dry weight of corneocytes. Filaggrin immunoreactivity was determined in the extract of each sample by western blotting with an antihuman filaggrin polyclonal antibody. Total immunoreactivity was determined by image analysis using Phoretix software. (From Refs. 70 and 71.)

ated with the stratum compactum–to–stratum disjunctum conversion [2,67]. The precise nature of the biochemical change resulting in this altered reaction to TRITC is unknown, although the isothiocyanate group is known to interact with free amino groups to produce a thiourea [68]. Hence increased TRITC binding in mature CEr may represent steric changes in the CE structure which allow interaction of the dye with previously masked areas of the CE structure. Certainly, from the morphological observations, it appears that the CEf transforms to become a less convoluted structure. Virtually nothing is known about the mechanisms that drive this morphological change, or indeed whether the morphological change is only detectable once the corneocytes are separated from the constraints of the tissue. We can speculate that this transformation is along the planar axes, owing to there being no apparent alteration in corneocyte thickness. In doing so, the decreased crenellation resulting from this change is likely to reduce the corneocyte–corneocyte contacts, aiding in the general dyshesion which occurs during stratum corneum maturation, and hence may play a role in desquamation. Cornified envelope transformation can only occur if there is a significant degradation of the restraining corneodesmosomes that attach each corneocyte to its neighbors. Interestingly, it is known that the predominant degradation of corneodesmosomes occurs at the planar faces of the corneocytes during the earlier phases of SC maturation [69], the loss of which would accommodate a planar two-dimensional change. It can be further speculated that the keratin intermediate filaments play a role in this maturation event, possibly even driving the transformation; however, precisely what role keratins play is unknown.

Since TGases are crucial for the production of the CE, it is conceivable that they are also involved in the CEf-to-CEr maturation process. Supporting this concept is the observation that total γ-glutamyl-ε-lysine cross-links increase in successive layers of the stratum corneum (Fig. 6) [70,71]. This suggests that the continued activity of stratum corneum TGases is important for correct maturation. Three pools of TGase activity can be found associated with the stratum corneum: a water-soluble TGase (Tris-buffer), a nonionic (Triton X100) detergent-soluble form, and a particulate form that cannot be liberated from the corneocyte. Ion exchange chromatography indicates that the water-soluble enzyme fraction is composed of both TGase 1 and 3 (Fig. 7). The Triton-soluble form represents bound enzyme, possibly associated with the covalently bound lipid, and is predominantly TGase 1; whereas the insoluble form may represent a pool of enzyme that is trapped within the CE. The importance of TGases to the CE maturation process can also be seen in TGase 1–deficient lamellar ichthyosis patients, where the CE are structurally much weaker than in normal corneocytes and the maturation process is prevented [18,64].

As with the protein components of the CE, the covalently bound lipid also appears to change during stratum corneum maturation. The deeper, less mature CE show increased cross-reactivity with involucrin antibodies and less staining

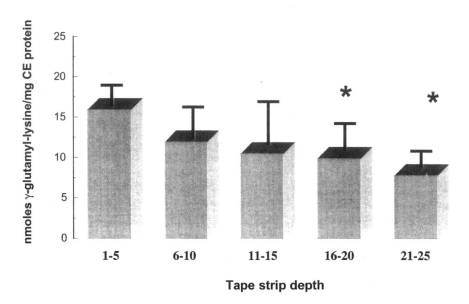

FIGURE 6 Distribution profile of ε-(γ-glutamyl)lysine cross-links in CE recovered from human stratum corneum. Consecutive tape strips were taken, pooled in groups of five and the corneocytes were exhaustively extracted in SDS/β-mercaptoethanol. γ-Glutamyl(lysine) cross-links were isolated from the CE by exhaustive protease digestion. The isolated ε-(γ-glutamyl)lysine dipeptide cross-links were quantified by reverse phase HPLC.* $p < 0.001$ compared to the surface γ-glutamyl(lysine) cross-link content ($n = 9$). (From Refs. 70 and 71.)

with the lipid stain Oil Red O. In contrast, the mature, peripheral CEr show less involucrin cross-reactivity and increased Oil Red O staining [72]. If confirmed, the increase in Oil Red O staining indicates that the CE progressively build up their covalently bound lipid. Furthermore, it suggests that the esterifying enzymes retain activity throughout the SC, presumably supplied with ω-hydroxyceramides from the intercellular space lipid lamellae. If indeed TGase 1 functions in this capacity, this would be consistent with the detection of TGase activity in the Triton X100 extracts of SC. The progressive reduction of involucrin labeling supports the continued enlargement of the covalently bound lipid covering due to sterical inhibition of antibody binding. However this could also be explained by an increase in involucrin cross-linking with maturation [73].

4 CORNIFIED ENVELOPES AND SKIN CONDITION

In considering the role of CE in skin condition, the necessity of isolating these structures with SDS and reducing agent has meant that they are devoid of the oth-

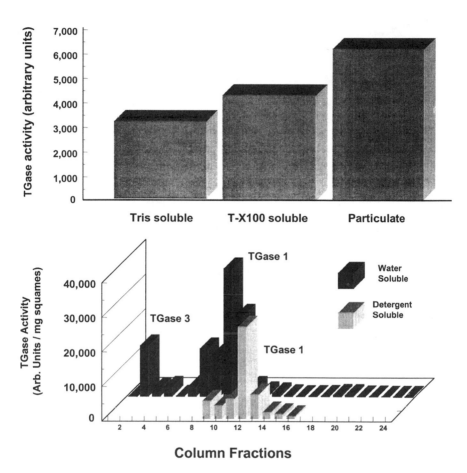

FIGURE 7 TGase enzymes in human stratum corneum. TGase activity was determined by putrescine cross-linking to dimethylcasein in extracts of stratum corneum. Panel A shows TGase activity determined from sequential extract of stratum corneum by 0.1 M Tris-HCl, pH 8, 10 mM EDTA (tris soluble); 0.1 M Tris-HCl, pH 8, 10 mM EDTA containing 1% (v/v) Triton X100 (T-X100 soluble); and in the remaining particular fraction. Panel B shows ion exchange chromatography of the Tris and T-X100 fractions on a MonoQ anion exchange column (SMART system; Pharmacia). (From Refs. 70 and 71.)

er main structural elements, particularly the keratin intermediate filaments and corneodesmosomal linkages. When viewed under the microscope, isolated unextracted corneocytes cannot readily be classified as CEf or CEr (Fig. 8). Therefore both the corneodesmosomes and keratin intermediate filaments must introduce structural constraints upon the CE as a whole. However, the corneodesmosomes

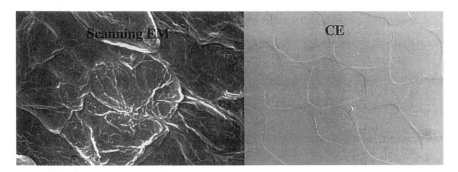

FIGURE 8 Comparison of peripheral CE and corneocytes. Peripheral corneocytes were harvested by tape-stripping and either exhaustively extracted
with SDS/β-mercaptoethanol and visualized using Normarski phase contrast
microscopy or analyzed directly by scanning electron microscopy. Although
the CE were predominantly CEr, scanning electron microscopy revealed a
ruffled appearance of the surface corneocytes. (From D. Atkins and A.
Watkinson, unpublished data.)

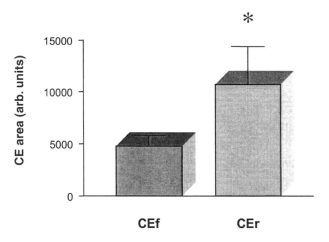

FIGURE 9 Comparison of CEr and CEf surface area. Corneocytes from upper
arm were harvested by tape-stripping and exhaustively extracted with
SDS/β-mercaptoethanol. After visualization using Normarski phase contrast
microscopy, electronically captured images were analyzed for cell surface
area. The results show the mean value ± s.d. for five samples, which in turn
were derived from measurements of at least 22 CE per sample, containing
approximately equal numbers of CEr and CEf (*p < 0.001). (From J. Richardson, unpublished data.)

and keratin intermediate filaments are not the sole determinants of CE shape. Area determination of CE shows that CEf are significantly smaller than CEr (Fig. 9). Therefore, within the CEf structure there must be physiochemical factors that constrain the structure to its ruffled appearance; moreover, subsequent modification of these factors during maturation allows the more open conformation of the CEr to form. Depth analysis of CE by TRITC labeling (Fig. 5) demonstrates that significant conversion of CEf to CEr occurs either at or immediately after the stratum compactum/disjunctum boundary. Conceivably, the ability of the CE to adopt a more open confirmation may contribute to the more open structure of the stratum disjunctum, and ultimately to the desquamatory process. Even in the presence of the keratin intermediate filaments, the hydrolysis of the corneodesmosomes during desquamation may allow the CE structure some freedom to open up, physically reducing corneocyte–corneocyte interactions.

When the CEf and CEr were named there was no reported evidence of their mechanical strength. Using micromanipulation of individual CE to measure the compressional mechanical component it was shown that the force required to maximally compress the CE is significantly different for the two types (Fig. 10): CEr were significantly stronger than CEf [70,71]. In addition, the CEr were considerably more heterogeneous in their mechanical behavior than CEf. Hence the terminology, based on appearance, does not represent a misnomer. It would therefore seem that CE maturation is a process necessary to create a much-strengthened outer layer to the stratum corneum. Since the stronger CEr structures normally arise in the more peripheral stratum corneum, we can speculate that they are involved in resisting the mechanical forces imposed on the tissue as a result of desiccation.

The rate at which the maturation event occurs appears to dictate the conversion of CEf to CEr. Environmentally exposed body sites have an increased rate of epidermal proliferation and smaller cell size [74,75]. Interestingly these sites also appear to have a decrease in the CEr content, compared to more protected body sites (Fig. 11). Cyanogen bromide cleavage of CE also suggests that CE from various body sites have slight structural differences [76], which may in part account for the variation in maturation. As a result it appears that increases in epidermal proliferation, with their knock-on effect of increasing stratum corneum maturation rate, also perturb the conversion of CEf to CEr.

A major body site difference in CE maturation is seen with palmo-plantar stratum corneum. Palmo-plantar stratum corneum is a specialized skin variant that is designed to withstand sheer and compressional forces. Structurally, it differs from normal interfollicular stratum corneum by corneodesmosomal retention and an increase in cell layers [77,78]. Analysis of CE reveals that palmo-plantar stratum corneum contains predominantly CEf in the more superficial layers (Fig. 12). Moreover, the cyanogen bromide cleavage peptides are different from those of interfollicular SC [76]. Hence, in the palmo-plantar stratum corneum the mat-

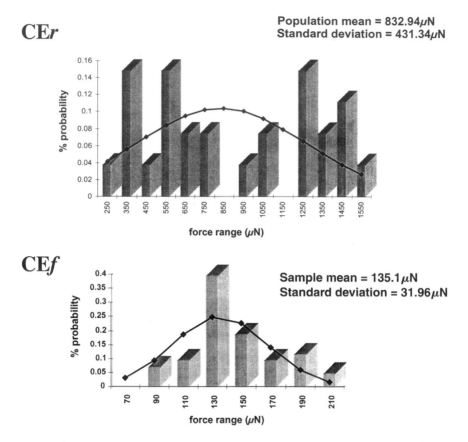

CE*r*

Population mean = 832.94μN
Standard deviation = 431.34μN

CE*f*

Sample mean = 135.1μN
Standard deviation = 31.96μN

Figure 10 Distribution profile of the maximal compressional forces (μN) of individual CE. Top panel shows the force range for CEr and the bottom panel for CEf. The maximal compression force for CEr was significantly different from that of CEf (p < 0.0001). (From Refs. 70 and 71).

uration process is either delayed or perturbed. Perceivably, one explanation for this lack of CE maturation is the structural constaints imposed on the CE due to the extensive corneodesmosomal content throughout the palmo-plantar stratum corneum. Interestingly, the preponderance of the weaker CEf in this tissue is at odds with its mechanical requirement. It can only be assumed that in this specialized stratum corneum structure the ruffled surface of the CEf maximizes the corneocyte–corneocyte interactions, strengthening the tissue.

Implicitly, one would expect that the platelike structure of the CE would contribute to skin texture. However, if the CE is not the major determinant of the

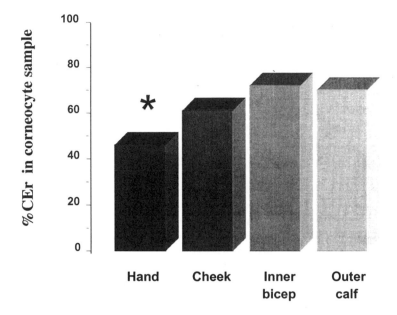

Figure 11 CE maturation in different body sites. Peripheral corneocytes were harvested by tape-stripping and exhaustively extracted with SDS/β-mercaptoethanol. The resultant CE were then visualized using Normarski phase contrast microscopy, and the CEr/CEf ratio was determined by Normarski phase contrast microscopy. The hand demonstrated significantly reduced levels of CE maturation (p < 0.001, cf. outer calf; n = 10). (From Ref. 70.)

surface of the corneocyte, the overall contribution of these structures to texture is debatable. However, skin smoothness is inversely related to friction and directly related to hardness, or resistance to deformation [79]. Measurement of skin texture using profilometry reveals that the greatest texture appears in areas with the highest proliferative rate [80,81], and consequently the greatest content of ruffled CEf. Therefore, the surface CEr may, by being mechanically stronger/harder, impart a smoother texture to the skin surface, despite the restraining function of the intermediate filaments. As such, normalization of stratum corneum maturation, with an increase in the CEr-containing corneocytes, would have beneficial effects upon skin smoothness.

5 CONCLUSION

In the last decade there have been significant advances in the understanding of the formation and structure of the CE. Several studies have shown the CE to be com-

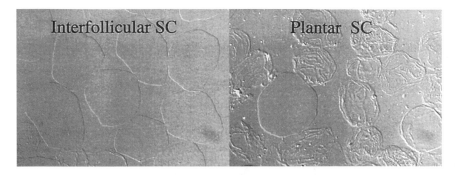

FIGURE 12 Comparison of peripheral CE from plantar and interfollicular stratum corneum. Peripheral corneocytes from either the sole of the foot or the axilla were harvested by tape-stripping and exhaustively extracted with SDS/β-mercaptoethanol. Normarski phase contrast microscopy revealed that the interfollicular CE were predominantly CEr, whereas the plantar CE were predominantly CEf. (From J. Richardson and A. Watkinson, unpublished data.)

posed of highly specialized structural proteins, which are laid down in a coordinated fashion to produce a robust protein cage encompassing the corneocyte. It has also been shown that once formed, the CE then undergoes a maturation process as it migrates through the stratum corneum, until it is eventually lost during desquamation. Our understanding of how this maturation process occurs and what this means for interaction with other structural elements of the stratum corneum is far from complete. It is inconceivable that the morphological and biochemical changes associated with the maturation event do not influence the condition of the skin. Indeed, perturbations of CE maturation invariably are associated with pathological skin conditions. A major challenge for the future research remains a more complete understanding of this maturation process and how it impinges on stratum corneum structure and skin condition.

ACKNOWLEDGMENT

I would like to thank Mrs. J. Richardson for her invaluable assistance in producing this manuscript. In addition I would like to thank Mr. P. Coan and Mr. D. Atkins for technical assistance with the TRITC analysis and SEM, respectively.

REFERENCES

1. Elias PM. Epidermal lipids, barrier function and desquamation. J Invest Dermatol 1983; 80(Suppl):44–49.
2. Harding CR, Watkinson A, Rawlings AV, Scott IR. Dry skin, moisturization and corneodesmolysis. Int J Cosmet Sci 2000; 22:21–52.
3. Marks R, Barton SP. The significance of the size and shape of corneocytes. In: Marks R, Plewig G, eds. Stratum Corneum. Berlin: Springer-Verlag, 1983:161–170.
4. Plewig G, Scheuber E, Reuter B, Waidelich W. Thickness of corneocytes. In: Marks R, Plewig G, eds. Stratum Corneum. Berlin: Springer-Verlag, 1983:171–174.
5. Zhen YX, Suetake T, Tagami H. Number of cell layers of the stratum corneum in normal skin—relationship to the anatomical location on the body, age, sex and physical parameters. Arch Dermatol Res 1999; 291:555–559.
6. Allen TD, Potten CS. Desmosomal form, fate and function in mammalian epidermis. J Ultrastruct Res 1975; 5:94–105.
7. Chapman SJ, Walsh, A. Desmosomes, corneosomes and desquamation. An ultrastructural study of adult pig epidermis. Arch Dermatol Res 1990; 282:304–310.
8. Holbrook KA. Biologic structure and function: perspectives on morphologic approaches to the study of the granular layer keratinocytes. J Invest Dermatol 1989; 92:84S–104S.
9. Matolsky AG, Balsamo CA. A study of the components of the cornified epithelium in skin. J Biophys Biochem Cytol 1955; 1:339–360.
10. Brody I. The modified plasma membranes of the transition and horny cells in normal human epidermis as revealed by electron microscopy. Acta Derm Venereol 1969; 49:128–138.
11. Farbman AI. Plasma membrane changes during keratinization. Anat Rev 1966; 156:269–282.
12. Haftek M, Serre G, Mils V, Thivolet J. Immunocytochemical evidence for a possible role of cross-linked keratinocyte envelopes in stratum-corneum cohesion. J Histochem Cytochem 1991; 39:1531–1538.
13. Lavker RM. Membrane coating granules: the fate of the discharged lamellae. J Ultrastruct Res 1976; 55:79–86.
14. Swartzendruber DC, Wertz PW, Madison KC, Downing DT. Evidence that the corneocyte has a chemically bound lipid envelope. J Invest Dermatol 1987; 88:709–713.
15. Rice RH, Green H. Cornified envelope of terminally differentiated human epidermal keratinocytes consists of cross-linked protein. Cell 1977; 11:417–422.
16. Martinet N, Beninati S, Nigra TP, Folk JE. N-(1,8)-bis(γ-Glutamyl)spermidine cross-linking in epidermal-cell envelopes—comparison of cross-link levels in normal and psoriatic cell envelopes. Biochem J 1990; 271:305–308.
17. Steinert PM. Structural-mechanical integration of keratin intermediate filaments with cell peripheral structures in the cornified epidermal keratinocyte. Biol Bull 1998; 194:367–368.
18. Reichert U, Michel S, Schmidt R. The cornified envelope: a key structure of terminally differentiating keratinocytes. In: Darmon M, Blumenberg M, eds. Molecular Biology of the Skin: The keratinocyte. New York: Academic Press, 1993:107–150.

19. Sun TT, Green H. Differentiation of epidermal keratinocyte in cell culture—formation of cornified envelope. Cell 1976; 9:511–521.
20. Robinson NA, LaCelle PT, Eckert RL. Involucrin is a covalently crosslinked constituent of highly purified epidermal corneocytes: evidence for a common pattern of involucrin crosslinking in vivo and in vitro. J Invest Dermatol 1996; 107:101–107.
21. Robinson NA, Lapic S, Welter JF, Eckert RL. S100A11, S100A10, annexin I, desmosomal proteins, small proline-rich proteins, plasminogen activator inhibitor-2, and involucrin are components of the cornified envelope of cultured human epidermal keratinocytes. J Biol Chem 1997; 272:12035–12046.
22. Steinert PM, Marekov LN. Direct evidence that involucrin is a major early isopeptide crosslinked component of the keratinocyte cornified cell envelope. J Biol Chem 1997; 272:2021–2030.
23. Mehrel T, Hohl D, Rothnagel JA, Longley MA, Bundman D, Cheng C, Lichti U, Bisher ME, Steven AC, Steinert PM, Yuspa SH, Roop DR. Identification of a major keratinocyte cell-envelope protein, loricrin. Cell 1990; 61:1103–1112.
24. Hohl D, Mehrel T, Lichti U, Turner ML, Roop DR, Steinert PM. Characterization of human loricrin—structure and function of a new class of epidermal-cell envelope proteins. J Biol Chem 1991; 266:6626–6636.
25. Hohl D, Roop D. Loricrin. In: Darmon M, Blumenberg M, eds. Molecular Biology of the Skin: The Keratinocyte. New York: Academic Press, 1993: 151–179.
26. Steinert PM, Marekov LN. The proteins elafin, filaggrin, keratin intermediate filaments, loricrin, and small proline-rich protein-1 and protein-2 are isodipeptide crosslinked components of the human epidermal cornified cell-envelope. J Biol Chem 1995; 270:17702–17711.
27. Hohl D, Deviragh PA, Amiguetbarras F, Gibbs S, Backendorf C, Huber M. The small proline-rich proteins constitute a multigene family of differentially regulated cornified cell-envelope precursor proteins. J Invest Dermatol 1995; 104:902–909.
28. Jarnik M, Kartasova T, Steinert PM, Lichti U, Steven AC. Differential expression and cell envelope incorporation of small proline-rich protein 1 in different cornified epithelia. J Cell Sci 1996; 109:1381–1391.
29. Steinert PM, Candi E, Kartasova T, Marekov L. Small proline-rich proteins are cross-bridging proteins in the cornified cell envelopes of stratified squamous epithelia. J Struct Biol 1998; 122:76–85.
30. Steinert PM, Kartasova T, Marekov LN. Biochemical evidence that small proline-rich proteins and trichohyalin function in epithelia by modulation of the biomechanical properties of their cornified cell envelopes. J Biol Chem 1998; 273:11758–11769.
31. Zettergren JG, Peterson LL, Wuepper KD. Keratolinin—the soluble substrate of epidermal transglutaminase from human and bovine tissue. Proc Natl Acad Sci 1984; 81:238–242.
32. Takahashi M, Tezuka T, Katunuma N. Phosphorylated cystatin-alpha is a natural substrate of epidermal transglutaminase for formation of skin cornified envelope. FEBS Lett 1992; 308:79–82.
33. Takahashi M, Tezuka T, Katunuma N. Filaggrin linker segment peptide and cystatin-α are parts of a complex of the cornified envelope of epidermis. Arch Biochem Biophys 1996; 329:123–126.

34. Ruhrberg C, Hajibagheri MAN, Simon M, Dooley TP, Watt FM. Envoplakin, a novel precursor of the cornified envelope that has homology to desmoplakin. J Cell Biol 1996; 134:715–729.

35. Ruhrberg C, Hajibagheri MAN, Parry DAD, Watt FM. Periplakin, a novel component of cornified envelopes and desmosomes that belongs to the plakin family and forms complexes with envoplakin. J Cell Biol 1997; 139:1835–1849.

36. Tezuka T, Takahashi M. The cystine-rich envelope protein from human epidermal stratum-corneum cells. J Invest Dermatol 1987; 88:47–51.

37. Richards S, Scott IR, Harding CR, Liddel JE, Powell GM, Curtis CG. Filaggrin—a novel component of the cornified envelope of the newborn rat. Biochem J 1988; 253(1):153–160.

38. Simon M, Haftek M, Sebbag M, Montezin M, Girbal-Neuhauser E, Schmitt D, Serre G. Evidence that filaggrin is a component of cornified cell envelopes in human plantar epidermis. Biochem J 1996; 317:173–177.

39. Folk JE. Transglutaminases. Ann Rev Biochem 1980; 49:517–531.

40. Thacher SM, Rice RH. Keratinocyte-specific transglutaminase of cultured human epidermal cells—relation to cross-linked envelope formation and terminal differentiation. Cell 1985; 40:685–695.

41. Kim IG, McBride OW, Wang M, Kim SY, Idler WW, Steinert PM. Structure and organization of the human transglutaminase-1 gene. J Biol Chem 1992; 267:7710–7717.

42. Kim SY, Chung SI, Yoneda K, Steinert PM. Expression of transglutaminase-1 in human epidermis. J Invest Dermatol 1995; 104:211–217.

43. Kim SY, Chung SI, Steinert PM. Highly-active soluble processed forms of the transglutaminase-1 enzyme in epidermal keratinocytes. J Biol Chem 1995; 270:18026–18035.

44. Ogawa H, Goldsmith LA. Human epidermal transglutaminase—preparation and properties. J Biol Chem 1976; 251:7281–7288.

45. Ogawa H, Goldsmith LA. Human epidermal transglutaminase. 2. Immunological properties. J Invest Dermatol 1977; 68:32–35.

46. Negi M, Colbert MC, Goldsmith LA. High molecular-weight human epidermal transglutaminase. J Invest Dermatol 1985; 85:75–78.

47. Kim IG, Gorman JJ, Park SC, Chung SI, Steinert PM. The deduced sequence of the novel protransglutaminase-E (TGase3) of human and mouse. J Biol Chem 1993; 268:12682–12690.

48. Reichert U, Fesus L. Programmed cell death. Retinoids Today and Tomorrow 1991; 24:31–34.

49. Steinert PM, Marekov LN. Initiation of assembly of the cell envelope barrier structure of stratified squamous epithelia. Mol Biol Cell 1999; 10:4247–4261.

50. Nemes Z, Marekov LN, Steinert PM. Involucrin cross-linking by transglutaminase 1—binding to membranes directs residue specificity. J Biol Chem 1999; 274:11013–11021.

51. Ishida-Yamamoto A, Tanaka H, Nakane H, Takahashi H, Izuka H. Antigen retrieval of loricrin epitopes at desmosomal areas of cornified cell envelopes: an immunoelectron microscopic analysis. Exp Dermatol 1999; 8:402–406.

52. Raknerud N. The ultrastructure of the interfollicular epidermis of the hairless (hr/hr)

mouse. III. Desmosomal transformation during keratinization. J Ultrastruct Res 1975; 52:32–51.

53. Candi E, Melino G, Mei G, Tarcsa E, Chung SI, Marekov LN, Steinert PM. Biochemical, structural, and transglutaminase substrate properties of human loricrin, the major epidermal cornified cell-envelope protein. J Biol Chem 1995; 270:26382–26390.

54. Yamada H, Takamori K, Ogawa H. Localization and some properties of skin sulfhydryl oxidase. Arch Dermatol Res 1987; 279:194–197.

55. Takamori K, Thorpe JM, Goldsmith LA. Skin sulfhydryl oxidase—purification and some properties. Biochim Biophys Acta 1980; 615:309–323.

56. Wertz PW, Downing DT. Covalently bound α-hydroxyacylsphingosine in the stratum corneum. Biochim Biophys Acta 1987; 917:108–111.

57. Wertz PW, Madison KC, Downing DT. Covalently bound lipids of human stratum corneum. J Invest Dermatol 1989; 92:109–111.

58. Wertz PW, Downing DT. Epidermal lipids. In: Goldsmith LA, ed. Physiology, Biochemistry and Molecular Biology of the Skin. Oxford: Oxford University Press, 1991:205–236.

59. Wertz PW, Swartzendruber DC, Kitko DJ, Madison KC, Downing DT. The role of corneocyte lipid envelopes in cohesion of the stratum corneum. J Invest Dermatol 1989; 93:169–172.

60. Marekov LN, Steinert PM. Ceramides are bound to structural proteins of the human foreskin epidermal cornified cell envelope. J Biol Chem 1998; 273:17763–17770.

61. Downing DT, Stewart ME, Lazo N. Forty per cent of porcine corneocyte envelope α-hydroxyceramides are bound to protein through their α-hydroxyl and sixty percent through their sphingosine 1-hydroxyl. J Invest Dermatol 1999; 112:575.

62. Stewart ME, Lazo LD, Downing DT. Modeling the topology of the corneocyte. J Invest Dermatol. 2000; 114:838.

63. Nemes Z, Marekov LN, Fesus L, Steinert PM. A novel function for transglutaminase 1: attachment of long-chain omega-hydroxyceramides to involucrin by ester bond formation. Proc Natl Acad Sci 1999; 96:8402–8407.

64. Elias PM, Uchida Y, Rice RH, Komuves L, Holleran WM. Formation of partial cornified envelopes and replete corneocyte-lipid envelope in patients with lamellar ichthyosis. J Invest Dermatol. 2000; 114:758.

65. Michel S, Schmidt R, Shroot B, Reichert U. Morphological and biochemical characterization of the cornified envelopes from human epidermal-keratinocytes of different origin. J Invest Dermatol 1988; 91:11–15.

66. Michel S, Reichert U. L'enveloppe cornee: une structure caracteristique des corneocytes. Rev Eur Dermatol. MST 1992; 4:9–17.

67. Bowser PA, White RJ. Isolation, barrier properties and lipid analysis of stratum compactum, a discrete region of the stratum corneum. Br J Dermatol 1985; 112:1–14.

68. Haugland RP. In: Handbook of Fluorescent Probes and Research Chemicals. 8th ed. Molecular Probes Inc.

69. Chapman SJ, Walsh A. Desmosomes, corneosomes and desquamation. An ultrastructural study of adult pig epidermis. Arch Dermatol Res 1990; 282:304–310.

70. Harding C, Long S, Rogers J, Banks J, Zhang Z, Bush A. The cornified cell enve-

lope: an important marker of stratum corneum maturation in healthy and dry skin. J Invest Dermatol 1999; 112:306.

71. Harding C, Rawlings AV, Long S, Rogers J, Banks J, Zhang Z, Bush A. The cornified cell envelope: an important marker of stratum corneum maturation in healthy and dry skin. In: Lal M, Lillford PJ, Niak VM, Prakash V, eds. Supramolecular and Colloidal Structures in Biomaterials and Biosubstances. London: Imperial College Press and The Royal Society, 2000:389–406.

72. Hirao T, Denda M, Takahashi M. Regional heterogeneity in hydrophobicity of cornified envelopes from human stratum corneum. J Invest Dermatol 1999; 113:460.

73. Ishida-Yamamoto A, Eady RAJ, Watt FM, Roop DR, Hohl D, Iizuka H. Immunoelectron microscopic analysis of cornified cell envelope formation in normal and psoriatic epidermis. J Histochem Cytochem 1996; 44:167–175.

74. Grove GL, Kligman AM. Corneocyte size as an indirect measure of epidermal proliferative activity. In: Marks R, Plewig G, eds. Stratum Corneum. Berlin: Springer-Verlag, 1983:191–195.

75. Corcuff P, Delesalle G, Schaffer H. Quantitative aspects of corneocytes. J Soc Cosmet Chem 1983; 34:177–190.

76. Legrain V, Michel S, Ortonne JP, Reichert U. Intraindividual and interindividual variations in cornified envelope peptide composition in normal and psoriatic skin. Arch Dermatol Res 1991; 283:512–515.

77. Skerrow CJ, Clelland DG, Skerrow D. Changes to desmosomal and lectin binding sties during differentiation in normal human epidermis: a quantitative ultrastructural study. J Cell Sci 1989; 92:667–677.

78. King IA, Wood MJ, Fryer PR. Desmoglein II–derived glycopeptides in human epidermis. J Invest Dermatol 1989; 92:22–26.

79. Cussler EL, Zlotnick SJ, Shaw MC. Texture perceived with fingers. Perception & Psychophysics. 1977; 21:504–512.

80. Schrader K, Bielfeldt S. Comparative studies of skin roughness measurements by image analysis and several in vivo skin testing methods. J Soc Cosmet Chem 1991; 42:385–391.

81. Fiedler M, Meier WD, Hoppe U. Texture analysis of the surface of the human skin. Skin Pharmacol. 1995; 8:252–265.

6

Dry and Xerotic Skin Conditions

Anthony V. Rawlings

Unilever Research, Port Sunlight Laboratory, Bebington,
Wirral, United Kingdom

Clive R. Harding and Allan Watkinson

Unilever Research, Colworth Laboratory, Sharnbrook, Bedford,
United Kingdom

Ian R. Scott

Unilever Research, Edgewater Laboratory, Edgewater, New Jersey

1 INTRODUCTION

"Dry skin" is a term used by consumers, cosmetic scientists, and dermatologists. Although this condition remains one of the most common of human disorders, it has never been defined unambiguously [1]. Usually it is described in terms of symptomatology, its physical signs, and its etiology with names such as xerosis, dermatitis, winter itch, rough skin, dry skin, and chapping. Moreover, dry skin is sometimes mistakenly considered as the opposite end of the spectrum to oily skin, and indeed early investigators believed dry skin to be a result of reduced sebum secretion. However, dry skin is characterized by a rough, scaly and flaky skin surface, especially in low humidity conditions and is often associated with the somatory sensations of tightness, itch, and pain [2].

Winter itch was first described in 1874 by Duhring [3], and its seasonal nature was confirmed in later studies. Decades later, Gaul [4] related the problem to the presence of dry air as measured by dew points, and the early work of Irwin

Blank in the 1950s proved that the low moisture content of the skin is a prime factor in precipitating this condition [5]. Low temperature and humidity are not the only factors that induce a dry skin condition; dry skin also occurs after excessive sun exposure or after the use of soaps and surfactants. Indeed, dry scaly skin is a characteristic feature in a wide range of more serious pathological conditions that affect the underlying epidermis.

During the last 50 years many scientists have tried to unravel the complex biological and physical perturbations that occur in this vexing condition, and in recent years our understanding of the biochemistry of the stratum corneum has advanced enormously [6]. It is now generally acknowledged that the stratum corneum is a dynamic tissue in which many enzymatic reactions are carefully regulated to ensure the proper maturation of the tissue to enable it to be fully functional. It has also become apparent that skin scaling is the result of a perturbation of the stratum corneum maturation process and especially that of desquamation. Many factors contribute to aberrant desquamation, although in winter dry skin this is primarily a result of environmental stresses. In this chapter, we will consider how perturbation of the normal functioning of the stratum corneum can precipitate the formation of dry skin.

2 DRY SKIN—THE CLINICAL CONDITION

Irrespective of body site, dry skin is characterized clinically by its rough look and feel. Several studies have been conducted to describe the visual condition on the face, hands, and legs. Indeed, the clinical severity of the dry skin (Fig. 1) is normally graded according to the following criteria of Kligman [7]:

> Grade 1   Normal skin.
> Grade 2   Mild xerosis characterized by small flakes of dry skin and whitening of dermatoglyphic triangles.
> Grade 3   Moderate xerosis, small dry flakes giving a light powdery appearance to the hand. Corners of dermatoglyphic triangles have started to uplift.
> Grade 4   Well-defined xerosis, the entire length of a number of dermatoglyphic triangles have uplifted to generate large dry skin flakes. Roughness is very evident.

This type of analysis, however, is subjective, and to give a more objective assessment of dry skin a variety of noninvasive instruments are used to characterize the condition. Leveque et al. [8] have used a variety of instrumental techniques. In these studies dramatic decreases in facial stratum corneum flexibility and conductance have been observed as skin dryness scores increase (Fig. 2). As expected trans-epidermal water loss also increases with increasing dryness.

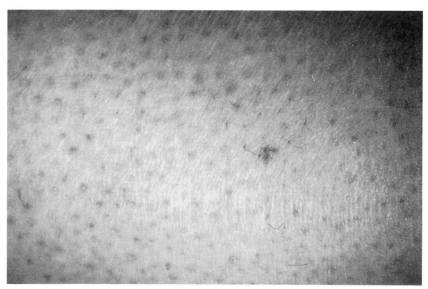

Grade 0

Grade 1

FIGURE 1 Photographs of typical dry skin conditions. Grade 0: normal, healthy. Grade 1: slight dryness; white borders. Grade 2: moderate dryness; raised edges, dry powdery appearance. Grade 3: marked dryness; definite uplift, visible flaking. Grade 4: extreme dryness; severe uplift and flaking.

Grade 2

Grade 3

FIGURE 1 Continued

Grade 4

FIGURE 1 Continued

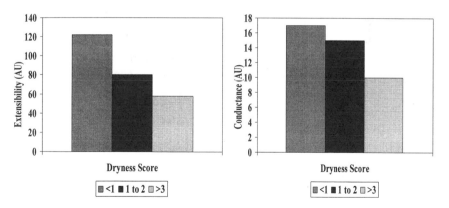

FIGURE 2 Relationship between skin extensibility and conductance with increasing dry skin. (Modified from Ref. 8.)

Crucial to the stratum corneum condition is the state of proliferation/differentiation of the underlying epidermis. Leveque et al. [8] demonstrated that corneocyte size decreased with increasing dry skin indicating that the perturbation of the stratum corneum is associated with an increase in epidermal proliferation. This is consistent with the work of Elias et al. [9], who demonstrated increases in epidermal proliferation following barrier damage, i.e., increased transepidermal water loss. Increases in epidermal proliferation are known to lead to smaller corneocytes [10]. Others have shown that the stratum corneum is thicker and reveals cracks in dry skin conditions [11]. Thus, compromised stratum corneum in dry skin leads to an increase in epidermopoiesis, a less flexible tissue (a property linked to both stratum corneum water content and thickness) together with a reduced barrier to water loss. These changes are associated with altered skin surface morphology [12]. Surface sebum does not appear to be a factor in dry skin since sebum secretion rates were shown not to correlate with the dry skin scores. Collectively these results indicate that the normal functioning of the stratum corneum is compromised in dry skin.

3 BIOLOGY OF STRATUM CORNEUM IN NORMAL AND DRY SKIN

Normal desquamation occurs following complete but gradual destruction of corneodesmosomes [13] leading to the imperceivable loss of individual cells from the surface of the stratum corneum. The process is intimately dependent upon the composition and organization of the intercellular lipids, levels and activity of stratum corneum glycosidases, and proteases together with effective tissue hydration. Early biochemical studies comparing the differences between normal and dry stratum corneum focused exclusively on changes in stratum corneum barrier lipids [14,15]. We believed, however, that a more holistic approach needed to be taken to properly understand the condition [6,16,17]. In the following sections we describe changes in stratum corneum morphology, lipid levels, corneodesmosome persistence, protease activity, corneocyte envelope morphology and natural moisturizing factor levels associated with the appearance of dry skin.

3.1 Stratum Corneum Morphology in Normal and Dry Skin

There is evidence that stratum corneum lipid lamellae and corneodesmosomes are modified during the normal desquamation process and these changes are essential to reduce cohesion in the peripheral layers [18,19]. In contrast, in dry skin the lipid structure becomes totally disorganized and corneodesmosomes persist into the outer layers of the stratum corneum. This is best exemplified by electron microscope studies [16].

Sequential tape-stripping of the surface of the stratum corneum of normal and dry skin together with subsequent electron microscopical analysis following ruthenium tetroxide staining revealed changes in stratum corneum lipid organization and corneodesmosome morphology between the inner and outer layers of the stratum corneum. In deeper cellular layers (third tape strip down) intact electron-dense corneodesmosomal structures were seen (Fig. 3D) in direct contact with the intercellular lipid lamellae. The corneodesmosomes appeared to undergo degradation and a reduction in number in the upper layers of the stratum corneum. During their degradation, corneodesmosomes showed digestion of their internal elements with vacuolation of their structures (Fig. 3C) before detaching from the corneocyte envelopes. Corneodesmosomal remnants often appear to be surrounded by intercellular lipids (Fig. 3B) before their total degradation (Fig. 3A). The lipid lamellae in the deeper tissue regions of soap-induced winter xerotic stratum corneum resembled normal tissue. However, in contrast to observations in normal skin, corneodesmosomes persisted to the surface layer of the stratum corneum (Fig. 4).

Additionally, in the deeper layers of normal stratum corneum, lipids were present as typical lamellae bilayer structures between the corneocytes (Fig. 5C). However, toward the surface layers of the stratum corneum, the bilayer structures were no longer present and appeared to have taken on a more amorphous-like structure (Fig. 5A,B). In severe xerosis (grade 4; see Fig. 6), normal intercellular lipid structures were still evident in the lower layers of the stratum corneum (Fig. 6C). However, in the peripheral layers of stratum corneum the normal lipid bilayer structure was replaced by large amounts of disorganized intercellular lipids with a structure completely different to that of normal healthy skin (Fig. 6A,B).

Other workers [20,21] have reported similar morphological changes on other body sites. Interestingly, Warner et al. [21] have provided further insights into these morphological changes examining the effects of aging, dryness, and soap use. They report an enormous variation in the lipid lamellae structure. In young individuals a normal lipid lamellae structure is observed, but is not apparent over the age of 40 years. It is speculated that this is probably due to the known age-related reduction in epidermal lipid biosynthesis, although the reported decrease in stratum corneum lipids levels during this period are relatively small.

The perturbation of the lipid lamellae in the peripheral layer could be due to the adverse effects of sebum lipids released on the surface of the skin. However, Sheu et al. [22] have clearly shown that deranged lipid lamellae are still found in the upper layers of plantar skin, which is a sebum-free body site. Nevertheless, biochemical degradation of lipid lamellae cannot be excluded especially as ceramide 1, a lipid thought to be "riveting" the lipid bilayers and controlling lipid phase behavior, is reported to be degraded in the stratum corneum [23]. Equally degradation of cholesterol sulfate is known to be in association with desquamation which may also influence the morphology of the lipid lamellae [19].

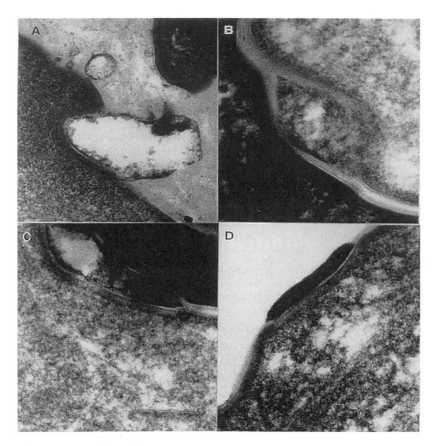

Fɪɢᴜʀᴇ 3 Electron micrographs of tape strippings of normal skin (grade 1), degradation of corneodesmosomes toward the surface of the stratum corneum. (A) First strip, corneodesmosome fully degraded. (B) Second strip, corneodesmosome partially degraded and encapsulated by lipid lamellae. (C) Second strip, corneodesmosome partially degraded, vacuolation of structure. (D) Third strip, normal corneodesmosome, lipid envelopes in direct contact with corneodesmosome. (X200,000; Bar = 0.05 μm.) (Modified from Ref. 16.)

   Overall, the data show that in healthy skin the periodic nature of the intercellular lipids become amorphous toward the surface layer. In contrast, in dry skin, a state of intercellular lipid disorganization, with a structure completely different to that in the surface layers of healthy skin, extends much deeper down into skin. This disorganized lipid structure is likely to influence both intercorneocyte

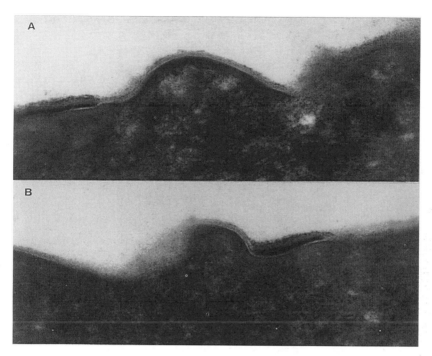

FIGURE 4 Electron micrographs of tape strippings of subjects with severe xerosis (grade 4), persistence of corneodesmosomes in outermost layers of the stratum corneum. First tape stripping from two subjects (A,B). (X200,000; Bar = 0.05 µm.) (Modified from Ref. 16.)

cohesion and corneodesmolysis and adversely affect the latter stages of desquamation, as can be observed from the increased levels of intact corneodesmosomes in the surface layers of the stratum corneum in dry skin.

3.2 Stratum Corneum Lipid Biochemistry in Normal and Dry Skin

The picture has emerged from the morphological studies mentioned that stratum corneum lipids influence the expression of dry skin. Nevertheless, early studies by Saint-Leger et al. [14] using a turbine agitated solvent extraction procedure found no differences in the levels of polar lipids (ceramides, cholesterol sulfate) between normal and dry skin. However, decreased levels of sterol esters and triglycerides, and increased fatty acid levels, were observed in dry skin. Similarly, Fulmer and Kramer [15] analyzing stratum corneum lipids recovered from skin biopsies concluded that the total amount of stratum corneum lipids is not af-

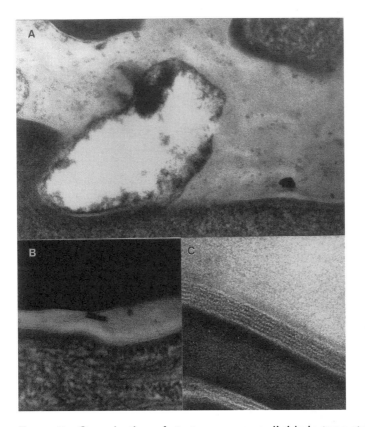

Figure 5 Organization of stratum corneum lipids in tape strippings of individuals with clinically nornal skin. Transmission electron micrographs of tape strippings. Ultrastructural changes in lipid organization toward the surface of the stratum corneum. (A) First strip, absence of bilayers and presence of amorphous lipidic material. (B) Second strip, disruption of lipid lamellae. (C) Third strip, normal lipid lamellae. (X200,000.) (Modified from Ref. 16.)

fected in surfactant-induced dry skin. However, increases in ceramides 2 and 4 together with cholesterol and decreases in cholesterol esters, ceramide 3, and fatty acids were seen in dry skin compared with normal skin.

Due to the apparent changes in stratum corneum lipid ultrastructure between normal and dry skin we decided to measure absolute levels of the major

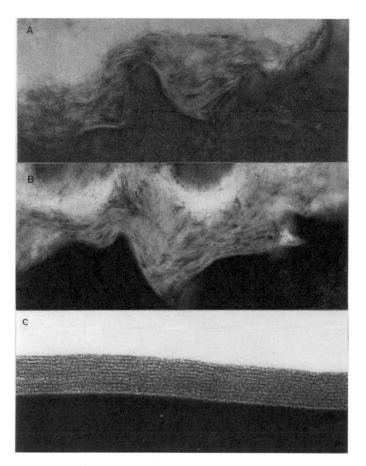

FIGURE 6 Organization of stratum corneum lipids in tape stripping of subjects with winter xerosis. Transmission electron micrographs of tape strippings of individuals with severe xerosis. Perturbation in lipid organization toward the surface of the stratum corneum. (A) First strip, disorganized lipid lamellae. (B) Second strip, disorganized lipid lamellae. (C) Third strip, normal lipid lamellae (X200,000.) (Modified from Ref. 16.)

stratum corneum lipid species in the two conditions, and also to compare lipid profiles in the inner and outer layers of the stratum corneum [16]. This approach was facilitated using a sequential tape-stripping procedure to recover corneocytes from progressively deeper layers and chromatographic removal of the tape adhesive from the lipid species before conducting high performance thin layer chromatography ensured optimal resolution of the major lipid species. However, cholesterol sulfate levels still could not be determined due to tape adhesive contaminants.

An initial analysis of stratum corneum lipid composition from normal and xerotic skin was performed on corneocytes pooled from all of the tape strippings. Compared with normal skin, statistically significant decreases in the mass levels of ceramides were seen in severe xerosis conditions (Table 1). However, the relative levels of the different ceramide species remained unchanged.

Of the other lipid species investigated, the relative and mass amounts of fatty acids tended to increase in the outer layers of the stratum corneum, but these observations were not statistically significant. However, cholesterol levels were significantly increased in outer compared with inner stratum corneum in dry skin. These changes are totally consistent with the observed changes in lipid ultrastructure.

The reasons for the aberration in stratum corneum lipid structure in winter xerosis is unknown, but they are probably related to diminishing ceramide and increasing fatty acid levels. Although the latter do not show statistical differences in their concentrations between the inner and outer layers of the stratum corneum due to the large interindividual variation, their mass levels were nearly doubled in subjects with xerosis.

TABLE 1   Relationship of Skin Xerosis and Stratum Corneum Lipid Composition

Lipid species	Skin xerosis grade			
	Grade 1	Grade 2	Grade 3	Grade 4
	Lipid Levels (ng lipid/µg protein)			
Ceramides	64.9 ± 34.4	68.6 ± 30.4	39.2 ± 14.9*	37.5 ± 14.1*
Fatty acids	62.1 ± 34.6	67.4 ± 32.7	60.5 ± 37.0	54.9 ± 28.1
Cholesterol	3.9 ± 2.1	7.7 ± 4.2	4.4 ± 2.0	4.6 ± 2.3
	Relative Lipid Levels (% of total lipids)			
Ceramides	47.1 ± 17.4	48.3 ± 8.6	40.2 ± 13.2	38.3 ± 11.2
Fatty acids	49.7 ± 18.6	46.2 ± 9.8	55.0 ± 12.0	56.0 ± 10.8
Cholesterol	2.0 ± 1.9	5.5 ± 2.6	4.8 ± 2.4	5.2 ± 3.2

Notes: Values represent mean standard deviation. Grade 1, n = 8; Grade 2, n = 8; Grade 3, n = 12; Grade 4, n = 12.
*Significantly different to Grade 1 ($p < 0.05$).

The increased fatty acids observed in dry skin may be derived from the soap used for bathing, result from the hydrolysis of ceramides by a ceramidase [24], or be of sebaceous origin. Excess fatty acids have been found in the lipid fractions derived from low humidity–induced dry skin samples of pigs [25], indicating intrinsic origins rather than extraneous sources. Whatever their source, it is therefore possible that the alteration of the ratio of the three major lipid components—fatty acids, sterols, and ceramides—causes phase separation of lipids at the surface of the stratum corneum. The excess fatty acid levels may further exacerbate the structural defects of the intercellular lipid; fatty acids alter the phase properties of phospholipid bilayers [26]

3.3 Stratum Corneum Corneodesmosomal Protein in Normal and Dry Skin

The main cohesive force within the stratum corneum is the corneodesmosome (or corneosome) [27], a specialized desmosome. The cohesion of the classical desmosome structure is provided by two heterogeneous families of proteins called cadherins (desmogleins, or dsg, and desmocollins, or dsc), each of which occur as three distinct isoforms [28,29]. The predominant cadherins in the corneodesmosome are dsg1 and dsc1, which are specifically modified for their specialized role within the lipid-rich intercellular spaces. The cadherins dsc1 and dsg1 span the corneocyte envelopes and bind homophilically, in the intercellular space, to their counterparts on adjacent cells. A potentially critical difference between epidermal desmosomes and the stratum corneum corneodesmosomes is the inclusion in the latter of the protein corneodesmosin [30]. This protein, recently identified as S protein, is a late differentiation antigen which co-localizes with the extracellular domains of the corneodesmosomes. The glycoprotein nature of this protein and its location have suggested that it is involved in cohesion, although this remains to be confirmed [31]. Corneodesmosomes are extensively cross-linked into the cornified envelope during late differentiation increasing the overall mechanical strength of the stratum corneum, but also dictating that corneodesmosomal degradation must occur to allow desquamation to proceed.

As demonstrated by electron microscopy on studies of winter- and soap-induced xerosis, corneodesmosomes are retained in the upper layers of the stratum corneum [16]. Biochemically, this increased retention is reflected in the increased levels of intact dsg1, dsc1, and corneodesmosin [16,32] in the superficial layers, indicating that hydrolysis of these molecules is inhibited (Fig. 7). The major consequence of this decreased hydrolysis and corneodesmosomal retention is that the predominant intercorneocyte linkages are not broken and the peripheral cells do not detach during desquamation. Hence, instead of the imperceptible loss of surface corneocytes, large clumps of cells accumulate on the surface of the skin.

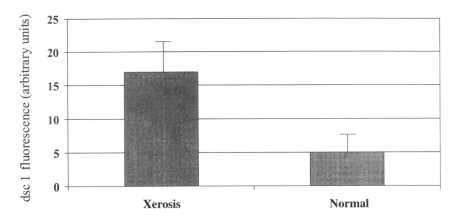

FIGURE 7 Histogram showing the increased levels of desmocollin 1 in stratum corneum of subjects with severe xerosis (grade 4) compared with normal stratum corneum (grade 1).

3.4 Stratum Corneum Enzymes and Enzyme Inhibitors in Normal and Dry Skin

The degradation of corneodesmosomal proteins during stratum corneum maturation points to the role of enzymes in the desquamatory process. These proteases, along with specific lipases, are delivered to their site of action through lamellar bodies' extrusion into the intercellular space during epidermal differentiation [33]. The stratum corneum is an extremely rich repository of proteases (Fig. 8), and the identification of desquamatory enzymes is complicated by the fact that much of the proteolytic activity extractable from this tissue is likely to represent redundant activity responsible for the intensely autolytic process of stratum corneum formation. Nevertheless, although the definitive identification of the proteases involved in corneodesmosome hydrolysis remains a challenge, the pioneering studies of Egelrud and others [34] have provided strong circumstantial evidence that the enzyme stratum corneum chymotryptic enzyme (SCCE) plays a critical role in desquamation. Protease inhibition studies have revealed similar profiles for SCCE, corneodesmosome, and dsg1 degradation as well as corneocyte release in vitro [35]. Moreover, immunolocalization studies demonstrate its occurrence in lamellar bodies in the stratum granulosum and in the intercellular spaces in the stratum corneum, localizations consistent with a role in desquamation [36]. More recently we have shown that pro-SCCE resides in significant amounts throughout the stratum corneum. This localization is exclusively to the intercellular space and in association with the cornified envelope of the corneocyte (Fig. 9). Interestingly, SCCE, the active protease, is found in the intercellular

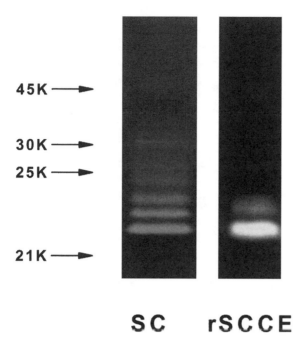

45K ➤

30K ➤
25K ➤

21K ➤

SC   rSCCE

Figure 8   Casein zymography of human stratum corneum extracts and recombinant SCCE. Samples of rSCCE and 1M NaCl extracts of human were fractionated on 12% polyacrylamide gels containing 0.2% casein and caseinolytic activity determined.

space but is also associated with desmosomal plaques and even in the corneocytes themselves. From this it is speculated that pro-SCCE activation occurs within the intercellular space, and the active SCCE slowly diffuses into the corneodesmosomal compartment and into the cell, degrading the cadherin-binding proteins as it does [37].

A potential causative factor in reduced corneodesmosomal degradation in xerosis is a reduction in SCCE and other proteolytic activity. Although several studies have been performed on SCCE and desquamation, precisely what changes in enzyme activity occur in perturbed desquamation are still poorly understood. Alternatively, extrinsic factors may lead to reduced enzyme activity. In soap-induced xerosis we have shown a reduction in extractable SCCE activity from the peripheral layers of the stratum corneum (Fig. 10). Nevertheless, immunoblotting has revealed no apparent alteration in pro-SCCE levels between normal and soap-induced dry skin, however there was a decrease in the levels of the active enzyme and an apparent increase in the levels of an SCCE degradative fragment. This loss

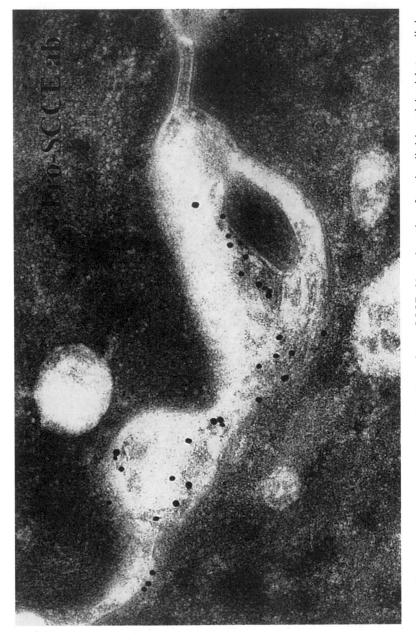

FIGURE 9 Electron microscopic localization of pro-SCCE. Note location for the lipid-enriched intercellular spaces.

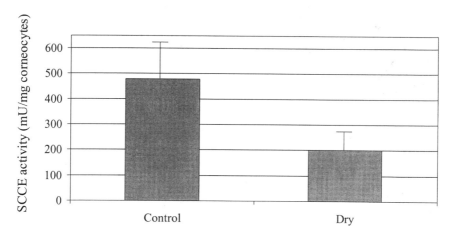

FIGURE 10 Stratum corneum chymotrypic enzyme activity levels in normal and soap-induced dry skin.

in active SCCE was attributed to the action of the soap since in deeper layers SCCE activity was unchanged. Moreover, the soap may be contributing to or accelerating the degradation of the active enzyme.

In addition to the desquamatory proteases, glycosidases present within the stratum corneum may be required for corneodesmosome degradation and desquamation. Corneodesmosomal glycoproteins may require deglycosylation to deprotect the proteins, rendering them more susceptible to proteolysis [38]. However, as yet no precise desquamatory glycosidase has been identified.

One consequence of xerosis is the potential exacerbation of the condition due to localized inflammatory action. Indeed, water barrier disruption promotes the synthesis and release of a range of proinflammatory cytokines, such as IL-1 and TNF, in the epidermis. In most cases, acute low level trauma probably does not initiate an inflammatory reaction due to innate anti-inflammatory mechanisms. Yet with chronic water barrier damage, such as in xerosis, there may be a more marked release of pro-inflammatory cytokines. Consequently, phagocytotic immune cells, especially the neutrophils, will be attracted into the xerotic site; on arrival, the neutrophils will secrete leukocyte elastase, cathepsin G, proteinase 3, and collagenase into the surrounding tissue, producing a protease burden on the keratinocytes. Additionally, the hyperproliferative epidermal cells will contribute to this protease burden by secretion and activation of a range of proteases such as plasminogen activator and the matrix metalloproteases.

The front line of epidermal antiproteinase defence, especially protection against antineutrophil elastase,is due to locally produced small proteinase inhibitors. Keratinocytes produce two low molecular weight protein protease inhibitors, primarily directed against elastase, called elafin (a.k.a. skin-derived antileukoprotease; SKALP) and secretory leukocyte protease inhibitor (SLPI) (a.k.a. antileukoprotease). Neutrophil elastase protection is also provided by 1 antitrypsin (a.k.a. 1 antiproteinase), derived from the plasma. Similarly, the proteases involved in hyperproliferation/wound repair are controlled by epidermally produced inhibitors; plasminogen activator inhibitors (PAI-1 and -2) and the tissue matrix metalloproteinase inhibitors (TIMPs) are all synthesized within the epidermis.

In normal healthy epidermis, these protein protease inhibitors closely regulate protease activity, containing activity close to the cell producing the proteases. In xerosis, however, it is possible that the inhibitors can become overwhelmed by the protease burden, whether produced by epidermal cells or infiltrating phagocytes. The potential consequences of excessive protease activity are (1) cellular damage, (2) pro-inflammatory cytokines release, and (3) premature degradation of cell–cell linkages promoting cell mitogenesis. Xerotic proteolytic activity may also potentially affect the sensory nerves innervating the epidermis, contributing to pruritus and pain associated with the condition. Evidence that proteolytic activity can contribute to the symptoms of xerosis comes from the effectiveness of topical applications of transexamic acid and 1 antitrypsin as treatment for xerosis [39].

3.5 Stratum Corneum Corneocyte Envelopes in Normal and Dry Skin

As explained in Chapter 5 there are two morphological forms of corneocyte envelopes, namely, a fragile (CEf) and a rigid form (CEr). Deep within the stratum corneum the corneocytes contain CE that are exclusively of the CEf type, whereas as the corneocytes migrate up through the stratum corneum CEr are increasingly formed. This maturation event, with the conversion of CEf to CEr, appears to occur after the hydrolysis of filaggrin, indicating an association with or after the formation of the stratum disjunctum. Quantification of envelope phenotype following 3 weeks of exaggerated soap washing to induce a dry skin condition reveals a significant change in the CEr-to-CEf ratio (Fig. 11). The dramatic decrease in CEr indicates that the process of CE maturation is impaired in dry skin compared with normal skin. The perturbation of CE maturation coincides with the reduced hydrolysis of corneodesmosomes as revealed by staining intact corneocytes with the dsc1 antibody. Soap-induced winter dry skin is also characterized by a significantly decreased activity of Tranglutaminase (TGase) activity, throughout the SC layers examined. These results indicate that soap-induced dry skin is associated with an altered and incomplete maturation of the CE, as indicated by the increased proportion of CEf, and, although circumstantial, the corresponding decrease in TGase activity is consistent with this enzyme playing a critical role in the process.

% Corneocytes

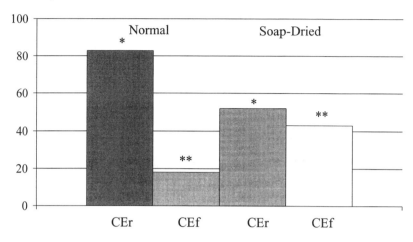

Figure 11 Percentage distribution of rigid (CEr) and fragile (CEf) envelopes recovered from normal (untreated) and soap-dried SC. Dry skin was generated on the volar forearm of six individuals by the exaggerated daily use of a harsh soap bar for 3 weeks. The other forearm remained untreated throughout this time and served as a control site. Samples of CE recovered after this time were stained with TRITC and viewed under fluorescent microscope. The proportion of the two envelope types were averaged following examination of photographs taken from five separate fields/sample. $^*p < 0.05$; $^{**}p < 0.001$.

Perturbation of CE maturation is also evident in more serious skin pathologies. In the hyperproliferative diseases such as psoriasis and ichthyoses the conditions are characterized by an increase in the content of the immature CEf, demonstrating further correlation of hyperproliferation with CE maturation. These occur due to altered epidermal hyperproliferation and differentiation. However, in some (e.g., lamellar ichthyosis) no TGase 1 activity is apparent.

In conclusion, however, regardless of the underlying mechanisms perturbed in these conditions it is clear that reduced CE maturation and reduced corneodesmosomal hydrolysis are common features of dry, flaky skin conditions.

3.6 Stratum Corneum Natural Moisturizing Factor

As already discussed by Harding and Scott [40], natural moisturizing factors (NMF) are critically important for maintaining the hydration and flexibility of the stratum corneum, and reduced NMF levels are implicated in the appearance and persistence of dry skin conditions. A significant correlation exists between hydration state of the SC and its amino acid content in elderly individuals with skin xerosis [41], but is less clear in others [44]. Free amino acid levels have been reported to decrease significantly in dry, scaly skin induced experimentally by repetitive tape-stripping [43] or by surfactant damage [44].

In our own laboratory we have found that aged skin has intrinsically lower NMF levels compared with young skin, and this reflects a general reduced synthesis of profilaggrin. These conclusions are supported by electron microscopy studies which indicate that a decreased number of keratohyalin granules [45], occupying a reduced volume within the cell, is found in senile xerosis. The decline in NMF production appears to reflect the cumulative effects of actinic damage as it was observed in SC recovered from the back of the hand (photodamaged), but not from the inner aspect of the biceps (photoprotected). It is likely that in aged skin, loss of NMF may become more pronounced as elderly individuals also show an age-related decline in water barrier repair which may lead to increased leaching of the water-soluble compounds from the surface layers [46].

Although decreased synthesis of profilaggrin and increased leaching from surfactant-damaged skin [47] are undoubtedly major factors leading to decreased levels of NMF in the superficial SC, the direct impact of sudden changes in environmental humidity on NMF generation should not be ignored. As we have already described elsewhere, the hydrolysis of filaggrin is critically regulated by the external relative humidity. The rapid decrease in environmental humidity and temperature, commonly associated with the onset of winter xerosis, is likely to result in a transient but acute perturbation of filaggrin proteolysis, as the proteases responsible are not fully activated. Similarly, a chronic perturbation in the efficiency of filaggrin proteolysis due to frequent and rapid changes in environmental humidity is also likely to contribute to the poor skin condition prevalent in certain individuals who endure constantly changing humidity conditions (e.g., flight attendants).

The classical, transient dry skin associated with newborn infants [48] can also be explained by the delay in production of NMF as the SC slowly equilibrates from the aqueous environment of the womb (where, of course, filaggrin, although synthesized, is not hydrolyzed to the ambient external humidity when proteolysis is initiated).

The dry flaky skin which characteristically appears several days after acute UVB damage is NMF deficient [49]. Studies suggest that this reflects initial damage to the granular layer and a subsequent decreased synthesis of profilaggrin, rather than any dramatic loss of hydrolysis of existing filaggrin. Indeed the characteristic skin flaking seen following UV damage can, under histological examination, be seen to occur through the layer of NMF-deficient corneocytes formed prematurely during the initial UV insult. As we have described, many elements of normal SC maturation are disrupted in xerosis, and increased NMF leaching from cornecytes may also occur due to parallel perturbations in lamellar granule synthesis and associated damage to the water barrier [50].

An inability to retain water due to defective NMF production/retention will of course not only impact the mechanical properties of the SC—a critical, and often overlooked role of water in the SC is in ensuring the activity of a variety of hydrolytic enzymes involved in various aspects of SC maturation and desquamation. When the tissue is desiccated a loss of intrinsic hydrolytic enzyme activity leads to ineffective corneodesmosomal degradation and consequent skin scaling.

The various processes leading from profilaggrin synthesis to conversion to filaggrin and then to NMF are under tight control. However, these controls are perturbed in different ways by a range of factors including UV light, exposure to surfactants, and, of course, changes in environmental humidity processes. These very different causes can all lead to reduced NMF levels and contribute to the complex phenomenon known as dry skin.

4 SUMMARY

A dry skin condition is the result of a range of environmental and pathological factors that disrupt the normal epidermal differentiation and stratum corneum maturation processes. It is a complex phenomenon involving several interdependent biochemical events in the stratum corneum. Morphologically, dry skin differs from normal due to a retention of corneodesmosomes in the peripheral desquamating layers of the stratum corneum. This retention of corneodesmosomes is the cause of the skin flaking associated with the xerotic condition; the abnormal retention of intercorneocyte links results in large clumps of corneocytes breaking off, i.e., scale, as opposed to the imperceptible loss of single cells. In addition, degradation or disruption of the stratum corneum multiple lipid bilayers occurs in several layers at the tissue periphery, rather than in the final desquamating layer. This results in a collapse of the bilayer structure to give a disorganized lipid matrix, which may be due to an observed decrease in ceramide levels and increase in fatty acid levels in peripheral layers of dry skin. Another component of the stratum corneum intercellular region, the putative desquamatory enzyme, SCCE, has been shown to be decreased in the outer layers of the stratum corneum in dry skin. Finally, the perturbations that cause dry skin even affect the structure of the corneocytes. We have similarly found aberrant maturation of the cornified envelopes, with increases in the fragile morphology in dry skin. Also there is a decrease in the production or proteolytic processing of filaggrin to produce the natural moisturizing factors; decreased levels of these hydroscopic molecules will result in a reduced ability to retain water within the tissue.

Each of these elements of stratum corneum maturation are crucial to the process as a whole. Hence, perturbation of one element is likely to have knock-on effects to other aspects of maturation. As such, disruption of the lipid bilayers is likely to allow greater leaching of the NMFs, reducing the water content of the tissue. This in turn will reduce the activity of enzymes such as SCCE and TGase, perturbing corneodesmosomal degradation and CE maturation, respectively. The decreased water content will also reduce the elasticity of the corneocyte structures, increasing the likelihood of the skin cracking.

The most common cause of stratum corneum maturation disruption is the affect of the environment and bathing habits. Some surfactants are known to effect the stratum corneum lipids and enzymes resulting in dry skin. However the major contributor to xerosis is the environmental humidity. This regulates the water content of the peripheral stratum corneum, influencing the enzymes involved in the final stages of maturation and desquamation. It is this crucial requirement of water in the peripheral stratum corneum that results in moisturizing agents still being the most frequently used treatment for common dry skin.

REFERENCES

1. Pierard GE. What does dry skin mean? Int J Dermatol 1987; 23:167–168.
2. Rudikoff D. The effect of dryness on skin. Clin Dermatol 1998; 16:99–107.
3. During LA. Pruritis himalis an undescribed form of pruritis. Phila Med Times 1874; 4:225–230.
4. Gaul LE, Underwood GB. Relation of dewpoint and barometric pressure to chapping of normal skin. J Invest Dermatol 1952; 19:9–19.
5. Blank IH. Further observations on factors which influence the water content of the stratum corneum. J Invest Dermatol 1953; 21:259–271.
6. Harding CR, Watkinson A, Scott IR, Rawlings AV. Dry skin, moisturisation and corneodesmolysis. Int J Cosmet Sci 2000; 22:21–52.
7. Kligman A. Regression method for assessing the efficacy of moisturizers. Cosmet Toil 1978; 93:27–35.
8. Leveque JL, Grove G, de Rigal J, Corcuff P, Kligman AM, Saint-Leger D. Biophysical characterisation of dry facial skin. J Soc Cosmet Chem 1987; 82:171–177.
9. Proksch E, Feingold KR, Man MQ, Elias PM. Barrier function regulates epidermal DNA synthesis. J Clin Invest 1991; 87:1668–1673.
10. Grove GL. Exfoliative cytological procedures as a non-intrusive method for dermatological studies. J Invest Dermatol 1979; 73:67–74.
11. Grove GL, Lavker RM, Holzle E, Kligman AM. Use of non-intrusive tests to monitor age associated changes in human skin. J Soc Cosmet Chem 1980; 32:15–26.
12. Sato J, Yanai M, Hirao T, Denda M. Water content and thickness of the stratum corneum contribute to skin surface morphology. Arch Dermatol Res 2000; 292:412–417.
13. Sato J. Desquamation and the role of stratum corneum enzymes in skin moisturization. In: Leyden J, Rawlings AV, eds. Skin Moisturization. New York: Marcel Dekker (in press).

14. Saint-Leger D, Francois AM, Leveque JL, Stuudemeuyer T, Kligman AM, Grove GL. Stratum corneum lipids in winter xerosis. Dermatologica 1989; 178:151–155.

15. Fulmer AW, Dramer GJ. Stratum corneum abnormalities in surfactant induced dry scaly skin. J Invest Dermatol 1989; 80:598–602.

16. Rawlings AV, Watkinson A, Rogers J, Mayo AM, Hope J, Scott IR. Abnormalities in stratum corneum structure, lipid composition and desmosome degradation in soap-induced winter xerosis. J Cosmet Chem 1994; 45:203–220.

17. Harding CR, Long S, Rogers J, Banks J, Zhang Z, Bush A. The cornified cell envelope: an important market of stratum corneum maturation in healthy and dry skin (abstr). J Invest Dermatol 1999; 112:306.

18. Chapman SJ, Walsh A, Jackson SM, Friedmann PM. Lipids, proteins and corneocyte adhesion. Arch Dermatol Res 1991; 283:1729–1732.

19. Ranasinghe AW, Wertz PW, Downing DT, McKenzie I. Lipid composition of cohesive and desquamated corneocytes from mouse ear. J Invest Dermatol 1985; 94:216–220.

20. Berry N, Charmeil C, Goujon C, Silvy A, Girard P, Corcuff P, Montastier A. A clinical, biometrological and ultrastructural study of xerotic skin. Int J Cosmet Sci 1999; 21:241–252.

21. Warner RR, Boissy YL. Effect of moisturising products on the structure of lipids in the outer stratum corneum of human. In: Loden M, Maibach HH, eds. Dry Skin and Moisturisers: Chemistry and Function. CRC Press, 2000; 349–372.

22. Sheu H, Chao S, Wong T, Lee Y, Tsai J. Human skin surface lipid film: an ultrastructural study and interaction with corneocytes and intercellular lipid lamellae of the stratum corneum. Br J Dermatol 1999; 140:385–391.

23. Bowser P. Essential fatty acids and their role in correcting skin abnormalities. Cosmetic Dermatol 1993; (suppl):11–12.

24. Wertz PW, Downing DT. Epidermal ceramide hydrolase. J Invest Dermatol 1990; 94:590.

25. Bissett DC, McBride JF. Use of the domestic pig as an animal mode of human dry skin. In: Maibach H, Lowe P, eds. Model in Dermatology. Vol. 1. Basel: Karger, 1985:159–168.

26. McKersie BD, Grove JH, Gowe LM. Free fatty acid effects on leakage, phase properties and fusion of fully hydrated model membranes. Biochim Biophys Acta 1989; 982:156–160.

27. Chapman S, Walsh A. Desmosomes, corneosomes and desquamation. Arch Dermatol Res 1990; 283:1729–1732.

28. King IA, O'Brien TJ, Buxton RS. Expression of the skin type desmosomal cadherins DSC1 is closely linked to the keratinisation of epithelial tissues during mouse development. J Invest Dermatol 1996; 107:531–538.

29. King IA, Dryst BD, Hunt DM, Kruger M, Arnemann J, Buxton RS. Hierarchical expression of desmosomes and cadherins during stratified epithelial morphogenesis in the mouse. Differentiation 1997; 62:83–96.

30. Montezin M, Simon M, Guerrin M, Serre G. Corneodesmosin, a corneodesmosome-specific basic protein is expressed in the cornified epithelia of the pig, guinea pig, rat and mouse. Exp Cell Res 1997; 231:132–140.

31. Simon M, Montezin M, Guerrin M, Durieu X, Serre G. Characterisation and purifi-

cation of human corneodesmosin, an epidermal basic glycoprotein associated with corneocyte specific modified desmosomes. J Biol Chem 1997; 272:31770–31776.

32. Bernard D, Camus C, Nguyen QL, Serre G. Proteolysis of corneodesmosomal proteins in winter xerosis. J Invest Dermatol 1995; 105:176.

33. Mennen GK, Ghadially R, Williams ML, Elias P. Lamellar bodies as delivery systems of hydrolitc enzymes, implications for normal and abnormal desquamation. Br J Dermatol 1992; 126:337–345.

34. Egelrud T. Purification and preliminary characterisation of stratum corneum chynotriptic enzymes—a proteinase that may be involved in desquamation. J Invest Dermatol 1993; 101:200–204.

35. Lundstrom A, Egelrud T. Evidence that cell shedding from plantar stratum corneum in vitro involves endegenous proteolysis of the desmoglein 1. J Invest Dermatol 1990; 94:216–220.

36. Sondell B, Thornall LE, Egelrud T. Evidence that stratum corneum chymotryptic enzyme is transported to the stratum corneum extracellular space via lamellar bodies. J Invest Dermatol 1995; 104:891–823.

37. Watkinson A, Smith C, Coan P, Wiedow O. The role of pro-SCCE and SCCE in desquamation. IFSCC Magazine 2000; 3:45–49.

38. Walsh A, Chapman S. Sugars protect desmosomal proteins from proteolysis. Br J Dermatol 1990; 122:289.

39. Denda M, Kitamura K, Elias PM, Feingold KR. *trans*-4-(Aminomethyl) cyclohexane carboxylic acid (T-AMCHA), an anti-fibrinolytic agent, accelerates barrier recovery and prevents the epidermal hyperplasia induced by epidermal injury in hairless mice and humans. J Invest Dermatol 1997; 109:84–90.

40. Harding CR, Scott IR. Natural moisturing factor. In: Leyden J, Rawlings AV, eds. Skin Moisturization. New York: Marcel Dekker (in press).

41. Horii I, Nakayama Y, Obata M, Tagami H. SC by hydration and amino acid content in xerotic skin. Br J Dermatol 1989; 121:587–592.

42. Jacobsen TM, Yuksel KU, Geesin JC, Gordon JS, Lane AT, Gracy RW. Effects of ageing and xerosis on the amino acid composition of human skin. J Invest Dermatol 1990; 95:296–300.

43. Denda M, Horii J, Koyama J, Yoshida S, Nanba R, Takahashi M, Horii I, Yamamoto A. SC Sphingolipids and free amino acids in experimentally induced scaly skin. Arch Dermatol Res 1992; 285:363–367.

44. Koyama J, Horii I, Kawasaki K, Nakayama Y, Morikawa Y, Mitsui T, Kumagai H. Free amino acids of stratum corneum as a biochemical marker to evaluate dry skin. J Soc Cosmet Chem 1984; 35:183–195.

45. Tezuka T. Electron microscopical changes in xerotic senilis epidermis. Its abnormal membrane coating granule formation. Dermatologica 1983; 166:57.

46. Zetterson EM, Ghadially R, Feingold KR, Crumrine D, Elias PM. Optimal ratios of topical stratum corneum lipids improve barrier recovery in chronologically aged skin. J Am Acad Dermatol 1997; 37:403–408.

47. Scott IR, Harding CR. A filaggrin analogue to increase natural moisturising factor synthesis in skin (abstr). Dermatology 2000 1993; 773.

48. Saijo S, Tagami H. Dry skin of newborn infants: functional analysis of the stratum corneum. Petiatr Dermatol 1991; 8:155–159.

49. Tsuchiya T, Horii I, Nakayama Y. Interrelationship between the change in the water content of the stratum corneum and the amount of natural moisturising factor of the stratum corneum after UVB irradiation. J Soc Cosmet Chem Japan 1998; 22:10–15.

50. Holleran WM, Uchida Y, Halkier-Sorensen L, Haratake A, Hara M, Epstein JH, Elias PM. Structural and biochemical basis for the UVB-induced alterations in epidermal barrier function. Photodermatol Photoimmunol Photomedicine 1997; 13:117–128.

7

Sensitive Skin and Moisturization

Paolo U. Giacomoni

Clinique Laboratories, Inc., Melville, New York

**Neelam Muizzuddin,
Rose Marie Sparacio, Edward Pelle,
Thomas Mammone,
Kenneth Marenus, and Daniel Maes**

Estee Lauder, Melville, New York

1 INTRODUCTION

Skin moisturization is a state of the surface of the skin, which is more often recognized by the individuals when moisturization is lacking, and when one has skin conditions that can be called dry, very dry, rough, or even ichthyotic. The moisturization of the upper part of the skin is likely to be dictated by the presence of lipids, water, urea, and other compounds. It can also be considered to be the consequence of how well the outer envelope of the skin opposes the evaporation. Several authors have undertaken to measure the water content of the outer surface of the skin. Other authors have emphasized the importance of the so-called transepidermal water loss (TEWL), expressed as grams of water per square meter per hour. The capability of the skin to oppose water evaporation can be equated to its capability to provide an overall barrier. The measure of TEWL provides information on the changes in moisturization induced by a treatment, which does not affect the barrier, and on changes of the barrier properties induced by a treatment, which does not affect moisturization.

Skin sensitivity is a self-assessed diagnosis of a physiological state that lacks rigorous clinical definition, complete etiological analysis, and accurate diagnostic tools. This undesirable state of the skin is characterized by a disagreeable feeling on the surface of the skin or by the observation of hyper-reactivity of the skin when it is exposed to mild environmental conditions such as water, wool fabrics, or cosmetics. According to Draelos [1], approximately 40% of the population believes it possesses the characteristics of sensitive skin, as determined by consumer marketing surveys. The characteristics of sensitive skin are the ones felt when, in response to topical application of cosmetics and toiletries, stinging, burning, pruritus, erythema, and desquamation are observed. Yet, as late as in 1997, Draelos noted, "Given the current incomplete knowledge of the sensitive skin condition, it is impossible to arrive at a consensus regarding the definition and origins of sensitive skin" [1].

The definitions of sensitive skin and of skin moisturization are partially subjective, and different people do react differently to the feeling of dry skin. It has been therefore particularly difficult to design experimental protocols and to interpret the results of experiments in the field of skin sensitivity and moisturization. These experiments are generally aimed at pointing out physiological and molecular properties able to allow one to better understand the phenomenon of sensitive skin.

Skin sensitivity and skin dryness are also encountered in mature individuals, and questions have been asked about the correlation between the appearance of skin sensitivity and the onset of those physiological phenomena that characterize aging in women.

In this chapter we summarize some of the experimental results obtained in this field and the interpretations that have been proposed.

2 TESTING METHODS

2.1 Testing for Sensitive Skin

Many tests are available to determine whether the sensitive behavior is the consequence of specific skin conditions, such as rosacea, contact dermatitis, acne, and dry skin, or the consequence of the etiologically undefined skin sensitivity of a given population to topically applied compounds. Among these, we would like to recall the cumulative irritancy test [2], repeat insult patch test [3], chamber scarification test [4], and the soap chamber test [5]. All these tests are performed by topical application of compounds after a penetration-enhancing treatment of the skin.

2.2 Testing for Skin Moisturization

Instruments for measuring skin moisturization do exist. They measure the numerical values of physical parameters of the surface of the skin which can somehow be correlated to the content of water of the upper part of the epidermis and of the stratum corneum. The dermal content of water can be assessed by nuclear magnetic resonance or by high frequency ultrasound [6], but these techniques hardly provide information about the state of hydration of the surface. This can be assessed by electrical devices able to measure the electrical impedance of the outer part of the skin (less than 0.1 mm deep) [7] as it is understood that the conductivity increases with the content of water on the surface of the skin. It has been reported that these instruments do not provide consistent results [8] and have to be calibrated with one another.

In addition to the direct measurement of the water concentration in the top layers of the skin, some techniques allow for the evaluation of the indirect consequence of the presence of water in the stratum corneum. Measurements of the pliability of the horny layer in vivo using the gas bearing electrodynamometer [9] have been shown to correlate directly with the water content of the stratum corneum. The advantage of this technique is that it is not subjected to all the interference known to affect the direct measurement of the water content of the skin by conductimetry (presence of hydroxyl anions or metal cations, for example).

Interestingly enough, the measure of the amount of water molecules (in the gaseous state) above the surface is in good correlation with the electrical measurements. Indeed when the conductivity is low (low content of water in the outer surface of the skin), the TEWL is high. It is thus not unreasonable to consider that a high value of the concentrations of water above the skin is the consequence of high concentrations of water below the surface (as in the case of an edema). One could also conclude that high TEWL is associated with a poor skin barrier function. If this conclusion holds, then one can suggest that a barrier unable to keep the water inside will also be less efficient in maintaining molecules to which we are continuously exposed out of the skin. Since environmental factors are often associate to phenomena of irritation or sensitivity, it might be interesting to look for a correlation, if any, between barrier function and skin sensitivity.

3 PROPERTIES OF SENSITIVE SKIN

Experiments performed in our laboratories have allowed us to recognize that there is a negative correlation between the self-assessed sensitivity of the skin and the barrier function of the skin of the same individuals, measured as susceptibility to respond to standard irritant treatment [10]. Observations were performed by comparing the results obtained in two cohorts of volunteers, one of people estimating themselves as having nonsensitive skin, the other formed by people estimating themselves to have sensitive skin. Female volunteers were included in the studies, if they were in normal health, with no evidence for acute or chronic diseases, including of course dermatologic and ophthalmologic problems. The test sites were devoid of nevi, moles, scars, warts, sunburn, suntan, and active dermal lesions. Pregnant or lactating women were not included in the study. The volunteers answered a questionnaire pertaining to the reactivity and sensitivity of their skin and were then separated in two groups, sensitive and normal, according to the answers to the questions in the questionnaire. On the day of the test, the volunteers were instructed to refrain from applying any kind of product to the face. All the tests took place in a controlled environment at 20°C +/– 1°C and 40% relative humidity.

3.1 Stripping and TEWL

In one experiment with about 100 volunteers per group, TEWL was measured on the cheek for every other volunteer, then a sticky tape (Tesa, Rochester, NY) was applied on the site, made to adhere with gentle strokes, and removed with an even pulling. After measuring the TEWL in the stripped site, sticky tape was applied to the same site and the operation repeated. In this way, the upper layers of the stratum corneum were removed. The TEWL was measured after every stripping. The average number of tape strippings necessary for doubling the TEWL was about 10 for the "sensitive skin" cohort and about 20 for the "nonsensitive skin" cohort. The results are summarized in Fig. 1.

3.2 Stinging Test

Another experiment with two cohorts of about 40 volunteers each was performed by randomly applying to the nasolabial fold on the two sides of the face equal volumes of lactic acid (10% in phosphate buffered saline) or of saline alone. Reactions (itching, burning, or stinging) were recorded 2.5 and 5 min after application. The intensity of stinging was graded by the volunteers, as nil, mild, moderate, or severe (scored as 0, 1, 2, or 3). The results indicated that the sting score upon lactic acid challenge was 0 or 1 for more than 80% of the volunteers in the "nonsensitive skin" group, whereas it was 2 or above 2, for 75% of the individuals in the "sensitive skin" group. The results are plotted in Fig. 2.

3.3 Balsam of Peru and Blood Flow

In a third experiment, balsam of Peru, which provokes a nonimmunogenic immediate contact urticaria, was applied to the skin of the cheek of the volunteers. The blood flow was assessed before the application and at determined time intervals after the application with a laser Doppler capillary blood flow detector. The aver-

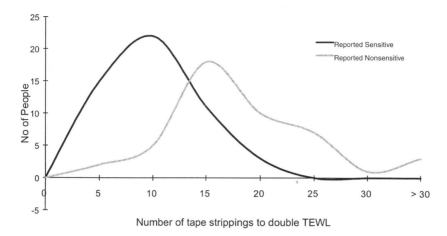

FIGURE 1 Trans-epidermal water loss versus stripping. Self-assessed sensitive and nonsensitive individuals were stripped and the TEWL was measured. The graph plots the distribution of the number of strippings necessary to double the TEWL in sensitive and nonsensitive individuals. (From Ref. 10.)

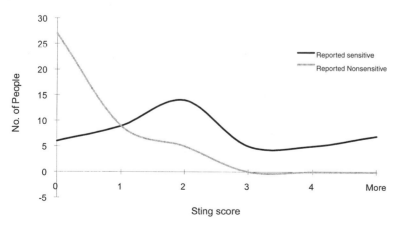

FIGURE 2 Sting score and sensitivity. Self-assessed sensitive and nonsensitive individuals were exposed to lactic acid. The graph plots the distribution of the sting score in the two cohorts. (From Ref. 10.)

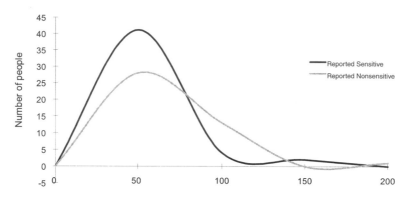

Time (min) to double blood flow

Figure 3 Time course of response to balsam of Peru. The distribution of the time interval necessary to double blood flow upon application of balsam of Peru is plotted for two cohorts of self-assessed sensitive and nonsensitive individuals. (From Ref. 10.)

age time interval necessary for doubling blood flow in the skin was slightly shorter in individuals with sensitive skin than in individuals with normal skin. The results are displayed in Fig. 3.

From these experiments it was concluded that skin sensitivity might be associated with impaired barrier function. An alternative possibility is that sensitive skin is associated with specific neural response, which induces more severe pain in the stinging test and slight edema upon stripping

4 CONDITIONS ASSOCIATED WITH SENSITIVE SKIN

4.1 Skin Sensitivity and Psychological Stress

Since there seems to be a relationship between a defective barrier and a sensitive skin condition, it was reasonable to ask whether or not the sensitive skin conditions observed on people under emotional stress are the consequence of an abnormal barrier function.

To answer that question we undertook a study to evaluate the role played by acute stress on the barrier function of the skin. Twenty-seven university students participated in a barrier recovery study. The study was organized during a period of vacation and repeated during a period of examinations. The second period was confirmed by an appropriate questionnaire to be more stressful than the vacation period. Barrier function was disrupted by tape stripping until the TEWL was about 20–30 g/m²/hr, and then was measured at 3, 6, and 24 hr poststripping. The rate of change of TEWL was used as an indicator of the recovery of barrier function. The results indicate that the recovery of barrier function is more rapid in a nonstressful than in a stressful situation. These results point out that psychological stress plays a role on the kinetics of recovery of disrupted barrier [11].

4.2 Skin Sensitivity and Age

Data published in the literature indicate that skin sensitivity declares itself or increases in the years of the onset of menopause [12]. This increase in sensitivity cannot be attributed to the thickness of the stratum corneum, which is known not to change with age [18]. It is not even the consequence of a change in skin thickness, since in three groups of premenopausal, perimenopausal, and early postmenopausal women, the average skin thickness did not change in a significative way (2.28 +/– 0.39, 2.18 +/– 0.35, and 2.02 +/– 0.36 mm, respectively) [14]. It is indeed known that skin becomes thinner in the years *after* the onset of menopause [15]. Other authors have explored the percutaneous absorption of xenobiotics such as hydrocortisone or testosterone on the forearm of pre- and postmenopausal women [16] and in two groups of young and old men [17]. They did not observe differences in the percutaneous absorption in the two groups of women [16], but observed that permeation of hydrocortisone, benzoic acid, acetyl salicylic acid, and caffeine were significantly lower in the group of old men [17]. They concluded: "It is a common misconception that older skin has a diminished barrier capacity, and that percutaneous absorption is therefore greater" [16].

In a study performed in our laboratory, we have analyzed the TEWL of 223 women aged between 21 and 79. The results are reported in Table 1. From these data it appears that the TEWL is low for young women, it increases by more than 25% for women in their maturity, and returns to lower values above the age of 50. These data can be interpreted by saying that the older individuals have functional barrier, as already suggested by the studies of Howard Maibach [16,17], whereas women in their maturity have impaired barrier because they live a more stressful life, in agreement with published data [11,18]. Thirty-eight out of the 223 panelists reported themselves as having sensitive skin. Measurements of TEWL on these "sensitive skin" panelists are reported in Table 2. It appears that in the age groups between 31 and 50, the vast majority of the individual levels of TEWL are above the average of each group (see Table 1). This allows one to conclude that sensitive skin can be associated with high trans-epidermal water loss.

5 DISCUSSION

Understanding the link between skin moisturization and skin sensitivity is of particular interest not only to the physiologist and the dermatologist, but also to the supplier of skin care products for cosmetics.

TABLE 1   Trans-Epidermal Water Loss Versus Age

Age group	Average TEWL	S.E.	S.D.	N
21–25	7.95	0.96	2.89	9
26–30	7.60	0.57	2.14	14
31–35	9.98	0.55	2.93	28
36–40	9.67	0.59	3.18	29
41–45	9.46	0.51	2.94	33
46–50	9.09	0.45	2.71	36
51–55	7.88	0.50	2.46	24
56–60	7.10	0.54	2.84	27
61–65	6.43	0.66	2.11	10
66–79	7.20	0.63	2.27	13

Notes: A Group of 223 women participated in the study. TEWL was measured with a Servomed EPI vaporimeter on the same region of the face (left jaw) for all the panelists.
N, number of panelist in each age group; S.E., standard error of the mean; S.D., standard deviation.

Data collected in our and in other laboratories indicate that sensitive skin is associated with increased TEWL, increased penetrability, and higher susceptibility to irritants. These parameters can be measured independently and, taken together, the data agree with the hypothesis that sensitive skin is a clinical state associated with impaired barrier function. The results of the stress/barrier repair study add to our understanding and allow us to conclude that stress impairs skin barrier, thus providing an explanation insofar as why many stressed individuals claim to have sensitive skin.

TABLE 2   Trans-Epidermal Water Loss and Sensitive Skin

Age group	Individual TEWL	Average TEWL
21–25		
26–30	6.37, 6.57, 8.69, 7.03, 5.40	6.81
31–35	8.5, 12.33, 11.33, 13.77, 4.77, 15.0, 11.33, 5.1	10.2
36–40	12.33, 15.9, 14.21, 6.87, 10.0, 7.6	11.15
41–45	13, 6.4, 11.44, 6.33, 14.67, 9.77, 10.8, 8	10.05
46–50	8.97, 13.67, 9.33, 9.57, 10.33, 9.5, 10	10.19
51–55	11.33, 5	
56–60	10	
61–65		
66–79	8.1	

When it comes to skin moisturization, not all the results published in the literature can be interpreted in such an unambiguous way. This is the consequence of the nature of the experimental devices at hand. They allow one to measure quantities that generally vary with more than one single variable. For instance, conductivity values can be the consequence of more or less water on the surface of the skin, or of more or less electrolytes in the same water content. Larger TEWL values can be the consequence of worse barrier if moisturization is constant, or of better moisturization if the barrier is constant. Paradoxically, the fact that sensitive skin requires less tape stripping for achieving a predetermined value of TEWL could be interpreted by saying that the two types of skin have the same barrier, but that sensitive skin is characterized by a higher state of water secretion upon stripping than nonsensitive skin. This kind of paradoxical reasoning can be carried out for all experiments in which quantities are measured that depend on variables which cannot be varied or measured independently one at the time. It is of concern here to point out that the lack of unambiguous wording adds to the difficulty in interpreting results. When it comes to skin moisturization, difficulties are encountered because hydration is only one of the parameters playing a role in moisturization; suppleness of the stratum corneum, smoothness of the outer surface, and elasticity of the dermis are parameters which contribute to the individual evaluation of one's own skin moisturization.

The biochemical nature of the difference between sensitive and nonsensitive skin is not yet understood. It is tempting to speculate that the relative amount of lipid molecules participating in the build-up of the barrier might be different in the two skin types. Preliminary experiments performed in our laboratory failed to point out significative differences as far as total ethanol-extractable lipids are concerned, as well as for squalene, free fatty acids, palmitate (16:0), palmitoleic acid (16:1), oleic acid (18:1), and stearic acid (18:0) (unpublished).

The results reviewed in this chapter confirm the positive correlation between self-assessed skin sensitivity and increased trans-epidermal water loss. Circumstantial evidence justifies interpreting this correlation by concluding that skin sensitivity is associated with impaired barrier function. Interestingly enough, this correlation is particularly true for mature women. On the other hand, the question concerning the impairment of barrier function with age remains open, and more experimental work is needed before a clear-cut conclusion can be drawn.

6 REFERENCES

1. Draelos ZD. Sensitive skin: perceptions, evaluation and treatment. Am J Cont Dermat 1997; 8:67–78.
2. Partick E, Maibach HI. Predictive skin irritation tests in animal and humans in dermato-toxicology. In: Marzulli FN, Maibach HI, eds. Dermatotoxicology, 4th Ed. New York: Hemisphere, 1991:211–212.

3. Shelanski HV, Shelanski MV. A new technique of human patch test. Proc Sci Sec Toilet Good Assoc 1953; 19:46–49.
4. Frosch PJ, Kligman AM. The chamber scarification test for assessing irritancy. Cont Dermat 1976; 2:314–324.
5. Agner T, Serup J. Quantification of the DMSO response: a test for assessement of sensitive skin. Clin Exp Dermatol 1989; 14:214–217.
6. Gniadecka M, Quistorff B. Assessment of dermal water by high-frequency ultra-sound: comparative studies with nuclear magnetic resonance. Br J Dermatol 1996; 135:218–224.
7. Blichmann CW, Serup J. Assessment of skin moisture. Measurement of electric con-ductance, capacitance and transepidermal water loss. Acta Der Venereol 1988; 68:284–290.
8. Van Neste D. Comparative study of normal and rough human skin hydration in vivo: evaluation with four different instruments. J Dermatol Sci 1991; 2:119–124.
9. Maes D, Short J, Turek B, Reinstein J. In vivo measuring of skin softness using the gas bearing electrodynamometer. Int J Cosmet Sci 1983; 5:189–200.
10. Muizzuddin N, Marenus KD, Maes DH. Factors defining sensitive skin and its treat-ment. Am J Cont Dermat 1998; 9:170–175.
11. Garg A, Chren MM, Sands LP, Matsui MS, Marenus KD, Feingold KR, Elias PM. Psychological stress perturbs epidermal permeability barrier homeostasis. Arch Der-matol 2001; 137:53–59.
12. Paquet F, Pierard-Franchimont C, Fumal I, Goffin V, Paye M, Pierard GE. Sensitive skin at menopause; dew point and electrometric properties of the stratum corneum. Maturitas 1998; 28:221–227.
13. Gilchrest BA. Aging of skin. In: Fitzpatrick TB, Eisen ZA, Wolff K, Freedberg IM, Austen KF, eds. Dermatology in General Medicine. New York: McGraw-Hill, 1993:150–157.
14. Panyakhamlerd K, Chotnopparatpattara P, Taechakraichana N, Kukulprasong A, Chaikittisilpa S, Limpaphayom K. Skin thickness in different menopausal status. J Med Assoc Thai 1999; 82:352–356.
15. Brincat MP. Hormone replacement therapy and the skin. Maturitas 2000; 35:107–117.
16. Oriba HA, Bucks DA, Maibach HI. Percutaneous absorption of hydrocortisone and testosterone on the vulva and on the forearm: effect of menopause and site. Br J Der-matol 1996; 134:229–233.
17. Roskos KV, Maibach HI, Guy RH. The effect of aging on percutaneous absorption in man. J Pharmacokinet Biopharm 1989; 17:617–630.
18. Denda M, Tsuchiya T, Elias PM, Feingold KR. Stress alters cutaneous permeability barrier homeostasis Am J Physiol Regul Integr Comp Physiol 2000; 278:367–372.

8

Photodamage and Dry Skin

James J. Leyden and Robert Lavker
University of Pennsylvania School of Medicine,
Philadelphia, Pennsylvania

Over the past 40 years, considerable evidence has been accumulated from a wide range of experimental studies in animals and humans to clearly indicate that ultraviolet radiation (UVR) from sun exposure has multiple profound effects on skin. Both acute and chronic effects are well described [1]. Ultraviolet radiation is responsible for skin cancer, photoaging, and photosensitivity diseases. In addition, profound immunological effects have been identified which account in part for the beneficial effects of UVR in many diseases such as psoriasis, atopic dermatitis, mycosis fungoid, and vitiligo.

Ultraviolet light is artificially divided into very short wave UVC (none currently reaches the earth's surface), UVB (290 to 320 nm), and UVA, which is divided into UVA II (320 to 340 nm) and UVA I (340 to 400 nm). Ultraviolet A makes up approximately 95% of the UVR to which we are exposed. Until relatively recently, the main focus of research had been directed toward UVB and its role in cancer and immune modulation; UVB wavelengths are far more energetic than UVA and clearly are the dominant factor in squamous cell formation and play an important role in basal cell cancer. In the past decade, in vivo studies in human volunteers have shown that repeated low doses of UVA II and I comparable to those obtained during everyday activities can also have profound effects in skin. Table 1 summarizes the work of many investigators and indicates all

155

wavelengths have profound biological effects on all components and cell types in skin.

1 EFFECTS OF PHOTODAMAGE

Photoaging and photodamage are terms used to describe the consequences of chronic exposure to ultraviolet light. Cumulative injury results in a constellation of histological and clinical findings (Table 2). Kligman first described the hallmark of chronically sun damaged skin viz. the accumulation of disorganized, coarse bundles of fibers which stain like normal elastic tissue [2]. He coined the

TABLE 1   Relative Effects of UVA on Skin Components and Cell Types

	UVA II	UVA I
Stratum corneum thickness (dry skin)	+++	+++
Epidermal thickness	++	++
Apoptosis	+++	+
Langerhans cell depletion	+++	+
Damage to elastin	++	+++
Sebaceous gland hypertrophy	++	++
Telangiectasias	++	?

TABLE 2   Histological and Clinical Manifestations of Photoaging

	Clinical signs
Stratum corneum thickening and microfissures	"Dry," flaky rough skin
DNA damage to basal cells and keratinocytes; dysplasia, neoplasia	Actinic keratosis; basal and squamous cell cancer
Melanocytic hyperplasia, dysplasia	Lentigos (age spots)
Epidermal inclusion cysts	Milia
Follicular epithelial hyperkeratosis	Solar comedones
Thickened, disorganized elastic fibers; decrease collagen	Wrinkling
Telangiectactic vessels; decrease in papillary dermis	Telangiectasis; sallowness
Sebaceous gland hypertrophy	Sebaceous hypertrophy

term elastosis to describe this material which replaced the normal mixture of collagen, elastin, and glycosaminoglycans. In the 30 years since that seminal observation, a variety of clinical and histological changes have come to be associated with chronic ultraviolet damage in skin. The clinical consequences of photodamage are responsible for the majority of undesired changes associated with aging and so-called premature skin aging, the clinical and histological hallmarks of photoaging [3].

1.1 Stratum Corneum

A prominent feature of photodamaged skin is a pronounced thickening of the stratum corneum (Fig. 1). This thickening is the result of faulty degradation of stratum corneum desmosomes. As the stratum corneum thickens, the outer layers become somewhat dehydrated. As a result, the outer stratum corneum becomes stiffer and microfissures develop (Fig. 2). Micro fissuring leads to clumps of stratum corneum cells partially tearing away. These clumps of uplifted cells are visible as flaking and feel rough to the touch. Many years ago, we inspected the skin of large numbers of individuals ranging from teenagers to those over 90. It is apparent, even in teenagers, that the sun-exposed arms are rougher and often show flaking, clearly different than sun-protected skin such as the upper inner forearm near the axilla.

1.2 Epidermis—Keratinocytes

Sun-exposed skin typically shows a thickened epidermis. This increase in the viable epidermal compartment indicates a hyperproliferative state, possibly indicat-

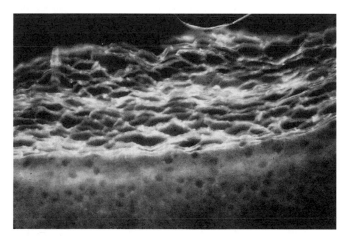

FIGURE 1 A markedly thickened stratum corneum resulting from the hyperplastic response of the epidermis to chronic UVA injury.

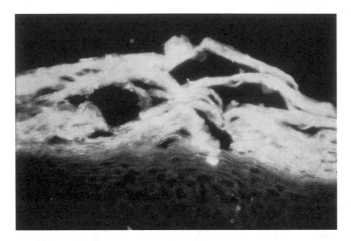

FIGURE 2 Microfissures develop as the thickened stratum corneum becomes stiff and fractures. The skin appears flaky and feels rough as clumps of cells uplift.

ing a chronic woundlike condition and a chronic attempt at repair. Epidermal DNA damage can be seen in the form of dysplasia and basal and squamous cell carcinoma. Another histological hallmark of photodamage are so-called sunburn cells [4]. These cells show pyknotic nuclei and a necrotic, eosinophilic cytoplasm. These cells are now referred to apoptotic cells, i.e., cells engaged in a programmed cell death or suicide presumably because sufficient DNA damage has occurred.

In a more subtle fashion, DNA damage can be seen by use of a monoclonal antibody to the p53 enzyme system—the so-called guardian of the genome. When epidermal DNA is damaged this system is activated to initiate repair. Defects in this system in the form of mutations lead to an increased risk for cancer. In addition to precancerous dysplasia and cancer, benign hyperproliferative lesions such as seborrhoic keratosis can develop [5].

Recently, we have come to realize that epidermal inclusion cysts (milia) may also be a sign of chronic ultraviolet damage. The index case was a 45-year-old male with the basal cell nevis syndrome who had hundreds of milia on his face without any history of dermabrasion or other resurfacing procedures. We examined more than 500 women who had previously been involved in clinical trials for photodamage and found a high correlation between their photodamage grade and the presence and number of milia. In that group, there were three women who had numerous milia with mild photodamage. These women had siblings and/or parents who also had large numbers of milia, suggesting a possible genetic factor. Follicular epithelial retention hyperkeratosis and comedone formation is another well-recognized feature of chronic photodamage.

1.3   Epidermis—Melanocytes

Increased numbers of melanocytes and melanocytic hyperplasia resulting in solar lentigos, age spots, and sunburn freckles are well-recognized consequences of chronic ultraviolet damage. The role of ultraviolet light in melanoma remains unsettled in terms of which wavelengths are involved and how central to melanoma development UV is, but none doubt its importance.

1.4   Dermis—Matrix

A histological hallmark of photoaging is a replacement of the normal dermal matrix of collagen, elastin, and glycosaminoglycans by large bundles of coarse elastic fibers and decreased collagen. The clinical consequence of elastosis is pronounced wrinkling and in advanced cases a yellowish cobblestone appearance associated with pronounced sagging. This process is often accompanied by a brisk neutophilic infiltrate which often can be appreciated clinically and is referred to as heliodermatitis or dermatoheliosis [6]. Neutrophil elastases may play a prominent role in damage to elastin and the subsequent wrinkling or sagging. The role of UV in the degeneration of surrounding collagen is now more fully understood and is the consequence of both UVA and UVB and the effect of ultraviolet light increasing the activity of metalloproteinases [7]. This family of 14 different proteinases can act on a broad range of substrates and can be activated in vivo by a single exposure to UV. The mechanism(s) of elastosis remain unclear. The major consequence of these changes in the dermal matrix is wrinkling. Wrinkles don't have a histological marker but rather can be best thought of as stress fractures from material which has aged. The radiating quality of wrinkles is similar to that seen in materials such as buildings and bridges. With more pronounced changes, skin "settles," which is seen clinically as sagging.

1.5   Dermis—Vasculature

Two changes can occur. Some patients show loss of the papillary plexus, flattening of the rete ridges, and loss of the papillary dermis. Clinically, these individuals have a sallow washed-out appearance. The other finding is that of a proliferative response producing dilated, enlarged vessels in the papillary and mid-dermis. Clinically, these are seen as telangiectasis.

1.6   Dermis—Sebaceous Gland

Sebaceous gland enlargement is another feature of chronic ultraviolet damage. Clinically, this can be seen as small, yellowish nodules or in more advanced cases as a thick, coarsening of skin with large, dilated follicular openings from which sebaceous material can be squeezed out.

2   VULNERABLE PHENOTYPES

It has been known for many years that fair skinned individuals, particularly those of Celtic ancestry, are particularly vulnerable to the acute adverse effects of ultraviolet light, i.e., sunburn. More recently, we have come to realize that there is a phenotype who appears to be more vulnerable to the chronic adverse effects of UV. These individuals have red hair, blue eyes, and have a Celtic background, but have the ability to tan often fairly deeply, after suffering initial burning. Typically, they have a very fair Celtic parent who burns and tans little or not at all, while the other parent tans easily and rarely burns. The vulnerable offspring is able to sustain more exposure because their tan prevents burning. Usually, these individuals are infrequent users of high-SPF sunscreens and pride themselves on their ability to tan while family members can't. These individuals develop dry skin, a leathery wrinkling, and pigmentary changes at a relatively early age (late 20s to early 30s) and by their mid-40s they tend to look older and are extremely unhappy.

"Dry skin" is a prominent feature of actinically damaged skin. It is such a prominent feature that the lay public has, with the help of many cosmetic companies, come to view dry skin as the causative agent for other signs of photodamage, most notably wrinkling. As is detailed in other chapters, dry skin is really an abnormally thickened stratum corneum which becomes stiff and cracks. The resulting uplifted clumps of cells become visible as flakes and skin develops a rough texture.

3   SKIN TEXTURE IN EXPOSED AND PROTECTED SITES

Some years ago, we examined a large number of people ranging from 11 to 70 years in age. The outer, exposed area of both forearms and the upper inner, sunprotected arm were graded using a visual analog scale. The results are summarized in Table 3. In all age groups the exposed sites clearly were rougher to touch, and visible differences were also common. Even in teenagers and young adults,

TABLE 3   Surface Texture in Sun-Exposed and -Protected Skin

	Exposed	Protected
Young (mean 29)	15 ± 6	5 ± 3
Middle age (mean 45)	40 ± 10	10 ± 6
Older (mean 65)	65 ± 13	30 ± 7

Note: Visual analog score 0 = none; 100 = very severe "dry skin."

the exposed areas were clearly drier. The magnitude of dryness in general paralleled other signs of photodamage such as freckling and other forms of melanocyte damage as well as wrinkling in the older age groups. In the teenagers and those in their 20s, while there was a definite difference in exposed and protected skin, the patient was typically unaware of the difference.

In sun-protected skin, there was an increase in "dryness" associated with age, and texture changes are a recognized change associated with the process of biological aging. It was striking, however, to note that the mean dryness score for the older group (mean age of 65) was significantly lower than the sun-exposed sites for middle-aged individuals (mean age 45). These findings suggest that chronic sun damage may be a more important factor in the pathophysiology of dry skin than is the inherent process of biological aging.

4 EFFECT OF REPEATED UV EXPOSURE ON THE STRATUM CORNEUM

In a series of studies, Lavker et al. as well as Lowe have defined the effects of UVB, UVA I, and UVA II in the stratum corneum of humans [8–11]. In their first study, repeated exposures of 0.5 MED of UVB or UVA produced thickening of the stratum corneum (Table 4). Previous work had shown this effect for UVB, but not for UVA. More surprisingly, the effect of repeated low-dose UVA was greater than that found with UVB. In a subsequent study, they showed that UVA I (340–400 nm) was as effective as the entire UVA band (320–400 nm) for a battery of markers of damage. Subsequently, the wavelength dependence for UVA-induced cumulative damage was investigated. The UVA wavelengths between 320 and 345 nm were more effective than longer (360–400 nm) wavelengths for epidermal and stratum corneum thickening (Table 4). All UVA bands were equally effective in inducing dermal changes. These results clearly implicate chronic damage by UVA as a major factor in the pathophysiology of dry skin. The implications for broad UV protection are clear. As few as nine exposures of UVA result in stratum corneum thickening.

TABLE 4   Effect of Repetitive Ultraviolet Light Exposure

	Stratum corneum thickness
25 doses of 20 J/cm^2 UVA (0.5 MED)	15.0 ± 0.7
25 doses of UVB (0.5 MED)	11.8 ± 0.9
9 doses of 35 J UVA	13.2 ± 0.6

In studies in which the biological effectiveness of various bands within the UVA spectrum were compared for the effects of cumulative damage, both the shorter UVA II wavelengths and longer UVA I are found to be responsible for stratum corneum thickening. Thus at equivalent suberythematogenic doses, UVA appears to be more effective than UVB in inducing stratum corneum thickening. The findings of Lavker et al. suggest that cumulative doses greater than 315 J/cm^2 result in stratum corneum thickening.

It is important to note that the doses of UVA used in these experiments are relative to daily exposure for many people. A few hours exposure will permit accumulation of comparable doses of UVA.

Recent evidence accumulating from a variety of phenotypes of dry skin such as seen in atopic dermatitis, inherited metabolic disorders, and detergent-chapped skin all point to a disturbance in the balance of intracellular lipids of the stratum corneum.

Permeability barrier function and orderly corneocyte desquamation require the organization of three nonpolar lipids, ceramides, free fatty acids, and cholesterol into extracellular lamellar membrane structure within the intercellular spaces of the stratum corneum. These lipids are delivered through the secretion of epidermal lamellar bodies. Although present in approximately equimolar ratios, ceramide predominates by weight, accounting for approximately 50%. In addition, lamellar bodies secrete hydrolytic lipid hydrolases such as β-glucocerebrosidase and secretory phospholipase, which process glucosylceramide, phospholipids, ceramide, and free fatty acids. Sphingomyelin is another source of ceramide through hydrolysis by sphingomyelinase. In Gaucher's disease, deficiency in β-glucocerebrosidase is associated with dry skin and defective stratum corneum function [12]. Likewise in Niemann–Pick disease deficiency in acid-sphingomyelinase is associated with similar findings [13]. In atopic dermatitis, there is abnormal expression of sphingomyelin deacylase, resulting in decreased levels of ceramide by competing for glucocerebroside and sphingomyelin [14]. The result is abnormal stratum corneum in terms of barrier and desquamation. Chronic exposure to detergents results in extraction of intracellular lipids and the formation of dry skin [15]. In all of these studies, the final pathway points to a decrease in ceramides, particularly ceramide 1. Ceramide 1 is rich in linoleic acid and is believed to play an important role in regulating water content. Decrease in this capacity may play a crucial role in the desquamation process. In hereditary icthyosis a deficiency of cholesterol sulfatase results in an extreme expression of abnormal desquamation viz. severely thickened stratum corneum.

The mechanisms by which repeated low-dose UVB and UVA induce abnormal desquamation are unknown. In recent studies (R Lavker, unpublished observations) using a monoclonal antibody to lamellar bodies, an increase secretion of these lamellae was found. Any molecular or biochemical aberrations remain to be elucidated. However, it is likely that an abnormality in one or more pathways leading to ceramide formation may be involved in UVR-induced dry skin.

Another possible pathway that may play a role in UVR-induced dry skin could involve the recently described mitochondrial DNA (mt DNA) mutations [16]. Such mutations have been linked with other chronic degenerative diseases such as Alzheimer's, progressive external opthalmoplegia, and Keans–Sayre syndrome. In addition, mitochondrial DNA mutations have been proposed to play a role in the biological process of aging.

Higher mutation frequency of mt DNA has been found in chronically sun-exposed skin, and more recent work has established a direct link between UVA radiation–induced oxidative stress and the most frequent mt DNA mutation [17]. This interesting story is currently viewed as most relevant to dermal fibroblast and dermal matrix changes. However, the possibility of such changes playing a role in epidermal changes remains a possibility.

Current evidence developed over the last 10 years clearly implicates chronic ultraviolet damage as a key factor in the development of dry skin. Both UVB and UVA are implicated, with the latter probably the more important causative factor. Studies indicate that cumulative low-dose UVB and UVA induce stratum corneum changes after as few as nine exposures. While the skin possesses capability to repair UV damage—best seen in the photodamage mouse model—the accumulation of UV damage clearly overwhelms repair mechanisms. Even in young adults, the clinical consequences of chronic UV damage can be appreciated. The implications for prevention are clear—broad spectrum UV protection, possibly in combination with blends of anti-oxidants to mute oxidative stress not prevented by UV-absorbing agents.

REFERENCES

1. Gilchrest BA. Skin aging and photoaging: an overview. J Am Acad Dermatol 1989; 21:610–613.
2. Kligman A. Early destruction effects of sunlight in human skin. J Am Med Assoc 1969; 210:2377–2380.
3. Kligman AM, Lavker RM. Cutaneous aging: the differences between intrinsic aging and photoaging. J Cutan Aging Cosmet Dermatol 1988; 1:5–11.
4. Gilchrest BA, Soter NA, Stoff JS, Mihm MC. The human sunburn reaction: histologic and biochemical studies. J Am Acad Dermatol 1981; 5:411–422.
5. Granstein RD, Sober AJ. Current concepts in ultraviolet carcinogenis. Proc Soc Exp Biol Med 1982; 170:115–125.
6. Lavker RM. Structural alteration in exposed and unexposed human skin. J Invest Dermatol 1979; 73:59–66.
7. Kligman LH, Akin FJ, Kligman AM. The contribution of UVA and UVB to connective tissue damage in hairless mice. J Invest Dermatol 1985; 84:272–276.

8. Lavker R, Kaidbey K. The spectral dependence for UVA-induced cumulating damage in human skin. J Invest Dermatol 199; 108:17–21.

9. Lavker RM, Gerberick GF, Veres D, Irwin CJ, Kaidby KH. Cumulative effects from repeated exposures to sunerythemal doses of UVB and UVA in human skin. J Am Acad Dermatol 1995; 32:53–62.

10. Lavker RM, Veres DA, Irwin CJ, Kaidbey KH. Quantitative assessment of cumulative damage from repetitive exposures to suberythemogenic doses of UVA in human skin. Photochem Photobiol 1995; 62:348–352.

11. Lowe NJ, Meyerd DP, Wieder JM, Luftman D, Borget T, Lehman MD, Johnson AW, Scott IR. Low doses of repetitive ultraviolet A induce morphologic changes in human skin. J Invest Dermatol 1995; 105:739–743.

12. Hulleran WM, Ginns EI, Menon GK, et al. Consequences of beta-glucocerebrosidase deficiency in epidermis: ultrastructure and permeability barrier alterations in Gaucher's disese. J Clin Invest; 93:1756–1764.

13. Schmuth M, Man M, Weber F, et al. Permeability barrier disorder in Niemann–Pick disease: sphingomyelin-ceramide processing required for normal barrier homeostasis. J Invest Dermatol 2000; 115:459–466.

14. Hara J, Higachi K, Okamoto R, et al. High expression of sphingomyelin deacylase is an important determinant of ceramide deficiency leading to barrier disruption in atopic dermatitis. J Invest Dermatol 2000; 115:406–413.

15. Rawlings AV, Watkinson A, Rogers J, et al. Abnormalities in stratum corneum structure, lipid composition and desmosome degredation in soap induced winter xerosis. J Cosmet Chem 1994; 45:203–220.

16. Berneburg M, Gattermann N, Stege H, et al. Chronically ultraviolet-exposed human skin shows a higher mutation frequency of mitochondrial DNA. Photochem Photobiol 1997; 66:271–275.

17. Bernburg M, Grether-Bech S, Kurten V, et al. Singlet oxygen mediates UVA-induced generation of photoaging-associated mitochondrial corneum deletum.

9

Atopic Dermatitis

Anna Di Nardo
University of Modena, Modena, Italy

Philip W. Wertz
Dows Institute for Dental Research, University of Iowa, Iowa City, Iowa

1 ATOPIC DERMATITIS

Widespread regions of dry itchy skin is one of the prominent clinical features of atopic dermatitis [1]. The intense itch is the most characteristic feature of this disease, and the consequences include scratching and eczematous lesions, as illustrated in Figure 1. Scratching can lead to disruption of the stratum corneum and infection. This disease is generally associated with asthma, allergic rhinitis, and elevated levels of IgE. There is frequently a family history of atopic dermatitis, indicating a genetic component in the etiology of the disease. All of these factors are taken into account in arriving at a clinical diagnosis.

The onset of atopic dermatitis most frequently occurs during the first year of life, and most cases become evident before age 5 [2]. Only rarely is there an adult onset. In most patients atopic dermatitis spontaneously resolves by about age 20, although it can be a lifelong disease. Adults who have been atopic often have unusually sensitive skin.

The differentiation process in atopic epidermis is notably altered. At a histologic level the intercellular spaces in the viable portion of the atopic epidermis appear to be swollen with fluid, and the spinous layer is thickened. In the vicinity

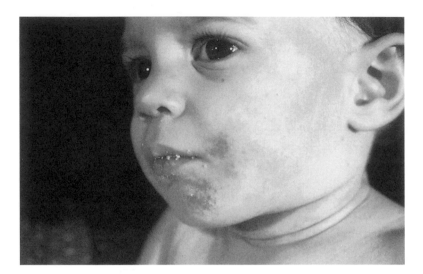

FIGURE 1 An infant with active atopic dermatitis. Note the eczematous lesions on the chin and cheek.

of eczematous lesions mononuclear cells are present within the viable epidermis, and the stratum corneum may be parakeratotic. In such areas the dermis becomes infiltrated mainly with lymphocytes. The altered keratinization process evident in the histopathology leads ultimately to altered stratum corneum lipid composition and possibly to reduced production of natural moisturizing factor in the stratum corneum. Both of these alterations could contribute to the dry skin of the atopic.

2 STRATUM CORNEUM LIPIDS

The dry skin of individuals with atopic dermatitis displays impaired barrier function as indicated by increased trans-epidermal water loss [3,4], illustrated in Figure 2, and diminished water-holding properties [5]. Both of these biophysical anomalies can be related to altered composition of the lipids of the stratum corneum [6–8]. While not the primary defect, the impaired barrier function and surface roughness associated with dryness may render the skin more susceptible to irritation.

The lipids found in normal stratum corneum consist mainly of a series of ceramides, cholesterol, and fatty acids, with small proportions of cholesterol sulfate and cholesterol esters [9–11]. Representative structures of the major lipids from human stratum corneum are given in Figure 3 [3,13–17]. This lipid mixture is biologically unusual in that it does not include phospholipids, which are the

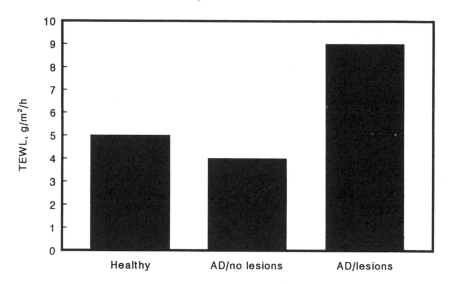

Figure 2 Trans-epidermal water loss (TEWL) from healthy subjects and from uninvolved skin of atopic patients with and without active lesions. Trans-epidermal water loss is not significantly different between healthy and uninvolved skin of atopic patients without active lesions; however, it is significantly elevated in uninvolved skin of atopic patients with active lesions. (Based on data from Ref. 4.)

major components of most biological membrane systems. It is thought that this unusual lipid mixture was selected by the forces of evolution to produce a relatively impermeable protective barrier that was sufficiently flexible to permit movement [11]. The development of such a protective layer was a critical step in the evolution of life on dry land [18].

2.1 Ceramides

Historically, ceramides were first identified as polar lipids of the stratum corneum by Nicolaides [19]. Later, Gray and White [20] showed that the ceramides and precursor glucosylceramides were structurally heterogeneous. They identified normal fatty acids and α-hydroxyacids as well as sphingosine and phytosphingosine as components of the epidermal sphingolipids. They also identified one glucosylceramide which contained ester-linked linoleic acid and an unusual amide-linked hydroxyacid that was subsequently shown to be an ω-hydroxyacid. The structures of the ceramides from pig epidermis were then determined [12]. These consisted of six chromatographically separable fractions. The least polar of these

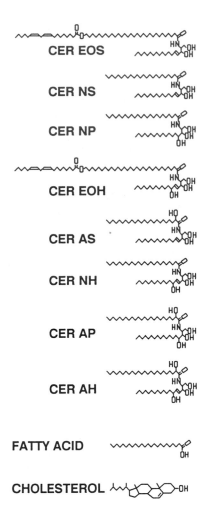

FATTY ACID

CHOLESTEROL

Figure 3 Representative structures of the major lipids from human stratum corneum. (From Refs. 9 and 13–17).

was designated ceramide 1, or acylceramide. This contains the ω-hydroxyacid, originally noted by Gray and White [20], amide-linked to a mixture of sphingosine and dihydrosphingosine bases with linoleic acid ester-linked to the ω-hydroxyl group. The next fraction, ceramide 2, consists of long, mostly 24- through 28-carbon, normal fatty acids amide-linked to sphingosine bases. Ceramide 3 contains the same long chain, normal fatty acids found in ceramide 2 but amide-linked to phytosphingosines: Ceramides 4 and 5 both contain α-hydroxyacids amide-linked to a mixture of sphingosines and dihydrosphingosines. They differ in that the chromatographically more mobile ceramide 4 contains mainly 24- through 28-carbon hydroxyacids, whereas ceramide 5 contains mostly α-hydroxypalmitic acid. The most polar of the porcine ceramides, ceramide 6, consists of α-hydroxyacids amide-linked to phytosphingosines.

Subsequently, covalently bound lipids on the outer surface of the cornified envelope were identified in porcine [21] and human [22] stratum corneum. These consist primarily of an ω-hydroxyceramide related to ceramide 1 along with smaller amounts of free fatty acids and free ω-hydroxyacids. It was proposed that this layer of covalently bound lipid on the outer surface of the cornified envelope may provide a template on which the free intercellular lipids spread and which may play an important role in organization of the intercellular lipids.

All of the ceramides identified in porcine stratum corneum, including the covalently bound hydroxyceramide, were subsequently identified among the human stratum corneum lipids [13,22]. In the human, a second covalently bound hydroxyceramide was also present which had an extra hydroxyl group on the long chain base component but was not a simple phytosphingosine [22]. This subsequently was shown to be 6-hydroxysphingosine [14]. The identification of this new long chain base led to the discovery of three new components among the free ceramides [14,15]. One of these contains normal fatty acids amide-linked to 6-hydroxyceramide. A second consists of α-hydroxyacids amide-linked to 6-hydroxysphingosine, and there is a minor amount of a ceramide analogous to ceramide 1 but containing 6-hydroxyceramide as the base component.

2.2 Ceramide Nomenclature

With the initially studied ceramides from porcine epidermis, nomenclature was analogous to the chromatographic separation with one ceramide structural type corresponding to each chromatographic fraction [12]. Numerous investigators have used this system and it is still in use.

When human stratum corneum ceramides were first subjected to analysis by thin layer chromatography using the same development regimen used to resolve the porcine ceramides, a similar but somewhat different chromatographic profile was obtained [13]. Fractions chromatographically identical to porcine ceramides 1, 2, and 3 were present and were named accordingly. A single broad band found in the region of the chromatogram corresponding to pig ceramides 4 and 5 was labeled ceramide 4/5. Material corresponding in chromatographic mobility to pig ceramide 6 split into an incompletely resolved doublet, the components of which were labeled as ceramide 6I and ceramide 6II. This system of ceramide nomenclature has been used in a number of reports. It is now recognized that in the human, the fraction originally labeled ceramide 3 actually contains, in addition to the normal fatty acid–phytosphingosine conjugate analogous to ceramide 3 in the pig, a small proportion of a ceramide analogous to pig ceramide 1 but containing 6-hydroxysphingosine as the base component. Ceramide 4/5 contains in addition to α-hydroxyacid-sphingosines the ceramide consisting of normal fatty acids conjugated to 6-hydroxysphingosine; and ceramide 6I consists of α-hydroxyacids amide-linked to 6-hydroxyceramide.

Given the diversity of ceramide structures and the differences between the human and porcine ceramides a nomenclature system based on structure rather than chromatographic mobility has been proposed by Motta [16]. In this system ceramides are designated, in general, as CER FB, where F indicates the type of amide linked fatty acid and B indicates the base. When an ester-linked fatty acid is also present a prefix of E is added, as in CER EFB. Normal fatty acids, α-hydroxyacids, and ω-hydroxyacids are indicated by N, A, and O, respectively, and sphingosines, phytosphingosines, and 6-hydroxysphingosine are indicated by S, P, and H. Within this system, ceramide 1, for example, becomes CER EOS. Ceramide 2 is CER NS, and so on. Table 1 summarizes the corresponding chromatographic fractions and names according to the Motta system.

2.3 Free Fatty Acids

In both the pig and human stratum corneum the major free fatty acids are straight-chained saturated species of 20 through 28 carbons [17,23]. In the human, fatty acids derived from sebaceous triglycerides can confound fatty acid analysis [24]; however, the sebaceous fatty acids are mainly 16 and 18 carbons long, with C16:1Δ6 being the most abundant [25]. The free fatty acids along with a minor amount of cholesterol sulfate are the only ionizable lipids in the stratum corneum,

TABLE 1 Ceramide Fractions and Identities

Porcine		Human	
Chromatographic fraction	Motta (16) nomenclature	Chromatographic fraction	Motta (16) nomenclature
1	CER EOS	1	CER EOS
2	CER NS	2	CER NS
3	CER NP	3	CERs EOH + NP
4	CER AS[a]	4/5	CERs AS + NH
5	CER AS[a]	6I	CER AH
6	CER AP	6II	CER AP

[a]CER AS in porcine fraction 4 contains 24- through 28-carbon α-hydroxyacids, whereas CER AS in fraction 5 contains almost exclusively α-hydroxypalmitic acid.
Source: Based on Refs. 11–14 and 20.

and it has been suggested that this is important for the formation of a lamellar phase [24].

2.4 Cholesterol and Derivatives

Cholesterol is a major lipid component and the sole sterol in both porcine and human stratum corneum [17]. Cholesterol sulfate is a minor stratum corneum component, but it has been implicated in the regulation of desquamation. Both with an organ culture model and with human skin in vivo, it has been demonstrated that hydrolysis of cholesterol sulfate accompanies the desquamation process while all other lipids survive cell shedding intact [13,26]. In addition, there is a genetic disease, recessive X-linked ichthyosis, in which the sulfatase that would normally hydrolyze cholesterol sulfate is defective [27] and cholesterol sulfate is present at abnormally high levels in the stratum corneum and elsewhere [28]. In this disease desquamation does not proceed normally and the skin surface can become rough and scaly. Degradation of the desmosomes between corneocytes is a necessary step leading to desquamation, and several serine proteases have been implicated. It has been suggested that hydrolysis of cholesterol sulfate may be required to permit proteolysis of the desmosomes [29], and recently it has been demonstrated that cholesterol sulfate is a serine protease inhibitor [30–32]. Cholesterol esters have been considered a marker of keratinization [33]. The principal fatty acid found in epidermal cholesterol esters is oleate [23]. Cholesterol esters are not themselves membrane-forming lipids and are generally not well incorporated into membranes formed from other lipids. It has been suggested the cholesterol esters phase separate from other lipids within the intercellular spaces of the stratum corneum. This could provide a mechanism for keeping oleate, a known permeability enhancer [34], out of the membrane domains, thereby preserving barrier function [11,24].

2.5 Phase Behavior and Organization

All of the ceramides and free fatty acids in epidermal stratum corneum are rodlike or cylindrical in shape, which makes them ideal for the formation of highly ordered gel phase membrane domains [11,24]. Cholesterol is capable of either decreasing or increasing the fluidity of membranes, depending upon the proportions and natures of the other lipids. It has been suggested that cholesterol serves to provide a degree of plasticity to what would otherwise be highly rigid and possibly brittle membranes. In this view the ceramides and fatty acids are essential for the barrier function of the skin, and the cholesterol is required to permit flexing without cracking the stratum corneum. A model that has been advanced and that is consistent with these suggestions is the domain mosaic model [35]. In this model the intercellular lamellae consist of gel phase domains within a continuous liquid crystalline domain. Molecules crossing these membranes would penetrate through the more fluid liquid crystalline domains more readily than through the gel phase, and the greatest flux would occur at the phase boundaries.

Examination of stratum corneum by transmission electron microscopy following treatment with ruthenium tetroxide has revealed that the number of lamellae across the intercellular space varies widely, but in most regions there are multiples of three lamellae with a broad–narrow–broad spacing [36,37]. The overall thickness of one broad–narrow–broad unit is 13 nm [36]. This lamellar spacing has also been confirmed by x-ray diffraction [38]. Near the ends of the corneocytes there is frequently one broad–narrow–broad unit. It has been proposed that this consists of the covalently bound lipid layers on either side of the intercellular space with an intervening layer formed by eversion of the sphingosine tails of the hydroxyceramides [11,24]. Some of the spaces would be filled by free lipid. In this model, the central narrow lamella is highly interdigitated and serves to effectively link adjacent corneocytes at their ends. Between the broad flat surfaces there are generally six or more lamellae, and it is thought that the linoleate-containing acylceramide (ceramide 1, CER EOS) plays an essential role in formation of the lamellar arrangements with six bands and higher multiples of three. In the six-band pattern it is thought that there is a central pair of bilayers that are linked together through the action of acylceramide. The ω-hydroxyacyl portion of the molecule is thought to span one bilayer, while the linoleate tail inserts into the second bilayer. On either side of the intercellular space is the covalently bound lipid, and between the central pair of bilayers are narrow lamellae that are thought to contain sphingosine chains from the covalently bound hydroxyceramides and linoleate chains from acylceramides in the central pair of bilayers. In accord with this proposed role for acylceramide a 13-nm lamellar phase has been reconstituted from extracted stratum corneum lipid and appears to require acylceramide [38]. It should be noted that the interactions of the covalently bound lipids and acylceramides link adjacent corneocytes in the vertical direction.

3 STRATUM CORNEUM LIPIDS IN ATOPIC DRY SKIN

Based on similarities between atopic dry skin and experimental essential fatty acid deficiency, Melnik et al. [39] investigated the ceramide content of atopic dry skin compared to age- and gender-matched normal controls. The skin in essential fatty acid–deficient animals, like that in atopic dermatitis patients, is rough and dry and displays increased trans-epidermal water loss [40]. Ceramide proportions and structures are known to be altered as essential fatty acid deficiency develops [41,42]. It was found that the proportion of total ceramides is significantly lower in the stratum corneum of atopic subjects [39]. A subsequent more-detailed study demonstrated reduced total ceramides in both lumbar and plantar stratum corneum in atopic subjects [43]. In addition, the proportion of free fatty acids was reduced in the lumbar stratum corneum and nails of the atopic subjects, but not in the plantar stratum corneum. In the nails there was a lower level of ceramides in atopics compared to controls, but the difference did not achieve statistical significance. No significant differences were seen between the atopic subjects compared to normal controls in the levels of cholesterol sulfate or of several sebaceous lipids. Cholesterol was not analyzed. It was suggested that alteration of the keratinization process leading to impaired ceramide synthesis may underlie atopic dry skin and increased trans-epidermal water loss in atopic dermatitis patients.

A more recent study by Yamamoto et al. [44] examined six chromatographically separable fractions of ceramides collected from the volar forearms of atopic subjects and normal control subjects. This study demonstrated that proportions of acylceramide were significantly reduced in atopic subjects compared to controls. No other differences in ceramide proportions were noted; however, it should be pointed out that although six fractions were reported, several pairs of fractions were incompletely resolved on the chromatograms precluding their accurate quantitation. Acylceramide fractions were isolated from the atopic and control subjects, and the compositions of the ester-linked fatty acids were determined by gas–liquid chromatography and compared. The only significant difference that was found was a higher proportion of C18:1 in the acylceramide from atopic subjects. Interestingly, in essential fatty acid deficiency the proportion of oleic acid in the acylceramide does increase; however, it does so at the expense of linoleic acid. In the case of atopic dermatitis there appears to be nonspecific replacement of ester-linked fatty acids.

The finding that atopic dry skin has a reduced proportion of acylceramide was confirmed by Matsumoto et al. [45], and it was found that "normal" regions of skin on atopic subjects had a ceramide profile that did not significantly differ from that found for control subjects.

In another recent study, it was confirmed that the amount of acylceramide per unit weight of stratum corneum was lower in atopic dermatitis patients with active lesions than in control subjects [4]. In this study the levels of ceramide fractions 2 and 3 as well as cholesterol sulfate were also found to be lower. In addition the total ceramide-to-cholesterol ratio was lower in atopic skin compared to normal controls. This suggests that the stratum corneum lipid anomalies may correlate with the severity of disease.

The total ceramide content of atopic stratum corneum from several studies is summarized in Figure 4. The reduced ceramide content of atopic stratum corneum may, at least in part, reflect increased activity of sphingomyelin deacylase in the viable portion of the epidermis [46].

4 MANAGEMENT OF DRY SKIN IN ATOPIC DERMATITIS

Dry skin reflects lower water content at the skin surface which is assessed either by measurement of conductance or capacitance of the skin surface [1]. Studies

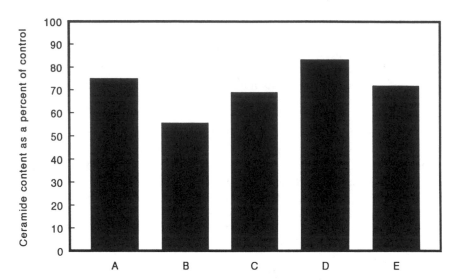

Figure 4 Ceramide content of stratum corneum from atopic subjects. (A) Sole [43]; (B) lumbar skin [43]; (C) volar forearm [45]; (D) volar forearm of atopic subjects without active lesions [4]; (E) volar forearm of subjects with active lesions [4].

have implicated both stratum corneum lipids [6–8] and amino acids [47–49] in the water-holding capacity of the skin. The free amino acids in the stratum corneum are produced primarily from degradation of filaggrin [49], and the concentration of free amino acids within corneocytes is approximately 2M, which produces a high osmotic strength and thereby provides a strong humectant effect. Sebaceous lipid is not a factor in holding water within the stratum corneum in young children since sebum production is very low prior to the onset of puberty [50]. The possibility that sebum may help to trap moisture at the skin surface in postpubertal individuals cannot be ruled out, although one study found no link between sebum secretion rate and xerosis in an elderly population [51].

There is no cure for atopic dermatitis, and therapy consists of addressing the symptoms on an empirical basis. A traditional standard treatment for the dry skin is frequent bathing without soap followed by application of a water-trapping agent. Two of the most commonly used trapping agents are petrolatum and mineral oil. A variety of emollients, or moisturizing creams and lotions, have been developed for the management of atopic dry skin [52], but no one topical formulation emerges as superior to others.

More recently a moisturizer cream containing canola oil and a canola fraction enriched in sterols and 5% urea has been tested on the dry skin of atopic subjects [53]. Overall, after twice daily treatment for 20 days subjects showed increased water content as judged by skin capacitance and improved barrier function as indicated by decreased trans-epidermal water loss. The subjects also became less susceptible to irritation by sodium dodecyl sulfate. In another recent study, it was found that after a mineral oil–based moisturizer containing glycerol and several humectants had been applied twice daily to atopic dry skin for 5 consecutive days there was substantially increased high-frequency conductance, indicating increased water content, that persisted for several days after the cessation of moisturizer application [54]. Interestingly, the treatment had no effect on transepidermal water loss.

A second approach to treatment of atopic dermatitis is the use of topical steroids [55]. During times of flaring a mid-strength anti-inflammatory steroid ointment should be applied within 3 min after bathing for best results. This should be done twice daily. Corticosteroids represent the only medication proven to be effective for management of atopic dermatitis.

A reasonable therapeutic strategy would be to attempt to normalize the defective lipid and humectant components of the xerotic stratum corneum; however, most approaches to date have mainly relied upon providing a variety of topical humectants in a water-trapping vehicle. The more detailed knowledge of the nature of the lipid defects associated with atopic dry skin should make it possible to arrive at formulations that would normalize this aspect of the stratum corneum. The increased commercial availability of different types of ceramides [56] should also facilitate this approach. In fact, it has been shown that topically applied lipid mixtures can accelerate barrier recovery after barrier disruption by different means, and this effect depends upon the proportions of the lipids in the formulation [57]. More research is necessary on the free amino acids in stratum corneum of atopic subjects before it could become possible to exploit this area therapeutically.

REFERENCES

1. Loden M. Biophysical properties of dry atopic and normal skin with special reference to effects of skin care products. Acta Derm Venereol 1995; 192(Suppl):1–48.
2. Leung DYM, Rhodes AR, Geha RS, Schneider L, Ring J. Atopic dermatitis (atopic eczema). In: Fitzpatrick TB, Eisen AZ, Wolf K, Freedberg IM, Austen KF, eds. Dermatology in General Medicine. 4th ed. New York: McGraw-Hill, 1993:1543–1564.
3. Werner Y, Lindberg M. Transepidermal water loss in dry and clinically normal skin in patients with atopic dermatitis. Acta Derm Venereol 1985; 65:102–105.
4. Di Nardo A, Wertz P, Giannetti A, Seidenari S. Ceramide and cholesterol composition of the skin of patients with atopic dermatitis. Acta Derm Venereol 1998; 78:27–30.
5. Thune P. Evaluation of the hydration and water-holding capacity in atopic skin and so-called dry skin. Acta Derm Venereol 1989; 144(Suppl):133–135.

6. Akimoto K, Yoshikawa N, Higaki Y, Kawashima M, Imokawa G. Quantitative analysis of stratum corneum lipids in xerosis and asteatotic eczema. J Invest Dermatol 1993; 20:1–6.

7. Imokawa G, Kuno H, Kawai M. Stratum corneum lipids serve as a bound-water modulator. J Invest Dermatol 1991; 96:845–851.

8. Imokawa G, Akasaki S, Minematsu Y, Kawai M. Importance of intercellular lipids in water-retention properties of the stratum corneum: induction and recovery study of surfactant dry skin. Arch Dermatol Res 1989; 281:45–51.

9. Gray GM, Yardley HJ. Different populations of pig epidermal cells: isolation and lipid composition. J Lipid Res 1975; 16:441–447.

10. Schurer NY, Elias PM. The biochemistry and function of stratum corneum lipids. Adv Lipid Res 1991; 24:27–56.

11. Wertz PW. Lipids and barrier function of the skin. Acta Derm Venereol 2000; 208(Suppl):1–5.

12. Wertz PW, Downing DT. Ceramides of pig epidermis: structure determination. J Lipid Res 1983; 24:759–765.

13. Long SA, Wertz PW, Strauss JS, Downing DT. Human stratum corneum polar lipids and desquamation. Arch Dermatol Res 1985; 277:284–287.

14. Robson KJ, Stewart ME, Michelsen S, Lazo ND, Downing DT. 6-Hydroxy-4-sphingenine in human epidermal ceramides. J Lipid Res 1994; 35:2060–2068.

15. Stewart ME, Downing DT. A new 6-hydroxy-4-sphingenine–containing ceramide in human skin. J Lipid Res 1999; 40:1434–1439.

16. Motta SM, Monti M, Sesana S, Caputo R, Carelli S, Ghidoni R. Ceramide composition of the psoriatic scale. Biochim Biophys Acta 1993; 1182:147–151.

17. Wertz PW, Downing DT. Epidermal lipids. In: Goldsmith L, ed. Physiology, Biochemistry and Molecular Biology of the Skin. New York: Oxford University Press, 1991:205–238.

18. Attenborough D. Life on Earth. Boston: Little, Brown & Company, 1980.

19. Nicolaides N. Skin lipids. II. Lipid class composition of samples from various species and anatomical sites. J Am Oil Chem Soc 1965; 42:691–702.

20. Gray GM, White RJ. Glycosphingolipids and ceramides in human and pig epidermis. J Invest Dermatol 1978; 70:336–341.

21. Wertz PW, Downing DT. Covalently bound ω-hydroxyacylsphingosine in the stratum corneum. Biochim Biophys Acta 1987; 917:108–111.

22. Wertz PW, Madison KC, Downing DT. Covalently bound lipids of human stratum corneum. J Invest Dermatol 1989; 91:109–111.

23. Wertz PW, Downing DT. Composition and morphology of epidermal cyst lipids. J Invest Dermatol 1987; 89:419–425.

24. Wertz PW, van den Bergh BAI. The physical, chemical and functional properties of lipids in the skin and other biological barriers. Chem Phys Lipids 1998; 91:85–96.

25. Nicolaides N, Fu HC, Ansari MNA, Rice GR. The fatty acids of wax esters and sterol esters from vernix caseosa and from human skin surface lipid. Lipids 1972; 7:506–517.

26. Ranasinghe AW, Wertz PW, Downing DT, Mackenzie IC. Lipid composition of cohesive and desquamated corneocytes from mouse ear skin. J Invest Dermatol 1986; 86:187–190.

27. Shapiro LJ, Weiss R, Buxman MM, Vidgoff J, Dimond RL. Enzymatic basis of typical X-linked ichthyosis. Lancet 1978; ii:756–757.
28. Williams ML. The ichthyoses—pathogenesis and prenatal diagnosis: a review of recent advances. Pediatr Sermatol 1983; 1:1–24.
29. Wertz PW, Squier CA. Cellular and molecular basis of barrier function in oral epithelium. Crit Rev Therap Drug Carrier Syst 1991; 8:237–269.
30. Iwamori M, Iwamori Y, Ito N. Regulation of the activities of thrombin and plasmin by cholesterol sulfate as a physiological inhibitor in human plasma. J Biochem 1999; 125:594–601.
31. Ito N, Iwamori Y, Hanaoka K, Iwamori M. Inhibition of pancreatic elastase by sulfated lipids in intestinal mucosa. J Biochem 1998; 123:107–114.
32. Iwamori M, Iwamori Y, Ito N. Sulfated lipids as inhibitors of pancreatic trypsin and chymotrypsin in epithelium of the mammalian digestive tract. Biochem Biophys Res Comm 1997; 237:262–265.
33. Yardley HJ, Summerly R. Lipid composition and metabolism in normal and diseased epidermis. Pharmacol Ther 1981; 13:357–383.
34. Mak VHW, Potts RO, Guy RH. Oleic acid concentration and effect in human stratum corneum: non-invasive determination by attenuated total reflectance infrared spectroscopy in vivo. J Control Rel 1990; 12:67–75.
35. Forslind B. A domain mosaic model of the skin barrier. Acta Derm Venereol 1994; 74:1–6.
36. Madison KC, Swartzendruber DC, Wertz PW, Downing DT. Presence of intact intercellular lamellae in the upper layers of the stratum corneum. J Invest Dermatol 1987; 88:714–718.
37. Swartzendruber DC, Manganaro A, Madison KC, Kremer M, Wertz PW, Squier CA. Organization of the intercellular spaces of porcine epidermal and palatal stratum corneum: a quantitative study employing ruthenium tetroxide. Cell Tissue Res 1995; 279:271–276.
38. Bouwstra JA, Gooris GS, Dubbelaar FE, Weerheim AM, Ijzerman AP, Ponec M. Role of ceramide 1 in the molecular organization of the stratum corneum lipids. J Lipid Res 1998; 39:186–196.
39. Melnik B, Hollmann J, Plewig G. Decreased stratum corneum ceramides in atopic individuals—a pathobiochemical factor in xerosis? Br J Dermatol 1988; 119:547–549.
40. Holman RT. Essential fatty acid deficiency. Prog Chem Fats Other Lipids 1968; 9:275–248.
41. Wertz PW, Cho ES, Downing DT. Effects of essential fatty acid deficiency on the epidermal sphingolipids of the rat. Biochim Biophys Acta 1983; 753:350–355.
42. Melton JL, Wertz PW, Swartzendruber DC, Downing DT. Effects of essential fatty acid deficiency on epidermal ω-acylsphingolipids and transepidermal water loss in young pigs. Biochim Biophys Acta 1987; 921:191–197.
43. Melnik B, Hollmann J, Hofmann U, Yuh M-S, Plewig G. Lipid composition of outer stratum corneum and nails in atopic and control subjects. Arch Dermatol Res 1990; 282:549–551.
44. Yamamoto A, Serizawa S, Ito M, Sato Y. Stratum corneum lipid abnormalities in atopic dermatitis. Arch Dermatol Res 1991; 283:219–223.

45. Matsumoto M, Umemoto N, Sugiura H, Uehara M. Difference in ceramide composition between "dry" and "normal" skin in patients with atopic dermatitis. Acta Derm Venereol 1999; 79:246–247.

46. Hara J, Higuchi K, Okamoto R, Kawashima M, Imokawa G. High-expression of sphingomyelin deacylase is an important determinant of ceramide deficiency leading to barrier disruption in atopic dermatitis. J Invest Dermatol 2000; 115:406–413.

47. Tanaka M, Okada M, Zhen YX, Inamura N, Kitano T, Shirai S, Sakamoto K, Inamura T, Tagami H. Decreased hydration state of the stratum corneum and reduced amino acid content of the skin surface in patients with seasonal allergic rhinitis. Br J Dermatol 1998; 139:618–621.

48. Yamamura T, Tezuka T. The water-holding capacity of the stratum corneum measured by ^{1}H-NMR. J Invest Dermatol 1989; 93:160–164.

49. Scott IR, Harding CR. Filaggrin breakdown to water binding compounds during development of the rat stratum corneum is controlled by the water activity of the environment. Dev Biol 1986; 115:84–92.

50. Strauss JS, Pochi PE. The hormonal control of the pilosebaceous unit. In: Toda K, ed. Biology and Disease of the Hair. Baltimore: University Park Press, 1975:231–245.

51. Frantz RA, Kinney CK, Downing DT. Variables associated with skin dryness in the elderly. Nursing Res 1986; 35:98–100.

52. Burr S. Emollients for managing dry skin conditions. Prof Nurse 1999; 15:43–48.

53. Loden M, Anderson AC, Lindberg M. Improvement in skin barrier function in patients with atopic dermatitis after treatment with a moisturizing cream (Canoderm). Br J Dermatol 1999; 140:264–267.

54. Tabata N, O'Goshi K, Zhen YX, Kligman AM, Tagami H. Biophysical assessment of persistent effects of moisturizers after their daily applications: evaluation of corneotherapy. Dermatology 2000; 200:308–313.

55. Sidbury R, Hanifin JM. Old, new, and emerging therapies for atopic dermatitis. Dermatol Clin 2000; 18:1–9.

56. Michniak BB, Wertz PW. Ceramides and lipids. In: Barel A, Maibach HI, Paye M, eds. Handbook of Cosmetic Science and Technology. New York: Marcel Dekker 2000:45–56.

57. Zettersten EM, Ghadially R, Feingold KR, Crumrine D, Elias PM. Optimal ratios of topical stratum corneum lipids improve barrier recovery in chronologically aged skin. J Am Acad Dermatol 1997; 37:403–408.

10

Psoriasis and Ichthyoses

Ruby Ghadially
Veterans Administration Medical Center and University of
California School of Medicine, San Francisco, California

1 INTRODUCTION

Dramatic changes in epidermal differentiation and stratum corneum structure and
function occur in psoriasis and in the ichthyoses. In this chapter the differences in
epidermal structure, composition, and function will be discussed, together with a
summary of relevant topical technologies to improve the skin conditions discussed.

Mammalian stratum corneum comprises a two-compartment system of
lipid-depleted corneocytes embedded in a lipid-enriched intercellular matrix (reviewed in Ref. 1). These intercellular lipids are organized into a series of broad
lamellar bilayers that regulate permeability barrier function and participate in the
cohesion and desquamation of the stratum corneum (reviewed in Ref. 2). The diseases discussed in this chapter are all characterized by a mild to severe compromise in epidermal permeability barrier function, basally or in response to stresses
to the barrier.

In normal stratum corneum, poorly understood changes occur in the stratum corneum interstices that lead to the orderly detachment of individual corneocytes at the skin surface. Alterations in lipid composition [3], the physical-chem-
ical state of the lamellar bilayers [4], and degradation of nonlipid constituents
such as desmosomes [5] have all been implicated as mediators of normal desqua-

179

mation. The extent to which one or more of these processes is responsible for the abnormal desquamation of the disorders of cornification is still not known [2,6].

Epidermal permeability barrier integrity requires the organization of stratum corneum lipids into extracellular lamellar bilayers, following the secretion of epidermal lamellar body contents at the stratum granulosum–stratum corneum interface [6]. With the advent of ruthenium tetroxide postfixation it is possible to obtain ultrastructural images of the stratum corneum interstices on a routine basis [7–10], and a detailed tableau is emerging of the intercellular bilayer system in normal and diseased stratum corneum.

Ultrastructural examination of normal stratum corneum reveals that the lamellae within the intercellular domains of normal human stratum corneum exhibit a similar organization and substructure to previous descriptions of porcine [7] and murine [8] stratum corneum. In optimal cross-sections, these membranes can be seen to comprise three types of electron-lucent lamellae that alternate with a single type of electron-dense lamella (Fig. 1). From the corneocyte envelope outward, the electron-lucent lamellae comprise, first, a continuous sheet immediately exterior to the cornified envelope [7,8,11]. The succeeding lamellae are organized external to adjacent lamellae with the center of the interrupted, lucent lamellae serving as the plane of symmetry. Each series of four electron-lucent lamellae alternating with five electron-dense lamellae, comprises the basic unit (Fig. 1 inset). At many points in the interstices this basic unit expands incrementally and suddenly by the addition of arrays of continuous electron-dense and -lucent lamellae. A "doublet" comprises two basic units minus one interrupted, electron-lucent lamella and two electron-dense lamellae, which result from sharing of these structures by two adjacent basic units. "Triplets" are the largest units observed in normal human stratum corneum.

Staining of lamellar bodies in the stratum granulosum with standard osmium tetroxide fixation provides excellent preservation of lamellar body structure. Briefly, cross-sectional images of lamellar bodies in normal epidermis demonstrated a trilaminar limiting membrane, and internal lamellar disklike structures, consisting of prominent dense lamellae separated by an electron-lucent band and divided centrally by a minor, striated electron-dense band (Fig. 2 inset).

Acute perturbations of the permeability barrier; e.g., solvent applications or tape-stripping, stimulate a sequence of homeostatic mechanisms, including (1) rapid secretion of pre-formed lamellar body contents; (2) generation of nascent lamellar bodies; (3) accelerated intercellular deposition of newly formed lamellar body contents; and (4) extracellular processing of lamellar body contents by co-localized hydrolytic enzymes into lamellar basic unit structures [12]. The lamellar body secretory response to barrier disruption is both fueled by and requires a burst in lipid synthesis [13–15]. Likewise, in the essential fatty acid–deficient mouse (a chronic barrier perturbation model often used as an analog for psoriasis), increased numbers of defective lamellar bodies, decreased extracellular

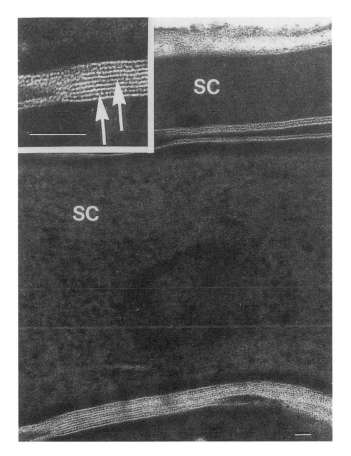

Figure 1 Normal human stratum corneum ruthenium tetroxide postfixation shows intercellular domains featuring intercellular bilayer structures with repeat pattern of lucent and dense bands. Inset: high power of same. Note single basic unit pattern (arrows). Scale bars = 0.06 μm. (From Ref. 31.)

lamellar bilayers [16], and increased lipid synthesis [17] occur. Many of the diseases discussed here (e.g., psoriasis, congenital ichthyosiform erythroderma, and epidermolytic hyperkeratosis) represent conditions of chronic barrier impairment such as essential fatty acid deficiency (EFAD).

2 PSORIASIS

Clinically, psoriasis is characterized by sharply demarcated erythematous plaques with a positive Auspitz sign (fine bleeding points when superficial scale is re-

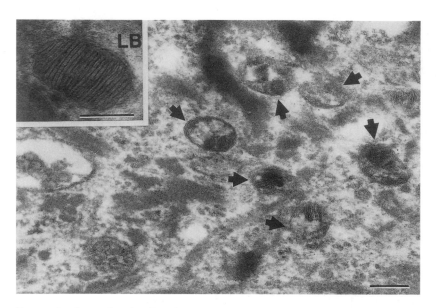

Figure 2 Lamellar bodies in the epidermis of normal skin and congenital ichthyosiform erythroderma. Vesicular lamellar bodies (arrows) are seen in the cytosol of all patients with congenital ichthyosiform erythroderma. Inset: lamellar body from normal epidermis shows disklike internal structures. Scale bars = 0.1 μm. (From Ref. 31.)

moved). Clinical types vary with activity of the disease which range from a chronic stationary phase to a resolving process, or to flares of disease that may be associated with sudden onset of a generalized exfoliative erythema, occasionally associated with sterile pustules [18].

The histology of psoriasis varies greatly depending on the clinical type of lesion. In a fully developed lesion at the margin of the plaque there is parakeratosis, Munro microabscesses (collections of neutrophils in the stratum corneum), absence of the granular layer, elongation of rete ridges, thinning of the suprapapillary epidermis acanthoses, and dilated and tortuous capillaries [19].

Although previous morphological studies reported either normal [20] or increased numbers [21,22] of lamellar bodies and lamellar body–like remnants within corneocytes in psoriasis, morphological abnormalities were not correlated with disease phenotype. More recent findings demonstrate that the extent of lamellar body formation correlates with the degree of defective barrier function [23,24]. Thus, the apparently conflicting prior reports of either normal or increased numbers of lamellar bodies could be attributable to phenotypic differences. Although the epidermis of both erythrodermic and active plaque psoriasis generates large numbers of lamellar bodies, in these phenotypes many lamellar bodies remain entombed in the corneocyte cytosol (Fig. 3) [23]. Thus, while normal homeostatic mechanisms appear to be operative in the acute psoriatic phenotypes (i.e., enhanced lamellar body formation), delivery of lamellar body–derived lipids to the intercellular spaces is defective, impeding the ability to form functional intercellular bilayer structures (Fig. 3). Thus, in the erythrodermic stratum corneum there are retained lamellar structures visible within the corneocytes (Fig. 3), and even with ruthenium postfixation the intercellular spaces appear strikingly devoid of lamellar bilayers. In contrast, in less acute psoriatic phenotypes; i.e., chronic plaque and sebopsoriasis, lamellar body contents are both formed and secreted almost normally, and as a result, barrier repair is relatively complete (Fig. 4). Fewer retained lamellar bodies are visible within corneocytes, and the numbers of extracellular lamellar bilayers are correspondingly greater than in erythrodermic lesions. Normal bilayers with normal dimensions are seen, although many lamellae maintain the unfurled elongated pattern characteristic of secreted lamellar body contents in the lower stratum corneum (Fig. 4). Thus, it is possible that improvement in barrier function is not only a consequence of this change in phenotype, but that it may actually drive this phenotypic shift, a conclusion supported by occlusion studies; i.e., artificial restoration of the barrier by occlusion results in lesion regression [25–27].

Failure of lamellar body secretion, with the persistence of lamellar body remnants in the corneocyte cytosol also occurs in lovastatin-treated epidermis [28], as well as in other hyperproliferative human dermatoses, including harlequin ichthyosis [29]. Although the decreased lamellar body secretion in acute forms of psoriasis could be a consequence of hyperproliferation alone, in another hyperproliferative dermatosis (essential fatty acid deficiency), which displays comparable abnormalities in barrier function and lamellar body formation to psoriasis [16], lamellar bodies are secreted normally rather than being retained within corneocytes [30]. However, the lamellar bodies in EFAD display abnormal lamellar contents, and a defective barrier results from incomplete formation of extracellular lamellar bilayers [8,16]. Thus, despite the hyperproliferative component of EFAD, retention of lamellar bodies does not occur. Likewise, in congenital ichthyosiform erythroderma, another hyperproliferative disorder, lamellar bodies are secreted normally and not retained within corneocytes [31], and despite the hyperproliferation, increased rather than decreased numbers of intercellular lamellae are found [31]. Thus, hyperproliferation alone may not be the cause of lamellar body retention in the acute psoriatic phenotypes.

The increase in proliferation is a key component of psoriasis and is accompanied by an increase in the epidermal growth factor receptor [32] and an increase in transforming growth factor alpha [33], one of the ligands for the epidermal growth factor receptor. Also there is an increase in ornithine decarboxylase [34] and in the transcription factor AP-1 [35]

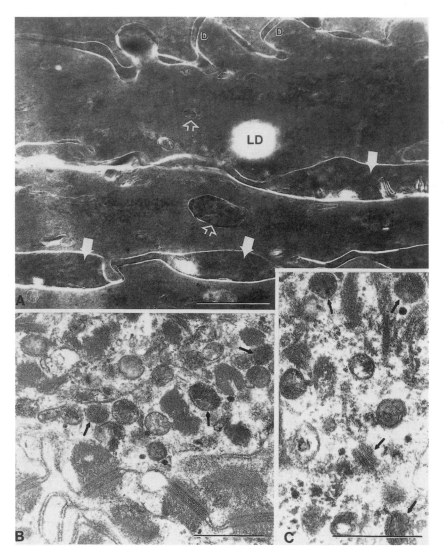

FIGURE 3 Erythrodermic psoriasis displays extensive abnormalities in the lamellar body secretory system. (A) Stratum corneum in erythrodermic psoriasis. Note the virtual absence of intercellular lamellae (white arrowheads). In addition, retained lamellar body structures (open arrowheads) are present. (B and C) Stratum granulosum in erythrodermic psoriasis. The number of lamellar bodies within the cytosol are dramatically increased, resembling the appearance of mice 3–6 hr after acetone wiping to remove the epidermal permeability barrier. Lamellar bodies are of normal size and internal structure. Scale bars = (A) 20 μm; (B) 17.5 μm; (C) 22.5 μm. (From Ref. 23.)

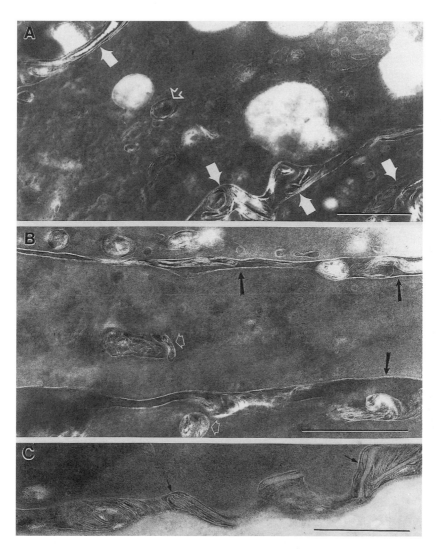

Figure 4 Chronic plaque psoriasis displays less extensive abnormalities in the lamellar body secretory system. (A and B) Stratum corneum in chronic plaque psoriasis. A paucity of intercellular lamellae are observed throughout the stratum corneum interstices (arrows). The membrane structures present retain the unfurled pattern of the lower stratum corneum and the mature pattern of bilayers usually observed in the upper stratum corneum is not evident (c.f. Fig. 1). (C) The stratum corneum in sebopsoriasis. The intercellular spaces contain more bilayers than in the other forms of psoriasis, but even in the upper stratum corneum, the membranes do not reveal a basic lamellar unit pattern. Scale bars = (A) 20 μm; (B,C) 25 μm. (From Ref. 23.)

The expression of the markers of epidermal differentiation are also altered. There is an increase in keratinocyte transglutaminase type 1, which catalyzes a critical step in formation of the cornified envelope [36]. In association with loss of the granular layer, filaggrin is underexpressed in psoriasis [37]. Involucrin, which is crosslinked to form the cornified envelope, is increased. Finally, keratins K6 and K16 (hyperproliferative keratins) are increased in the suprabasal layers of psoriatic lesions, while K1 and K10 (used as markers of terminal differentiation) are decreased [38].

In psoriatic skin trans-epidermal water loss levels are increased 1- to 20-fold [24,39–43]. Few prior studies have correlated trans-epidermal water loss with lesion phenotype. Whereas Grice et al. [41] found no significant functional differences between erythrodermic and plaque psoriasis, trans-epidermal water loss levels decreased as the disease became less active, consistent with data showing that barrier function correlates better with disease activity than with lesion phenotype; i.e., the highest trans-epidermal water loss levels occurred in erythroderma and active plaque psoriasis, while chronic plaque and sebopsoriasis displayed trans-epidermal water loss levels between these and uninvolved skin (Table 1) [23]. Moreover, epidermal morphology was comparable in worsening active plaque psoriasis to acute erythroderma. In contrast, epidermal structure in stable erythroderma patients closely resembled active plaque psoriasis [23].

TABLE 1 Abnormality in Barrier Function in Psoriasis Correlates with the Severity of Psoriatic Phenotype

	Trans-epidermal water loss (g/m²/hr)	p value
Erythroderma (n = 3)	36.4 ± 2.26	p = 0.001[a]
Uninvolved skin	3.5 ± 0.99	p < 0.001[b]
Active plaque (n = 8)	16.1 ± 0.97	p < 0.001[a]
Uninvolved skin	3.9 ± 0.41	p = 0.005[c]
Chronic plaque (n = 12)	9.0 ± 1.93	p = 0.019[a]
Uninvolved skin	4.1 ± 0.51	

Notes: Trans-epidermal water loss was measured in patients with different psoriatic phenotypes. Measurements were taken from the affected area and an adjacent area of uninvolved skin. The most severe phenotype (erythroderma) displays the highest trans-epidermal water loss, approximately 10 times the uninvolved skin. Results are mean ± SEM.
[a]Affected versus nearby uninvolved skin.
[b]Erythroderma versus active plaque.
[c]Active plaque versus chronic plaque psoriasis.
Source: Ref. 23.

These results suggest that barrier repair mechanisms are operative in psoriasis; and they appear to be, in part, successful at normalizing barrier function, perhaps leading to more chronic psoriatic phenotypes. Likewise, with artificial barrier restoration by occlusion alone, psoriatic lesions usually regress [25–27].

Much indirect evidence, including the data summarized here, supports the hypothesis that the primary trigger for psoriasis may arise in the epidermis, and that the disease-specific inflammatory infiltrate may be recruited secondarily [44,45]. Psoriatic epidermis transplanted onto nude mice retains its psoriatic morphology, as well as its increased labeling index [46]. A similar persistence of phenotype occurs in transplants of the flaky skin mouse model of psoriasis [47]. Moreover, although some studies suggest that psoriatic fibroblasts drive the disease [48], others have found that psoriatic fibroblasts do not direct hyperproliferation, nor do normal fibroblasts inhibit psoriatic hyperproliferation [49]. Furthermore, barrier abrogation stimulates DNA synthesis [50], as well as provoking a rapid increase of both epidermal cytokine mRNA and protein generation [44,51]. Finally, Nickoloff et al. [45] showed that epidermal production of cytokines following barrier abrogation precedes movement of inflammatory cells from the circulation into the dermis or epidermis. Together, these findings suggest that the dermal inflammatory components of psoriasis may be recruited subsequent to primary events arising in the epidermis. These findings also are consistent with the occurrence of the Koebner phenomenon [52] and the observation that occlusion alone clears many psoriatic lesions [25–27].

3 ICHTHYOSIS VULGARIS

Ichthyosis vulgaris, the most common of the ichthyotic conditions discussed here, is an autosomal dominant condition that usually starts in childhood and presents as fine white scales on the extensor surfaces of the extremities and the trunk.

Ichthyosis vulgaris is characterized histologically by mild hyperkeratosis and reduced or absent keratohyalin granules. Ultrastructural evaluation has shown that although the stratum corneum is thicker than normal, and keratohyalin granules are absent, the typical keratin pattern of normal skin is seen suggesting that filaggrin is not essential for keratin filament aggregation [53]. There is abnormal persistence of desmosomes in the stratum corneum [54].

Biochemically, profilaggrin (a major component of keratohyaline granules) and filaggrin are reduced or absent. Little profilaggrin mRNA was detected by in situ hybridization in vivo, and in keratinocytes profilaggrin was less than 10% of normal, while the mRNA was 30–60% of controls. Furthermore, expression of keratin K1 and loricrin (other markers of epidermal differentiation) were not affected [55]. The degree of biochemical abnormality correlated with the ultrastructural quantitation and with the severity of the clinical disorder [53]. Trypsin-like and chymotrypsin-like serine proteases are involved in the degradation of desmoglein [56], a transmembrane protein within desmosomes. The enzymatic activities of trypsin-like and chymotrypsin-like serine proteases were significantly decreased in ichthyosis vulgaris [56].

Basal trans-epidermal water loss shows a small but significant increase in ichthyosis vulgaris [40,57]. Furthermore, a loss of pH gradient occurs, reflected by a higher skin surface pH, and a neutral pH of 7 obtained with removal of only half of the stratum corneum, as compared to normal skin where the "acid mantle" penetrates deep into the skin [58]. This could be explained by the depletion of acidic proteins urocanic acid and pyrrolidone carboxylic acid due to filaggrin deficiency, which results in a delay in the accumulation of protons and moves the pH gradient outward in ichthyosis vulgaris [58].

4 RECESSIVE X-LINKED ICHTHYOSIS

Recessive X-linked ichthyosis is characterized by a generalized desquamation of large, adherent, dark brown scales, more extensive on the extensor aspects of the limbs. Extracutaneous manifestations include corneal opacities and cryptorchidism [59]. This condition is caused by a deficit in steroid sulfatase [60,61]. The deletion or mutation of the gene encoding for the enzyme steroid sulfatase has been localized to the distal short arm of the X chromosome (Xp22.3) [62].

Histology shows compact hyperkeratosis, with a normal or slightly thickened stratum granulosum [59]. This is a retention hyperkeratosis with a normal rate of cell turnover [59]. Ultrastructural studies reveal an increase in the number and volume of keratohyalin granules. Desmosomal disks are visible even in the most superficial layers of the epidermis, suggesting increased intercellular cohesiveness. Cells of the stratum corneum contain large numbers of melonosomes, probably due to decreased degradation, and resulting in the dark scale seen clinically [63,64]. Examination of the intercellular lamellar domains of the stratum corneum [65] reveals lamellae that are fragmented and disrupted, with extensive nonlamellar domains within the extracellular space (Fig. 5). In a study of lipid mixtures using small angle x-ray diffraction, it was found that both an increase in pH (7.4 at the stratum granulosum–stratum corneum interface versus 5 at the skin surface) and an increase in cholesterol sulfate promote the formation of a normal lamellar phase as seen in vivo, suggesting that cholesterol sulfate may be required to dissolve cholesterol in the lamellar phases and to stabilize stratum corneum lipid organization. Therefore, a drop in cholesterol sulfate content in the superficial layers of the stratum corneum is expected to destabilize the lipid lamellar phases and facilitate the desquamation process [66].

The epidermal permeability barrier is slightly impaired in recessive X-linked ichthyosis despite the great hyperkeratosis. Whereas a single study of 13 patients with recessive X-linked ichthyosis found no statistical change in basal trans-epidermal water loss [67], basal trans-epidermal water loss was slightly but significantly increased in other studies [40,57,65]. This increase in trans-epider-

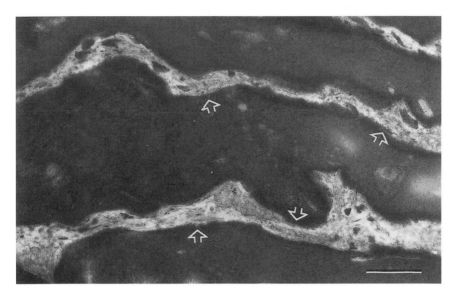

Figure 5 Stratum corneum from a patient with recessive X-linked ichthyosis. Lamellae are fragmented and disrupted (arrows) with extensive nonlamellar domains present within the extracellular spaces. Scale bar = 0.5 μm. (From Ref. 65.)

mal water loss can be reproduced in murine epidermis by the application of topical cholesterol sulfate [65]. The hyperkeratosis may be compensatory to the barrier defect or reflect decreased desquamation. There was a decreased response to sodium lauryl sulfate in terms of increased trans-epidermal water loss and erythema [67] and a delay in barrier recovery after tape-stripping (n = 15).

Many recent findings regarding the effects of cholesterol sulfate on epidermis make it possible to speculate about why the normal shedding of corneocytes is delayed in recessive X-linked ichthyosis [68]. Although cholesterol sulfate is normally present in epidermis, it accumulates in recessive X-linked ichthyosis, is growth inhibitory to human keratinocytes, activates protein kinase C (which phosphorylates transglutaminase 1), induces transcription of the transglutaminase gene, inhibits certain proteases in stratum corneum, and is reduced in the epidermis following retinoid therapy [68]. Furthermore, treatment with steroid sulfatase under occlusion [69], 19% cholesterol [70] or 2% cholesterol [65], improves scaling.

5 LAMELLAR ICHTHYOSIS

Lamellar ichthyosis is a term that applies to a heterogeneous group of autosomal recessive disorders [71–73] that are often divided into two disorders, lamellar ichthyosis and congenital ichthyosiform erythroderma. Lamellar ichthyosis is known by multiple terms including DOC 4 (lamellar-recessive type), nonbullous congenital ichthyosiform erythroderma, nonertyhrodermic autosomal recessive lamellar ichthyosis, ichthyosis congenita, and classic lamellar ichthyosis. Congenital ichthyosiform erythroderma is sometimes referred to as nonbullous congenital ichthyosiform erythroderma, DOC 5 (congenital erythrodermic type), ichthyosis congenita, and erythrodermic autosomal recessive lamellar ichthyosis [74]. Here, lamellar ichthyosis will be divided into classic lamellar ichthyosis, to differentiate the term from the all-inclusive term of lamellar ichthyosis, and congenital ichthyosiform erythroderma.

5.1 Classic Lamellar Ichthyosis

These patients are often preterm, collodion babies that shed their membranes to reveal their underlying phenotype in the first few weeks of life. Clinically there are dark platelike scales involving the entire body including flexor surfaces. Ectropion is common.

Classic lamellar ichthyosis is a retention hyperkeratosis. Histopathology reveals compact orthokeratosis and slight acanthosis. Lamellar ichthyosis was previously thought to be a hyperproliferative condition. However, on division of patients into classic lamellar ichthyosis versus congenital ichthyosiform erythroderma it is seen that the mitotic rate of classic lamellar ichthyosis is only slightly increased, while that of congenital ichthyosiform erythroderma is markedly increased [75].

Ultrastructural studies have shown that the intercellular domains in classic lamellar ichthyosis often appear to be decreased in quantity due to their separation by extensive, largely empty lacunae or clefts within the electron-dense lamellae of membrane stacks (Fig. 6). Furthermore, the intercellular lamellae in classic lamellar ichthyosis also showed an abnormal banding pattern, with an absence of the interrupted lamella that is invariably present in normal human stratum corneum (cf. Fig. 1) and usually present in congenital ichthyosiform erythroderma samples (cf. Fig. 6). This results in alternating lucent and dense bands that are evenly spaced (Fig. 5 inset), an observation confirmed by computer transforms of optical diffraction. Large numbers of desmosomes persist within the intercellular spaces, even within the outermost layers of the hyperkeratotic stratum corneum [31]. The numbers, size, and internal contents of lamellar bodies in classic lamellar ichthyosis are normal. Small angle x-ray diffraction peak showed smaller repeated distances of lipid bilayers in stratum corneum samples of the patients compared with healthy volunteers [31,72].

Transglutaminase and the marginal band may be present or absent [71–73]. Transglutaminase-deficient mice exhibit a phenotype similar to lamellar ichthyosis with a collodion membrane–like taut and wrinkled skin [76]. Absence of the

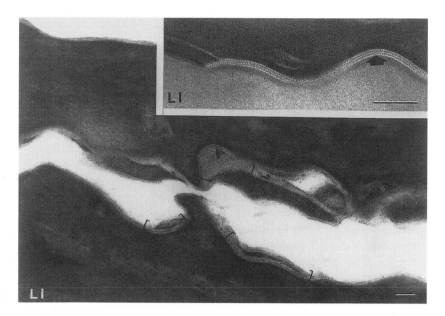

FIGURE 6 Stratum corneum from patients with classic lamellar ichthyosis (LI). The numbers of intercellular lamellae appear decreased in number (brackets) due to separation artifacts and/or clefts within electron-dense lamellae. Inset: absence of an interrupted band, with even spacing of lucent and dense bands. Ruthenium tetroxide. Scale bars = 0.1 μm. (From Ref. 31.)

marginal band and deposition of electron-dense aggregates along the cell membrane were demonstrated in such knockout mice, as well as intracellular aggregation of loricrin [76]. Because of the lack of clear clinical descriptions in some series, a study was done in some patients with congenital ichthyosiform erythroderma clinically versus some with classic lamellar ichthyosis [77]. In this study patients with congenital ichthyosiform erythroderma were shown to have abnormal transglutaminase versus those with classic lamellar ichthyosis who had absent transglutaminase [77].

Frost showed an increase in trans-epidermal water loss in four patients with lamellar ichthyosis [40]. However, no distinction was made between classic lamellar ichthyosis and congenital ichthyosiform erythroderma at the time of this study. In another study lamellar ichthyosis demonstrated increased trans-epidermal water loss rates, significantly elevated in relation to those of ichthyosis vulgaris or of recessive X-linked ichthyosis [57]. This study included 10 patients, eight with the phenotype of classic lamellar ichthyosis and two with a phenotype compatible with congenital ichthyosiform erythroderma. Barrier properties were also studied in two patients with the clinical picture of classic lamellar ichthyosis and one with the picture of congenital ichthyosiform erythroderma (a sibling of one of the classic lamellar ichthyosis type subjects) [72]. Trans-epidermal water loss was significantly increased in all. Stratum corneum lipid profiles showed significant differences in the relative ceramide fractions in these patients [72].

5.2 Congenital Ichthyosiform Erythroderma

Often born as collodion babies, these patients have erthroderma and fine white scales. They may also have ectropion. In contrast to classic lamellar ichthyosis, this is a hyperproliferative state.

Histology shows features of hyperproliferation including some parakeratosis (not seen in classic lamellar ichthyosis) and much greater acanthosis than that seen in classic lamellar ichthyosis [78]. Also in contrast to classic lamellar ichthyosis, the degree of hyperkeratosis is much less severe. Ultrastructurally, using ruthenium tetroxide postfixation, chracteristic findings for congenital ichthyosiform erythroderma (CIE) included (1) foci containing excessive numbers of lamellae in stacks (Fig. 6; cf. Fig. 1); (2) a predominance of incompletely formed and/or disorganized lamellar arrays (Fig. 6C); (3) shortened arrays of lamellar body–derived membranes (Fig. 6C); (4) variations in the substructure of individual lamellae, both within the lucent and dense bands (Fig. 6D,E) and abnormal interlamellar dimensions by x-ray diffraction; (5) electron-lucent domains, presumably representing nonlamellar phases because of the presence of flocculent, amorphous material (Fig. 6B) (such domains occurred interspersed between stacks of lamellar bilayers); and (6) desmosomes, which normally deteriorate above the first six to eight layers of normal stratum corneum, persisting in abundance in all of the 25-plus layers of the stratum corneum [31]. Increased numbers of lamellar bodies of decreased size were observed in the stratum granulosum in all CIE patients. Moreover, the internal contents of lamellar bodies from congenital ichthyosiform erythroderma epidermis were distinctly abnormal, most appearing empty or containing only fragments of lamellar structures (Fig. 2), creating a vacuolated appearance [31].

Studies of barrier function have been in combination with patients with classic lamellar ichthyosis (see preceding).

6 EPIDERMOLYTIC HYPERKERATOSIS

Epidermolytic hyperkeratosis (also known as bullous congenital ichthyosiform erythroderma) is an autosomal dominant condition, although 50% of cases are sporadic and probably new mutations [74]. Patients develop blistering on the extensor surfaces and later localized areas of severe hyperkeratosis. However, epidermolytic hyperkeratosis is clinically heterogeneous [79]. After studying 52 patients with epidermolytic hyperkeratosis DiGiovanna and Bale divided the

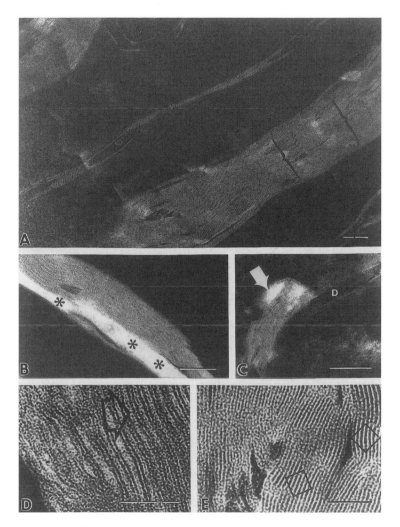

FIGURE 7 Stratum corneum from patients with congenital ichthyosiform erythroderma. (A) Between corneoctes stained densely with ruthenium, note increased numbers of lamellae in stacks (brackets). (B) Apparent phase separation of lipids into lamellar and nonlamellar domains (*). (C) Disorganization and fragmentation of lamellar arrays as well as shortened lamellar arrays (white arrow). (D and E) In some congenital ichthyosiform erythroderma patients an abnormal or diminished interrupted lamella is seen. Also the interrupted bands are dense rather than lucent (D, arrow), a reversal of the normal pattern. Another phenotype shows a complete absence of interrupted lamellae within an expanded stack (E, box). Ruthenium tetroxide. Scale bars = (A,B) 0.1 μm; (C) 0.5 μm; (D,E) 0.04 μm. (From Ref. 31.)

patients into those with palm and sole involvement and those without. Each of these two groups was divided further into three groups. Epidermolytic hyperkeratosis occurs as a result of mutations in conserved regions of keratins K1 and K10. There appears to be some correlation between the type of epidermolytic hyperkeratosis and the mutation; most patients with palm and sole involvement have keratin 1 mutations near the beginning of the 1A rod domain, while most without palm and sole involvement display keratin 10 mutations [79,80].

Histological and ultrastructural examination of the epidermis shows a thickened stratum corneum and marked vacuolation of the suprabasal layer. Electron microscopy shows tonofilament clumping around the nucleus of suprabasal keratinocytes. Thus, it seems that in some patients there is a point mutation in K1 or K10 that appears to weaken the suprabasal keratin network and impair the mechanical stability of the epidermis resulting in the hyperkeratosis, fragility, and blister formation [81].

Frost et al. [40] demonstrated a marked increase in trans-epidermal water loss in seven patients with epidermolytic hyperkeratosis. In a mouse model of epidermolytic hyperkeratosis [82] electron microscopy using ruthenium tetroxide postfixed skin samples demonstrated normal extrusion and morphology of lamellar bodies as well as the formation of normal lamellar layers [83]. However, there were significant changes in ceramide subpopulations of the stratum corneum lipids. The total amount of ceramide 2 was elevated, whereas ceramides 1, 3, 4, and 5 were decreased among total stratum corneum lipids. The amount of the ceramide precursors sphingomyelin and glucosylceramide was reduced in the stratum corneum without accompanying changes in the mRNA for acid sphingomyelinase [83].

7 TREATMENT

Most of these conditions are lifelong disturbances that rely on the use of continuous treatment throughout life. Broad aims are to moisturize, effect keratolysis, prevent evaporation, and humidify the environment. These conditions may be disabling conditions requiring extensive treatment multiple times daily or may be mild, with only occasional emollient use needed. In treating chronic conditions the cosmetic acceptability of the creams prescribed is of utmost importance to ensure compliance with therapy. The selection of the cream base (hydrophilic versus lipophilic, nonocclusive versus semi-occlusive) is key not only for the pharmacological effect, but for compliance. Also, the presence of erosions or fissures may preclude the use of certain more irritating creams.

Little specific treatment is available for ichthyosis vulgaris, although it might seem obvious to replace the lack of natural moisturizing factor (NMF) composed of hygroscopic, amino acid–derived breakdown products from filaggrin and keratohyalin [84].

The milder forms of recessive X-linked ichthyosis improve with emollients and keratolytics. Commonly used agents include urea, 2–10%, lactic acid, 12%, and propylene glycol, 10–25% [68]. Cholesterol-containing creams improved recessive X-linked ichthyosis in a mouse model [65] as well as in human subjects [65,70]. Topical isotretinoin may help in recessive X-linked ichthyosis [85]. Liarazole is a newer agent that may be ueful for recessive X-linked ichthyosis and lamellar ichthyosis and seems to work by increasing the endogenous levels of retinoic acid [86]. Recessive X-linked ichthyosis gets better in the summer months and may be improved by UV or climate therapy. It also improves with age. Treatment focuses on prevention by genetic counselling and prenatal diagnosis. However, single gene recessive genetic skin disorders offer attractive prototypes for the development of therapeutic cutaneous gene delivery. For example, Jensen et al. transfected recessive X-linked ichthyosis keratinocytes with the steroid sulfatase gene and induced the enzyme activity of the cells and a normal phenotype in culture [87]. Furthermore, a new retroviral expression vector was produced and utilized to effect steroid sulfatase gene transfer to primary keratinocytes from recessive X-linked ichthyosis patients. Transduced and uncorrected recessive X-linked ichthyosis keratinocytes, along with normal controls, were then grafted onto immunodeficient mice to regenerate full thickness human epidermis. Unmodified recessive X-linked ichthyosis keratinocytes regenerated a hyperkeratotic epidermis lacking steroid sulfatase expression with defective skin barrier function, effectively recapitulating the human disease in vivo. Transduced recessive X-linked ichthyosis keratinocytes from the same patients, however, regenerated epidermis histologically indistinguishable from that formed by keratinocytes from patients with normal skin. Transduced recessive X-linked ichthyosis epidermis demonstrated steroid sulfatase expression in vivo by immunostaining as well as a normalization of histologic appearance at 5 weeks postgrafting. The resulting transduced recessive X-linked ichthyosis epidermis also demonstrated a return of barrier function parameters to normal [88].

Although the introduction of systemic retinoids in the late 1970s helped many lamellar ichthyosis patients, the mainstay of therapy remains external and will probably do so until gene therapy finds its way into the therapeutic repertoire [68]. It has been shown that by combining two or more keratolytic agents and moisturizers in the same base it is usually possible to achieve additive or even synergistic effects without using irritating concentrations of either ingredient [89]. In a double-blind trial of four different cream mixtures in 20 patients with lamellar ichthyosis a mixture of 5% lactic acid and 20% propylene glycol was significantly more effective than either product alone in the same vehicle [90]. However, interestingly in these studies trans-epidermal water loss was further increased, revealing one issue with treating a symptom rather than the disease itself. Treatment regimens differ from country to country and center to center. For example, whereas urea-containing lipophilic creams are popular in many European countries, mixtures containing propylene glycol or alpha-hydroxyacids seem to be the first choice in the United States and many other countries [68]. Specific drugs have been used topically including retinoids, liarozole, and calcipotriol. However the risks of extensive use of these drugs topically in a defective barrier state is obvious.

Prenatal diagnosis is now possible for lamellar ichthyosis [91,92]. Choate et al. [93,94] grafted transglutaminase-deficient lamellar ichthyosis skin onto immunodeficient mice. They then transfected the keratinocytes with transglutaminase and showed restored involucrin cross-linking and normal epidermal architecture with restored cutaneous barrier function. These findings suggest that not only lipids, but also structural proteins are important for the normal function of the epidermal permeability barrier.

The aim in treating epidermolytic hyperkeratosis is to reduce the hyperkeratosis without aggravating the erosive component. This is certainly the concern when topical [95] or oral retinoids are used for this condition. However, used correctly topical tretinoin may be effective in some patients with epidermolytic hyperkeratosis [68]. The mainstay of therapy for many patients includes bland emollients, topical antiseptics, and intermittent use of antibiotics. The antibiotic preparations prevent and treat the bacterial overgrowth that occurs in this condition. Prenatal diagnosis is available for this condition [96].

REFERENCES

1. Elias PM, Menon GK. Structural and lipid biochemical correlates of the epidermal permeability barrier. Adv Lipid Res 1991; 24:1–23.
2. Williams ML. Lipids in normal and pathological desquamation. Adv Lipid Res 1991; 24(3):211–262.
3. Lampe MA, Williams ML, Elias PM. Human epidermal lipids: characterization and modulations during differentiation. J Lipid Res 1983; 24(2):131–140.
4. Rehfeld SJ et al. Calorimetric and electron spin resonance examination of lipid phase transitions in human stratum corneum: molecular basis for normal cohesion and abnormal desquamation in recessive X-linked ichthyosis. J Invest Dermatol 1988; 91(5):499–505.
5. Egelrud T, Hofer PA, Lundström A. Proteolytic degradation of desmosomes in plantar stratum corneum leads to cell dissociation in vitro. Acta Derm Venereol 1988; 68(2):93–97.
6. Williams ML, Elias PM. Genetically transmitted, generalized disorders of cornification. The ichthyoses. Dermatol Clin 1987; 5(1):155–178.
7. Swartzendruber DC, et al. Molecular models of the intercellular lipid lamellae in mammalian stratum corneum. J Invest Dermatol 1989; 92(2):251–257.
8. Hou SY, et al. Membrane structures in normal and essential fatty acid–deficient stratum corneum: characterization by ruthenium tetroxide staining and x-ray diffraction. J Invest Dermatol 1991; 96(2):215–223.

9. Fartasch M. Epidermal barrier in disorders of the skin. Microsc Res Tech 1997; 38(4):361–372.

10. Fartasch M, Williams ML, Elias PM. Altered lamellar body secretion and stratum corneum membrane structure in Netherton syndrome: differentiation from other infantile erythrodermas and pathogenic implications. Arch Dermatol 1999; 135(7):823–832.

11. Swartzendruber DC, ct al. Evidence that the corneocyte has a chemically bound lipid envelope. J Invest Dermatol 1987; 88(6):709–713.

12. Menon GK, Feingold KR, Elias PM. Lamellar body secretory response to barrier disruption. J Invest Dermatol 1992; 98(3):279–289.

13. Menon GK, et al. De novo sterologenesis in the skin. II. Regulation by cutaneous barrier requirements. J Lipid Res 1985; 26:418–427.

14. Grubauer G, Feingold KR, Elias PM. The relationship of epidermal lipogenesis to cutaneous barrier function. J Lipid Res 1987; 28(6):746–752.

15. Holleran WM, et al. Sphingolipids are required for mammalian epidermal barrier function. Inhibition of sphingolipid synthesis delays barrier recovery after acute perturbation. J Clin Invest 1991; 88(4):1338–1345.

16. Elias PM, Brown BE. The mammalian cutaneous permeability barrier: defective barrier function in essential fatty acid deficiency correlates with abnormal intercellular lipid deposition. Lab Invest 1978; 39(6):574–583.

17. Feingold KR, et al. The effect of essential fatty acid deficiency on cutaneous sterol synthesis. J Invest Dermatol 1986; 87:588–591.

18. Christophers E, Sterry W. In: Fitzpatrick TB, Eizen AZ, Wolff K, Freedberg IM, Auskn KF, eds. Dermatology in General Medicine. New York: McGraw-Hills 1993:490–514.

19. Toussaint S, Kamino H. In: Elder, DEA, ed. Lever's Histopathology of the Skin. Philadelphia: Lippincott-Raven, 1997:151–184.

20. Bonneville MA, Weinstock M, Wilgram GF. An electron microscope study of cell adhesion in psoiatic epidermis. J Ultrastr Res 1968; 23(1):15–43.

21. Mottaz JH, Zelickson AS. Keratinosomes in psoriatic skin. Acta Derm Venereol 1975; 55(2):81–85.

22. Lupulescu AP, Chadwick JM, Downham TFD. Ultrastructural and cell surface changes of human psoriatic skin following Goeckerman therapy. J Cutan Pathol 1979; 6(5):347–363.

23. Ghadially R, Reed JT, Elias PM. Stratum corneum structure and function correlates with phenotype in psoriasis. J Invest Dermatol 1996; 107(4):558–564.

24. Motta S, et al. Abnormality of water barrier function in psoriasis. Role of ceramide fractions. Arch Dermatol 1994; 130(4):452–456.

25. Baxter DL, Stoughton RB. Mitotic index of psoriatic lesions treated with anthralin, glucocorticosteriod and occlusion only. J Invest Dermatol 1970; 54(5):410–412.

26. Friedman SJ. Management of psoriasis vulgaris with a hydrocolloid occlusive dressing. Arch Dermatol 1987; 123(8):1046–1052.

27. Shore RN. Clearing of psoriatic lesions after the application of tape [letter]. N Engl J Med 1985; 312(4):246.

28. Feingold KR, et al. Cholesterol synthesis is required for cutaneous barrier function in mice. J Clin Invest 1990; 86:1738–1745.

29. Hashimoto K, Khan S. Harlequin fetus with abnormal lamellar granules and giant mitochondria. J Cutan Pathol 1992; 19(3):247–252.
30. Menon GK, et al. Lamellar bodies as delivery systems of hydrolytic enzymes: implications for normal cohesion and abnormal desquamation. Br J Dermatol 1992; 126:337–345.
31. Ghadially R, et al. Membrane structural abnormalities in the stratum corneum of the autosomal recessive ichthyoses. J Invest Dermatol 1992; 99(6):755–763.
32. Nanney LB, et al. Altered [^{125}I] epidermal growth factor binding and receptor distribution in psoriasis. J Invest Dermatol 1986; 86:260–265.
33. Elder JT, et al. Overexpression of transforming growth factor a in psoriatic epidermis. Science 1989; 243:811–814.
34. Kagramanova AT, Tishchenko LD, Berezov TT. [The ornithine decarboxylase activity of the epidermis in psoriasis as a biochemical index of the hyperproliferative process]. Biulleten Eksperimentalnoi Biologii i Meditsiny 1993; 115(6):618–620.
35. Nagpal S, Athanikar J, Chandraratna RA. Separation of transactivation and AP1 antagonism functions of retinoic acid receptor alpha. J Biol Chem 1995; 270(2):923–927.
36. Schroeder WT, et al. Type I keratinocyte transglutaminase: expression in human skin and psoriasis. J Invest Dermatol 1992; 99(1):27–34.
37. Bernard BA, et al. Abnormal sequence of expression of differentiation markers in psoriatic epidermis: inversion of two steps in the differentiation program? J Invest Dermatol 1988; 90(6):801–805.
38. Thewes M, et al. Normal psoriatic epidermis expression of hyperproliferation-associated keratins. Arch Dermatol Res 1991;283(7):465–471.
39. Felsher Z, Rothman S. The insensible perspiration of the skin in hyperkeratotic disorders. J Invest Dermatol 1945; 6:271–278.
40. Frost P, et al. Ichthyosiform dermatoses. 3. Studies of transepidermal water loss. Arch Dermatol 1968; 98(3):230–233.
41. Grice KA, Bettley FR. Skin water loss and accidental hypothermia in psoriasis, ichthyosis, and erythroderma. Br Med J 1967; 4(573):195–198.
42. Grice K, Sattar H, Baker H. The cutaneous barrier to salts and water in psoriasis and in normal skin. Br J Dermatol 1973; 88(5):459–463.
43. Tagami H, Yoshikuni K. Interrelationship between water-barrier and reservoir functions of pathologic stratum corneum. Arch Dermatol 1985; 121(5):642–645.
44. Wood LC, et al. Cutaneous barrier perturbation stimulates cytokine production in the epidermis of mice. J Clin Invest 1992; 90(2):482–487.
45. Nickoloff BJ, Naidu Y. Perturbation of epidermal barrier function correlates with initiation of cytokine cascade in human skin. J Am Acad Dermatol 1994; 30:535–546.
46. Fraki JE, Briggaman RA, Lazarus GS. Transplantation of psoriatic skin onto nude mice. J Invest Dermatol 1983; 80(3)(Suppl): 31s–35s.
47. Sundberg JP, et al. Full-thickness skin grafts from flaky skin mice to nude mice: maintenance of the psoriasiform phenotype. J Invest Dermatol 1994; 102(5):781–788.
48. Saiag P, et al. Psoriatic fibroblasts induce hyperproliferation of normal keratinocytes in a skin equivalent model in vitro. Science 1985; 230(4726):669–672.
49. Priestly GC, Lord R. Fibroblast–keratinocyte interactions in psoriasis: failure of pso-

riatic fibroblasts to stimulate keratinocyte proliferation in vitro. Br J Dermatol 1990; 123(4):467–472.

50. Proksch E, et al. Barrier function regulates epidermal DNA synthesis. J Clin Invest 1991; 87(5):1668–1673.

51. Wood LC, et al. Barrier function coordinately regulates epidermal IL-1 and IL-1RA mRNA levels. Exp Dermatol 1994; 3:56–60.

52. Eyre RW, Krueger GG. Response to injury of skin involved and uninvolved with psoriasis, and its relation to disease activity: Koebner and 'reverse' Koebner reactions. Br J Dermatol 1982; 106(2):153–159.

53. Sybert VP, Dale BA, Holbrook KA. Ichthyosis vulgaris: identification of a defect in synthesis of filaggrin correlated with an absence of keratohyaline granules. J Invest Dermatol 1985; 84(3):191–194.

54. Elsayed-Ali, H, Barton S, Marks R. Stereological studies of desmosomes in ichthyosis vulgaris. Br J Dermatol 1992; 126(1):24–28.

55. Nirunsuksiri W, et al. Decreased profilaggrin expression in ichthyosis vulgaris is a result of selectively impaired posttranscriptional control. J Biol Chem 1995; 270(2):871–876.

56. Suzuki Y, et al. The role of two endogenous proteases of the stratum corneum in degradation of desmoglein-1 and their reduced activity in the skin of ichthyotic patients. Br J Dermatol 1996; 134(3):460–464.

57. Lavrijsen AP, et al. Barrier function parameters in various keratinization disorders: transepidermal water loss and vascular response to hexyl nicotinate. Br J Dermatol 1993; 129(5):547–553.

58. Ohman H, Vahlquist A. The pH gradient over the stratum corneum differs in X-linked recessive and autosomal dominant ichthyosis: a clue to the molecular origin of the "acid skin mantle"? J Invest Dermatol 1998; 111(4):674–677.

59. Hernández-Martín A, González-Sarmiento R, De Unamuno P. X-linked ichthyosis: an update. Br J Dermatol 1999; 141(4):617–627.

60. Koppe G, et al. X-linked icthyosis. A sulphatase deficiency. Arch Disease Childhood 1978; 53(10):803–806.

61. Webster D, et al. X-linked ichthyosis due to steroid-sulphatase deficiency. Lancet 1978; 1(8055):70–72.

62. Ballabio A, et al. Isolation and characterization of a steroid sulfatase cDNA clone: genomic deletions in patients with X-chromosome-linked ichthyosis. Proc Natl Acad Sci USA 1987; 84(13):4519–4523.

63. Feinstein A, Ackerman AB, Ziprkowski L. Histology of autosomal dominant ichthyosis vulgaris and X-linked ichthyosis. Arch Dermatol 1970; 101(5):524–527.

64. Mesquita-Guimarães, J. X-linked ichthyosis. Ultrastructural study of 4 cases. Dermatologica 1981; 162(3):157–166.

65. Zettersten E, et al. Recessive X-linked ichthyosis: role of cholesterol-sulfate accumulation in the barrier abnormality. J Invest Dermatol 1998; 111(5):784–790.

66. Bouwstra JA, et al. Cholesterol sulfate and calcium affect stratum corneum lipid organization over a wide temperature range. J Lipid Res 1999; 40(12):2303–2312.

67. Johansen JD, et al. Skin barrier properties in patients with recessive X-linked ichthyosis. Acta Derm Venereol 1995; 75(3):202–204.

68. Vahlquist A. Ichthyosis—an inborn dryness of the skin. In: Dry Skin and Moisturizers: Chemistry and Function Boca Raton: CRC Press, 2000:121–133.

69. Yoshiike T, et al. The effect of steroid sulphatase on stratum corneum shedding in patients with X-linked ichthyosis. Br J Dermatol 1985; 113(6):641–643.

70. Lykkesfeldt G, Høyer H. Topical cholesterol treatment of recessive X-linked ichthyosis. Lancet 1983; 2(8363):1337–1338.

71. Hohl D, Huber M, Frenk E. Analysis of the cornified cell envelope in lamellar ichthyosis [see comments]. Arch Dermatol 1993; 129(5):618–624.

72. Lavrijsen AP, et al. Reduced skin barrier function parallels abnormal stratum corneum lipid organization in patients with lamellar ichthyosis. J Invest Dermatol 1995; 105(4):619–624.

73. Huber M, et al. Lamellar ichthyosis is genetically heterogeneous—cases with normal keratinocyte transglutaminase [see comments]. J Invest Dermatol 1995; 105(5):653–654.

74. Ammirati CT, Mallory SB. The major inherited disorders of cornification. New advances in pathogenesis. Dermatol Clin 1998; 16(3):497–508.

75. Hazell M, Marks R. Clinical, histologic, and cell kinetic discriminants between lamellar ichthyosis and nonbullous congenital ichthyosiform erythroderma. Arch Dermatol 1985; 121(4):489–493.

76. Matsuki M, et al. Defective stratum corneum and early neonatal death in mice lacking the gene for transglutaminase 1 (keratinocyte transglutaminase). Proc Natl Acad Sci USA 1998; 95(3):1044–1049.

77. Choate KA, Williams ML, Khavari PA. Abnormal transglutaminase 1 expression pattern in a subset of patients with erythrodermic autosomal recessive ichthyosis. J Invest Dermatol 1998; 110(1):8–12.

78. Williams ML, Elias PM. Heterogeneity in autosomal recessive ichthyosis. Clinical and biochemical differentiation of lamellar ichthyosis and nonbullous congenital ichthyosiform erythroderma. Arch Dermatol 1985; 121(4):477–488.

79. DiGiovanna JJ, Bale SJ. Clinical heterogeneity in epidermolytic hyperkeratosis. Arch Dermatol 1994; 130(8):1026–1035.

80. Yang JM, et al. Arginine in the beginning of the 1A rod domain of the keratin 10 gene is the hot spot for the mutation in epidermolytic hyperkeratosis. J Dermatol Sci 1999; 19(2):126–133.

81. Smack DP, Korge BP, James WD. Keratin and keratinization. J Am Acad Dermatol 1994; 30(1):85–102.

82. Porter RM, et al. The relationship between hyperproliferation and epidermal thickening in a mouse model for BCIE. J Invest Dermatol 1998; 110(6):951–957.

83. Reichelt J, et al. Normal ultrastructure, but altered stratum corneum lipid and protein composition in a mouse model for epidermolytic hyperkeratosis. J Invest Dermatol 1999; 113(3):329–334.

84. Scott IR, Harding CR, Barrett JG. Histidine-rich protein of the keratohyalin granules. Source of the free amino acids, urocanic acid and pyrrolidone carboxylic acid in the stratum corneum. Biochim Biophys Acta 1982; 719(1):110–117.

85. Steijlen PM, et al. Topical treatment of ichthyoses and Darier's disease with 13-*cis*-retinoic acid. A clinical and immunohistochemical study. Arch Dermatol Res 1993; 285(4):221–226.

86. Lucker GP, et al. Oral treatment of ichthyosis by the cytochrome P-450 inhibitor liarozole. Br J Dermatol 1997; 136(1):71–75.

87. Jensen TG, et al. Correction of steroid sulfatase deficiency by gene transfer into basal cells of tissue-cultured epidermis from patients with recessive X-linked ichthyosis. Exper Cell Res 1993; 209(2):392–397.

88. Freiberg RA, et al. A model of corrective gene transfer in X-linked ichthyosis. Hum Mol Gene 1997; 6(6):927–933.

89. Gnemo A, Vahlquist A. Lamellar ichthyosis is markedly improved by a novel combination of emollients [letter]. Br J Dermatol 1997; 137(6):1017–1018.

90. Ganemo A, Virtanen M, Vahlquist A. Improved topical treatment of lamellar ichthyosis: a double-blind study of four different cream formulations. Br J Dermatol 2000; 141(6):1027–1032.

91. Perry TB, et al. Prenatal diagnosis of congenital non-bullous ichthyosiform erythroderma (lamellar ichthyosis). Prenatal Diagnosis 1987; 7(3):145–155.

92. Akiyama M, Holbrook KA. Analysis of skin-derived amniotic fluid cells in the second trimester; detection of severe genodermatoses expressed in the fetal period. J Invest Dermatol 1994; 103(5):674–677.

93. Choate KA, et al. Transglutaminase 1 delivery to lamellar ichthyosis keratinocytes. Hum Gene Ther 1996; 7(18):2247–2253.

94. Choate KA, et al. Corrective gene transfer in the human skin disorder lamellar ichthyosis. Nat Med 1996; 2(11):1263–1267.

95. Schorr WF, Papa CM. Epidermolytic hyperkeratosis. Effect of tretinoin therapy on the clinical course and the basic defects in the stratum corneum. Arch Dermatol 1973; 107(4):556–562.

96. Holbrook KA, et al. Epidermolytic hyperkeratosis: ultrastructure and biochemistry of skin and amniotic fluid cells from two affected fetuses and a newborn infant. J Invest Dermatol 1983; 80(4):222–227.

11

Solvent-, Surfactant-, and Tape Stripping–Induced Xerosis

Mitsuhiro Denda

Shiseido Life Science Research Center, Yokohama, Japan

1   INTRODUCTION

Dry skin is commonly observed in various dermatoses such as atopic dermatitis, psoriasis, ichthyosis, and xenile xerosis [1]. Dermatitis induced by environmental factors such as exposure to a detergent, organic solvent, low humidity, and UV irradiation also show skin surface dryness [1]. Dry, scaly skin is characterized by a decrease in the water-retention capacity of the stratum corneum [2] with water content decreased to less than 10%. Hyperkeratosis, abnormal scaling, and epidermal hyperplasia are usually observed in dry skin [3]. Patients often suffer from itching. In some cases, the skin barrier function of the stratum corneum is decreased and trans-epidermal water loss (TEWL) is increased because of abnormality in barrier homeostasis [3]. In modern life, various environmental factors might induce the xerosis. For example, dry scaly skin has been reported among industrial painters in Japan [4]. People working in the industry also had irritated skin without any specific reason. Household detergents have also been reported to induce dry skin in Japan. Imabayashi reported [5] that 26.7% of the 1861 female university students in her survey had suffered from impaired skin due to the use of household detergents, and 74.6% of the subjects who claimed of having skin problems showed dry scaly skin. There were some seasonal changes in the occurrence of dry skin induced by detergents. A previous study suggested that environmental dryness itself induces xerotic skin [6].

This chapter describes several model systems of dry skin for clinical research of dermatitis associated with skin surface dryness. The recently reported methods to improve skin barrier homeostasis, which play a crucial role in protecting the body from environmental factors, are also reviewed.

2 ROLE AND FUNCTION OF STRATUM CORNEUM

The stratum corneum has two functions for protecting internal organs from environmental dryness. One is a water-impermeable barrier function and the other is a buffer function against dryness [7]. The water impermeability is due to the intercellular lipid bilayer structure and also the order of the corneocytes [8]. The cornified envelope, which is formed on the surface of the corneocytes, plays an important role in the structure of the barrier [9]. The buffer function of the stratum corneum is due to water molecules in the corneocytes [7]. Hydrophilic molecules such as amino acids hold water in the stratum corneum. Decrease of free amino acids in the corneocytes is commonly observed in various kinds of dermatitis which are characterized by dry scaly skin [10–13]. Decline of these functions leads to deterioration of the skin condition (Table 1).

Although the lipid structure itself was previously suggested to absorb huge amounts of water [14], this was disputed later. Cornwell et al. [15] demonstrated the effect of hydration on the intercellular lipid structure of the human stratum corneum using wide-angle x-ray diffraction. They monitored the packing arrangement of the lipid bilayers on the stratum corneum and found no effects of the hydration on the lipid structure. The lipid bilayer structure contains some water molecules, but it is a relatively small amount in comparison with the amount of water in the cornified cells. Moreover, in dry skin induced by detergent or tape-stripping, the total amount of stratum corneum ceramide, which is a major component of the intercellular lipids, did not change, athough the skin surface conductance and barrier function decreased and the amino acid content decreased [11]. Tanaka et al. [13] reported that the amino acid content was reduced in the stratum corneum in atopic respiratory disease and the trans-epidermal water loss did not change. They suggested that the free amino acid content is a crucial factor in the dry scaly features of not only experimentally induced dry skin, but also atopic dermatitis. Water in the stratum corneum is mainly held in the corneocytes by hydrophilic molecules like amino acids [10]. Intercellular lipids protect the corneocytes and prevent leakage of water, amino acids, and other water-soluble molecules (Fig. 1).

The ultrastructure of the intercellular lipids in the stratum corneum contributes to the barrier function of healthy skin, but the decline of the barrier function in dermatoses might be caused by various other factors. We previously eval-

TABLE 1 Alteration of Physiological and Biochemical Factors in Stratum Corneum of Xerotic Skin

	TEWL	Hydration	Free amino acids	Ceramides
Experimentally induced xerosis				
Repeated barrier disruption (Ref. 11,27)	Increased	Decreased	Decreased	No change
SDS treatment (Ref. 11)	Increased	Decreased	Decreased	No change
Low humidity (Ref. 52)	Decreased	Decreased	Decreased (unpublished)	Increased
Chronic xerosis				
Atopic dermatitis (Ref. 12)	Increased	Decreased	Decreased	Decreased
Hemodialysis (Ref. 12)	Increased	Decreased	Decreased	Increased
Senile xerosis (Ref. 10,12)	Decreased	Decreased	Decreased	Decreased

uated the intercellular lipid alkyl chain conformation by attenuated total reflectance infrared spectroscopy on healthy skin and surfactant-induced scaly skin of human subjects [16]. In normal, healthy skin, there was a correlation between the lipid conformation and the trans-epidermal water loss. However, no difference was observed in the surfactant-induced scaly skin. Menton et al. reported [17] that the arrangement of corneocytes became disordered during high mitotic activity. Menon et al. demonstrated [18] that inhibition of cholesterol synthesis, which plays a crucial role in barrier function, induced a deposition of abnormal lamellar body contents and formation of clefts in the intercellular domains. Disorder of the corneocytes or clefts of the lipid domain might cause barrier dysfunction.

The hydrophobic envelope formed on the surface of the corneocytes plays an important role in the stabilization of the intercelluar lipid bilayer structure (See chapter in this volume by A. Watkinson). The cross-linked protein structure on the corneocyte is mainly composed of involucrin, loricrin, and filaggrin [9]. Then ω-hydroxyceramide molecules covalently attach to the protein envelope. Abnormality of the formation of this protein/lipid envelope on the surface of the corneocytes induces barrier abnormalities even when other lipid synthesis and processing systems are normal. Behne et al. [19] demonstrated that an inhibition of

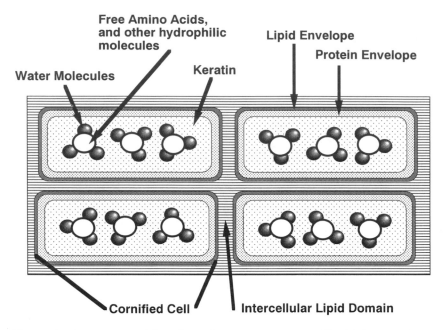

FIGURE 1 Structure and function of stratum corneum. The high water imper-meability is due to specific "brick and mortar" structure constructed by cor-neocytes and intercellular lipid domain. The buffer function is held by water molecules in the corneocytes. Hydrophilic molecules such as free amino acids play a crucial role to hold water in the stratum corneum.

ω-hydroxyceramide induced the delay of the barrier repair after tape-stripping. Segre et al. [20] reported a transcription factor, Klf4, is required for the skin bar-rier formation. Klf4-/- mice showed absence of the barrier and its abnormal corni-fied envelope, whereas the mutant mice showed a normal lipid profile.

    These results suggest that various factors contribute to the skin barrier func-tion. Thus, dry scaly skin might be induced by a variety of causes.

3   XEROSIS INDUCED BY ACETONE AND TAPE-STRIPPING

Damage of the stratum corneum barrier function can be repaired [21]. Immedi-ately after barrier disruption, repair responses, including epidermal lipid synthe-sis, lipid processing, and lipid secretion into the intercellular domain between the stratum corneum and epidermal granular layer, are accelerated [22].

    However, recent studies suggested that environmental or intrinsic factors affect cutaneous barrier homeostasis. Psychological stress delays barrier recovery after artificial barrier disruption (Fig. 2) [23,24]. Glucocorticoid in serum might

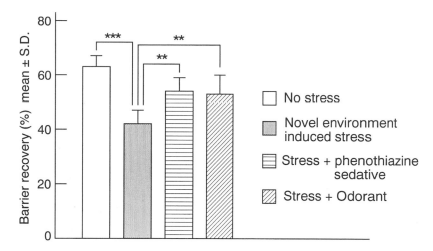

FIGURE 2 Psychological stress induced by novel environment delayed the skin barrier recovery after the barrier disruption. Reduction of the stress by application of phenotheiazine sedative or inhalation of specific odorant improve the barrier homeostasis. **p < 0.01; ***p < 0.001.

mediate skin homeostasis through the central nervous system [24]. There is a circadian rhythm in the stratum corneum barrier homeostasis [25]. On the other hand, the barrier becomes fragile and recovery is delayed with aging [26]. Moreover, when the barrier disruption is repeated, epidermal hyperplasia and inflammation are induced even when the level of the disruption is relatively small [27]. Under low humidity, the hyperplastic response induced by barrier disruption is amplified [6].

Barrier disruption is observed in variously induced scaly skin [3] and is known to cause changes in epidermal biochemical processes, DNA synthesis [28], calcium localization [29], and cytokine production [30]. Upregulation of specific keratin molecules and adhesion molecules associated with an inflammatory response are also observed [31]. Because a decline of the stratum corneum barrier function is observed in various types of skin diseases, xerosis induced by barrier disruption might be a good model of those dermatoses.

In our daily life, the stratum corneum barrier is potentially perturbed by chemicals such as surfactants, detergents, and organic solvents. Gruneward et al. demonstrated [32] damage of the skin by repeated washing with surfactant solutions. They treated skin following the repeated use of sodium dodecyl sulfate (SDS) and N-cocoyl protein condensate sodium as a mild washing substance for one week. In their report, they suggested that repeated washing with even a mild surfactant damaged the skin.

Skin on the back or forearm skin is used for the experiments [11]. It was easier to induce scaly skin on the back than on the forearm. After stripping the stratum corneum on the back nine times with adhesive cellophane tape, the TEWL value was over 10 mg/cm^2/hr, and most of the stratum corneum was removed. But to induce dry scaly skin on the forearm, stripping up to 30–50 times was needed. One week after the treatment, TEWL increased, skin surface conductance decreased, and the cell area in the stratum corneum also decreased. The skin surface became scaly and flaky. Abnormal scaling is observed on the surface of the skin after tape-stripping. These phenomena are commonly observed in natural dry skin, such as in atopic dermatitis and psoriasis.

Acetone treatment is also used for barrier disruption [33]. Compared to tape-stripping, this treatment breaks the stratum corneum barrier homogeneously. On the other hand, it takes a longer period of time to break the barrier than by tape-stripping. Thus, the barrier disruption by acetone treatment is more useful for studies using hairless mice than human subjects because the mouse has a thin stratum corneum.

Treatment with surfactants is another way to break the barrier [32]. The efficacy varies with each surfactant. Yang et al. suggested [34] some kind of anionic surfactant such as sodium dodecyl sulfate, affecting not only the stratum corneum barrier, but also the nucleous layer of the epidermis. Fartasch demonstrated [35] that the topical application of SDS caused damage to the nucleated cells of the epidermis and that acetone treatment disrupted the lipid structure only in the stratum corneum. Some surfactants induce an inflammatory response of the epidermis. These effects of surfactants will be described in the next section.

The degree of epidermal hyperplasia correlated with the level and duration of barrier disruption [27]. Using hairless mice, we investigated the effects of repeated barrier disruption [27]. Not only epidermal hyperplasia, but also cutaneous inflammation was observed with a longer and higher level of repeated barrier disruption by tape-stripping and acetone treatment. Flank skin of hairless mice is often used for the study, but ears of other types of hairy mice can also be used for the study. In our previous study [27], ear skin of ICR mice showed more obvious inflammation after repeated barrier disruption than that of flank skin of hairless mice. Since neither the increase in epidermal cytokine production nor the described changes in cutaneous pathology were prevented by occlusion, this model should not be attributed to increased water loss, but rather to epidermal injury resulting in the production and release of epidermal cytokines.

The xerosis induced by repeated barrier disruption would be a very useful model for the dry scaly skin induced by environmental factors such as detergents or organic solvents. However, although repeated barrier disruption induces inflammation, epidermal hyperplasia, and abnormal keratinization, there are several histological differences between this model and psoriasis. Gerritsen et al. reported [36] the absence of some characteristic features of psoriasis in the dry skin induced by repeated tape-stripping. They also demonstrated the difference of filaggrin expression between the model system and psoriasis. The different features of these chronic skin diseases and the model system should be investigated for further understanding of the diseases.

4 SURFACTANT-INDUCED XEROSIS

In our daily life, surfactants, i.e., detergents, are a potential cause of dermatitis [4,5]. Thus, the dry skin induced by surfactants has been studied not only as a model system of dry skin, but also for clinical study of skin trouble in our daily life. As described, the surfactant could damage not only stratum corneum barrier function, but also other skin properties.

The effect of the surfactant on skin is dependent on the type of the surfactant. Wilhelm et al. demonstrated the irritation potential of anionic surfactants [37]. They evaluated the effects of sodium salts of n-alkyl sulfates with various carbon chain lengths on TEWL and found the maximum response on the C12 analog. In this report, they suggested that the mechanisms responsible for the hydration of the stratum corneum are related to the irritation properties of the surfactants. Leveque et al. also suggested [38] the occurrence of the hyperhydration of the stratum corneum consecutive to the inflammation process. They demonstrated that the increase of TEWL was induced by SDS without removal of lipids in the stratum corneum. Sodium dodecyl sulfate might influence not only stratum corneum barrier function, but also the nucleated layer of the epidermis and/or dermal system associated with inflammation [38]. A previous study revealed no correlation between the level of epidermal hyperplasia and TEWL increase on the SDS-irritated skin [39]. Ruissen et al. demonstrated [40] different effects of various types of detergents on keratinocyte culture and human intact skin. As a hyperproliferative/inflammatory marker, they monitored SKALP, a protease inhibitor that is found in hyperproliferative skin. In their in vitro system, anionic SDS induced SKALP expression, SDS also induced upregulation of involucrin and downregulation of cytokeratin 1 expression, which are associated with epidermal inflammation and hyperplasia. On the other hand, a cationic detergent, cetyltrimethylammonium bromide (CTAB), and nonionic detergents, Nonident P-40 and TritonX-100, did not induce the expression of the proliferative markers observed by the SDS treatment. Different detergents showed different features of cytotoxicity of human keratinocyte. CTAB, Triton X-100, and Nonident-P40 showed strong, SDS showed moderate, and Tween-20 showed no cytotoxicity. Thus, cytotoxicity was not correlated with the potential of epidermal proliferation. They also compared the induction of erythema and skin barrier disruption by different detergents. In both parameters, SDS showed the most obvious effects; Triton X-100 showed the smallest; and CTAB showed a moderate effect on human skin. Other reports demonstrated an induction of intercellular adhesion molecule-1 (ICAM-1) [41] or vascular endothelial growth factor (VEGF) [42] by

SDS treatment. These results suggest that anionic detergents such as SDS have a high potential to induce epidermal hyperplasia or inflammation. Thus, SDS has often been used in dry scaly skin model systems.

In our previous study [16], we used human forearm skin or back skin. The forearm skin was treated with a 5% aqueous solution of SDS and an occlusive dressing applied. After the treatment, we washed the surfactant solution with water and then we continuously measured TEWL, skin surface conductance, and lipid morphology in the stratum corneum by ATR-IR for 14 days (Fig. 3). The lipid morphology in the stratum corneum was disordered by the treatment, but recovered to normal within a couple of days. On the other hand, both TEWL and skin surface conductance were abnormal even 2 weeks after the SDS treatment. In the case of a single application of the barrier disruption by tape-stripping and acetone treatment, these parameters recovered to normal within a couple of days. Thus, the occlusive dressing of the surfactant affected skin not only on the stratum corneum, but also the nucleated layer of the epidermis and dermis. Potentially this method damages the skin too much. One must pay attention to the concentration of the surfactant solution and the period of the occlusive dressing. The skin damage varies with the individual. The subsequent occlusion substantially increases the irritant response of the skin to repeated short-term SDS treatment.

5   OTHER SUBSTANCES WHICH COULD INDUCE XEROSIS

In addition to surfactants, several chemical substances also induce dry scaly skin. Chiba et al. demonstrated [43] that topical application of squalene-monohydroperoxide, a product of UV-peroxidated squalene, induced dry skin on hairless mice. In this model, they showed hyperkeratosis and epidermal proliferation. Peroxidized lipid by UV irradiation might be a cause of xerotic skin.

Sato et al. [44] demonstrated that cholesterol sulfate inhibited both trypsin type and chymotrypsin type protease and suggested the inhibition of these protesases reduced degradation of desmosomes, which play a crucial role in the adhesion of corneocytes and, as a consequence, abnormal scales were induced. Abnormality of cholesterol sulfate processing also induced serious skin abnormalities [45]. The content of cholesterol sulfate in total lipids is 5% in the healthy epidermis and about 1% in the stratum corneum. Steroid sulfatase catalyzes the desulfation of cholesterol sulfate to cholesterol. In recessive X-linked ichthyosis, which displays a large amount of abnormal scales, the level of cholesterol sulfate in the stratun corneum was increased 10-fold because of the absence of steroid sulfatase. Moreover, Nemes et al. [46] reported another potential negative role of cholesterol sulfate in the stratum corneum. Involucrin cross-linking and involucrin esterification with ω-hydroxyceramides are crucial for cornified envelope formation. They demonstrated that both reactions were inhibited by cholesterol sulfate.

A

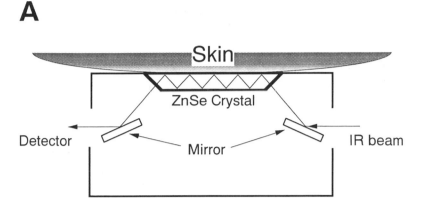

B

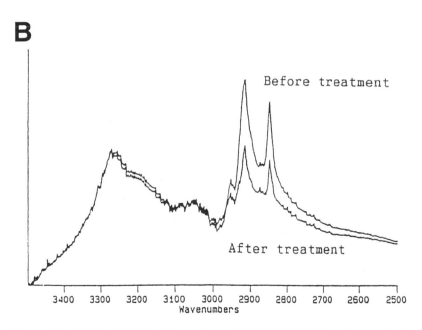

FIGURE 3 (A) Model of optic system of ATR IR. (B) The change in the C–H stretching frequency before and after acetone treatment.

Perturbation of stratum corneum desquamation by environmental factors also induces scaly skin (see chapter in this volume by J. Sato)

6   XEROSIS INDUCED UNDER LOW ENVIRONMENTAL HUMIDITY

Low humidity affects the condition of normal skin and may trigger various cutaneous disorders [47]. Various skin diseases which are characterized by a dry scaly condition such as atopic dermatitis and psoriasis tend to worsen during the winter season [48,49] (See chapter titled "Winter Xerosis" by A. V. Rawlings). In common dermatitis, a decline in barrier function often parallels increased severity of clinical symptomology. These conditions all tend to worsen during the winter season when humidity is low [48,49]. Abundant indirect evidence has suggested that decreased humidity precipitates these disorders, while increased skin hydration appears to ameliorate these conditions [6]. The mechanisms by which alterations in relative humidity might influence cutaneous function and induce cutaneous pathology are poorly understood.

We previously demonstrated [6] that low humidity stimulates the epidermal hyperproliferative and inflammatory response to barrier disruption. Low humidity affected stratum corneum morphology [50] and caused abnormal desquamation (Fig. 4) [51]. These findings suggest that this model system, i.e., dry skin in-

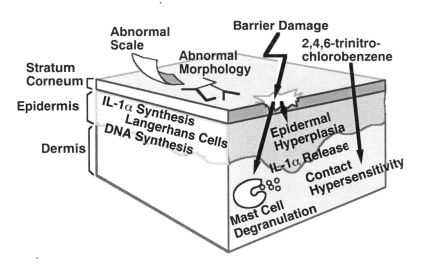

Figure 4   Alteration of the skin under dry environment. Dry environment induces epidermal DNA and cytokine synthesis, and the skin becomes more sensitive to physical or chemical insults from outside.

duced by low humidity, is also an important model for clinical research of skin diseases associated with skin surface dryness.

In these studies we used hairless mice [6,50–52]. Before the experiments, the mice were caged separately for at least 4 days. These cages were kept in a room with temperature maintained at 22–25°C and relative humidity (RH) of 40–70%. Then the mice were kept separately in 7.2-L cages in which the relative humidity was maintained at either 10% (low humidity) with dry air or 80% (high humidity) with humid air. The temperature was 22–25°C with fresh air circulated 100 times per hour, and the animals were kept out of the direct stream of air. The level of NH_3 was always below 1 ppm.

Under low humidity, epidermal DNA synthesis increased within 12 hr [53]. Abnormal scaling and increase of stratum corneum thickness were also observed within 2–3 days [51]. Obvious epidermal hyperplasia and mast cell degranulation were observed 48 hr after the treatment of flank skin with acetone in the animals that had been kept in low humidity for 48 hr [6]. Contact hypersensitivity to 2,4,6-trinitrochlorobenzene also increased after exposure to low humidity for 2 days [54]. An immunohistochemical study showed that the amount of interleukin 1α (IL-1α) in the epidermis was higher in animals kept in low humidity than in those kept in high humidity [7]. The release of IL-1α from skin immediately after tape-stripping was significantly higher in the animals kept in low humidity than kept in high humidity. Moreover, epidermal IL-1α mRNA increased significantly in the animals kept in low humidity for 24 hr. These studies provide evidence that changes in environmental humidity contribute to the seasonal exacerbation/amelioration of cutaneous disorders such as atopic dermatitis and psoriasis, diseases which are characterized by a defective barrier, epidermal hyperplasia, and inflammation. Because these responses were prevented by occlusion with a plastic membrane, petrolatum, and humectant [6], this dry skin model is a good model to evaluate the clinical methods to treat skin problems.

7 NEW ROUTES TO TREAT XEROSIS

As described, repeated barrier disruption induces epidermal hyperplasia and inflammation. Even slight damage of the barrier resulted in epidermal hyperplasia under low humidity. We previously reported [55,56] several methods to accelerate skin barrier repair by regulation of nonlipid factors such as enzymes and ions. We also demonstrated that the acceleration of the barrier repair improved those skin conditions [55]. Thus, studies on the biochemical and biophysical functions associated with the epidermal barrier homeostasis should be important for clinical dermatology (Table 2).

Damaged barrier function can be restored by topical application of a water-impermeable substance such as petrolatum [57]. In this case, the petrolatum stays in the stratum corneum and forms a water-impermeable membrane. However,

TABLE 2 List of Applications which Accelerate Stratum Corneum
Barrier Recovery

Lipids (Ref. 57)	Petrolatum
	Optimized mixture of ceramide, cholesterol, and fatty acid (single lipid application delayed the barrier recovery)
Protease inhibitors (Ref. 55)	Trypsin-like serine protease inhibitor
	Plasminogen activator inhibitor
Ions (Ref. 56)	Some magnesium salts (not all)
	Mixture of magnesium and calcium chloride
Histamine receptor antagonists (Ref. 73)	H1 receptor antagonist
	H2 receptor antagonist (H3 receptor antagonist did not affect the barrier recovery)
Nuclear hormone receptor activator (Ref. 72)	PPARα activator

Man et al. demonstrated that a topically applied mixture of stratum corneum lipids, i.e., ceramide, cholesterol, and free fatty acids, was incorporated in nucleated layer of epidermis and accelerated repair of the barrier function after its being damaged [58]. Their studies first demonstrated a method to accelerate barrier recovery by regulating endogeneous factors in the epidermis.

We previously demonstrated [55] that *trans*-4-(aminomethyl) cyclohexane carboxylic acid (t-AMCHA), an antifibrinolytic agent which activates plasminogen, improved the barrier homeostasis and whole skin condition. After barrier disruption; proteolytic activity in the epidermis increased within 1–2 hr. This increase was inhibited by t-AMCHA. Topical application of t-AMCHA or trypsin-like serine protease inhibitors accelerated the barrier recovery. Moreover, topical application of t-AMCHA improved epidermal hyperplasia induced by repeated barrier disruption. These findings suggested that manipulations that injure the stratum corneum activate the plasminogen/plasmin system and the increase of the extracellular protease activity is detrimental to barrier repair and may induce pathologic changes in the skin. Kitamura et al. also reported [59] the efficacy on this agent to dry skin. The protease balance might be important for the barrier homeostasis and skin pathology.

Lipid metabolism is regulated by a series of enzymes in the epidermis [22] and each of them has their optimal conditions such as pH [66] and other ion balance [56]. For example, the pH value of the healthy stratum corneum is kept acidic because the lipid-processing enzymes have an acidic optimal pH. Mauro et al. [66] demonstrated that topical application of basic buffer after barrier disruption delayed the repair process because the basic condition perturbates the lipid processing.

Other ions such as calcium and magnesium [56,61] also play important roles in lipid metabolism in the epidermis. We demonstrated that the topical application of calcium or potassium reduced barrier repair, and magnesium and a mixture of calcium and magnesium salts accelerated the repair process [56]. Topical application of 10 mM magnesium chloride, magnesium sulfate, and magnesium lactate aqueous solution accelerated barrier repair. Application of magnesium bis(dihydrogen phosphate) or magnesium chloride in PBS solution did not affect the barrier recovery rate. Application of 10 mM calcium chloride aqueous solution delayed the barrier repair, but a mixture of calcium chloride and magnesium chloride accelerated barrier recovery when the calcium-to-magnesium molar ration was lower than 1. Application of the mixture also improved the condition of dry scaly skin induced by SDS treatment (Fig. 5). These results suggest an important role for these ions in barrier homeostasis.

We demonstrated a heterogeneous distribution of calcium, magnesium, and potassium in the human epidermis [62]. Both calcium and magnesium were localized in the glanular layer, while potassium was localized in the spinous layer. Immediately after the barrier function, this distribution disappeared. Calcium plays various roles in the formation of the stratum corneum barrier [61]. It induces terminal differentiation [63], carnified envelope formation, and epidermal lipid synthesis [64]. Menon et al. demonstrated that alteration of the calcium gradient affects the exocytosis of the lamellar body at the interface between the stratum corneum and epidermal granular layer [65]. Vicanova demonstrated [66] the improvement of the barrier function in the reconstructed human epidermis by the normalization of epidermal calcium distribution. The heterogeneous field which is formed by ions such as calcium, magnesium, and potassium might be crucial for the terminal differentiation and the barrier formation in the epidermis. Rab plays an important role in the exocytosis and endocytosis after modification with hydrophobic molecules [67]. Magnesium is required for the activity of Rab-geranylgeranyl transferase, which modifies Rab [68]. For barrier formation, exocytosis of the lamellar body is an important process. Previous studies have indicated that Rab is modified by Rab-geranylgeranyl transferase during the terminal differentiation of the epidermis [69]. Regulation of ion gradation in the epidermis might be important to improve barrier homeostasis and skin pathology.

Feingold and coworkers demonstrated an important role of nuclear hormone receptor on epidermal differentiation and stratum corneum barrier formation. Activation of PPARα by farnesol also stimulated the differentiation of epidermal keratinocytes [70,71]. And in carnified envelope formating, involucrin and transglutaminase protein mRNA levels were also increased by the activation of PPARα [72]. Interestingly, DNA synthesis was inhibited by the treatment [72].

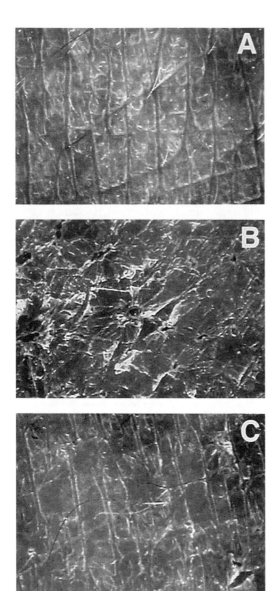

FIGURE 5 Effect of magnesium and calcium salts mixture solution on SDS-induced xerosis. (A) Microscopic picture of healthy human skin. (B) Microscopic picture of skin surface 1 week after SDS treatment. Obvious scales are observed. (C) Skin surface of skin treated by SDS and application of equimolar mixture of MgC_{12} and CaC_{12}. Most of the abnormal scales observed in (B) were reduced.

They also showed that topical application of PPARα activators accelerated the barrier recovery after tape-stripping or acetone treatment and prevented the epidermal hyperplasia induced by repeated barrier disruption [72]. Regulation of the nuclear hormone receptor would open a new possibility for improvement of the cutaneous barrier.

Recently, Ashida et al. presented the relationship between histamine receptor and skin barrier function [73]. Three different types of histamine receptors, H1, H2, and H3, have been reported. First, topical application of histamine H1 and H2 receptor antagonists accelerated the barrier repair. Histamine itself, H2 receptor agonist, and histamine releaser delayed the barrier repair. Histamine H3 receptor antagonist and agonist did not affect the barrier recovery rate. We demonstrated that topical application of the H1 and H2 receptor antagonists prevented the epidermal hyperplasia induced by barrier disruption under low humidity. The mechanism of the relationship between the histamine receptors and the barrier repair process has not yet been elucidated.

As described, psychological stress [23,24] and aging [26] disrupt the barrier homeostasis. The delay of barrier repair induced by psychological stress was prevented by application of a sedative drug or inhalation of specific odorants which had a sedative effect [74]. The delay of barrier recovery with aging was improved by topical application of cholesterol [75] or mevalonic acid [76], because the delay of the aged skin was caused by a decrease of cholesterol synthesis. Removal of each cause of the barrier abnormality is the basic idea to improve the barrier homeostasis. Thus, studies on the relationship between the barrier homeostasis and the physiology of the whole body system is important in clinical dermatology.

Regulation of epidermal lipid metabolism by eliminating other causative factors might be effective to improve skin pathology. Because it can improve the endogeneous homeostatic process, occlusion or moisturization with artificial material could improve the skin condition. However, such treatment potentially perturbs the homeostasis of the skin. On the other hand, recovery of the original, endogenous skin function by acceleration of its homeostatic process results in natural healthy skin without side effects. Methods to accelerate barrier repair might open new possibilities for future skin care systems.

8 CONCLUSION

In modern life, various environmental factors might induce xerotic skin. Skin surface dryness is caused by various factors. Decrease of free amino acid in the stratum corneum is commonly observed in different types of chronic and experimentally induced dry skin. Barrier abnormality is also often observed in xerotic skin, and improvement of the barrier homeostasis is effective to improve the whole skin condition. The series of experimentally induced xerosis presented here are useful for further understanding of the mechanistic study of xerosis. These models should be important to develop a new strategy to treat xerosis.

REFERENCES

1. Sauer GC, Hall JC. Manual of Skin Diseases. 7th ed. Philadelphia Lippincott-Raven, 1996.
2. Tagami H, Yoshikuni K. Interrelationship between water-barrier and reservoir functions of pathologic stratum corneum. Arch Dermatol 1985; 121:642–645.
3. Black D, Diridollou S, Lagarde JM, Gall Y. Skin care products for normal, dry and greasy skin. In: Baran R, Maibach HI, eds. Textbook of Cosmetic Dermatology, 2 ed. London: Martin Dunitz, 1998; 125–150.
4. Kishi R, Harabuchi I, Katakura Y, Ikeda T, Miyake H. Neurobehavioral effects on chronic occupational exposure to organic solvents among Japanese industrial painters. Environ Res 1993; 62:303–313.
5. Imabayashi Y. Skin surface lipids and sweat of hand in girl students who complained of impaired skin on the hand by using household detergents. Fukuoka Igaku Zasshi 1990; 81:359–369.
6. Denda M, Sato J, Tsuchiya T, Elias PM, Feingold KR. Low humidity stimulates epidermal DNA synthesis and amplifies the hyperproliferative response to barrier disruption: implication of seasonal exacerbations of inflammatory dermatoses. J Invest Dermatol 1998; 111:873–878.
7. Denda M. Influence of dry environment on epidermal function. J Dermatol Sci 2000; 24:522–528.
8. Elias PM, Menon GK. Structural and lipid biochemical correlates of the epidermal permeability barrier. In: Elias PM, ed. Advances in Lipid Research. Vol. 24. Skin Lipids. San Diego: Academic Press, 1991; 1–26.
9. Nemes Z, Steinert PM. Bricks and mortar of the epidermal barrier. Exp Mol Med 1999; 31:5–19.
10. Horii I, Obata M, Tagami H. Stratum corneum hydration and amino acid content in xerotic skin. Br J Dermatol 1989; 121:587–592.
11. Denda M, Hori J, Koyama J, Yoshida S, Namba R, Takahashi M, Horii I, Yamamoto A. Stratum corneum sphingolipids and free amino acids in experimentally induced scaly skin. Arch Dermatol Res 1992; 284:363–367.
12. Takahashi M, Ikezawa Z. Dry skin in atopic dermatitis and patients on hemodialysis. In: Loden M, Maibach HI, eds. Dry Skin and Moisturizers: Chemistry and Function. Boca Raton: CRC Press, 2000; 135–146.
13. Tanaka M, Okada M, Zhen YX, Inamura N, Kitano T, Shirai S, Sakamoto K, Inamura T, Tagami H. Decreased hydration state of the stratum corneum and reduced amino acid content of the skin surface in patients with seasonal allergic rhinitis. Br J Dermatol 1998; 139:618–621.
14. Imokawa G, Hattori M. A possible function of structural lipids in the water-holding properties of the stratum corneum. J Invest Dermatol 1985; 84:282–284.
15. Cornwell PA, Barry BW, Stoddart CP, Bouwstra JA. Wide-angle x-ray diffraction of human stratum corneum: effects of hydration and terpene enhancer treatment. J Pharm Pharmacol 1994; 46:938–950.

16. Denda M, Koyama J, Namba R, Horii I I. Stratum corneum lipid morphology and transepidermal water loss in normal skin and surfactant-induced scaly skin. Arch Dermatol Res 1994; 286:41–46.
17. Menton DN, Eisen AZ. Structural organization of the stratum corneum in certain scaling disorders of the skin. J Invest dermatol 1971; 57:295–307.
18. Menon GK, Feingold KR, Man MQ, Schande M, Elias PM. Structural basis for the barrier abnormality following inhibition of HMG CoA reductase in murine epidermis. J Invest Dermatol 1992; 98:209–219.
19. Behne M, Uchida Y, Seki T, de Montellano PO, Elias PM, Holleran WM. Omegahydroxyceramides are required for corneocyte lipid envelope (CLE) formation and normal epidermal permeability barrier function. J Invest Dermatol 2000; 114:185–192.
20. Segre JA, Bauer C, Fuchs E. Klf4 is a transcription factor required for establishing the barrier function of the skin. Nat Genet 1999; 22:356–360.
21. Elias PM, Holleran WM, Menon GK, Ghadially R, Williams ML, Feingold KR. Normal mechanisms and pathophysiology of epidermal permeability barrier homeostasis. Curr Opin Dermatol 1993; 231–237.
22. Elias PM, Feingold KR. Lipids and the epidermal water barrier: metabolism, regulation, and pathophysiology. Semin Dermatol 1992; 11:176–182.
23. Denda M, Tsuchiya T, Hosoi J, Koyama J. Immobilization-induced and crowded environment–induced stress delay barrier recovery in murine skin. Br J Dermatol 1998; 138:780–785.
24. Denda M, Tsuchiya T, Elias PM, Feingold KR. Stress alters cutaneous permeability barrier homeostasis. Am J Physiol 2000; 278:R367–R372.
25. Denda M, Tsuchiya T. Barrier recovery rate varies time-dependently in human skin. Br J Dermatol 2000; 142:881–884.
26. Ghadially R, Brown BE, Sequeira-Martin SM, Feingold KR, Elias PM. The aged epidermal permeability barrier. J Clin Invest 1995; 95:2281–2290.
27. Denda M, Wood LC, Emami S, Calhoun C, Brown BE, Elias PM, Feingold KR. Theepidermal hyperplasia associated with repeated barrier disruption by acetone treatment or tape stripping cannot be attributed to increased water loss. Arch Dermatol Res 1996; 288:230–238.
28. Proksch E, Feingold KR, Man MQ, Elias PM. Barrier function regulates epidermal DNA synthesis. J Clin Invest 1991; 87:1668–1673.
29. Menon GK, Elias PM, Lee SH, Feingold KR. Localization of calcium in murine epidermis following disruption and repair of the permeability barrier. Cell Tis Res 1992; 270:503–512.
30. Wood LC, Jackson SM, Elias PM, Grunfeld C, Feingold KR. Cutaneous barrier perturbation stimulates cytokine production in the epidermis of mice. J Clin Invest 1992; 90:482–487.
31. Nickoloff BJ, Naidu Y. Perturbation of epidermal barrier function correlates with initiation of cytokine cascade in human skin. J Am Acad Dermatol 1994; 30:535–546.
32. Gruneward AM, Gloor M, Gehring W, Kleesz P. Damage to the skin by repetitive washing. Contact Dermatitis 1995; 32:225–232.
33. Denda M, Brown BE, Elias PM, Feingold KR. Epidermal injury stimulates prenylation in the epidermis of hairless mice. Arch Dermatol Res 1997; 289:104–110.
34. Yang L, Man MQ, Taljebini M, Elias PM, Feingold KR. Topical stratum corneum

lipids accelerate barrier repair tape stripping, solvent treatment and some but not all types of detergent treatment. Br J Dermatol 1995; 133:679–685.

35. Fartasch M. Ultrastructure of the epidermal barrier after irritation. Microsc Res Tech 1997; 37:193–199.

36. Gerritsen MJP, van Erp PEJ, van Vlijmen-Willems IMJJ, Lenders LTM, van de Kerkhof PCM. Repeated tape stripping of normal skin: a histological assessment and comparison with events seen in psoriasis. Arch Dermatol Res 1994; 286:455–461.

37. Wilhelm KP, Cua AB, Wolff HH, Maibach HI. Surfactant-induced stratum corneum hydration in vivo: prediction of the irritation potential of anionic surfactants. J Invest Dermatol 1993; 101:310–315.

38. Leveque JL, de Rigal J, Saint-Leger D, Billy D. How does sodium lauryl sulfate alter the skin barrier function in man? A multiparametric approach. Skin Pharmacol 1993; 6:111–115.

39. Welzel J, Metker C, Wolff H, Wilhelm KP. SLS-irritated human skin shows no correlation between degree of proliferation and TEWL increase. Arch Dermatol Res 1998; 290:615–620.

40. Ruissen F, Le M, Carroll JM, Valk PGM, Schalkwijk J. Differential effects of detergents on keratinocyte gene expression. J Invest Dermatol 1998; 110:358–363.

41. Driesch P, Fartasch M, Huner A, Ponec M. Expression of integrin receptors and ICAM-1 on keratinocytes in vivo and in an in vitro reconstructed epidermis: effect of sodium dodecyl sulphate. Arch Dermatol Res 1995; 287:249–253.

42. Palacio S, Schmitt D, Viac J. Contact allergens and sodium lauryl sulphate upregulate vascular endothelial growth factor in normal keratinocytes. Br J Dermatol 1997; 137:540–544.

43. Chiba K, Sone T, Kawakami K, Onoue M. Skin roughness and wrinkle formation induced by repeated application of squalene-monohydroperoxide to the hairless mouse. Exp Dermatol 1999; 8:471–479.

44. Sato J, Denda M, Nakanishi J, Nomura J, Koyama J. Cholesterol sulfate inhibits proteases that are involved in desquamation of stratum corneum. J Invest Dermatol 1998; 111:189–193.

45. Zettersten E, Man MQ, Sato J, Denda M, Farrell A, Ghadially R, Williams ML, Feingold KR, Elias PM. Recessive X-linked ichthyosis: role of cholesterol-sulfate accumulation in the barrier abnormality. J Invest Dermatol 1998; 111:784–790.

46. Nemes Z, Demeny M, Marekov LN, Fesus L, Steinert PM. Cholesterol 3-sulfate in terferes with cornified envelope assembly by diverting transglutaminase 1 activity from the formation of cross-links and esters to the hydrolysis of glutamine. J Biol Chem 2000; 275:2636–2646.

47. Rycroft PJG, Smith WDL. Low humidity occupational dermatoses. Contact Dermatitis 1980; 6:488–492.

48. Wilkinson JD, Rycroft RJ. Contact Dermatitis. In: Champion RH, Burton JL, Ebling FJG, eds. Textbook of Dermatology, 5th ed. London: Blackwell Scientific, 1992:614–615.

49. Sauer GC, Hall JC. Seasonal skin diseasses. In: Sauer GC, Hall JC, eds. Manual of Skin Diseases. Philadelphia: Lippincott-Raven, 1996:23–28.

50. Sato J, Yanai M, Hirao T, Denda M. Water content and thickness of stratum corneum contribute to skin surface morphology. Arch Dermatol Res 2000; 292:412–417.

51. Sato J, Denda M, Nakanihi J, Koyama J. Dry conditions affect desquamation of stratum corneum in vivo. J Dermatol Sci 1998; 18:163–169.
52. Denda M, Sato J, Masuda Y, Tsuchiya T, Koyama J, Kuramoto M, Elias PM, Feingold KR. Exposure to a dry environment enhances epidermal permeability barrier function. J Invest Dermatol 1998; 111:858–863.
53. Sato J, Denda M, Ashida Y, Koyama J. Loss of water from the stratum corneum induces epidermal DNA synthesis in hairless mice. Arch Dermatol Res 1998; 290:634–637.
54. Hosoi J, Hariya T, Denda M, Tsuchiya T. Regulation of the cutaneous allergic reaction by humidity. Contact Dermatitis 2000; 42:81–84.
55. Denda M, Kitamura K, Elias PM, Feingold KR. *trans*-4-(Aminomethyl) cyclohexane carboxylic acid (T-AMCHA), an anti-fibrinolytic agent, accelerates barrier recovery and prevents the epidermal hyperplasia induced by epidermal injury in hairless mice and humans. J Invest Dermatol 1997; 109:84–90.
56. Denda M, Katagiri C, Hirao T, Maruyama N, Takahashi M. Some magnesium salts and a mixture of magnesium and calcium salts accelerate skin barrier recovery. Arch Dermatol Res 1999; 291:560–563.
57. Man MQ, Brown BE, Wu-Pong S, Feingold KR, Elias PM. Exogenous nonphysiologic vs physiologic lipids. Arch Dermatol 1995; 131:809–816.
58. Man MQ, Feingold KR, Thornfeld CR, Elias PM. Optimization of physiologic lipid mixtures for barrier repair. J Invest Dermatol 1996; 106:1096–1101.
59. Kitamura K, Yamada K, Ito A, Fukuda M. Research on the mechanism by which dry skin occurs and the development of an effective compound for its treatment. J Soc Cosmet Chem 1995; 29:133–145.
60. Mauro T, Grayson S, Gao WN, Man MQ, Kriehuber E, Behne M, Feingold KR, Elias PM. Barrier recovery is impeded at neutral pH, independent of ionic effects: implications for extracellular lipid processing. Arch Dermatol Res 1998; 290:215–222.
61. Lee SH, Elias PM, Proksch E, Menon GK, Man MQ, Feingold KR. Calcium and potassium are important regulators of barrier homeostasis in murine epidermis. J Clin Invest 1992; 89:530–538.
62. Denda M, Hosoi J, Ashida Y. Visual imaging of ion distribution in human epidermis. Biochem Biophys Res Commun 2000; 272:134–137.
63. Watt FM. Terminal differentiation of epidermal keratinocytes. Curr Opin Cell Biol 1989; 1:1107–1115.
64. Watanabe R, Wu K, Paul P, Marks DL, Kobayashi T, Pittelkow MR, Pagano RE. Upregulation of glucosylceramide synthase expression and activity during human keratinocyte differentiation. J Biol Chem 1998; 273:9651–9655.
65. Menon GK, Price LF, Bommannan B, Elias PM, Feingold KR. Selective obliteration of the epidermal calcium gradient leads to enhanced lamellar body secretion. J Invest Dermatol 1994; 102:789–795.
66. Vicanova J, Boelsma E, Mommas AM, Kempenaar JA, Forslind B, Pallon J, Egelrund T, Koerten HK, Ponec M. Normalization of epidermal calcium distribution profile in reconstructed human epidermis is related to improvement of terminal differentiation and stratum corneum barrier formation. J Invest Dermatol 1998; 111:97–106.
67. Novick P, Brennward P. Friends and family: the role of the Rab GTPases in vesicular traffic. Cell 1993; 75:597–601.

68. Seabra MC, Goldstein JL, Sudhof TC, Brown MS. Rab geranylgeranyl transferase. J Biol Chem 1992; 267:14497–14503.

69. Song HJ, Rossi A, Ceci R, Kim IG, Anzano MA, Jang SI, DeLaurenzi V, Steinert PM. The genes encoding geranylgeranyl transferase a-subunit and transglutaminase I are very closely linked but not functionally related in terminally differentiating keratinocytes. Biochem Biophys Res Commun 1997; 235:10–14.

70. Hanley K, Komuves LG, Ng DC, Schoonjans K, He SS, Lau P, Bikle DD, Williams ML, Elias PM, Auwerx J, Feingold KR. Farnesol stimulates differentiation in epidermal keratinocytes via PPARα. J Biol Chem 2000; 275:11484–11491.

71. Hanley K, Jiang Y, He SS, Friedman M, Elias PM, Bikle DD, Williams ML, Feingold KR. Keratinocyte differentiation is stimulated by activators of the nuclear hormone receptor PPARα. J Invest Dermatol 1998; 111:368–375.

72. Feingold KR. Role of nuclear hormone receptors in regulating epidermal diffrentiation. Program and Preprints of Annual Scientific Seminar. Soc Cosmet Chem 1999; 30–31.

73. Ashida Y, Denda M, Hirao T. Histamine H1 and H2 receptor antagonists accelerate skin barrier repair and prevent epidermal hyperplasia induced by barrier disruption in a dry environment. J Invest Dermatol 2001; 116:261–265.

74. Denda M, Tsuchiya T, Shoji K, Tanida M. Odorant inhalation affects skin barrier homeostasis in mice and humans. Br J Dermatol 2000; 142:1007–1010.

75. Ghadially R, Brown BE, Hanley K, Reed JT, Feingold KR, Elias PM. Decreased epidermal lipid synthesis accounts for altered barrier function in aged mice. J Invest Dermatol 1996; 106:1064–1069.

76. Haratake A, Ikenaga K, Katoh N, Uchiwa H, Hirano S, Yasuho H. Topical mevalonic acid stimulates de novo cholesterol synthesis and epidermal permeability barrier homeostasis in aged mice. J Invest Dermatol 2000; 114:247–252.

12

Clinical Effects of Emollients on Skin

Joachim Fluhr

University of Pavia, San Matteo, Pavia, Italy and
University of California, San Francisco, San Francisco, California

Walter M. Holleran

University of California, San Francisco, San Francisco, California

Enzo Berardesca

University of Pavia, San Matteo, Pavia, Italy

1 INTRODUCTION

Emollients play a central role in topical treatments in dermatology, with their protective and curative effects being of renewed interest. Different therapeutic functions of dermatological emollients are well recognized, and a review of such has recently been published [1]. Research has shown that the composition of emollients is of great importance for disease treatment. For example, the more chronic the cutaneous disease is regarded, the higher the emollient lipid content should be, as treatment efficacy is improved with the use of adequate emollients. However, the specific role of emollients in drug delivery systems for different skin diseases has not yet been studied in detail. In this chapter a number of features of emollients will be presented, including emollient composition, classification, and role in therapeutics; potential mechanisms of emollient function; and the role(s) of emollients in epidermal barrier function and specific diseases. Recent studies have shown that the use of an appropriate emollient for the treatment of specific skin disorders can have a significant impact on both the clinical outcome of treatment and, more importantly, on the relapse-free period. The chosen emollient should no longer be regarded simply as a drug carrier, vehicle, or delivery system, but rather as an essential component of successful topical treatment. Thus, it may be of importance to adapt the type and composition of emollients either as adjuvant treatment or as the delivery system, according to the disease status.

2 BASIC EMOLLIENT CLASSIFICATION

Emollients can be divided into different classes according their composition.

However, the classification of commercially available products is often difficult or impossible based solely upon product labeling. For example, the listed specification for the emulsion systems is commonly abbreviated either as O/W, to delineate oil in water, or W/O, to delineate water in oil. Thus, the amount of water, and conversely oil, in the different emulsion systems usually is not specified. Therefore, for the purposes of dermatological compounding, pharmacopoeia formulations are sometimes more suitable than commercially available emollients, as the specific components can be identified and modulated according to specific disease requirements. Some specific formulation examples are described throughout this text.

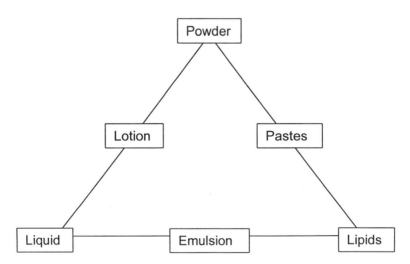

FIGURE 1 Shows a phase triangle regarding dermatological compounds. Such a classification has been useful in order to facilitate the choice of an emollient for specific skin diseases and the state of the disease, e.g., in atopic dermatitis.

2.1 Hydrogel Emollients

The first class of emollients, the hydrogels, itself can be divided into two groups: (1) surface-active hydrogels that produce a thin film at the surface and (2) carbomer-gels, which penetrate or act in deeper parts of the skin [1]. In general, the penetration rate of either type of hydrogel can be enhanced increasing the amount of isopropanol in the composition. However, the carbomer-hydrogels are rarely used as dermatological therapeutics, as they deliver the active compounds in deeper parts as, e.g., in heparin-containing sports-gels. For preservation reasons the carbomer-hydrogels also contain larger amounts of ethanol, isopropanol, or preservatives. Different amounts and types of polyethyleneglycol characterize an additional group of hydrogel emollients. These emollients are especially useful for antiseptic and antifungal preparations.

2.2 Oil-in-Water Emollients

Emollients usually are presented in the form of lotions (O/W emulsions) or creams which are characterized by a hydrophilic external phase. As such, O/W emulsions are the most frequently used emollient type for commercial topical dermatologics. They have excellent absorption qualities and are readily formulated into cosmetically elegant products. Due to their relatively high water content, the O/W emollients exert a cooling effect as free water is liberated following topical application.

2.3 Water-in-Oil Emollients

Conversely, W/O emulsions are characterized by a lipophilic external phase. In these preparations, the lipid phase consists primarily of petrolatum and/or paraffin oil to which other lipid fractions may or may not be added. The more lipid-rich formulations are used in chronic dermatological disease in the nonacute phase, skin conditions where a lack of skin hydration and skin plasticity as well as an increased scaling can be observed, e.g., in eczematous skin conditions.

2.4 Amphiphilic Emollients

Amphiphilic creams, which contain both W/O and O/W characteristics, can be mixed with either lipophilic or hydrophilic (e.g., aqueous) compounds and may be useful for a wider range of formulations. An example of a common amphiphilic creme is given in the German Pharmacopoeia (Deutscher Arzneimittel Codex; DAC) as follows [2]:

Base cream DAC	
Glycerol monostearate 60	4.0
Cetyl alcohol	6.0

Mid-chain triglycerides	7.5
White petrolatum	25.5
Macrogol-1000-glycerol monostearate	7.0
Propylene glycol	10.0
Purified water	40.0

3 SPECIFIC EFFECTS OF EMOLLIENTS

Emollients exert a number of effects in and on the skin, including skin hydration, skin cooling, and lipidization. As mentioned, the relative cooling effect of emollients can be attributed to the amount of water and/or alcohol in the emulsion system(s). This effect is more pronounced when an aqueous or alcohol phase is present within the external phase of the formulation, e.g., in lotions, hydrogels, or O/W emulsions. However, relatively nonstable W/O emulsions, like cold creams, also can exert mild cooling effect(s) when applied topically to the skin [3].

Emollients also are well known to influence the hydration of the stratum corneum, for which at least three different mechanism have been proposed:

1. The emollient can exert a direct hydrating effect by liberating water from the formulation itself [4]. In short-term applications, this hydrating effect is more pronounced with formulations containing a high percentage of water when compared with lipid-rich and low-water-containing preparations [5]. As expected, the hydrating effect of O/W systems in short-term applications depends primarily on the water content of the formulation [3], since only the presence of unbound water insures hydration of the stratum corneum. In contrast, long-term applications of either W/O or O/W emulsions with different water content revealed hydration of the stratum corneum with the W/O but not with the O/W emulsions [6]. Thus, although a W/O emulsion may be cosmetically less acceptable, such a formulation can be expected to achieve better stratum corneum hydration, especially with prolonged use.

2. The occlusive effect of the formulation can influence stratum corneum hydration, especially in long-term applications. A standard model for this occlusion effect is petrolatum [5], for which the highest occlusive effect was detected [3]. Water-in-oil emulsions with low water content have occlusive effects similar to petrolatum, while W/O emulsions with high water content have occlusive properties similar to O/W emulsions [3]. Interestingly, even O/W formulations with high water content can exert an occlusive effect after the unbound water evaporates. However, the occlusive effects of each of these formulations are not always desirable. For example, in atopic dermatitis, where a for-

mulation with high lipid content is desired, an occlusive effect may enhance discomfort and induce itching response. The occlusive effects also may enhance drug penetration, an effect that may or may not be desired.

3. A third mechanism by which emollients influence skin hydration is evident when highly hygroscopic compounds like glycerol are applied. By absorbing water either from the emollient itself, from surface water, or from water evaporation, these agents then are able to increase stratum corneum hydration [7,8].

In addition, emollients can exert a lipidizing or "greasing" effect that is of great importance in skin conditions were patients express discomfort due to cracked or rigid skin. It has been suggested that this lipidization effect be of major importance to the plasticity of the skin [9]. Moreover, lipid-rich formulations improve skin distensibility, while creams and gels with lower lipid content have a more pronounced effect on skin hydration, as previously discussed [9]. The emollient greasing effect appears to be limited to the application period and is not a long-term effect.

Finally, it should be noted that compounds with distinct dielectric constants have been shown to influence the electrophysical properties of the stratum corneum as measured by capacitance- or conductance-based instruments [10]. Thus, it is plausible that topically applied moisturizing creams might be a source of false-positive results using these instruments [11]. Although a good correlation between capacitance values and water content of the tested creams has been demonstrated [11], a sufficient time lag following application of compounds should be allotted before any such measurements are registered.

4 BARRIER PROTECTION AND BARRIER RECOVERY

A number of factors are involved with determining the effectiveness of emollients to protect skin barrier. Commonly used barrier creams, which are either W/O emulsions or emollients with lipophilic character, are claimed to protect against hydrophilic irritants. On the other hand, barrier creams that are O/W emulsion systems, or that act like hydrophilic systems, are thought to protect against lipophilic irritants. Dermatological skin protection (especially in work conditions) is based on different product groups in situations where barrier or protective creams are employed. For example, pre-exposure skin care includes the use of O/W and W/O emulsions, tannery substances, zinc oxide, talcum, perfluorpolyethers, chelating agents, and UV protectors [12]. However, cleansing products and postexposure skin care are two other important components of skin protection. Postexposure skin care is based on emollients, moisturizers, humectants, and lipid-rich formulations. Although claimed protective effects have been shown using specific test conditions, double-blind, placebo-controlled, randomized trials are still lacking, especially under conditions that approximate real workplace situations [12]. In fact, cumulative stress tests with repetitive application of irritants appear to be the best conditions for approximating work conditions [13–19].

The distinction between skin protection and skin care is not always clear. For example, in nurses a barrier cream was compared with its emollient vehicle for effects on clinical improvement. Interestingly, both clinical skin status and stratum corneum hydration improved significantly in each treatment group, without evidence of a difference between the emollient and the barrier cream groups [20]. Thus, the emollient or vehicle alone often shows a significant improvement of the clinical skin conditions as well as the stratum corneum hydration. Thus Berndt and colleagues proposed that a strict distinction between skin care and skin protection products should not be maintained [20]. Correct instructions for the consumer should be stressed with regard to regular and frequent application of a protection product in order to be effective [21]. In addition, a recent study discussed whether claims could be made with respect to protective and preventive properties of topically applied body lotions and barrier creams [22]. In this particular study, enhanced stratum corneum hydration, improved barrier function, as well as a faster barrier recovery were reported after sodium lauryl sulfate (SLS) barrier disruption [22].

Exposure to tensides represents a common potential workplace irritant. Protection against tensides seems to be more effective with lipid-enriched emollients, such as W/O emulsions [23,24]. In contrast, Held and colleagues showed that a 4-week pretreatment of normal skin with W/O emollients increases susceptibility to detergents (sodium lauryl sulfate) [25]. Thus the long-term application of barrier creams in working conditions where detergents are present should be carefully evaluated.

Clinical observations have established that skin irritants are more harmful in dry skin conditions. Thus emollients often are used to increase the water content of the stratum corneum as a preventive measure [26]. Moisturizer-containing emollients prevent irritant skin reactions induced by detergents and may also accelerate regeneration of barrier function in irritated skin [27]. Emollients with moisturizing properties usually contain either singly or in combination humectants, such as urocanic acid, ammonia, lactic acid, pyrrolidone carboxylic acid, urea, citrate, glycerol, sorbitol, and hydroxyacids. These agents belong to a group called natural moisturizing factors (NMF), or moisturizers. Their common properties include the increase of hydration and the enhancement of water-binding capacity in the upper stratum corneum. Reduced NMF content in the stratum corneum can diminish water-absorption capacity and may result in perturbation of corneodesmolysis leading to hyperkeratosis [28].

Emollients with barrier properties also can prevent certain types of epidermal damage. For example, Fartasch and colleagues have shown that alterations of the lower part of stratum corneum and damage to the nucleated layers of the epidermis are induced by sodium lauryl sulfate [29]. In this model, formation of lamellar lipid membrane structures was disturbed in the lower stratum corneum. In contrast, the upper stratum corneum showed intact intercellular lipid bilayers. The barrier disruption effect of SLS was prevented by the application of a barrier cream (discussed in more detail subsequently), with diminished sodium lauryl sulfate penetration as the likely mechanism [29].

4.1 Emollients in Atopic Dermatitis

The utility of emollients in the treatment of atopic dermatitis is well recognized. In atopic dermatitis stratum corneum, hydration and water-binding capacity are reduced [30–32], and impaired barrier function is readily observed in involved skin [30,33]. These patients also are more prone to develop an irritant contact dermatitis [34] and show less pronounced so-called hardening effect than healthy control patients, i.e., with repeated skin barrier disruption, the barrier deterioration stopped after a certain time, suggesting that the stratum corneum accommodates the barrier insults [35]. In atopic dermatitis stratum corneum, the content of barrier lipids is reduced, most prominently that of ceramide 1 and ceramide 3 [33,36]. This reduction of ceramide levels may result form the overaction of a sphingomyelin deacylase enzyme [37,38]. However, sebaceous gland activity, the role of which remains unknown, also is reduced in these patients [39]. Moreover, in atopic dermatitis stratum corneum the membrane-coating granules, or lamellar bodies, are incompletely extruded and organized. This, along with the altered stratum corneum lipid content, may partly explain the impaired barrier function in these patients [40].

Thus, ideal emollients for patients with atopic dermatitis should

Improve barrier function
Have protective properties
Improve stratum corneum hydration
Have an antibacterial active compound (e.g., *Staph. aureus*)

These demands can be met by emollients

Showing W/O emulsions properties with a high water content [24]
Containing a moisturizer (e.g., glycerol, urea) [7,41]
Having a physiological lipid mixture [42–44]
Containing an antiseptically active compound (e.g., triclosan) [45,46]

In this regard, urea-containing emollients were able to improve skin barrier function and to reduce skin susceptibility to irritants within patients suffering from atopic dermatitis [41]. Evening primrose oil (20%) in a W/O emulsion (but not in an amphiphilic emulsion system) also improved barrier function and stratum corneum hydration in atopic patients [47].

Some examples of useful formulations for water-rich W/O emollients for patients with atopic dermatitis are as follows [1]:

W/O emulsion I

Urea	5.0
Glycerol 85%	10.0
Triclosan	3.0
Eucerinum W/O emollient*	ad 100.0

W/O emulsion II

Urea	5.0
Glycerol 85%	10.0
Triclosan	3.0
Pionier KWH Pharm†	30.0
Citric acid anhydr.	0.07
Magnesium sulfate heptahydrate	0.5
Purified water	ad 100.0

W/O emulsion III

Glycerol 85%	22.0
Triclosan	4.4
Excipial U Lipolotio§	ad 220.0

These emollients have shown good stability for more than 3 months [1] and can be used for compounding other active ingredients like evening primrose oil or pale sulfonated shale oil (in W/O emulsion I). As a note of caution, formulations intended for facial use should avoid urea due to its irritative potency and potential [48].

For patients showing allergic reactions to constituents of emollients [49] (e.g., patients with a long history of leg ulcers [50]), fragrances, lanolin, cetyl-

---

*Beiersdorf, Hamburg, Germany.
†Hansen & Rosenthal, Germany: mineral oil 77.9%, polyglyceryl-3-isostearate 10.0%, isopropyl palmitate 8.0%, polyethylene 4.1%.
§Spirig AG, Egerkingen, Switzerland: containing 4% urea and Triclosan.

stearyle alcohol, and parabens should be avoided, if possible. In such instances, the following emollient can be recommended [1]:

Cold cream

Cytylwaxester	11.75
Bccswax	13.5
Paraffin oil	63.25
Purified water	11.50

5 ROLE OF LANOLIN IN EMOLLIENTS

Lanolin, or wool wax, is the secretion product of sebaceous glands of sheep and serves to impregnate and protect the wool fibres. Commercially available lanolin is commonly a mixture of wool wax (65–75%), water (20–30%), and paraffin (up to 15%). Wool wax contains mainly sterol esters, ester waxes, hydroxyesters, and lanolin alcohols (6–12%), with about 40% of the esters containing α-hydroxyesters. However, the exact number of different esters is yet unknown.

Moreover, the sensitization potential of lanolin remains still under discussion [51]. Clark has proposed a reduction or purification of lanolin alcohols in order to minimize the risk of sensitization [52,53]. Interestingly, an epidemiological study revealed that lanolin-induced allergies occur in less than 0.001% of individuals, i.e., less than ten per million [54], while a recent studies showed higher percentage of positive test reactions in children with atopic dermatitis (1.7 and 4.4%) [55,56]. The population of the pediatric studies [50,51] was much more selected than the population in the epidemiological study [50]. Kligman suggests that most of the lanolin sensitization cases represent false-positive results, and thus wool wax–containing products can be considered safe [51].

Lanolin has known moisturizing properties [57], similar to petrolatum, with long-term effects that can be detected up to 14 days after termination of treatment [57]. The hydrating effect of lanolin has been shown using electrophysical measurements [58,59]. While lanolin penetrates into the stratum corneum, it remains concentrated in the upper layers [60]. Compared with vehicle, topically applied lanolin accelerated barrier recovery following an acute barrier disruption with acetone [61]; 3% lanolin significantly reduced trans-epidermal water loss both 45 min and 4 hr following disruption. Moreover, the immediate effect of lanolin on barrier recovery was pronounced. In fact, the positive barrier effect of lanolin was comparable to that of an optimized ratio of stratum corneum lipids, i.e., a barrier formulation (to be discussed in more detail) including cholesterol, ceramides, essential fatty acids, and nonessential fatty acids in a ratio 3:1:1:1 [42,44,61]. Finally, skin roughness is positively influenced by formulations containing lanolin in a dose-dependent manner [62]. Thus, although the exact nature of contact sensitization against lanolin has not been revealed, the positive effects of this compound appear to far outweigh the allergic risk potential.

6 PETROLATUM AS EMOLLIENT MODEL

Petrolatum (petroleum jelly) is regarded as a standard emollient and is widely used in both therapeutic and cosmetic applications. Petrolatum is a purified material obtained from petroleum consisting of a variety of long chain aliphatic hydrocarbons. It has been used in skin care since the late 19th century, yet is still listed in the current pharmacopoeia (e.g., in the United States and Germany). In practical dermatology petrolatum is used either as vehicle for patch testing or drug delivery and as an adjuvant emollient.

Usually, petrolatum does not contain significant water and as such has a long stability. It is considered to be an inert emollient with no direct irritation effect. Petrolatum is frequently used as vehicle for patch testing, representing the classic vehicle for lipophilic compounds in this setting. Petrolatum-based formulations have shown excellent stability, as there is no or only little change in incorporated compound concentrations in petrolatum. The remarkable value and long shelf-life of petrolatum are derived both from its oxidation-resistant properties and from the minimal chemical degradation petrolatum compounds undergo [63].

Petrolatum can be used as drug delivery system especially for lipophilic agents, but also in liposomal formulations [64]. When applied topically, petrolatum itself penetrates only the very superficial layers of the stratum corneum. The most important property of petrolatum is its moisturization of the stratum corneum, attributable to its relative occlusive effects (as discussed previously) [3,65]. As such, petrolatum is considered a standard emollient for comparative testing of hydration and barrier repair [66].

The hydration effect of petrolatum on the stratum corneum has been measured by a number of noninvasive methods, including capacitance, conductance, optothermal infrared spectrometry, and trans-epidermal water loss [3,5,9,59,67, 68]. In many studies petrolatum is used as positive standard to demonstrate the reduction of trans-epidermal water loss. Petrolatum is regarded as one of the most potent occlusive emollients [3,5]. Ghadially and colleagues reported an accelerated barrier recovery after barrier disruption using topical petrolatum [69]. In this study, penetration of petrolatum throughout the stratum corneum interstices was evident, allowing normal or even accelerated barrier recovery despite its occlusive properties [69]. Figure 2 shows a significantly accelerated barrier recovery of petrolatum-treated human skin following acute barrier disruption at 6, 24, and 48 hr [69].

As seen in Fig. 3 petrolatum-treated skin revealed large quantities of flocculent, moderately electron-dense material limited to the stratum corneum inter-

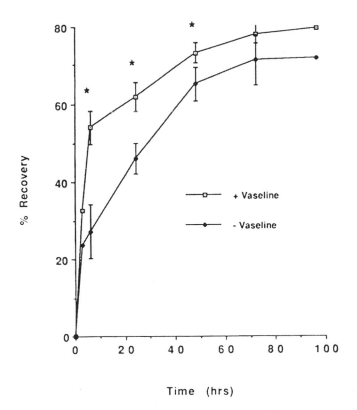

FIGURE 2 Petrolatum accelerates barrier recovery rates after repeated applications of petrolatum following acute barrier disruption with acetone in humans. Values are given in mean +/– standard error of the mean (n = 5); *p < 0.05 with the paired t test. (From Ref. 69.)

cellular spaces and extending to the lower layers of the stratum corneum. Figure 4 gives further information about the relation of topically applied petrolatum to the intercellular lamellar bilayers in the stratum corneum. In some cases lead-labeled petrolatum itself showed a lamellar structure [69].

In addition, a petrolatum-based barrier cream for hand dermatitis has shown positive results [70]. Moreover, a petrolatum-containing cream showed a decrease in bacteria colonization and a reduced frequency of dermatitis in premature infants [71]. The reported comedogenicity of petrolatum remains controversial, as the rabbit ear model used in the studies on this topic does not accurately predict skin conditions in humans [72–74]. Thus, it is clear that the dermatologic utility of petrolatum remains high, with new uses being developed regularly.

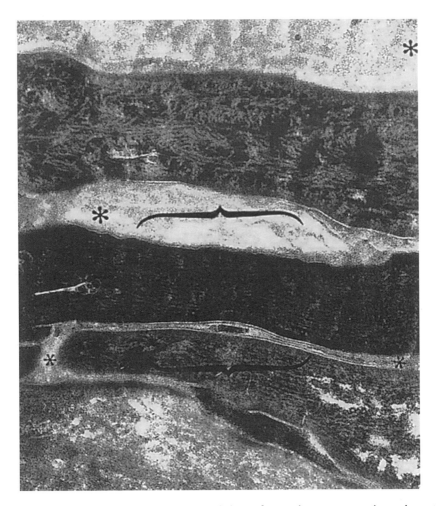

FIGURE 3 Ruthenium tetroxide staining of petrolatum treated murine stratum corneum. Expansion of intercellular space (brackets) is filled with flocculent, amorphous material at several levels within the stratum corneum (*). (×60,000). (From Ref. 69.)

For example, Morrison reports that a number of recent patents claim utility of petrolatum for different skin care products, including one for treatment of diaper rash, a moisturizing bar with soap containing petrolatum as a major component, a skin care product to reduce wrinkles, and products for moisturization and skin conditioning [63]. Recent publications using disposable diapers designed to deliver a petrolatum-based formulation continuously to the skin also have shown significant reductions in severity of erythema and diaper rash [75,76].

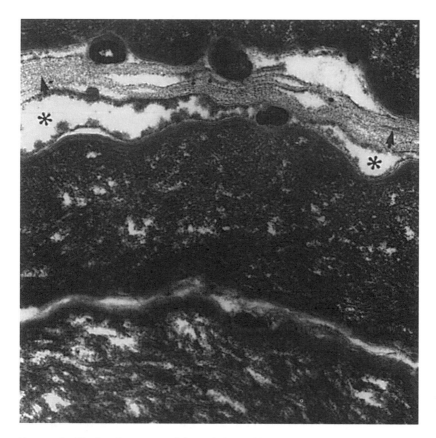

FIGURE 4   Ruthenium tetroxide staining of lead-containing, petrolatum-treated murine stratum corneum. Note expansion of intercellular space by large amounts of nonlamellar, flocculent material (*), with lamellar bilayers displaced to one side of intercellular spaces. Additionally lead deposits decorating lamellar bilayers can be noticed (arrows) (×80,000). (From Ref. 69.)

7   ROLE OF PHYSIOLOGICAL LIPIDS IN EMOLLIENT FORMULATIONS

The barrier function of the skin is mediated by intercellular bilayers in the stratum corneum. Cholesterol, ceramides, and essential and nonessential fatty acids play key roles in the formation of these bilayers [77,78]. Stratum corneum lipids are composed of about 40% ceramides, 25% cholesterol, and 20% free fatty acids (by weight) [78]. Taking the average molecular weight of these three lipid classes into account, the normal stratum corneum has an approximately equimolar physiologic ratio of ceramides, cholesterol, and free fatty acids. Following barrier disruption in hairless mice, epidermal cholesterol and fatty acid syntheses are immediately increased, while increased ceramide production is evident about 6 hr later [77,79–81]. These key barrier lipids are delivered to the intercellular space of the stratum corneum as a mixture of precursors by the extrusion of lamellar body content at the stratum granulosum–stratum corneum interface [82,83]. Fusion of the extruded lamellar contents within the lower stratum corneum leads to continuous membrane sheets, which ultimately form mature membrane bilayer structures [82,84]. The final membrane structural transformation correlates with changes in lipid composition, i.e., the polar lipid precursors (glycosphingolipids, phospholipids, and cholesterol sulfate) are metabolized to more nonpolar lipid products [77,83]. (See Fig. 5.)

Topical application of physiologic lipids has distinct effects from those of nonphysiologic lipids like petrolatum. For example, studies have shown that topical application of only one or two of the three physiologic lipids to a disrupted hairless mouse skin impedes rather than facilitates barrier recovery, evidenced by changes in trans-epidermal water loss [79]. However, if members of all three key lipid classes (i.e., cholesterol, ceramide, and free fatty acid or their precursors) are applied together to barrier-disrupted skin, normalized rates of barrier repair are observed [42,79]. The topically applied physiologic lipids not only are concentrated in the stratum corneum membrane domains, but also are delivered to the nucleated layers of the epidermis [42,79]. Depending on the composition of the lipid mixture, either normal or abnormal lamellar bodies are formed, ultimately resulting in either normal or abnormal lamellar membrane unit structures in the stratum corneum intercellular spaces [42,79]. The process of passive lipid transport across the stratum corneum as well as the uptake into nucleated cells (stratum granulosum). The subsequent reorganization of lamellar unit structures takes about 2 hr after acute barrier disruption in murine epidermis [79,82]. It appears

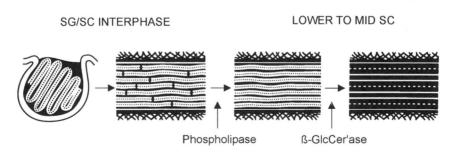

SG/SC INTERPHASE   LOWER TO MID SC

Phospholipase   ß-GlcCer'ase

FIGURE 5 Lamellar body exocytosis and end-to-end fusion of lamellar body–derived sheets to uninterrupted plasma membranes, and subsequent compaction of adjacent membrane sheets into lamellar bilayer unit structures. These changes correlate with extracellular lipid processing of polar lipids to nonpolar lipids. These steps are required in order to form the intercellular bilayer structures. (From Ref. 85.)

that the incorporation of applied physiologic lipids into barrier lipids follows two pathways: (1) direct incorporation into stratum corneum membrane domains and (2) lipids appear to traverse the intercellular route in the stratum corneum and ultimately get incorporated in at lower stratum granulosum cells. The intercellular lipids then appear able to enter the nucleated cells, incorporate into the appropriate lipid metabolic pathway(s), and ultimately utilize the lamellar body delivery system to re-enter the intercellular membrane domains [42]. Topically applied lipids to either intact or acetone-treated skin did not downregulate the physiological lipid synthesis [86,42]. These studies support the hypothesis that the epidermis can internalize and process physiologic lipids (Fig. 6).

In contrast, nonphysiologic lipids like petrolatum appear to simply form a bulk hydrophobic phase in the stratum corneum intercellular spaces to restore the barrier under similar conditions [42,69]. The same studies showed further enhancement of barrier recovery if the proportion of one of the fatty acids (linoleic

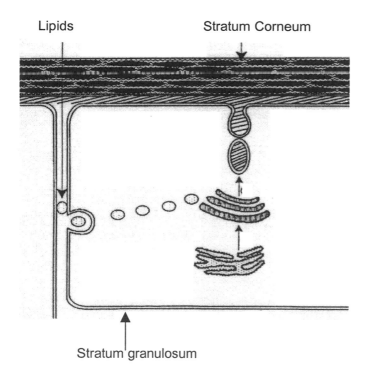

Lipids   **Stratum Corneum**

Stratum granulosum

FIGURE 6   Putative route of incorporation and processing of exogenous physiologic lipids within cells of the outermost granular layer. Exogenous lipids may be delivered by an endocytic pathway to the transgolgi complex. These lipids become available for the lamellar body formation. (From Ref. 42.)

acid, palmitic acid, or stearic acid) or the other key species was augmented to threefold in a four-component system, i.e. consisting of fatty acid, ceramide, cholesterol, and essential fatty acids in a 3:1:1:1 ratio [43]. Interestingly, the structural requirements of this lipid mixture are not restricted to essential fatty acids, findings that were confirmed in similarly disrupted human barrier [43]. Also interesting, acylceramides applied as a single agent delayed barrier recovery. However, acylceramides in a mixture with cholesterol (optimum ratio of 1:5:1 or 1:2) also revealed accelerated barrier recovery after acute barrier disruption [43]. Moreover, in another study stratum corneum hydration (measured by conductance) was increased 4 hr after topical application of cholesterol/acylceramide/petrolatum/glycerol-containing vehicle (propylene glycol/ethanol) [87]. These findings were confirmed as accelerated barrier repair was noted using a similar formulation after tape-stripping, solvent treatment, and some types of detergent treatment [88]. Specifically, topical application of the physiologic lipids cholesterol, ceramide, palmitate, and linoleate in the ratio of 4.3:2.3:1:1.08 showed enhanced barrier recovery. However, it must be noted that in barrier repair versus hydration studies, correlations between moisturizing properties and barrier repair mechanism of applied lipid mixtures are not always evident. Actually, the best hydrating lipid composition is often different from the optimal barrier repair formulation and vice versa [87].

8   CONCLUSIONS

In this chapter different roles of emollients have been presented, including emollient classification, with some examples of compounded emollients and specific effects of emollients with special focus on barrier protection and barrier recovery. An extended discussion was presented on the special functions of lanolin, petrolatum, and physiological lipids in emollient formulation. Choosing the appropriate emollient for the treatment of different skin diseases may have a high impact on the clinical outcome of a treatment and even more on the relapse-free period. The chosen emollient should no longer be regarded simply as a drug carrier or vehicle or drug delivery system but as an essential part of topical treatment. Thus it may be of importance to adapt type and composition of the emollient according to the evolution of the disease either as an adjuvant treatment or as drug delivery system, especially in dermatological prescriptions. This review may help in a better understanding of specific function(s) of emollients and enable an evidence-based use of different emollient types and compositions.

REFERENCES

1.   Gloor M, Thoma K, Fluhr J. Dermatologische Externatherapie. Berlin: Springer-Verlag, 2000.

2. Deutscher Arzneimittel-Codex. Eschborn: Govi Verlag, 1999.

3. Lehmann L, Gloor M, Schlierbach S, Gehring W. Stabilität und Okklusivität von Externagrundlagen auf der Haut. Z Hautkr 1997; 872:585–590.

4. Blichmann CW, Serup J, Winther A. Effects of single application of a moisturizer: evaporation of emulsion water, skin surface temperature, electrical conductance, electrical capacitance, and skin surface (emulsion) lipids. Acta Derm Venereol 1989; 69:327 330.

5. Loden M. The increase in skin hydration after application of emollients with different amounts of lipids. Acta Derm Venereol 1992; 72:327–330.

6. Fluhr JW, Vrzak G, Gloor M. Hydratisierender und die Steroidpenetration modifizierender Effekt von Harnstoff und Glycerin in Abhängigkeit von der verwendeten Grundlage. Z Hautkr 1997; 73:210–214.

7. Fluhr JW, Gloor M, Lehmann L, Lazzerini S, Distante F, Berardesca E. Glycerol accelerates recovery of barrier function in vivo. Acta Derm Venereol 1999; 79:418–421.

8. Batt M, Fairhust E. Haydration of the stratum corneum. J Cosmet Sci 1986; 8.

9. Jemec GB, Wulf HC. Correlation between the greasiness and the plasticizing effect of moisturizers. Acta Derm Venereol 1999; 79:115–117.

10. Fluhr JW, Gloor M, Lazzerini S, Kleesz P, Grieshaber R, Berardesca E. Comparative study of five instruments measuring stratum corneum hydration (Corneometer CM 820 and CM 825, Skicon 200, Nova DPM 90003, DermLab). Part I. In vitro. Skin Res Technol 1999; 5:161–170.

11. Jemec GB, Na R, Wulf HC. The inherent capacitance of moisturising creams: a source of false positive results? Skin Pharmacol Appl Skin Physiol 2000; 13:182–187.

12. Wigger-Alberti W, Elsner P. Barrier creams and emollients. In: Kanerva L, Elsner P, Wahlberg JE, Maibach HI, eds. Handbook of Occupational Dermatology. Berlin: Springer, 2000:490–496.

13. Grunewald AM, Gloor M, Gehring W, Kleesz P. Damage to the skin by repetitive washing. Contact Dermatitis 1995; 32:225–232.

14. Wigger-Alberti W, Hinnen U, Elsner P. Predictive testing of metalworking fluids: a comparison of 2 cumulative human irritation models and correlation with epidemiological data. Contact Dermatitis 1997; 36:14–20.

15. Wigger-Alberti W, Rougier A, Richard A, Elsner P. Efficacy of protective creams in a modified repeated irritation test. Methodological aspects. Acta Derm Venereol 1998; 78:270–273.

16. Wigger-Alberti W, Krebs A, Elsner P. Experimental irritant contact dermatitis due to cumulative epicutaneous exposure to sodium lauryl sulphate and toluene: single and concurrent application. Br J Dermatol 2000; 143:551–556.

17. Frosch PJ, Kurte A. Efficacy of skin barrier creams. IV. The repetitive irritation test (RIT) with a set of 4 standard irritants. Contact Dermatitis 1994; 31:161–168.

18. Frosch PJ, Kurte A, Pilz B. Efficacy of skin barrier creams. III. The repetitive irritation test (RIT) in humans. Contact Dermatitis 1993; 29:113–118.

19. Frosch PJ, Schulze-Dirks A, Hoffmann M, Axthelm I, Kurte A. Efficacy of skin barrier creams. I. The repetitive irritation test (RIT) in the guinea pig. Contact Dermatitis 1993; 28:94–100.

20. Berndt U, Wigger-Alberti W, Gabard B, Elsner P. Efficacy of a barrier cream and its vehicle as protective measures against occupational irritant contact dermatitis. Contact Dermatitis 2000; 42:77–80.
21. Wigger-Alberti W, Maraffio B, Wernli M, Elsner P. Self-application of a protective cream. Pitfalls of occupational skin protection. Arch Dermatol 1997; 133:861–864.
22. de Paepe K, Derde MP, Roseeuw D, Rogiers V. Claim substantiation and efficiency of hydrating body lotions and protective creams. Contact Dermatitis 2000; 42:227–234.
23. Grunewald AM, Gloor M, Gehring W, Kleesz P. Efficacy of barrier creams. Curr Probl Dermatol 1995; 23:187–197.
24. Bettinger J, Gloor M, Gehring W. Influence of a pretreatment with emulsions on the dehydrating effect of the skin by surfactants. Int J Cosm Sci 1994; 16:53–60.
25. Held E, Sveinsdottir S, Agner T. Effect of long-term use of moisturizer on skin hydration, barrier function and susceptibility to irritants. Acta Derm Venereol 1999; 79:49–51.
26. Zhai H, Maibach HI. Moisturizers in preventing irritant contact dermatitis: an overview. Contact Dermatitis 1998; 38:241–244.
27. Ramsing DW, Agner T. Preventive and therapeutic effects of a moisturizer. An experimental study of human skin. Acta Derm Venereol 1997; 77:335–337.
28. Harding CR, Watkinson A, Rawlings AV, Scott IR. Dry skin, moisturization and corneodesmolysis. Int J Cosmet Sci 2000; 22:21–52.
29. Fartasch M, Schnetz E, Diepgen TL. Characterization of detergent-induced barrier alterations—effect of barrier cream on irritation. J Invest Dermatol Symp Proc 1998; 3:121–127.
30. Loden M, Olsson H, Axell T, Linde YW. Friction, capacitance and transepidermal water loss (TEWL) in dry atopic and normal skin. Br J Dermatol 1992; 126:137–141.
31. Thune P. Evaluation of the hydration and the water-holding capacity in atopic skin and so-called dry skin. Acta Derm Venereol 1989; 144(Suppl):133–135.
32. Berardesca E, Fideli D, Borroni G, Rabbiosi G, Maibach H. In vivo hydration and water-retention capacity of stratum corneum in clinically uninvolved skin in atopic and psoriatic patients. Acta Derm Venereol 1990; 70:400–404.
33. Di Nardo A, Wertz P, Giannetti A, Seidenari S. Ceramide and cholesterol composition of the skin of patients with atopic dermatitis. Acta Derm Venereol 1998; 78:27–30.
34. Gehring W, Gloor M, Kleesz P. Predictive washing test for evaluation of individual eczema risk. Contact Dermatitis 1998; 39:8–13.
35. Grunewald AM, Gloor M, Kleesz P. Barrier recompensation mechanisms. Curr Probl Dermatol 1996; 25:206–213.
36. Imokawa G, Abe A, Jin K, Higaki Y, Kawashima M, Hidano A. Decreased level of ceramides in stratum corneum of atopic dermatitis: an etiologic factor in atopic dry skin? J Invest Dermatol 1991; 96:523–526.
37. Hara J, Higuchi K, Okamoto R, Kawashima M, Imokawa G. High expression of sphingomyelin deacylase is an important determinant of ceramide deficiency leading to barrier disruption in atopic dermatitis. J Invest Dermatol 2000; 115:406–413.
38. Higuchi K, Hara J, Okamoto R, Kawashima M, Imokawa G. The skin of atopic der-

matitis patients contains a novel enzyme, glucosylceramide sphingomyelin deacy-lase, which cleaves the N-acyl linkage of sphingomyelin and glucosylceramide. Biochem J 2000; 350:747–756.

39. Wirth H, Gloor M, Stoika D. Sebaceous glands in uninvolved skin of patients suffering from atopic dermatitis. Arch Dermatol Res 1981; 270:167–169.

40. Fartasch M, Diepgen TL. The barrier function in atopic dry skin. Disturbance of membrane coating granule exocytosis and formation of epidermal lipids? Acta Derm Venereol 1992; 176(Suppl):26–31.

41. Loden M, Andersson AC, Lindberg M. Improvement in skin barrier function in patients with atopic dermatitis after treatment with a moisturizing cream (Canoderm). Br J Dermatol 1999; 140:264–267.

42. Mao-Qiang M, Brown BE, Wu-Pong S, Feingold KR, Elias PM. Exogenous non-physiologic vs physiologic lipids. Divergent mechanisms for correction of perme-ability barrier dysfunction. Arch Dermatol 1995; 131:809–816.

43. Man MM, Feingold KR, Thornfeldt CR, Elias PM. Optimization of physiological lipid mixtures for barrier repair. J Invest Dermatol 1996; 106:1096–1101.

44. Man MQ, Feingold KR, Elias PM. Exogenous lipids influence permeability barrier recovery in acetone-treated murine skin. Arch Dermatol 1993; 129:728–738.

45. Gehring W, Forssman T, Jost G, Gloor M. Die keimreduzierende Wirkung von Erythromycin und Triclosan bei atopischer Dermatitis. Akt Dermatol 1996; 22:28–31.

46. Sugimoto K, Kuroki H, Kanazawa M, Kurosaki T, Abe H, Takahashi Y, Ishiwada N, Nezu Y, Hoshioka A, Toba T. New successful treatment with disinfectant for atopic dermatitis. Dermatology 1997; 195(Suppl 2):62–68.

47. Gehring W, Bopp R, Rippke F, Gloor M. Effect of topically applied evening prim-rose oil on epidermal barrier function in atopic dermatitis as a function of vehicle. Arzneimittelforschung 1999; 49:635–642.

48. Agner T. An experimental study of irritant effects of urea in different vehicles. Acta Derm Venereol 1992; 177(Suppl):44–46.

49. Gallenkemper G, Rabe E, Bauer R. Contact sensitization in chronic venous insuffi-ciency: modern wound dressings. Contact Dermatitis 1998; 38:274–278.

50. Pasche-Koo F, Piletta PA, Hunziker N, Hauser C. High sensitization rate to emulsi-fiers in patients with chronic leg ulcers. Contact Dermatitis 1994; 31:226–228.

51. Kligman AM. The myth of lanolin allergy: lanolin is not a contact sensitizer. In: The Lanolin Book. Hamburg: Beiersdorf, 1999:161–175.

52. Clark EW, Cronin E, Wilkinson DS. Lanolin with reduced sensitising potential: a preliminary report. Contact Dermatitis 1977; 3:69–73.

53. Clark EW. The history and evolution of lanolin. In: The Lanolin Book. Hamburg: Beiersdorf, 1999:15–50.

54. Clark EW. Estimation of general incidence of specific lanolin allergy. J Soc Cosmet Chem 1975; 26:323–335.

55. Dotterud LK, Falk ES. Contact allergy in relation to hand eczema and atopic dis-eases in north Norwegian schoolchildren. Acta Paediatr 1995; 84:402–406.

56. Giordano-Labadie F, Rance F, Pellegrin F, Bazex J, Dutau G, Schwarze HP. Fre-quency of contact allergy in children with atopic dermatitis: results of a prospective study of 137 cases. Contact Dermatitis 1999; 40:192–195.

57. Kligman A. Regression method for assessing the efficacy of moisturizers. Cosmet Toil 1978;93:27.
58. Moss J. The effect of three moisturisers on skin surface hydration. Skin Res Technol 1996; 2:32.
59. Petersen EN. The hydrating effect of a cream and white petrolatum measured by optothermal infrared spectrometry in vivo. Acta Derm Venereol 1991; 71:373–376.
60. Clark EW. Short term penetration of lanolin into human stratum corneum. J Soc Cosmet Chem 1992; 43:219.
61. Elias P, Mao-Quiang M, Thornfeldt CR, Feingold KR. The epidermal permeability barrier: effects of physiologic and non-physiologic lipids. In: The Lanolin Book. Hamburg: Beiersdorf, 1999:253–278.
62. Sauermann G, Schreiner V. The skin caring effect of topical products containing lanolin alcohols. In: The Lanolin Book. Hamburg: Beiersdorf, 1999:217–235.
63. Morrison DS. Petrolatum. In: Lodén M, Maibach HI, eds. Dry Skin and Moisturizers. Boca Raton: CRC, 2000:251–257.
64. Foldvari M. Effect of vehicle on topical liposomal drug delivery: petrolatum bases. J Microencapsul 1996; 13:589–600.
65. Lazar AP, Lazar P. Dry skin, water, and lubrication. Dermatol Clin 1991; 9:45–51.
66. O'Goshi KI, Tabata N, Sato Y, Tagami H. Comparative study of the efficacy of various moisturizers on the skin of the ASR miniature swine. Skin Pharmacol Appl Skin Physiol 2000; 13:120–127.
67. Loden M, Lindberg M. The influence of a single application of different moisturizers on the skin capacitance. Acta Derm Venereol 1991; 71:79–82.
68. Pellacani G, Belletti B, Seidenari S. Evaluation of the short-term effects of skin care products: a comparison between capacitance values and echographic parameters of epidermal hydration. Curr Probl Dermatol 1998; 26:177–182.
69. Ghadially R, Halkier-Sorensen L, Elias PM. Effects of petrolatum on stratum corneum structure and function. J Am Acad Dermatol 1992; 26:387–396.
70. Schleicher SM, Milstein HJ, Ilowite R, Meyer P. Response of hand dermatitis to a new skin barrier-protectant cream. Cutis 1998; 61:233–234.
71. Nopper AJ, Horii KA, Sookdeo-Drost S, Wang TH, Mancini AJ, Lane AT. Topical ointment therapy benefits premature infants [see comments]. J Pediatr 1996; 128:660–669.
72. Zimmermann R. [The rabbit ear model as comedogenic test. 3. Histologic and enzyme histochemical studies of the follicle and sebaceous gland epithelium]. Dermatol Monatsschr 1990; 176:55–61.
73. Fulton JE Jr, Pay SR, Fulton JED. Comedogenicity of current therapeutic products, cosmetics, and ingredients in the rabbit ear. J Am Acad Dermatol 1984; 10:96–105.
74. Frank SB. Is the rabbit ear model, in its present state, prophetic of acnegenicity? J Am Acad Dermatol 1982; 6:373–377.
75. Odio MR, O'Connor RJ, Sarbaugh F, Baldwin S. Continuous topical administration of a petrolatum formulation by a novel disposable diaper. 2. Effect on skin condition. Dermatology 2000; 200:238–243.
76. Odio MR, O'Connor RJ, Sarbaugh F, Baldwin S. Continuous topical administration of a petrolatum formulation by a novel disposable diaper. 1. Effect on skin surface microtopography. Dermatology 2000; 200:232–237.

77. Elias PM, Feingold KR. Lipids and the epidermal water barrier: metabolism, regulation, and pathophysiology. Semin Dermatol 1992; 11:176–182.
78. Schurer NY, Elias PM. The biochemistry and function of stratum corneum lipids. Adv Lipid Res 1991; 24:27–56.
79. Mao-Qiang M, Elias PM, Feingold KR. Fatty acids are required for epidermal permeability barrier function. J Clin Invest 1993; 92:791–798.
80. Holleran WM, Man MQ, Gao WN, Menon GK, Elias PM, Feingold KR. Sphingolipids are required for mammalian epidermal barrier function. Inhibition of sphingolipid synthesis delays barrier recovery after acute perturbation. J Clin Invest 1991; 88:1338–1345.
81. Feingold KR, Man MQ, Menon GK, Cho SS, Brown BE, Elias PM. Cholesterol synthesis is required for cutaneous barrier function in mice. J Clin Invest 1990; 86:1738–1745.
82. Menon GK, Feingold KR, Elias PM. Lamellar body secretory response to barrier disruption. J Invest Dermatol 1992; 98:279–289.
83. Elias PM, Menon GK. Structural and lipid biochemical correlates of the epidermal permeability barrier. Adv Lipid Res 1991; 24:1–26.
84. Fartasch M, Bassukas ID, Diepgen TL. Structural relationship between epidermal lipid lamellae, lamellar bodies and desmosomes in human epidermis: an ultrastructural study. Br J Dermatol 1993; 128:1–9.
85. Elias PM. Stratum corneum architecture, metabolic activity and interactivity with subjacent cell layers. Exp Dermatol 1996; 5:191–201.
86. Menon GK, Feingold KR, Moser AH, Brown BE, Elias PM. De novo sterologenesis in the skin. II. Regulation by cutaneous barrier requirements. J Lipid Res 1985; 26:418–427.
87. Thornfeldt C. Critical and optimal molar ratios of key lipids. In: Lodén M, Maibach HI, eds. Dry Skin and Moisturizers. Boca Raton: CRC, 2000.
88. Yang L, Mao-Qiang M, Taljebini M, Elias PM, Feingold KR. Topical stratum corneum lipids accelerate barrier repair after tape stripping, solvent treatment and some but not all types of detergent treatment. Br J Dermatol 1995; 133:679–685.

13

Humectants

Anthony V. Rawlings

Unilever Research, Port Sunlight Laboratory, Bebington, Wirral,
United Kingdom

Clive R. Harding and Allan Watkinson

Unilever Research, Colworth Laboratory, Sharnbrook, Bedford,
United Kingdom

Prem Chandar and Ian R. Scott

Unilever Research, Edgewater Laboratory, Edgewater, New Jersey

1 INTRODUCTION

Dry skin is a complex phenomenon in which the skin can feel rough, tight, and itchy and visibly look "dry" due to the appearance of macroscopic flakes or scale on the skin surface [1]. To understand dry skin, we must first understand the processes taking place both in the epidermis and the stratum corneum, but particularly within the superficial layers of the stratum corneum because this is ultimately where dry skin is manifest. Dry skin results from a perturbation in the process of desquamation, the progressive degradation of the cohesive forces binding the corneocytes of the stratum corneum [2]. In healthy skin, desquamation is a carefully regulated process in which the surface corneocytes are shed in careful balance with the underlying formation of new corneocytes at the stratum granulosum/corneum boundary, without compromising the overall integrity of this critical tissue. Desquamation is not only responsible for maintaining stratum

245

corneum thickness, but by ensuring a continual turnover of corneocytes it also protects against the ever-present damaging effects of the environment. The major event occurring in desquamation is the controlled degradation of the corneodesmosomes, rivet-like protein complexes that, by linking neighboring corneocytes, represent the principal cohesive element of the tissue. Less well-understood changes in lipid organization and phase behavior also play a role in facilitating this process. Under normal conditions, the corneodesmosomes are degraded by proteases, located in the stratum corneum intercellular space, which hydrolyze the binding regions of these structures. (For reviews see Refs. 3 and 4.)

Fundamentally, dry skin occurs when the desquamation process is perturbed and the peripheral corneodesmosomes are not degraded, resulting in an accumulation of cohesive rafts of corneocytes on the skin's surface [5]. These accumulations of surface corneocytes are manifest as dry flaky scale. Probably the major extrinsic factor involved in perturbation of the desquamation process is reduced humidity, although low temperature and UV damage can also precipitate this condition [6]. Low environmental humidity increases the desiccation stress on the outermost layers of the stratum corneum, leading to a reduction in water content. Since the desquamatory enzymes require water for functionality, the reduced water content then leads to a decrease in the activity of these hydrolytic enzymes, perturbed corneodesmosomal hydrolysis resulting in skin scale [7].

Due to the crucial importance of water to the desquamatory process, the most effective treatment for common dry skin ailments is moisturization, a fact initially demonstrated by Irwin Blank in the 1950s [8]. His demonstration that the low moisture content of the skin was the primary factor in causing the dry skin condition was the beginning of moisturization research as we know it.

2 WATER AND THE STRATUM CORNEUM

As the main barrier tissue against the environment, the major role of the stratum corneum is to prevent water loss. This is primarily achieved by the network of organized lipid lamellae surrounding the corneocytes, which are highly effective at reducing water flux through this tissue, although without question the physical presence of the multiple layers of corneocytes play a significant role [9]. Except during water immersion or with total skin occlusion, we are constantly losing water to the atmosphere. However in desiccating conditions, where the external humidity is less than 100%, water will be continuously transferred outward and be lost from the skin. This is referred to as trans-epidermal water loss (TEWL) and is general regarded as a measure of the barrier competency [10,11]. This water loss from the surface of the stratum corneum is replenished from the hydrated tissues below, resulting in a water flux across the skin [12].

Paradoxically, the stratum corneum must not only be an efficient barrier to water loss, but must itself retain water to allow the hydrolytic events essential for maturation together with desquamation and also to maintain tissue plasticity (see later discussion). Water retention in the stratum corneum is achieved primarily due to the presence of high concentration of small hygroscopic molecules, the natural moisturizing factors (NMF) [13]. In addition, it has also been suggested that the polar barrier lipids, the ceramides, also function to retain water within this tissue.

Compared with other "normal" aqueous tissues, the stratum corneum usually contains very little water (5–15% by weight), especially the outer layers. Due to the combined action of the hygroscopic molecules, the stratum corneum has the ability to imbibe five to six times its own weight in water resulting in a general swelling of the tissue. Moreover the resultant hydration of the stratum corneum is dependent on the ambient relative humidity (RH) in a logarithmic relationship. Typical hydration RH curves can be seen in Fig. 1 [14]. The water content of the stratum corneum is also temperature dependent. At a given RH, the water content of the stratum corneum was observed to increase by 50% when the temperature was raised from 20 to 35°C at RH below 60% RH.

The bonding of water within the stratum corneum varies depending on the water content of the tissue. Around 10–15% of water is tightly bound to the polar groups of the structural proteins and is essentially unavailable for hydrolytic

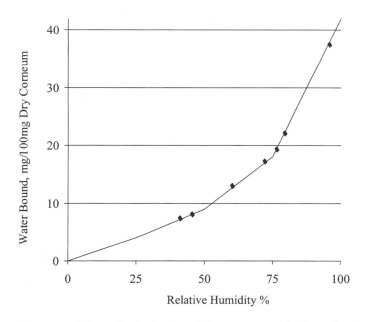

Figure 1 Effect of relative humidity on water binding of guinea pig footpad stratum corneum. (Modified from Ref. 14.)

processes. As the water content increases, the water is less tightly bound; and above about 40% it essentially acts as free bulk water [15].

3 MOISTURIZERS AND HUMECTANTS

It is not surprising, regarding the importance of water to the stratum corneum maturation process that moisturization is still the most effective treatment available for common dry skin. However, despite the importance of water to the desquamatory process and tissue plasticity, topically applied water is in fact a poor treatment for dry skin. It can initially alleviate the signs of dry skin; however, the effect of water in any moisturizing product only provides short-term relief of dry skin (minutes) as it quickly evaporates from the skin's surface and does not address the underlying problem of impaired enzyme activity.

As exogenous water alone is insufficient to moisturize the skin and correct the aberrant desquamatory process, cosmetic treatments to alleviate the condition are required, i.e., moisturizers.

Classically, three approaches can be used to moisturize the stratum corneum: (1) emolliency (to mask the rough scaly condition); (2) occlusion (to reduce water loss from the skin); or (3) humectancy (to help retain water in the skin). The last two routes work by retaining water in the stratum corneum, which would be naturally lost from the body by TEWL. The humectancy route can also attract water to the skin from the outside but only under high humidity conditions. In reality modern commercial moisturizers act by a combination of these effects, normalizing the water content of the upper layers of the stratum corneum and, by increasing enzyme activity, lead to an improvement in the natural exfoliation process and a smoother moisturized skin surface [7]. In this chapter we review the function of humectants and how, by helping to retain water, they affect the biology of the stratum corneum.

Humectants are water-soluble organic compounds, typically polyhydric alcohols (polyols) that can imbibe water. Indeed, these can be thought of as the cosmetic equivalents of the NMF. The most common is glycerol, but other examples include sorbitol, propylene glycerol, butylene glycol, urea, sodium lactate, and sodium pyrollidone carboxylic acid (PCA) (the last three being intrinsic moisturizers produced within the stratum corneum).

The efficacy of humectants can be determined using a simple hygroscopic measurement. The humectant is equilibrated in an atmosphere of defined constant relative humidity and weighed, and the final weight is compared to the value for the dry weight of the humectant, determined after treatment with phosphoric oxide (Table 1). Alternatively, a more realistic method of determining humectancy involves treating samples of stratum corneum with the agent and then incubating under defined humidities and determining water uptake [16]. In both of these assays, the sodium and ammonium salts of PCA and lactic acid are the most effec-

TABLE 1   Hygroscopicity and Water-Holding Capacities of Humectants
(25°C, 50% RH)

Humectant	Hygroscopicity (H_2O mg/100 mg)	Water-Holding Capacity (H_2O mg/100 mg)
DPG[1]	12	8
Sorbitol	1	21
PEG 200[2]	20	22
Glycerin	25	40
Na-PCA[3]	44	60
Na-lactate	56	84

[1]Dipropylene glycerol
[2]Polyethylene glycerol (MW 200)
[3]Sodium pyrrolidone carboxylate
Source: Modified from Ref. 16.

tive humectants, although glycerol is also extremely effective. Nevertheless, as will be outlined later in this chapter a simple humectancy assessment of glycerol fails to emphasise its true value as a highly effective conditioning agent for the skin.

4   EFFECT OF HUMECTANTS ON STRATUM CORNEUM FLEXIBILITY

Originally dry skin was thought to be the result of the mechanical cracking of a dehydrated stratum corneum, and therefore the purpose of water was to influence the plasticization of the skin [8]. We now know that this is a considerable simplification, and the primary precipitating event in the formation of dry skin is the impairment of several hydrolytic events, of which desquamation is the most critical. However, flexibility of the stratum corneum is essential if the permeability barrier is to remain intact. Furthermore, the level of hydration affects the pliability and overall mechanical properties of the stratum corneum. Blank [8] estimated that a concentration of 10% of water in the stratum corneum was the critical level of hydration for pliability and that this could be obtained at 60% relative humidity. We have also demonstrated that stratum corneum extensibility behavior is influenced by relative humidity and that optimal extensibility is related to the cohesive properties of the tissue, which are in turn influenced by the underlying desquamation process. Under low humidity conditions the flexibility of the stratum corneum can sometimes be compromised, and the tissue is potentially susceptible to damage due to mechanical stress [17].

It is the less tightly bound water or the free water, dependent on the presence of natural moisturizing factors and the intercellular lipids, that is responsible for the plasticizing effect on the stratum corneum. Topically applied water alone only provides a temporary effect as it is lost by evaporation from the skin (Fig. 2).

Takahashi et al. [16] have also investigated humectancy and stratum corneum plasticization. They determined that the higher the water-holding capacity, the more the plasticizing effect. In line with the known humectancy, the sodium salts of PCA and lactic acid were more effective than glycerol at 50% RH (Fig. 3). Urea was also effective at plasticizing the stratum corneum, a property which is believed to be related to its well-known hydrogen bond–breaking potential [18]. Similarly, Middelton [19] measured changes in stratum corneum extensibility and water-holding capacity and showed that at 81% RH sodium lactate and sodium PCA were as effective as other moisturizing agents. However, one potential problem with these simple salt humectants is that their imparted benefits are generally lost on washing.

Our own work has focused on the pleiotropic properties of the humectant glycerol. We have demonstrated that at 44% RH glycerol is an effective plasticizer of the stratum corneum (Fig. 4), although at higher humidities glycerol shows no advantage in plasticization effects compared with propylene glycol or sodium

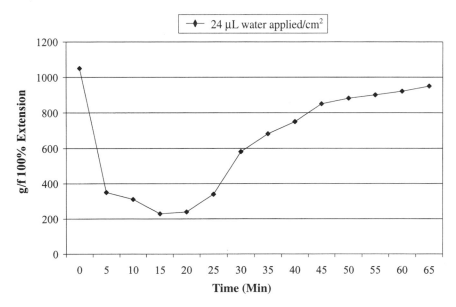

FIGURE 2 Temporary effect of water on plasticization of stratum corneum.

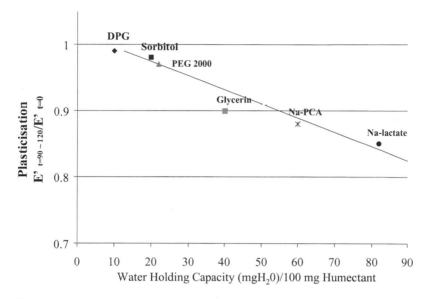

FIGURE 3 Relation between water-holding capacity of humectants and their stratum corneum plasticizing effects. (Modified from Ref. 16.)

lactate. The plasticization effects of glycerol could result from its effects on stratum corneum lipids, although it will also influence protein behavior. However, in our linear extensiometer method we are probably only measuring the influence of glycerol on the lipid lamellae [17]. These properties reflect the ability of glycerol to improve stratum corneum flexibility by breaking hydrogen bonding between the headgroups of adjacent ceramide within the highly organized lipid microenvironment.

5 EFFECT OF HUMECTANTS ON CORNEODESMOSOMES

The topical application of humectants is certainly effective in ameliorating the symptoms of dry skin, but do they function by normalizing the hydrolysis of corneodesmosomes? To examine the effect of glycerol upon this process, we have investigated changes in stratum corneum morphology, changes in the levels of desmoglein 1—a constituent protein of the corneodesmosome which is known to be degraded in desquamation [4]—and finally changes in the desquamatory potential of the stratum corneum following treatment [7].

Electron microscopy studies revealed that extensive corneodesmosome degradation occurred in the stratum corneum incubated under a variety of hu-

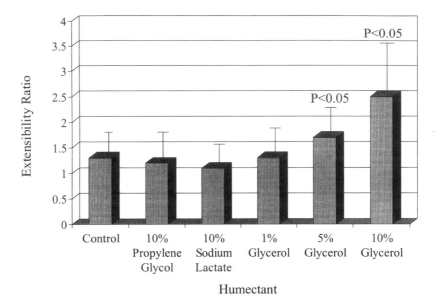

FIGURE 4   Effect of humectants on stratum corneum plasticization at 44% RH.

midities. At high humidity (Fig. 5b), corneodesmosomes were clearly in various stages of degradation, whereas at low humidity (Fig. 5a), degradation was less obvious. The application of lotions containing glycerol to tissue samples incubated at high humidity was seen to further increase corneodesmosomal degradation. In such samples it was difficult to locate the electron-dense corneodesmosomal structures within tissue sections (Fig. 5c), although such structures were readily observed in untreated tissue or tissue incubated at low humidity (Fig. 5a). However, glycerol lotions had no effect on increasing desmosomal degradation under conditions of low humidity (data not shown). To quantify corneodesmosome digestion, the number and type of corneodesmosomes (arbitrarily designated as either "fully-intact"—electron-dense structures closely associated with corneocyte envelopes—or "partially-degraded"—structures with electron-lucent areas and/or separated from corneocyte envelopes) were determined in 20 representative electron micrographs for each treatment. Although the total number of corneodesmosomes counted per unit area was not largely affected by the differing humidities, there was a clear indication of advanced corneodesmosomal digestion at the higher humidity. At 44% RH the mean number of intact electron-dense corneodesmosomes was found to increase three- to fourfold when compared to tissues incubated at 80% RH. In control versus glycerol-treated tissue the mean number of total corneodesmosomes was decreased from 14 corneodesmosomes per unit area

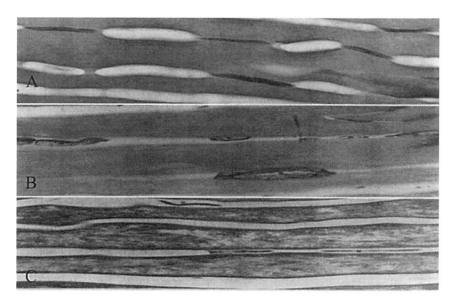

FIGURE 5 Osmium tetroxide– and potassium ferrocyanide–fixed stratum corneum. (A) Control tissue, no glycerol treatment, incubated at 44% RH for 7 days. Note intact electron-dense desmosomes attached to corneocyte envelopes (*). (B) Tissue incubated at 80% RH for 7 days (no glycerol treatment). Note partial degradation of corneodesmosomes, vacuolated structures beginning to be dissociated from corneocyte envelopes (*). (C) Tissue incubated at 80% RH for 7 days following 5% glycerol treatment. Note paucity and virtually complete degradation of corneodesmosomes no longer attached to corneocytes (*). Each micrograph shows the lower levels of the stratum corneum (stratum compactum) where corneodesmosomes are in greater abundance. Areas of corneocyte interdigitation can be seen in (B) (×200,000; bar = 0.05 mm). (Modified from Ref. 7.)

(control tissue) to 4 corneodesmosomes per unit area (glycerol). The numbers of intact electron-dense corneodesmosomes were also dramatically reduced to a mean of 1 per unit area (Fig. 6).

To examine desquamatory potential, a corneocyte release model was established where biopsied skin was incubated at a variety of humidities with or without pretreatment with a range of lotions. Following incubation for 24 hr at 20°C and 80% RH, each biopsy was placed into 0.1M Tris-HCl buffer, pH 8.0, and vortexed in microfuge tubes. This procedure detached functionally desquamated corneocytes from the surface of the biopsy. The corneocytes were then recovered by centrifugation and counted in a microhaematometer as a measure of desquamation.

As can be seen from Fig. 7, the desquamation rates for skin incubated at 80

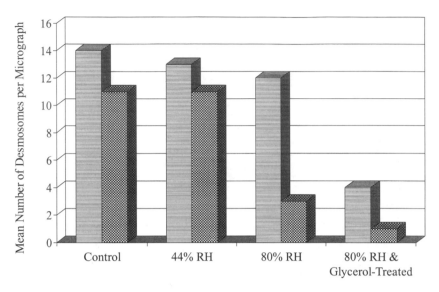

FIGURE 6 Comparison of the number of corneodesmosmes in control stratum corneum and stratum corneum incubated for 7 days at 44% RH, 80% RH, and 80% RH following 5% glycerol treatment. Note the decrease in intact ▤ and total ▨ corneodesmosomes (structures that are electron dense and attached to corneocyte envelopes) in glycerol-treated tissue incubated at 80% RH. (Modified from Ref. 7.)

and 100% humidity are essentially indistinguishable. However, at lower humidities the desquamation rate is very much reduced. These data suggest that even though the hydration of the skin is greater at 100% RH, this has no dramatic effect on desquamation compared with 80% RH, when the skin is losing a greater amount of water. This observation is consistent with the accepted scientific view that the stratum corneum only needs to contain 10–20% water to function properly. At the lower humidities in this experiment the skin is losing water to the atmosphere too quickly to function properly. This leads to a lowered desquamation rate in vitro, reflecting the likely formation of dry skin due to a reduction in the number of corneocytes released compared with the unwashed control. This is consistent with a perturbation of corneodesmosomal degradation (Fig. 8) [20]. Topical application of a glycerol-containing moisturizing lotion clearly increased the number of corneocytes released even for the soap-washed sample. These results suggest that the soap is not inhibiting the enzyme activity directly because it can be subsequently restored by glycerol. Rather it implies that the microenvironment within which the enzymes function to degrade the extracellular portion of the corneodesmosomes is perturbed following soap washing, but can be restored by the influence of glycerol. The result of this increased corneocyte release on the appearance of the skin surface is shown in Fig. 9. The soap-washed surface is

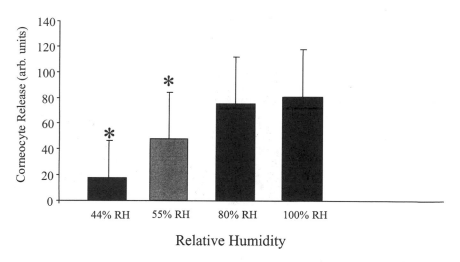

FIGURE 7 Relationship between corneocyte release and relative humidity (p < 0.05).

clearly more flaky compared to the soap-washed moisturizer treatment control. The effect of the moisturizer on corneocyte release in this regard is largely due to the presence of glycerol.

The degradation of corneodesmosomes was confirmed by immunochemically quantifying the levels of intact dsg 1, extracted from stratum corneum samples and resolved by electrophoresis. As can be seen from Fig. 10, compared with vehicle-treated stratum corneum the levels of dsg1 were dramatically reduced in the glycerol-treated stratum corneum when incubated at 80% RH.

6 MODE OF ACTION OF HUMECTANTS ON BARRIER LIPIDS

It is well established that the stratum corneum lipids are the major barrier to water loss from the skin. This property is highly dependent on the ability of these lipids to form multiple layers in a lamellar liquid crystallization arrangement. Friberg et al. [21] have proposed that the stratum corneum lipids are a mixture of solid and liquid crystalline states in which the latter permit liquidlike diffusion of water through the lipid bilayers, but the solid states allow rapid water loss due to cracks in the structure.

Disturbances in both the lipid ultrastructure and changes in lipid composition are now well described in dry skin [2,22–25]. It has been proposed that due to the elevated levels of fatty acid soaps in such conditions that a solid crystalline phase predominates in dry skin. Therefore, treatments that maintain a higher proportion of lipid in the liquid state may be effective moisturizers. Mattai et al. [26]

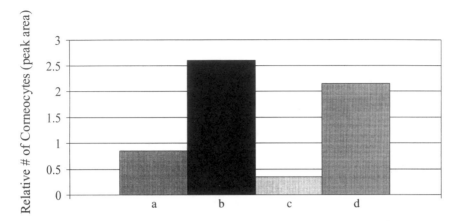

FIGURE 8 Relative corneocyte release in control and glycerol-treated tissues in normal and soap-washed skin. (a) Control: water washed, no product; (b) water washed, VICL treated; (c) control: Ivory soap washed, no product; (d) Ivory soap washed, VICL treated. $p < 0.05$ for (b) versus (a), (c) versus (a), and (d) versus (a). $p > 0.05$ for (b) versus (d).

have examined the effects of glycerol on the physical properties of model stratum corneum lipids at low (6% RH) and high (92% RH) relative humidity, using polarized light microscopy and differential scanning calorimetry. At high humidities a liquid crystalline state was maintained for the model lipids, whereas at low humidity significant crystallization occurred as the lipids became dehydrated. Hence, glycerol may condition the skin by an alternative mechanism to humectancy whereby at low humidity glycerol conditioner maintains the liquid crystalline state of the stratum corneum lipid.

In related studies Orth et al. [27] also demonstrated through electron microscopic evaluation of the stratum corneum that following use of glycerol-containing moisturizers the corneocytes and the stratum corneum intercellular spaces are expanded, and they further demonstrated that the glycerol reservoir was present throughout the stratum corneum.

7 EFFECT OF HUMECTANTS ON NORMAL AND DRY SKIN

7.1 Effect of Glycerol on Stratum Corneum Properties in Normal Skin

Using a variety of noninvasive instrumental techniques (measurement of TEWL, skin surface topography, and determination of the coefficient of friction and elec-

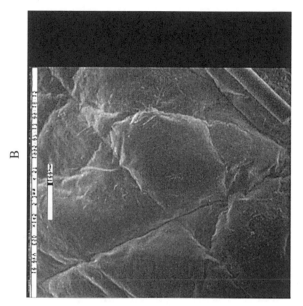

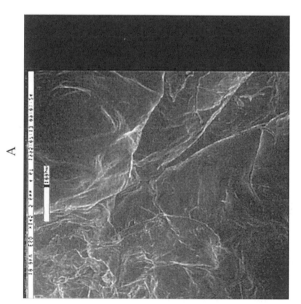

Figure 9 Visualization of surface morphology of (A) soap-washed stratum corneum and (B) soap-washed stratum corneum and then treated with glycerol, using environmental scanning electron microscopy.

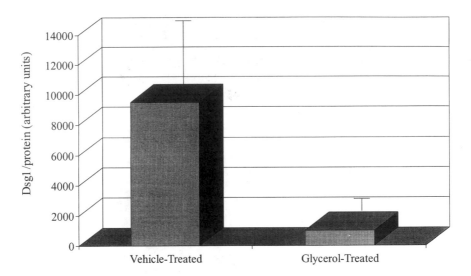

FIGURE 10 Comparison of the effect of glycerol on stratum corneum desmoglein 1 digestion at 80% RH. (Modified from Ref. 7.)

trical impedance), Batt et al. [28] examined the effects of water and glycerol on normal forearm volar skin. As expected, application of water produced a rapid but temporary response in all the instrumental techniques used, whereas topical application of glycerol-containing products delivered greater and sustained effects. For example, skin treated with glycerol- and non–glycerol-containing products initially shows an increase in TEWL, which was markedly decreased by the application of glycerol-containing emulsions following the evaporation of water. Similarly, there was an enhanced smoothing effect of the glycerol emulsion, as measured by change in coefficient of friction that was prolonged over the base lotion. Similar results were obtained using the other instrumental approaches. Interestingly, glycerol was retained in the stratum corneum over a long period of the time and such a reservoir would account for the persistence of its effects.

7.2 Effect of Glycerol on the Amelioration of Dry Skin

The effects of glycerol on the treatment of soap-induced dry skin have been studied by many investigators. In our own studies we have used a Kligman regression moisturizing efficacy test [29] as modified by Boisits [30] to understand the properties of this unique humectant. In these studies subjects induce a moderate dry skin on their lower legs by washing twice daily for seven days with a commercial soap [20]. Following this dry-down period subjects then apply a commercial moisturizer (2 mg/cm^2) to one leg and the same commercial moisturizer without glycerol to the contralateral site on their other leg twice daily. Dryness and erythema were evaluated by expert clinical assessment at study baseline, and then once every second day over the 2-week product application period using a standard visual grading system. As can be seen from Fig. 11 both the glycerol- and non–glycerol-containing formulations reduced mean dryness scores. However, the formulation that contained glycerol lowered dryness scores significantly greater than the formulations without glycerol. These observations are consistent with the hypothesis that the glycerol-containing lotion restored desquamation to normal quicker than nonglycerol formulations and thereby lowered the soap induced visual dryness score.

Using further modifications to the standard moisturizing efficacy testing method (a 7-day treatment followed by a 7-day regression) Appa [31] has demonstrated that moisturization efficacy increased with increasing concentrations of glycerol before reaching a plateau at 25 wt%. Equally these high-glycerol formulations gave significantly better relief of dryness than a low–glycerol-containing moisturizer.

Summers et al. [32] have demonstrated that low–glycerol-containing (1%) formulations alone are essentially ineffective in alleviating skin xerosis. In these

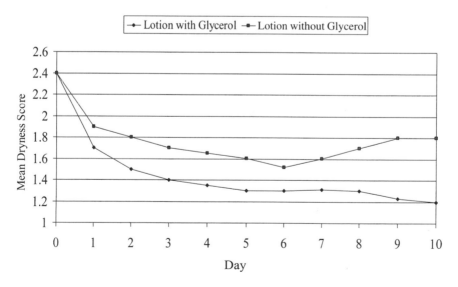

FIGURE 11 Effect of glycerol- and non–glycerol-containing lotions on the alleviation of dry skin clinically. Note faster amelioration of condition with lotion containing glycerol.

studies a combination of technologies, i.e., occlusive barrier technology in addition to glycerol, was essential in delivering the benefit.

Hence the onset of commonly occurring soap-induced xerosis starts with a perturbation of the skin desquamatory function. This is clearly seen in Fig. 12, which demonstrates the relative changes in cohesive strength of surface corneocytes following continued soap washing as well as soap washing followed by moisturizer treatment [20]. The methodology used, modified from Christiansen [33], allows an assessment of the cohesive strength of the surface layer of corneocytes based on the recovery of corneocytes using a low–adhesive strength polymeric gel. The use of a low-strength polymeric gel which is capable of only removing loose surface corneocytes is critical to the success of this method, giving greater discrimination of cohesive strength than using traditional more aggressive tape, which often removes layers of stratum corneum. Quantification of the number of cells removed can be accomplished by a simple protein analysis. As can be seen in Fig. 12 soap washing leads to an increased cell cohesion within 2 weeks. This result is interpreted as a persistence of desmosomal linkages and other adhesive elements between cells right up to the skin surface. Concomitant use of a humectant-based moisturizer leads to a normalization of desquamation and a subsequent reduction of the cell cohesion amongst surface cells as they become looser due to enhanced corneodesmosomal degradation. Interestingly, in this study the use of a glycerol-based moisturizer leads to a more rapid normal-

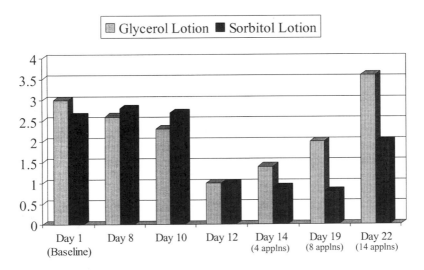

FIGURE 12 Effect of glycerol and sorbitol lotions on stratum corneum cell loss in vivo. Note faster amelioration of dry skin with glycerol lotion.

ization compared to a sorbitol-based moisturizer. Again these studies suggest that loss of effective hydration rather than any intrinsic loss of proteases, or proteolytic activity due to surfactant inhibition, is responsible for the perturbation in desquamation.

More recently we have demonstrated that glycerol lotions as well as improving skin quality also increase the maturation of stratum corneum corneoctye envelopes from a fragile morphology in dry skin to a more resilient morphology consistent with the repair of the skin to a more normal state [34]. The effect of moisturization on the improvement in these corneocyte phenotypes are shown in Fig. 13.

7.3 Effect of Glycerol on the Recovery of Barrier Function In Vivo

In recent studies Fluhr et al. [35] have demonstrated that glycerol accelerates the recovery of barrier function in vivo following damage by sodium lauryl sulfate (SLS) or repeated tape-stripping. In the first study volar forearms were tape-stripped 13 × using scotch tape until a TEWL level of 15 $g/m^2/hr$ was obtained. Glycerol (25 or 50 wt%) was then applied directly to the skin or under an occlusive patch. Although occlusion itself had no effect on barrier recovery, the glycerol-treated sites whether occluded or not resulted in a faster decrease in TEWL. Occlusion has been shown to delay barrier repair in mice, though the effect in hu-

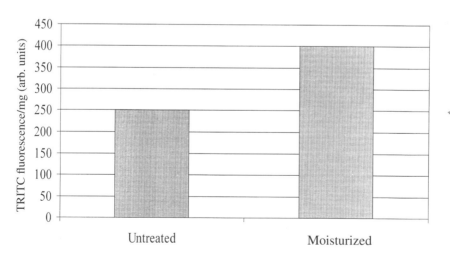

Figure 13 Effect of glycerol lotions on relative proportion corneocyte envelope types. Increased TRITC fluorescence relates to an increase of mature CEr. Note improvement in resilient phenotype following glycerol treatment.

mans is inconsistent and equivocal. In this study occlusion alone had no effect on barrier repair, but glycerol application under occlusion enhanced the moisturizing effect. In the second study, stratum corneum barrier function was perturbed by washing with 0.2% SLS with a foam roller, and creams containing glycerol were applied to forearms. After 3 days of treatment the use of the glycerol formulations was associated with lower TEWL and elevated capacitance. Significant improvement in moisturization was observed at 7 days. However, for the effects on TEWL, significant differences were not observed until after 2 weeks. These results suggest that glycerol creates a stimulus for barrier repair. The effect was long lasting, persisting for up to 7 days after the end of the treatment. Therefore, glycerol can also be regarded as a barrier-enhancing and stabilizing agent. Whether other polyols have this effect is unknown.

7.4 Effect of Other Humectants on Dry Skin

7.4.1 PCA

A vast amount of work has been performed examining the effects of PCA and its salts in vitro, but there has been little work in vivo except one study of Middleton and Roberts [36], demonstrating that PCA lotion were more effective at treating dry skin compared to a placebo lotion. As discussed previously [13], the precise mode of action of PCA and other low molecular weight free amino acids and their derivatives remains unclear.

7.4.2 Urea

Urea is a natural component of the stratum corneum moisturizing factor and it is commonly used in skin care. It has been proven to be an excellent skin humidifier and descaling agent, and it has been used effectively in hand creams for over half a century. Clinical studies have shown urea to be more effective than petroleum jelly and salicylic acid. Urea lotions have also been shown to reduce TEWL, increase skin capacitance, and reduce skin irritation. There is also some evidence urea may improve epidermal lipid biosynthesis and improve barrier performance [37].

7.4.3 Lactic Acid

Like glycerol, α-hydroxyacids (AHAs), and particularly the salts of lactic acid, have pleiotropic effects on the skin. The anti-aging effects will be reviewed by Johnson [38]. However lactic acid salts are well established as agents that can ameliorate the signs and symptoms of dry skin clinically [39–41]. Alpha-hydroxyacids, like glycerol, can promote desquamation in vivo. The precise mode of action is not well understood, but ultrastructural studies have demonstrated a corneodesmolytic activity, particularly in the stratum dysjunctum layers of the stratum corneum [42]. Equally important these agents also prevent the reappearance of dry skin when directly compared with lactic acid–free products [39]. Like urea, lactic acid has been shown to improve the barrier properties of the stratum corneum as exemplified by decreased TEWL and lower irritant reactions after exposure to SLS [43]. Studies from our own lab have indicated that this reflects an underlying stimulation of ceramide synthesis that serves to compensate for the loss of these critical barrier components in dry skin [44].

8 CONCLUDING COMMENTS

The term "moisturizer" was first coined to describe products that provided hydration for the skin thereby keeping it soft, supple, and smooth. However, water alone is not a panacea for dry skin, and indeed water can be damaging to the skin. Although water in a cosmetic product can have a short-term effect on the properties of the stratum corneum, it has become apparent that moisturizers deliver their primary benefits by maximizing the retention of water within the stratum corneum. This water then has the dual effect of providing the required hydration of the many hydrolyases involved in stratum corneum maturation and desquamation or enhancing stratum corneum flexibility.

As is evident from this synopsis, not all humectants are equivalent in their ability to improve skin condition, and we have seen that the mode of action of humectants at the molecular level may reflect an influence on an intracellular or an intercellular event within the stratum corneum. Within the range of humectants used in dry skin products, glycerol appears unique in providing more benefit to this tissue than can be explained by simple humectancy. This range of properties is not shared by other polyols, which nevertheless still remain common humectant ingredients in many formulations. Glycerol is capable of plasticizing the stratum corneum, manipulating the lyotropic nature of the lamellar lipids and thereby promoting the enzyme-mediated lysis of corneodesmosomes within the extracellular matrix. This latter finding indicates that glycerol is a true corneodesmolytic agent and enhances desquamation effectively to ameliorate dry and scaly skin. Understanding the mechanism by which this remarkable molecule can influence barrier repair remains to be elucidated.

REFERENCES

1. Pierard GE. What does dry skin mean? Int J Dermatol 1987; 23:167–168.
2. Rawlings AV, Watkinson A, Rogers J, Mayo AM, Hope J, Scott IR. Abnormalities in stratum corneum structure, lipid composition and desmosome degradation in soap-induced winter xerosis. J Cosmet Chem 1994; 45:203–220.
3. Rawlings AV, Scott IR, Harding CR, Bowser PA. Stratum corneum moisturisation at the molecular level. J Invest Dermatol 1994; 103:731–740.
4. Harding CR, Watkinson A, Scott IR, Rawlings AV. Dry skin, moisturisation and corneodesmolysis. Int J Cosmet Sci 2000; 22:21–52.

5. Rawlings AV, Harding CR, Watkinson A, Scott IR. Dry and xerotic skin conditions. In: Leyden J, Rawlings AV, eds. Skin Moisturization. New York: Marcel Dekker (in press).

6. Suzuki Y, Koyama J, Moro O, Horii I, Kukuchi K, Tanida M, Tagami H. Br J Dermatol 1996; 134:460–464.

7. Rawlings A, Harding CR, Watkinson A, Banks J, Ackerman C, Sabin R. The effect of glycerol and humidity on desmosome degradation in stratum corneum. Arch Dermatol Res 1995; 287:457–464.

8. Blank IH. Further observations on factors which influence the water content of the stratum corneum. J Invest Dermatol 1953; 21:259–271.

9. Lindberg M, Forslind B. The skin as a barrier. In: Loden M, Maibach HI, eds. Dry Skin and Moisturizers. Boca Raton: CRC Press, 2000:27–37.

10. Scheuplen PJ, Blank IH. Permeability of the skin. Physiol Rev 1971; 51:702–747.

11. Idson B. Water and the skin. J Soc Cosmet Chem 1973; 24:197–212.

12. Idson B. Biophysical factors in skin penetration. J Soc Cosmet Chem 1971; 22:615–34.

13. Harding CR, Scott IR. Natural moisturising factor. In: Leyden J, Rawlings AV, eds. Skin Moisturization. New York: Marcel Dekker (in press).

14. Middleton JC. The mechanism of water binding in the stratum corneum. Br J Dermatol 1968; 80:437–450.

15. Potts RO. Stratum corneum hydration: experimental techniques and interpretations of results. J Soc Cosmet Chem 1986; 37:9–33.

16. Takahashi M, Yamada M, Machida Y. A new method to evaluate the softening effects of cosmetic ingredients on the skin. J Soc Cosmet Chem 1984; 35:171–181.

17. Rawlings AV, Watkinson A, Harding CR, Ackerman C, Banks J, Hope J, Scott IR. Changes in stratum corneum lipid and desmosome structure together with water barrier function during mechanical stress. J Soc Cosmet Chem 1995; 46:141–151.

18. Takahashi M, Kawasaki K, Tanaka M, Ohta S, Tsuda Y. The mechanism of stratum corneum plasticisation with water. In Marks R, Pine PA, Bioengineering of the Skin. eds Lancaster: MTP Press, 1981 67–73.

19. Middleton JD. Development of a skin cream designed to reduce dry and flaky skin. J Soc Cosmet Chem 1974; 25:519–534.

20. Chander P, Harding CR, Watkinson A, Banks J, Sabin R, Hoyberg K, Rawlings AV. Superiority of glycerol containing moisturisers on desquamation and desmosome hydrolysis. J Invest Dermatol 1996; 106:919.

21. Friberg SE, Kyali I, Rhein LD. Direct role of linoleic acid in barrier function. Effect of linoleic acid on the crystalline structure of oleic acid/oleate model stratum corneum lipid. J Disp Sci Technol 1990; 11:31–47.

22. Saint-Leger D, Francois AM, Leveque JL, Stuudesmeuyer T, Kligman AM, Grove GL. Stratum corneum lipids in winter xerosis. Dermatologica 1989; 178:151–155.

23. Fulmer AW, Kramer GJ. Stratum corneum abnormalities in surfactant induced dry scaly skin. J Invest Dermatol 1989; 80:598–602.

24. Warner RR, Boissy YL. Effect of moisturising products on the structure of lipids in the outer stratum corneum of human. In: Loden M, Maibach HI, eds. Dry Skin and Moisturizers. Boca Raton: CRC Press, 2000: 349–372.

25. Berry N, Charmeil C, Goujon C, Silvy A, Girard P, Corcuff C. Moisturiser. A clini-

cal, biometrological and ultrastructural study of xerotic skin. Int J Cosmet Sci 1999; 21:241–252.

26. Mattai J, Froebe CL, Rhein LD, Simion A, Ohlmeyer DT, Friberg SE. Preventation of model stratum corneum lipid phase transitions in vitro by cosmetic additives. Differential scanning calorimetry optical microscopy and water evaporation studies. J Soc Cosmet Chem 1993; 44:89–100.

27. Orth DS, Appa Y, Contard P, Siegel E, Donnelly TA, Rhcins LA. Effect of high glycerin therapeutic moisturizers on the ultrastructure of the stratum corneum. Annual meeting of ADD 1995.

28. Batt MD, Davis WB, Fairhurst WA, Gerrard WA, Ridge BD. Changes in the physical properties of the stratum corneum following treatment with glycerol. J Soc Cosmet Chem 1988; 39:367–381.

29. Kligman A. Regression method for assessing the efficacy of moisturizers. Cosmet Toil 1978; 93:27–35.

30. Boisits EK, Nole GE, Cheney MC. The refined regression method. J Cutan Aging Cosmet Dermatol 1989; 1:155–163.

31. Orth D, Appa Y. Glycerine: a natural ingredient for moisturising skin. In: Loden M, Maibach HI, eds. Dry Skin and Moisturizers. Boca Raton: CRC Press, 2000:213–228.

32. Summers RS, Summers B, Chander P, Fernberg C, Gursky R, Rawlings AV. The effect of lipids, with and without humectant, on skin xerosis. J Soc Cosmet Chem 1996; 47:27–39.

33. Christensen MS, Nacht S, Kantor SL, Gans EH. A method for measuring desquamation and its use for assessing the effects of some common exfoliants. J Invest Dermatol 1978; 71:289–294.

34. Harding CR, Rawlings AV, Long S, Richardson J, Rogers J, Zhang Z, Bush A. The cornified cell envelope: an important marker of stratum corneum maturation in healthy and dry skin. In: Lal M, Lifford PJ, Waik VM, Prakash V, eds. Supramolecular and Celloidal Structures in Biomaterials and Biosubstrates. Proceedings of the 5th Roycal Society–Unilever Indo-UK forum in materials science and engineering. 1999:386–405.

35. Fluhr JW, Gloor M, Lehmann L, Lazzerini S, Distante F, Berardesca E. Glycerol accelerates the recovery of barrier function in vivo. Acta Derm Venereol 1999; 79:418–421.

36. Middleton JD, Roberts ME. Effect of a skin cream containing the sodium slat of pyrollidone carboxylic acid on dry and flaky skin. J Soc Cosmet Chem 1978; 29:201–205.

37. Loden M. Urea. In: Loden M, Maibach HI, eds. Dry Skin and Moisturizers. Boca Raton: CRC Press, 2000:243–257.

38. Johnson AW. Hydroxyacids. In: Leyden J, Rawlings AV, eds. Skin Moisturization. New York: Marcel Dekker (in press).

39. Bagatell FK, Smoot W. Observations on a lactate containing emollient cream. Cutis 1976; 18:591.

40. Dahl MV, Dahl AC. 12% lactate lotion for the treatment of xerosis. Arch Dermatol 1983; 119:27.

41. Wehr R, Krochmal L, Bagatell F, Ragsdale W. A controlled 2 center study of lactate

12% lotion and a petrolatum based cream in patients with xerosis. Cutis 1986; 23:205.

42. Leveque S. Salicylic acid and derivatives: which roles. In: Leyden J, Rawlings AV, eds. Skin Moisturization. New York Marcel Dekker (in press).

43. Berardesca E, Distante F, Vignol G, Oresajo C, Green B. Alpha-hydroxy acids modulate stratum corneum barrier function. Br J Dermatol 1997; 137:934.

44. Rawlings AV, Davies A, Carlomusto M, Pillai S, Zhang K, Kosturko R, Verdejo P, Feinberg C, Nguyen L, Chandar P. Keratinocyte ceramide synthesis, effect of lactic acid isomers on straturm corneum lipid levels and stratum corneum barrier function. Arch Dermatol Res 1996; 288:383.

14

Ceramides as Natural Moisturizing Factors and Their Efficacy in Dry Skin

Genji Imokawa

Kao Biological Science Laboratories, Haga, Tochigi, Japan

1 INTRODUCTION

The flexibility of the stratum corneum (SC) plays an important role in keeping the skin supple and in giving it a radiant appearance. Water present within the SC is essential for maintaining the flexibility of the SC, and is constitutively regulated by the water-holding capacity of the SC. Much evidence suggests that water-soluble materials, such as free amino acids, organic acids, urea, and inorganic ions determine the water-holding properties of the SC; these materials have been termed natural moisturizing factors [1]. Based upon this theory, many moisturizers have been designed and developed in the cosmetic field. Well-known removers of lipids, such as organic solvents, despite their poor ability to remove water-soluble materials, induce dry skin, which is characterized by a reduction in the water-holding function of the SC. Thus, we hypothesized that structural lipids, mainly comprised of ceramides, play a significant role in the water-holding potential of the SC. In this chapter, we introduce a new mechanism underlying the water-holding properties of the SC and elucidate the role of ceramides as natural moisturizing factors and their efficacy in the clinical treatment of dry skin.

2 MOISTURIZING MECHANISMS IN THE STRATUM CORNEUM

2.1 Lipid Removal and Dry Skin

In order to clarify the roles of lipids in holding water molecules within the SC, we have tried to specifically remove lipids from the SC and assessed the effects on its water-holding properties [2–5]. Treatment of human forearm skin with acetone/ether (1:1) for periods of 5 to 20 min induces an enduring (more than 4 days) chapped and scaly appearance of the SC with no inflammatory reaction in a time-dependent manner (Fig. 1). Under these conditions, a significant decrease in the water content, as measured by the conductance value, is observed in the treated areas (Fig. 2). The decreased conductance barely returns to the normal level until more than 4 days after the treatment. In contrast, such a persistent scaly skin, accompanied by a significant decrease in the conductance value, was not induced after only 1 min of treatment. Of considerable interest is the fact that the acetone/ether treatment did not induce a substantial release from the SC of any hygroscopic materials, such as free amino acids or lactic acid (Fig. 3) [3], which suggests a deep involvement of structural lipids in the induced deficiency of wa-

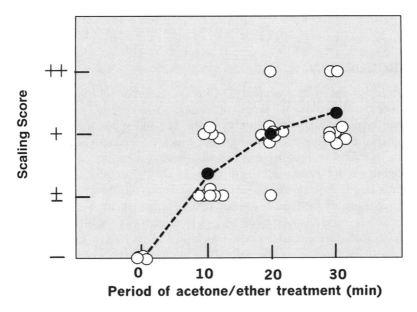

Figure 1 The induction of dry skin on the forearms of healthy volunteers following treatment with acetone/ether (1:1) in a time-dependent manner. The intensity of the induced dry skin is expressed as the scaling score.

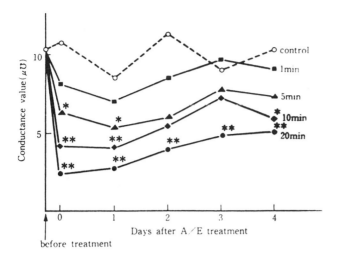

FIGURE 2 Different times of treatment of human forearm skin with acetone/ether (1:1) demonstrates a marked decrease in water content as measured by impedance meter. n = 6; **p < 0.01; *p < 0.05.

ter content. In order to clarify the mechanisms involved in the decrease of the conductance value, we compared the composition of lipids extracted by the solvent after varying periods [2–5]. One-dimensional thin-layer chromatography (TLC) analysis (Fig. 4) shows that, even after only 1 min of treatment, the amounts of sebaceous gland lipids extracted, such as squalene, triglycerides, and wax esters, have almost reached a plateau. Additional or prolonged treatments induce no further substantial release of those lipids. On the other hand, SC lipids (SCLs), such as cholesterol, cholesterol esters, and ceramides, are successively solubilized from the SC by the solvent in a time-dependent manner. These findings suggest that the defect in the water-holding properties of dry skin induced by acetone/ether treatment is directly associated with the depletion of intercellular lipids.

2.2 Intercellular Lipids and Bound Water

Since lipids by themselves have little or no affinity for water molecules, it is intriguing to determine how intercellular lipids are associated with the incorporation of water molecules. It is well known that water within the SC does not freeze readily, even at temperatures lower than $-40°C$, which suggests its existence as bound water within the SC. In order to examine the amounts of bound water in the SC which reflect the water-holding function, a SC sheet was taken from human forearm skin using a surgical knife with the help of tweezers, and was sub-

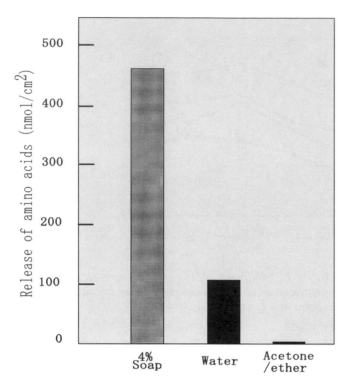

Figure 3 The release of amino acids from forearm skin following various treatments for 20 min.

jected to differential scanning calorimetry (DSC). This technique allows the amount of nonfreezable water to be calculated based on the melting behavior of the water in the SC. The DSC curve of the intact SC sheet shows one endothermic peak at –17 to –6°C with a much lower melting temperature of ice than 0°C (freezing point depression behavior) (Fig. 5) [6–8]. The plot of calculated transition enthalpy against the total water content in the SC sheet demonstrates that the intact SC sheet possesses approximately 33.3% bound water that never freezes, even below –40°C (Fig. 6). Since it is known that the healthy SC contains approximately 30% water under normal conditions, when measured for water content by the Karl–Fisher method, it is conceivable that all water within a healthy SC exists as bound (nonfreezable) water, and that this plays a pivotal role in the water-holding function of the healthy SC. On the other hand, treatment of the SC sheet with acetone/ether can selectively deplete SCLs, and such treatment elicited a marked difference in DSC thermograms where an endothermic peak appears even at 30% water content, indicating a decrease in the bound-water content (Fig.

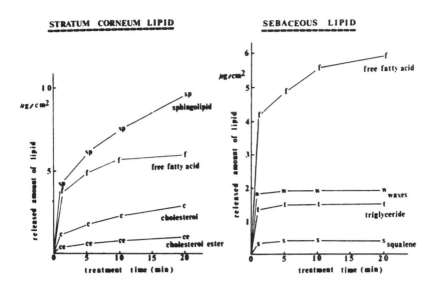

FIGURE 4 Thin-layer chromatographic analysis of lipids released by human forearm skin after different times of treatment with acetone/ether (1:1).

7). However, the melting temperature around which the endothermic peak is observed does not change even after acetone/ether treatment, which suggests that the acetone/ether treatment does not release any water-soluble materials, such as amino acids. The plot of the calculated transition enthalpy against the total water content in the acetone/ether-treated SC sheet demonstrates that the depletion of SCLs by acetone/ether treatment causes the SC bound-water content to decrease from 33.3 to 19.7% (Fig. 6).

2.3 Recovery of Dry Skin by Application of Lipid

It is well known that intercellular lipids contain several components, such as cholesterol, ceramides, and fatty acids, which by themselves possess no substantial capacity for holding water in vitro [4]. Therefore, it seems reasonable to assume that in vivo these lipids are specifically compartmentalized into the intercellular spaces to exert their water-holding properties. This led us to determine whether the various intercellular lipids have the potential to repair the disrupted water-holding properties when applied topically to dry skin. Hence, we tried to measure the therapeutic potential of topical application of extracted lipids to repair the water-holding properties of lipid-depleted SC in which a marked decrease in those properties had been observed. Two daily topical applications of a 10% SCL fraction in alkyl glyceryl ether (GE)/squalene base on the acetone/ether-treated SCL

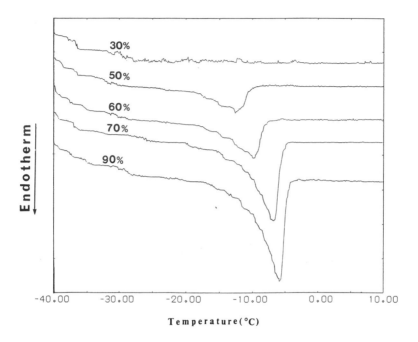

FIGURE 5 DSC thermal profiles obtained for intact human SC sheets with various levels of water content.

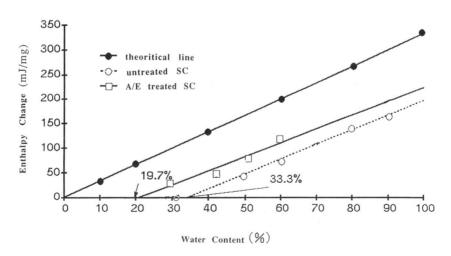

FIGURE 6 Calculation of bound water by plotting the melting enthalpy of ice against the total water content in intact and in acetone/ether-treated human SC. SC, stratum corneum sheet.

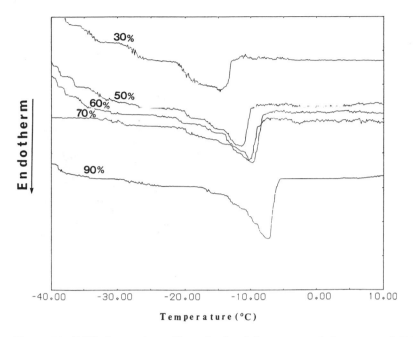

FIGURE 7 DSC thermal profiles obtained for acetone/ether-treated (20 min) human SC sheets in the presence of various levels of water content.

induced a significant recovery of the decreased conductance value compared with no treatment or treatment with the GE/squalene base only. In contrast, the seba-ceous lipid (SL) fraction does not elicit any significant recovery even when com-pared with GE/squalene (Fig. 8) [8–10]. The recovery level included by the SCL therapy is significantly higher than 10% glycerin in the same GE/squalene sol-vent. Nevertheless, when GE is not added to this system, there is no significant re-covery detectable with any of the lipid fractions. The recovery observed is specif-ic for a combined treatment with GE among the various surfactants tested. This specific action is based on the fact that GE has significant potential as a penetra-tion enhancer, and it is likely that such recovery requires substantial penetration of ceramides into the SC layers. Consistent with those changes in the conduc-tance value, the scaling that occurs after acetone/ether treatment significantly de-creases after the two daily applications with SCL compared with no application.

2.4   Recovery of Bound Water by Application of Lipid

The application of isolated SCLs to the lipid-depleted SC sheet restores the DSC thermograms almost to the level of the intact SC sheet (Fig. 9) [7,8]. The plot of

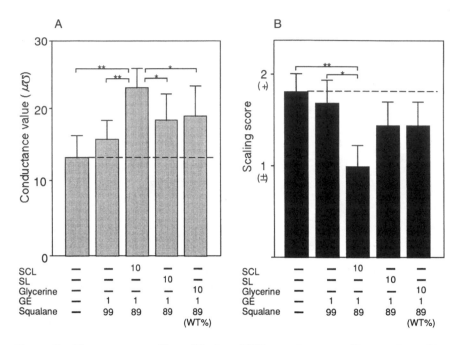

FIGURE 8 The recovery effect of isolated SCLs on forearm skin roughened by 30-min treatment with acetone/ether (1:1) as assessed by water content and scaling score on day 4 following daily treatment for 3 days. (A) Water content measured by impedance meter. (B) The intensity of scaly appearance. SCL, stratum corneum lipid; SL, sebaceous lipid; GE, glyceryl ether. n = 10; **p < 0.01; * p < 0.05.

calculated transition enthalpy against the total water content in the SCL-treated SC sheet demonstrates a marked increase in the bound-water content, from 19.7 to 26.8%, whereas the control treatment of squalene/1% GE has no effect on the bound-water content of the SC sheet (Fig. 10). Taken together, the evidence presented suggests that intercellular lipids in the SC serve as a bound-water modulator, providing it with radiance.

2.5 Major Lipid Components in the Water-Holding Mechanism

In order to determine which components are crucial for the water-holding function of intercellular lipids, the potential of each lipid component to repair dry skin

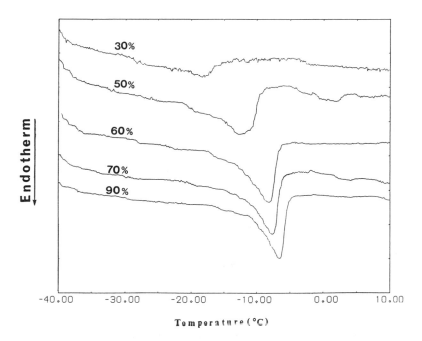

FIGURE 9 DSC thermal profiles obtained for human SC sheets treated with SCL following acetone/ether treatment in the presence of various levels of water content. SCL, stratum corneum lipid.

induced by acetone/ether treatment was examined in vivo [8–10]. Two daily topical applications of five chromatographically purified lipid fractions (cholesterol ester, free fatty acid, cholesterol, ceramide, glycolipid) from the SCL at 10% concentration were carried out in the same system after a 30-min treatment with acetone/ether. Of the five lipid fractions tested, the ceramide fraction induced the most significant increase in the conductance value compared with the GE/squalene base (Fig. 11). Furthermore, the glycolipid and cholesterol fractions also elicited a significant recovery compared with no application. In contrast, neither the free fatty acid nor the cholesterol ester elicited any significant increase in the conductance value. The marked recovery effects of the ceramide fraction on the water-holding function and its therapeutic value to scaly dry skin was also demonstrated by applying the water-in-oil (W/O) emulsion containing the ceramide fraction to lipid-depleted forearm skin (Fig. 12) [10]. Thus, ceramides play a central role as a water-modulator in the SC because of their predominant abundance and their relatively high capacity to hold water.

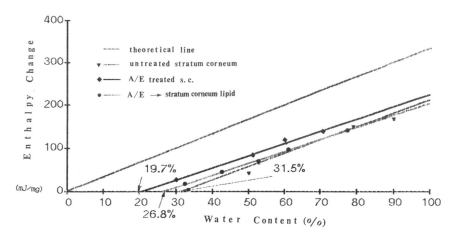

FIGURE 10 Calculation of bound water by plotting the melting enthalpy of ice against the total water content in SCL-treated human SC sheets following treatment with acetone/ether. A/E, acetone/ether; SC, stratum corneum.

2.6 The Role of Water-Soluble Materials in the Water-Holding Properties

To determine the role of water-soluble materials in the water-holding properties, forearm skin that had been acetone/ether treated was then treated with water (which efficiently releases amino acids) under various humidity conditions to evaluate changes in water content expressed as conductance. Although acetone/ether treatment elicited decreased water content on the skin surface under various humidity conditions, the removal of amino acids had no significant effect on the water-holding properties of the skin surface in vivo, except under high humidity (Fig. 13) [11,12]. In this connection, treatment of the lipid-depleted SC sheet with water released amino acids amounting to 0.13 mg/mg SC. In accordance with such a release of amino acids, water treatment caused DSC thermograms to delete the freezing point depression behavior (Fig. 14) [7,8]. Even under this condition, there was no substantial change in the degree of the endothermic peak with various water contents, suggesting that there was no involvement of water-soluble materials such as amino acids in the capacity of the SC to hold water. Furthermore, our ^{13}C-NMR study demonstrated that the depletion of water-extractable materials from the SC caused marked increases in the molecular interactions between the 10-nm filaments of keratin fibers [12,13]. This induced increase of molecular interaction could be reversed by the application of water-extractable materials, such as amino acids. Based on these facts, it is conceivable that water-extractable materials play an important role in curtailing the intermol-

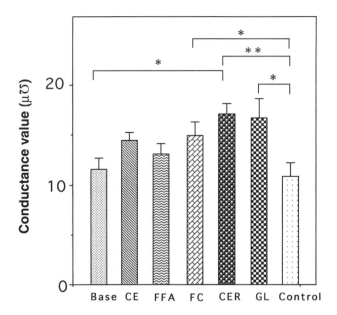

Figure 11 The effect of isolated SCL components on the recovery of forearm skin roughened by 30-min treatment with acetone/ether (1:1) as assessed by water content on day 4 following daily treatment for 3 days. Base: squalene (containing 1% glyceryl ether); CE, cholesterol fraction; FFA, free fatty acid fraction; CER, ceramide fraction; GL, glycolipid fraction; Control, nontreatment. **p < 0.01; *p < 0.05.

ecular forces between nonhelical regions of 10-nm filaments through interactions with water molecules, which probably provides the keratin fiber assembly with a high molecular mobility rather than the retention of water molecules.

3 THE MECHANISM OF DRY SKIN IN XEROSIS AND ATOPIC DERMATITIS

3.1 Xerosis

When a xerotic area of skin on the cheek was measured for its water content by an impedance meter and for its ceramide content by TLC analysis and compared with healthy skin, the xerotic area showed a decrease in water content as well as a decrease in ceramide content compared with the healthy skin (Fig. 15) [14]. This suggests that the decreased ceramide content is responsible for the decreased water content. Asteatotic eczema and its prototype, xerosis, have been thought to

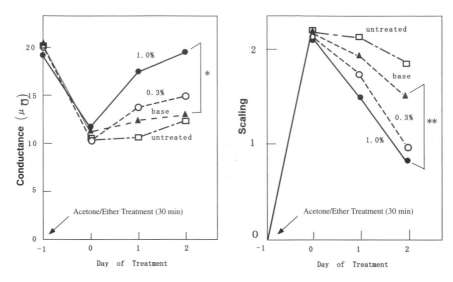

Figure 12 The effect of an isolated ceramide fraction on the recovery of forearm skin roughened by 30-min treatment with acetone/ether (1:1) as assessed by water content and scaling during the course of daily treatment for 3 days. Base: O/W cream containing 1% GE. n = 9; **p < 0.01; *p < 0.05.

be associated with deficient skin surface lipids, which are mainly supplied by sebaceous glands. This hypothesis is based on the fact that sebum-derived lipids play an important role in preventing the skin from water loss by forming lipid films on its surface. In contrast, our evidence presented here demonstrated that SCL produced by keratinocytes through the keratinization process serve as water modulators, by trapping moisture as bound water to the SC as well as by acting as permeability barriers by forming multilamellar structures between the SC cells. Of these lipids, ceramides comprise the major constituents of the SCL and perform both functions. Thus, quantitative analysis of ceramides in the SC provides useful information about the etiological involvement of ceramides in such dry skin disorders. Ceramides were quantified by TLC after n-hexane/ethanol extraction of resin-stripped SC and were evaluated as micrograms per milligram SC [15]. In healthy skin, there was an age-related decline in total ceramides (Fig. 16) [16], while xerosis of leg skin which had significantly reduced water-holding properties (Fig. 17) exhibited a decreased level of ceramides compared with the healthy young skin, but no significant decrease compared with healthy age-matched skin (Fig. 18). These data indicate that apparent slight increases in ce-

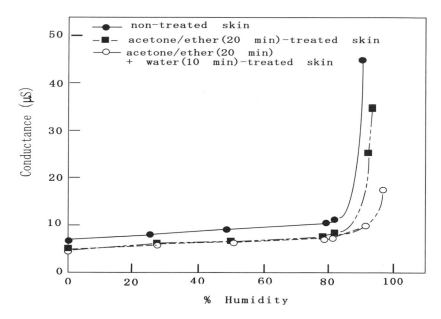

Figure 13 The water-holding profile of forearm skin following treatment with acetone/ether or with acetone/ether and water under different humidity conditions.

ramides are artifacts due to inflammatory processes or scratching, which results from susceptibility to dryness or itchiness. It is very likely that the observed decrease in the SCL explain the high incidence of dry skin in older people during the winter. The progression toward severe xerosis and asteatotic eczema can be ascribed to inflammation due to scratching or to environmental stimuli triggered by dry, itchy skin resulting from ceramide deficiency.

3.2 Atopic Dermatitis

Atopic dermatitis (AD) dry skin is characterized by a diminished water permeability barrier and deficient water-holding properties, as revealed by an evaporimeter to measure trans-epidermal water loss and by a capacitance conductance meter to measure skin surface water content, respectively (Fig. 19) [5,17,18]. Based upon the established relationship between ceramides and the water-holding properties of the SC, we have tried removing SC layers to assess the quantity of ceramides per unit mass of the SC. There was a marked reduction in the amount

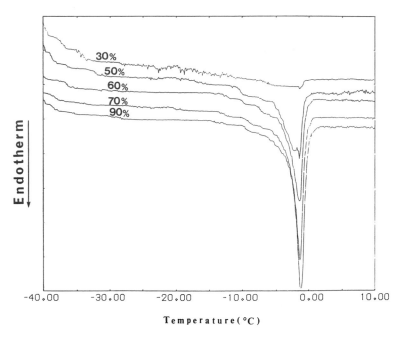

Figure 14 DSC thermal profiles obtained for water-treated human SC sheets following treatment with acetone/ether in the presence of various levels of water content. SC, stratum corneum sheet; AE, acetone/ether.

of ceramides in the lesional forearm skin of AD patients compared with the skin of healthy individuals of the same age (Fig. 20) [16]. Interestingly, the nonlesional skin of AD patients also exhibited a similar and significant decrease of ceramides. Among the six ceramide fractions, ceramide 1 was most significantly reduced in both the lesional and in the nonlesional skin [16]. These findings suggest that an insufficiency of ceramides in the SC is an etiologic factor in atopic dry skin. As a biological mechanism involved in the ceramide deficiency observed in AD, we have recently found that a hitherto undiscovered epidermal enzyme, sphingomyelin deacylase, is abnormally expressed in the epidermis of AD patients. This enzyme hydrolyzes the common substrate, sphingomyelin, at its acyl site to yield sphingosylphosphorylcholine rather than ceramide, which is the reaction product produced by sphingomyelinase, and this leads to the decreased generation of ceramides [19–21]. Consistent with the expression of sphingomyelin deacylase, we have recently confirmed that there is a marked accumulation of sphingosylphosphorylcholine in the upper SC of AD patients compared with healthy age-matched controls [22].

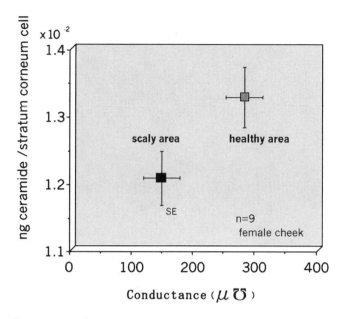

FIGURE 15 Comparison in the amounts of ceramide and water content between scaly and healthy skin measured by impedance meter. Ceramide content is expressed as ng/SC cell.

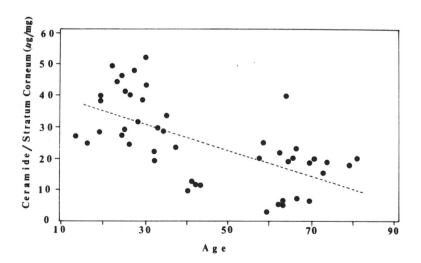

FIGURE 16 The age-dependent decrease in the amount of ceramides in the SC of healthy forearms. Ceramide content is expressed as µg/mg SC.

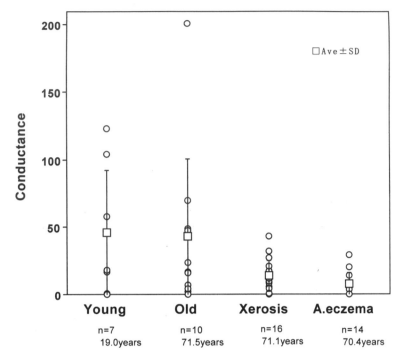

FIGURE 17 Water contents measured by impedance meter in the leg skin of young and old volunteers and of xerotic and asteatotic eczema patients.

4 DESIGN OF PSEUDOCERAMIDE AS A MOISTURIZER

4.1 Structural Analysis of Water-Holding Function Synthetic Pseudo-Ceramides

Since ceramides were found to be essential in providing the SC with water by forming lipid multilayers, it would be ideal to use ceramides as a new moisturizer. However, ceramides, whether natural or synthetic, are too expensive to make them commercially profitable. With reference to the chemical structures of natural ceramides (Fig. 21), we have designed simple approaches to synthesize various pseudoceramides at low cost to develop new moisturizers [23–26]. Following synthetic trials, their efficacy was assessed using experimentally induced dry skin. During these assessments, we concluded that (as depicted in Fig. 21), the structural features best suited for synthetic pseudoceramides are as follows: (1) a structure with a hydroxyethyl group at the amide residue, (2) the presence of two

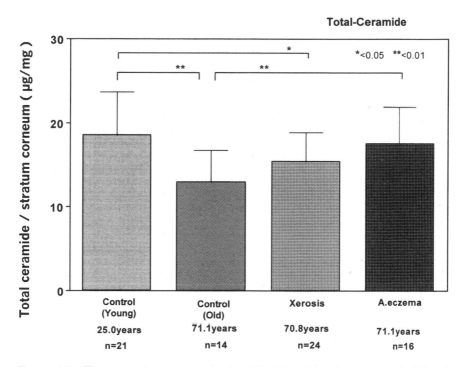

FIGURE 18 The ceramide content in the SC of leg skin of young and old volunteers and of xerotic and asteatotic eczema patients. Ceramide content is expressed as μg/mg SC.

saturated alkyl chains, (3) a structure having a total of 31 carbons in the sphingosine and free fatty acid bases.

4.2 Bound Water–Holding Capacity of Pseudoceramides in the SC Sheet

To clarify whether the restorative effect of optimized synthetic pseudoceramides on dry skin is based upon their bound water–holding capacity, we evaluated changes in bound-water content within the SC when the pseudoceramides were applied to lipid-depleted SC sheets. The application of synthetic pseudoceramides in combination with other intercellular lipids to lipid-depleted SC sheets restored the DSC thermograms almost to the levels of intact SC sheets (Fig. 22) [27,28]. The plot of calculated transition enthalpy against the total water content in the SC sheets demonstrates that application of synthetic pseudoceramides in combination with other intercellular lipids induces a marked increase in the bound-water content, form 19.7 to 26.8%. In contrast, treatment with the control

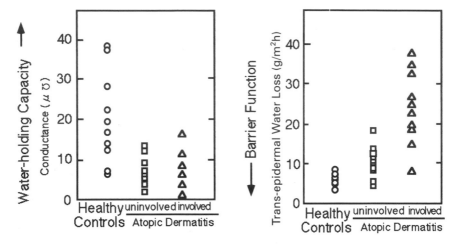

FIGURE 19 Characteristics of the skin of AD patients as revealed by decreased water content (left) and barrier function (right), measured by impedance meter and evaporimeter, respectively.

solution composed of squalene and 1% GE did not influence the bound-water content of SC sheets (Fig. 23) [27,28]. These findings suggest that the therapeutic effect of the optimized pseudoceramides on dry skin results from their restorative effect on the bound-water content within the SC and that ceramide is adequately suited with respect to its bound-water holding capacity.

5 EFFICACY IN CLINICAL USE

5.1 Use in Experimentally Induced Dry Skin

In order to clarify the time course and dose dependency of the recovery in skin conductance, the optimized pseudoceramide, at 3 or 5% concentration, was applied daily for three successive days (from day 0 to day 2), and its effect was evaluated daily. A significant increase relative to the base cream (control) was observed with both the 3 and the 5% pseudoceramide within two days after the first application, with the 5% concentration showing a higher recovery than the 3% (Fig. 24) [24]. In long term experiments [29] using an 8% pseudoceramide cream on dry forearm skin induced by washing with soap, visual evaluations (Fig. 25A) and instrumental readings (Fig. 25B) indicate that both samples examined (the 8% pseudoceramide cream and a commercially available American anti-aging cream P) showed significant improvement from the baseline. In addition, the 8% pseudoceramide-containing sample was significantly better in moisturizing the

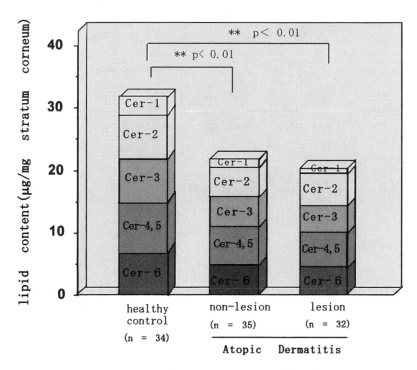

FIGURE 20 Quantitation of ceramides in the SC of patients with AD. Ceramide content is expressed as μg/mg SC. Cer, ceramide.

dry skin compared with the commercially available moisturizer cream. The within-treatment binomial analysis of the dryness scores indicate that both samples showed significant improvement from the baseline throughout the entire study, including the regression phase. The within-treatment binominal analysis of the dryness scores show both samples to be significantly better than baseline on days 21 and 28. The between-treatment binomial analysis of the dryness scores indicates that the pseudoceramide-containing cream was assigned the lower score significantly more often than was the control cream P on days 2, 7, 19, 21, 26, and 28. The analysis of variance of the dryness scores indicates a significant difference between the two samples. The overall sample mean for the pseudoceramide-containing cream was significantly lower, that is, it was less dry, than for the control cream P. The impedance readings reflect the skin's water content, and therefore the higher the value obtained, the more moist the skin. The pseudoceramide-containing cream impedance reading near the elbow was significantly higher on study days 2 through 23 than those values for the control cream P. Sim-

natural ceramides

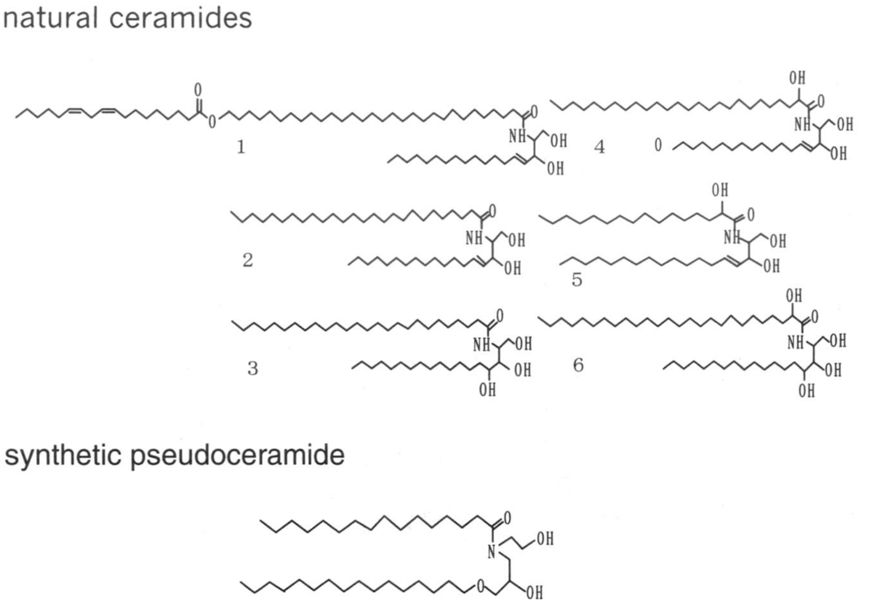

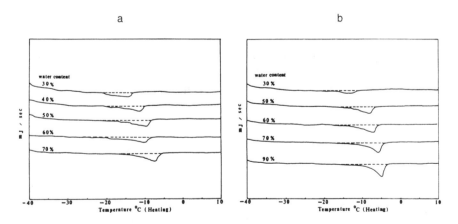

synthetic pseudoceramide

FIGURE 21 Species and structures of natural ceramides and synthetic pseudoceramide.

a   b

FIGURE 22 DSC thermal profiles obtained for synthetic pseudoceramide-treated human SC sheets after acetone/ether treatment. (a) Acetone/ether-treated SC sheet. (b) Pseudoceramide-treated SC sheet after acetone/ether treatment.

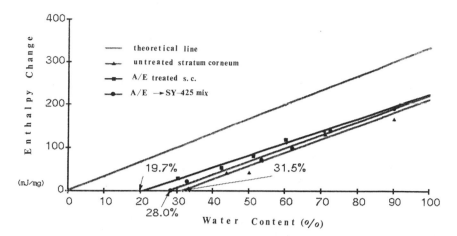

FIGURE 23 The melting enthalpy of ice plotted against the total water content in the SC sheets treated with a lipid mixture which included the synthetic pseudoceramide, based upon DSC analysis. SC, stratum corneum, SY-425 mix, pseudoceramide plus other intercellular lipids.

ilarly, the pseudoceramide-containing cream impedance readings taken near the wrist were significantly higher than for the control cream P on study days 2 through 26.

5.2   Clinical Use in Treatment of Xerosis

A 5% pseudoceramide-containing cream was applied twice daily for 3 weeks to aged facial skin (n = 35 females) which exhibits xerosis and was compared with the effects of the typical commercially available American anti-aging cream G (Fig. 26) [8,29]. The within-treatment binomial analysis of the dryness scores indicates that both samples showed significant improvement from the baseline throughout the entire study. The between-treatment binomial analysis of the dryness scores indicates that the pseudoceramide-containing cream was assigned the lower score significantly more often than was the control cream on weeks 1, 2, and 3. The analysis of variance of the dryness scores indicates a significant difference between the two samples. The overall sample mean for the pseudoceramide-containing cream was significantly lower, that is, it was less dry, than for the control cream. The impedance readings in another study of xerotic skin using the American anti-aging cream E as a control indicated that the pseudoceramide-containing cream impedance reading on the cheek was significantly higher on study weeks 1 through 3 than those values for the control cream (Fig. 27) [29].

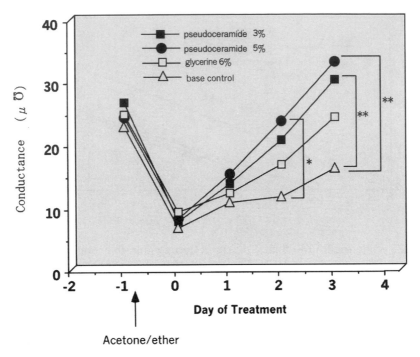

FIGURE 24 The time course and dose dependency of the effect of the optimized ceramide on human skin. The forearm skin of healthy male volunteers was treated with acetone/ether for 30 min on day –1. The sample, emulsified in W/O base cream at the indicated concentrations, was applied daily from day 0 to day 2. Conductance values were measured daily and compared with base only. *p < 0.05; **p < 0.01.

5.3 Clinical Use on Atopic Dry Skin

When an 8% pseudoceramide-containing cream was applied for 6 weeks to dry skin on one forearm of AD patients (n = 18) and compared with a control cream (which replaced the pseudoceramide with cholesterol ester at the same concentration, a typical anti-aging moisturizing cream) applied to the other forearm, the clinical appearance (including dryness, scaling, itching, and erythema) was improved with the ceramide cream being significantly or slightly more effective than the cholesterol ester cream (Fig. 28A) [28–30]. Evaluation by trans-epidermal water loss and water content analyses revealed that the ceramide cream significantly enhances the barrier function and water-holding property of atopic dry skin compared with the cholesterol ester cream (Fig. 28B). This result suggests that the ceramide cream has the distinct potential to repair the damaged barrier

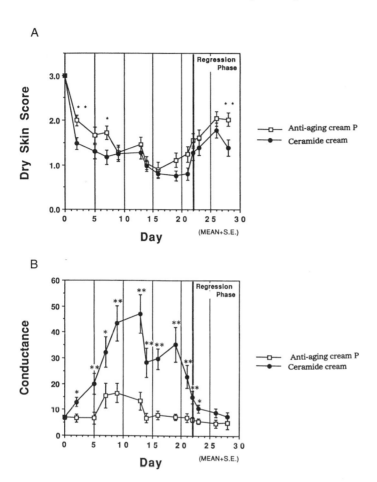

FIGURE 25 The effect of pseudoceramide cream on dry skin induced by washing with soap for 28 days. Candidates with dry skin on their forearms were selected from volunteers who had undergone a 1 week conditioning period using Ivory soap exclusively on the test areas. Test materials were assigned to the right or left arms according to a predetermined randomization. Test materials were applied twice daily for 21 consecutive days. A regression period of 1 week without moisturizer then followed before the start of treatment with 8% pseudoceramide cream. (A) Comparison of dry skin. Visual evaluations were conducted with the aid of a 7 diopter illuminated magnifying lens on 13 days over a 28-day period. By the same observer throughout the study n = 23, **p < 0.01; *p < 0.05. (B) Comparison of conductance. Instrumental evaluation with a Skicon 200 impedance meter was made on the same days as in (A) **p < 0.01; *p < 0.05.

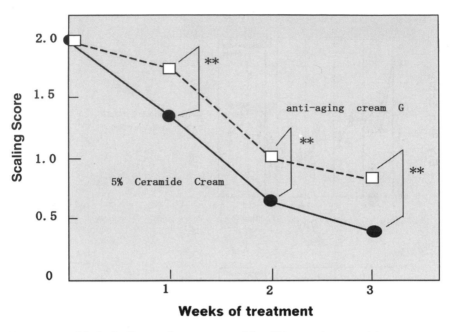

FIGURE 26   Clinical effects of treatment with a 5% pseudoceramide cream on xerotic skin (cheek) compared with an American anti-aging cream G over 3 weeks of treatment, as demonstrated by the scaling score. n = 35; **p < 0.01.

function in addition to its enhancement of the water-holding function. Comparison of clinical improvements elicited by the ceramide and the cholesterol ester creams (Fig. 28C) reveals that treatment with the ceramide cream provides a significantly better clinical improvement (p < 0.05 by the Wilcoxon test) than did the cholesterol ester cream.

Figure 29 shows another clinical study [31], which applied an 8% pseudoceramide-containing cream on the dry skin of AD patients (n = 19) and compared that with a 10% urea cream (which is recommended as a moisturizing cream for atopic dry skin by Japanese dermatologists). Treatment for 6 weeks with the pseudoceramide cream caused a significant decline in clinical symptoms, including dryness, scaling, itchiness, and redness, with a significantly higher efficacy than the 8% urea cream in scaling and redness scores. There were some cases in which the urea cream treatment elicited some side effects such as biting, burning, and redness, whereas no such side effects were observed with the pseudoceramide cream during this 6-week study. To determine the influence on barrier function, a closed patch test using a mite antigen extract was carried out on the forearm skin of AD patients (n = 4) who had positive allergic reactions before ap-

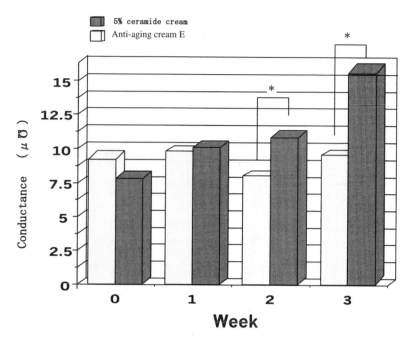

Figure 27 Clinical effects of treatment with a 5% pseudoceramide cream on xerotic skin (cheek) compared with an American anti-aging cream E during 3 weeks of treatment, as demonstrated by conductance value. n = 30; *p < 0.05.

plication of those creams. The skin treated with the pseudoceramide cream recovered its barrier function and became completely resistant against the mite allergy under the closed patch test, whereas the skin treated with the urea cream had a stronger positive allergic reaction (than before the application), which indicates that the barrier disruption still existed and may even have worsened (Table 1). This is consistent with the barrier recovery effect of the pseudoceramide cream observed in other studies [30] which measured the trans-epidermal water loss value. Comparison of clinical improvement between the pseudoceramide and the urea creams (Fig. 30) reveals that treatment with the 8% pseudoceramide cream provides a significantly better clinical improvement (p < 0.05 by Fisher test) than does treatment with the 10% urea cream.

Figure 31 shows different clinical studies [32] which applied an 8% pseudoceramide-containing cream on the dry skin of AD patients (n = 24) and compared that with a 20% urea cream. Treatment for 6 weeks with the pseudoceramide cream caused a significant decline in the clinical symptoms, including

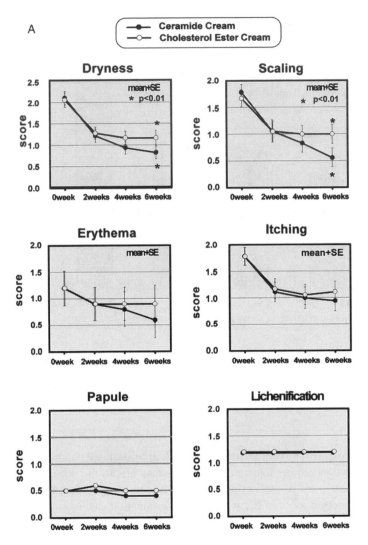

FIGURE 28 Clinical effects of an 8% pseudoceramide cream on dry forearm skin of AD patients compared with a cholesterol ester cream (which replaced the pseudoceramide with 5% cholesterol ester) as demonstrated (A) by clinical scores and (B) by water content and barrier function measured by Impedance meter and evaporimeter, respectively. (C) Clinical improvement between the 8% pseudoceramide and the cholesterol ester cream were also compared.

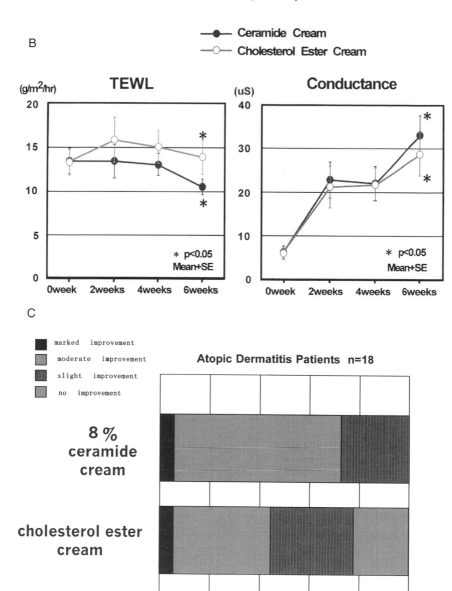

FIGURE 28 Continued

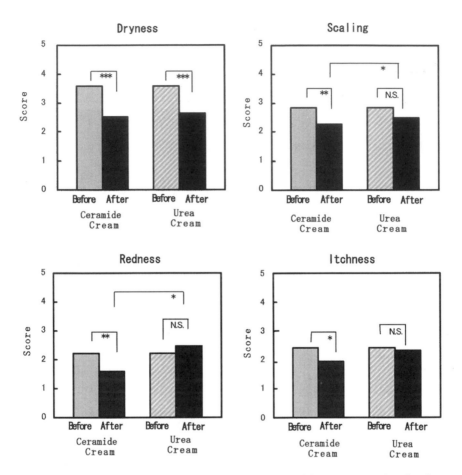

FIGURE 29 Clinical effects of an 8% pseudoceramide cream on the dry forearm skin of AD patients compared with a 10% urea cream, as demonstrated
by clinical scores. *p < 0.05; **p < 0.01; ***p < 0.001 by Wilcoxon test.

dryness, scaling, and itchiness, with an efficacy similar to the 8% urea cream.
Consistent with those clinical improvements, treatment with the pseudoceramide
cream significantly improved water content as well as barrier function (measured
by trans-epidermal water loss) to a significantly greater extent than did the urea
treatment (Fig. 31). Comparison of clinical improvement between the pseudoceramide and the urea creams (Fig. 32) reveals that treatment with the 8% pseudoceramide cream provides a significantly better clinical improvement (p < 0.05 by
the Wilcoxon test) than does the 20% urea cream.

Another comparative study [33] of an application of an 8% pseudoce-

TABLE 1 Effect of Pseudoceramide Cream on Recovery of Barrier Function

	Before treatment	Treated sample	
		8% ceramide cream–treated site	10% urea cream–treated site
–	0	4	0
+	4	0	1
++	0	0	3
Total	4	4	4

Notes: A 48-hr closed patch test was performed using a 5% mite antigen solution on forearm skin following 4 weeks of treatment with pseudoceramide cream or 10% urea cream.

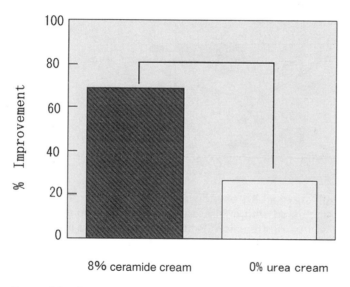

FIGURE 30 Comparison of clinical improvement in 19 AD patients following treatment with an 8% pseudoceramide cream and a 10% urea cream. *p < 0.05 by Fisher test.

ramide-containing cream with a heparin-containing cream (which is another typical moisturizing cream recommended by dermatologists for atopic dry skin) on atopic dry skin (nonlesional skin) of patients with AD for 6 weeks demonstrated that the pseudoceramide cream was significantly more effective in improving atopic dry skin with respect to dryness than was the heparin cream (Fig. 33). Con-

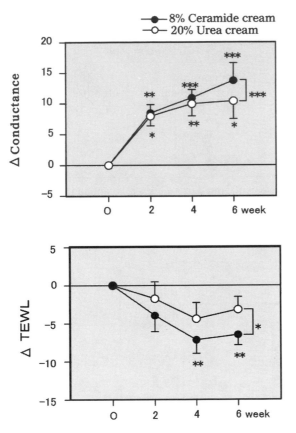

Figure 31 Clinical effects of an 8% pseudoceramide cream on dry forearm skin of AD patients compared with a 20% urea cream, as demonstrated by water content (Top) and barrier function (Bottom), measured by impedance meter and evaporimeter, respectively. *p < 0.05; **p < 0.01; ***p <0.005; ****p < 0.001.

sistent with such clinical improvement, the pseudoceramide cream–treated skin showed a significantly increased water content measured by an impedance meter to an extent similar to the heparin cream (Fig. 34). Interestingly, when comparing their influence on the barrier function measured by evaporimeter, the pseudoceramide cream was found to significantly improve the atopic dry skin with respect to its barrier function, whereas the heparin-containing cream did not show any significant effect on the barrier function (Fig. 35). A comparison of the clinical improvement between the pseudoceramide cream and the heparin cream (Fig. 36) reveals that treatment with the 8% pseudoceramide cream provides a significant-

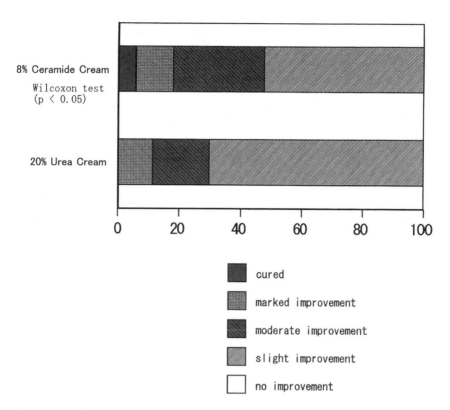

FIGURE 32   Comparison of clinical improvement in 24 AD patients following treatment with an 8% pseudoceramide cream and a 20% urea cream.

ly better clinical improvement (p < 0.05 by the Wilcoxon test) than does the heparin cream.

6 SUMMARY

After several efforts to clarify a new mechanism involved in holding water within the SC, we have reached a distinct principle by which the SC acquires the capacity to retain moisture. It is due to the intercellular lipids which comprise the multilamellar structures located between the SC cells. Thus, water molecules are incorporated into the multilamellar structures in a bound form that plays an essential role in retaining moisture in the SC, which thus acquires resistance to evaporation even under severe dry conditions. Ceramides are an integral component of intercellular lipids and play a major role in the multilamellar architecture.

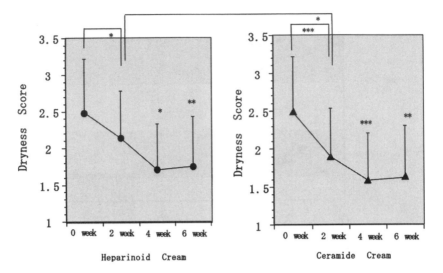

FIGURE 33 Clinical effects of an 8% pseudoceramide cream on dry forearm skin of AD patients compared with heparin cream, as demonstrated by dryness scores. *p < 0.05; **p < 0.01; ***p < 0.005.

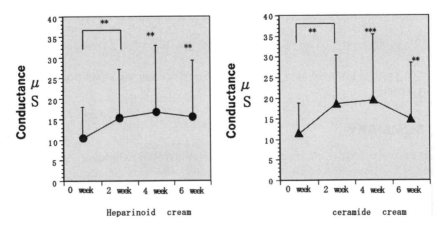

FIGURE 34 Clinical effects of an 8% pseudoceramide cream on dry forearm skin of AD patients compared with a heparin cream, as demonstrated by water content measured by impedance meter. **p < 0.01; ***p < 0.005.

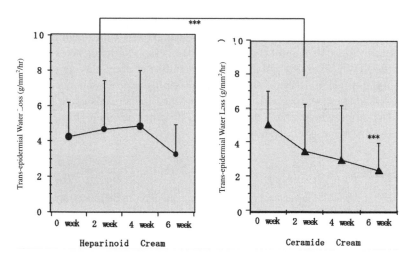

FIGURE 35 Clinical effects of an 8% pseudoceramide cream on dry forearm skin of AD patients compared with a heparin cream, as demonstrated by barrier function measured by evaporimeter. ***p < 0.005.

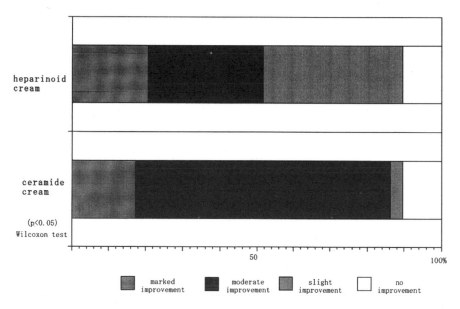

FIGURE 36 Comparison of clinical improvement in 29 AD patients following treatment with an 8% pseudoceramide and a heparin cream.

With the idea that ceramides are an ideal moisturizer when available, we have attempted to synthesize various pseudoceramides which exert water-holding properties similar to those of natural ceramides. Since ceramide deficiencies are observed in the SC in several dry skin symptoms and since they play an essential role in eliciting dry skin, it seems likely that the application of pseudoceramides to dry skin is an ideal approach for therapy. Several clinical trials using pseudoceramide-containing creams have demonstrated that their use is highly effective in preventing and treating dry skin conditions.

REFERENCES

1. Jacobi OT. About the mechanisms of moisture regulation in the horny layer of the skin. Pro Sci Sect Good Assoc 1959; 31:22–24.
2. Imokawa G, Hattori M. A possible function of structural lipid in the water-holding properties of the stratum corneum. J Invest Dermatol 1985; 84:282–284.
3. Imokawa G. Stratum corneum moisturizing effect and intercellular lipids. Fragrance J 1987; 15:35–41.
4. Imokawa G. Intercellular Lipids of the Stratum Corneum. Gendai Hifukagaku Taikei. Nakayama Publishing, 1990; 43–53.
5. Imokawa G. Properties and function of the stratum corneum lipids and its measurement. Rinshouhifuka 1990; 44:583–588.
6. Imokawa G, Akasaki S, Kuno O, Zama M, Kawai M, Minematsu Y, Hattori M, Yoshizuka N, Kawamata A, Yano S, Takaishi N. Function of lipids on human skin. J Dis Sci Tech 1989; 10:617–641.
7. Imokawa G, Kuno H, Kawai M. Stratum corneum lipids serve as a bound-water modulator. J. Invest. Dermatol. 1991; 96:845–851.
8. Imokawa G. Water and the stratum corneum. In: Elsner P, Berardesca E, Maibach HI, eds. Bioengineering of Skin. Vitro and in Vivo Models. Vol 1. CRC Press, 3. 1993:23–47.
9. Imokawa G, Akasaki S, Hattori M, Yoshizuka N. Selective recovery of deranged water-holding properties by stratum corneum lipids. J. Invest. Dermatol. 1986; 87:758–761.
10. Akasaki S, Minematsu Y, Yoshizuka N, Imokawa G. The role of intercellular lipids in the water-holding properties of the stratum corneum: recovery effect on experimentally induced dry skin. Jap. J. Dermatol. 1988; 98:40–51.
11. Imokawa G. Role of stratum corneum components in their moisturizing function. Fragrance J 2000; 17:27–39.
12. Imokawa G. Atopic dermatitis: dry skin mechanism. Japan Pediatr Dermatol 1997; 16:87–99.
13. Jokura T, Ishikawa Y, Tokuda H, Imokawa G. Molecular analysis of elastic properties of the stratum corneum by solid-state ^{13}C-nuclear magnetic resonance spectroscopy. J Invest Dermatol 1995; 104:806–812.
14. Imokawa G. Stratum corneum intercellular lipids: function and association with dry skin disorders. Rinsho Hifuka 1993; 35:1147–1161.
15. Akimoto K, Yoshikawa N, Higaki Y, Kawashima M, Imokawa G. Quantitative

analysis of stratum corneum lipids in xerosis and asteatotic eczema. J Dermatol (Tokyo) 1993; 20:1–6.

16. Imokawa G. Abe A, Kumi J, Higaki Y, Kawashima M, Hidano A. Decreased level of ceramides in stratum corneum of atopic dermatitis: an etiologic factor in atopic dry skin? J. Invest. Dermatol. 1991; 96:523–526.

17. Imokawa G. Atopic dermatitis and abnormality in sphingolipid metabolisms. The lipid 1996; 7:428–423.

18. Imokawa G, Kawashima M. Atopic dermatitis and the stratum corneum lipids. Tokyo Tanabe Quarterly 1997; 42:41–52.

19. Murata Y, Ogata J, Higaki Y, Kawashima M, Yada Y, Higuchi K, Tsuchiya T, Kawaminami S, Imokawa G. Abnormal expression of sphingomyelin acylase in atopic dermatitis: an etiologic factor for ceramide deficiency? J. Invest Dermatol. 1996; 106:1242–1249.

20. Hara J, Higuchi K, Okamoto R, Kawashima M, Imokawa G. High expression of sphingomyelin deacylase is an important determinant of ceramide deficiency leading to barrier disruption in atopic dermatitis. J Invest. Dermatol. 2000; 115:406–413.

21. Higuchi K, Hara J, Okamoto R, Kawashima M, Imokawa G. The skin of atopic dermatitis patients contains a novel enzyme, glucosylceramide sphingomyelin deacylase, which cleaves the N-acyl linkage of sphingomyelin and glucosylceramide. Biochem. J. 2000; 350:747–756.

22. Okamoto R, Hara J, Kawashima M, Takagi Y, Imokawa G. Quantitative analysis of sphingosylphosphorylcholine in the stratum corneum of atopic dermatitis patients [abstract]. J Dermatol Sci 1999; 21:221.

23. Imokawa G, Akasaki S, Zama M, Minematsu Y, Kawamata A, Yano Y, Takaishi N. Selective recovery of deranged water-holding properties in the stratum corneum by synthesized pseudo-ceramide derivatives. Proc Jpn Soc Invest Dermatol 1988; 12:126–127.

24. Imokawa G, Akasaki S, Kawamata A, Yano S, Takaishi N. Water-retaining function in the stratum corneum and its recovery properties by synthetic pseudo-ceramides. J Soc Cosmet Chem 1989; 40:273–285.

25. Imokawa G. Function of epidermal sphingolipids and their application. Fragrance J 1990; 4:26–34.

26. Imokawa G. Stratum corneum intercellular lipids: their function and application. Hifu to Biyo 1991; 23:3806–3818.

27. Imokawa G. Structure and function of intercellular lipids in the stratum corneum. Yukagaku 1995; 44:751–766.

28. Imokawa G. Moisturizers used in dermatology fields. J Clin Dermatol 1998; 56:87–96.

29. Imokawa G. Skin moisturizers: development and clinical use of ceramides. In: Loden M, ed. Dry Skin and Moisturizers. CRC Press, 1999:269–299.

30. Koizumi K, Noguchi K, Imokawa G, Etou T, Nakagawa H, Isibashi H. Clinical effects of synthetic pseudo-ceramides on the dry skin of atopic dermatitis patients [abstract]. Jpn J Dermatoallergol 1993; 2:66.

31. Mizutani J, Takahashi M, Shimizu M, Kariya N, Sato H, Imokawa G. Usage of pseudoceramide cream in atopic dry skin in comparison with 10% urea cream. Nishihihon Hifuka 2001; 63:457–461.

32. Yamanaka M, Ishikawa O, Takahashi M, Sato H, Imokawa G. Usage of pseudoceramide cream in atopic dry skin in comparison with 20% urea cream. Hifu 2001; 43:341–347.
33. Nakamura T, Honma D, Katusragi T, Sakai H, Hashimoto Y, Iizuka H. Usage of pseudoceramide cream in atopic dry skin in comparison with heparinoid cream. Nishinihon Hifu 1999; 61:671–681.

15

Phosphatidylcholine and Skin Hydration

Miklos Ghyczy
Nattermann Phospholipid GmbH, Cologne, Germany

Vladimir Vacata
University of Bonn, Bonn, Germany

Phosphatidylcholine (PC) is the most abundant phospholipid in animal cells. It possesses an intrinsic hydration force, and its metabolites are essential osmoprotectants. Phosphatidylcholine composed of saturated fatty acids (hydrogenated PC; HPC) possesses physical properties which are comparable with those of the components of the skin permeability barrier. When applied to skin, HPC is taken up by the stratum corneum (SC); it interacts with lipids of the permeability barrier, but it does not cause any irritation. Phosphatidylcholine, HPC, and their metabolites display preventive efficacy in pathological states caused by the redox imbalance and the ensuing genesis of free radicals. This phenomenon is taken advantage of in the drug formulations where PC ameliorates certain side effects of drugs. In human skin challenged by sodium lauryl sulfate (SLS), HPC increases skin hydration, but does not exhibit any effect on the trans-epidermal water loss (TEWL). In addition, HPC has the ability to counteract the inflammatory effects of SLS. And HPC is an industrially available, easy-to-handle and well-defined substance produced according to the cGMP standards. The favorable biological effects inspire a new approach to the development of topical formulations for the treatment and prevention of frequent skin problems connected with dry skin and the ensuing pathological states.

1 INTRODUCTION

Phospholipids, as components of lecithins, are the emulsifiers with perhaps the longest history in cosmetics and dermatology. Even the oldest cosmetic protocols recommend egg yolk (which contains 10% phospholipids) as a universal emulsifier. In the past 10 years, some 700 articles and patents have been published and/or registered concerning the use of phospholipids in skin products. However, despite the growing interest in this field, the mode of action and the function of phospholipids in skin are still subjects of critical discussion.

The data acquired during the past decade on skin hydration, skin barrier, and PC itself may help to explain and justify the long-lasting interest in phospholipids and particularly in PC and its applications. The new findings disclose the central role of skin hydration for healthy skin. There are two factors which control the water content in stratum corneum—the intracellular occlusion and the intercellular humectancy [1]. It was also shown that PC with saturated fatty acids (INCI definition: hydrogenated lecithin) possesses thermodynamic and structure-forming properties similar to those of the SC lipids [2]. Hydrogenated PC was found to be capable of penetrating into the SC lipid barrier, though at significantly lower rates than PC with unsaturated fatty acids [3,4]. Because skin contains phospholipases D and A, PC may also serve as a source of osmoprotectants such as choline, betaine, and glycerylphosphatidylcholine. In medicine PC is used as drug substance, and findings in related fields suggest that the mode of its action is based on redox regulation and prevention of formation of free radicals and the ensuing oxidative stress [5]. All these findings suggest that topically applied HPC may have the potential to control skin hydration and prevent the pathological states of dry skin.

2 CONTROL OF SKIN HYDRATION

It is now generally recognized that sufficient water content of SC is the basic prerequisite to healthy skin. This is based on the recent acknowledgment that the SC homeostasis depends on the activity of several enzymes for which stringently controlled water content is essential [6]. This water content is a function of two principles. The first is the permeability barrier, which controls the translocation of water from the lower to the to the upper layer of the SC and subsequently to the environment. The structure responsible for the control is a stack of continuous lipid bilayers in a gel state. Perturbation of this barrier by a diet deficient in linoleic acid or by an external insult such as extensive skin cleansing results in an increased TEWL. The second principle consists of the natural moisturizing factors (NMF) located in the corneocytes. The concentration of NMF in the corneocytes is controlled by NMF synthesis, which itself is feedback-controlled by the water content as well as by external noxae and aging [1].

In view of this knowledge the prevention of and the cure for dry skin syndrome by a topical product should strive for a normalization of both the intercellular occlusion by mitigating the lipid barrier damage and the hypo-osmolarity in the corneocytes.

3 PHOSPHATIDYLCHOLINE, PHOSPHOLIPIDS, AND LECITHIN

Phospholipids belong to the most versatile and to a large extent still enigmatic biomolecules. Not only do they form barriers between biological compartments and the environment, but they also provide the matrix for the all-important chemical reactions of photosynthesis and energy conversion. The metabolites of phospholipids are involved in the regulation of cell volume (the osmoprotectant function), in the signaling systems of cells and organs, as well as in the control of redox reactions. The underlying mechanisms of many of these functions, the redox reactions in particular, are still poorly understood [5].

This may help to explain why PC is used in so many diverse applications, e.g., as an excipient in cosmetics and drug formulations, as an active substance with distinct pharmacological efficacies in dietetics, and as an emulsifier in drugs and food.

Phospholipids can be categorized by their chemical structure. Because excellent reviews on this subject are available, only the aspects relevant for the subject of this chapter will be given here [7,8].

The chemical structure of phospholipids can differ both in the hydrophilic headgroups and the hydrophobic fatty acids which are esterified to the backbone glycerol moiety of the molecule. Figure 1 and Table 1 outline the general formulas of phospholipids and the variations in composition of their fatty acids and hydrophilic headgroups. Additionally, the melting point temperature of the fatty acids is given. The most important headgroups of phospholipids are choline, ethanolamine, inositol, serine, and glycerol. The fatty acids of phospholipids can be either saturated or unsaturated, with chain lengths of mainly 14, 16, and 18 carbons. Biological membranes of humans always consist of mixtures of phospholipids, but the most abundant and ever-present phospholipid is PC, most commonly with unsaturated fatty acids and, to a lesser extent, also with saturated fatty acids (HPC). There are at least two exceptions to this last rule. The first exception is the membrane of the lung–air interface, in which the most abundant phospholipid is HPC with two palmitic acids. A membrane formed of PC with such saturated fatty acids is more rigid, and it is often referred to as crystalline, or being in a gel state. The different composition of the membrane at the lung–air interface is a consequence of a different requirement put on the membrane that separates the aqueous and gaseous phases, as compared to most other biological membranes, which separate two aqueous phases. The second exception to the rule

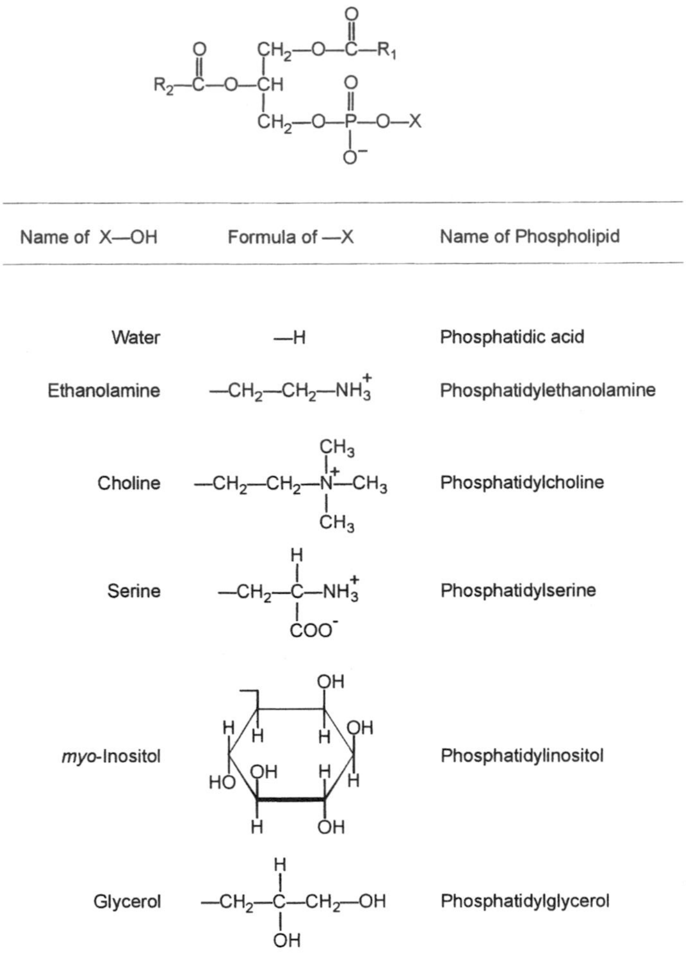

Name of X—OH	Formula of —X	Name of Phospholipid
Water	—H	Phosphatidic acid
Ethanolamine	$-CH_2-CH_2-NH_3^+$	Phosphatidylethanolamine
Choline	$-CH_2-CH_2-\overset{+}{N}(CH_3)_3$	Phosphatidylcholine
Serine	$-CH_2-\underset{COO^-}{\overset{H}{C}}-NH_3^+$	Phosphatidylserine
myo-Inositol		Phosphatidylinositol
Glycerol	$-CH_2-\underset{OH}{\overset{H}{C}}-CH_2-OH$	Phosphatidylglycerol

FIGURE 1 General chemical formulas of phospholipids.

is the membranous structure of SC, which separates the aqueous phase of the human body and the gaseous phase of its environment. Similar to the lung–air interface, its structure is composed of gel-state bilayers.

Lecithin originating from soybeans or eggs is a mixture of phospholipids (cf. Fig. 1), sterols, carbohydrates, glycolipids, fatty acids, and triglycerides. It is used in substantial quantities in the food, feed, and technical industries. Because the complete composition of lecithin is not known; and its components are subject to fluctuations in concentration, depending on the country of origin, extrac-

TABLE 1 The Most Common Fatty Acids in Phospholipids

Symbol	Common name	Systematic name	Structure	Melting point (°C)
Saturated fatty acids				
14:0	Myristic acid	Tetradecanoic acid	$CH_3(CH_2)_{12}COOH$	52,0
16:0	Palmitic acid	Hexadecanoic acid	$CH_3(CH_2)_{14}COOH$	63,1
18:0	Stearic acid	Octadecanoic acid	$CH_3(CH_2)_{16}COOH$	69,6
20:0	Arachidic acid	Eicosanoic acid	$CH_3(CH_2)_{18}COOH$	75,4
Unsaturated fatty acids				
18:1	Oleic acid	9-Octadecenoic acid	$CH_3(CH_2)_7(CH{=}CH)(CH_2)_7COOH$	13,4
18:2	Linoleic acid	9,12-Octadecadienoic acid	$CH_3(CH_2)_7(CH{=}CHCH_2)_2(CH_2)_3COOH$	−9,0
18:3	α-Linolenic acid	9,12,15-Octadecatrienoic acid	$CH_3(CH_2)_7(CH{=}CHCH_2)_3COOH$	−11,0
18:3	γ-Linolenic acid	6,9,12-Octadecatrienoic acid	$CH_3(CH_2)_4(CH{=}CHCH_2)_3(CH_2)_3COOH$	−10,0
20:4	Arachidonic acid	5,8,11,14-Eicosatetraenoic acid	$CH_3(CH_2)_3(CH{=}CHCH_2)_4(CH_2)_2COOH$	−49,5

tion process, storage conditions, and product age, lecithin itself cannot be recommended for use in modern cosmetic products.

Unfortunately, the term lecithin is often used rather loosely and imprecisely. Particularly in the English literature it is often used synonymously for PC and/or the complex mixture of lecithin as just outlined. This often leads to confusion and to incompatible findings achieved with PC, phospholipid mixtures, and lecithin.

It is also important to note that the only phospholipids documented in accordance with the requirements of cosmetic and drug applications are pure PC and fractions with a high content of PC, either in unsaturated or hydrogenated form, originating from soybeans.

An important factor of the use of lecithin and phospholipids in topical formulations is the presence of phosphatidylethanolamine (PE). This phospholipid possesses a primary amino group (cf. Fig. 1) which may react with aldehydes, ketones, and carbohydrates present in the topical formulation or in the skin. Such a chemical reaction may have two effects. It may cause a time-dependent deterioration of components such as perfumes and preservatives. Or, if the amino group of PE does interact with biomolecules which are components of the skin, it may lead to unpredicted pathological states. Because every lecithin and most phospholipid products contain PE, this aspect should be considered when designing a new formulation.

3.1 Phosphatidylcholine and Water

Phosphatidylcholine is hygroscopic—one molecule of PC binds approximately 20 molecules of H_2O. Each molecule of PC permeating into SC will drag along 20 molecules of water. Also, in contrast to other phospholipids present in lecithin, PC (and to a lesser extent also PE) is the only phospholipid with an intrinsic hydration force [9]. The water-binding capacity of PC is thus independent of the presence of ions. It can be assumed that if PC is taken up by the SC, the water content and the water-binding capacity of the SC will be elevated by virtue of the intrinsic hydration force of the PC taken up. Because in a disrupted permeation barrier the flow of ions from the inside to the outside of skin has a messenger function [10], the ion-independent hydration force of PC may be of importance in the treatment of damaged skin.

In the skin, PC is metabolized by the enzymes phospholipase A (PLA) and phospholipase D (PLD) into choline, betaine, and glycerylphosphatidylcholine (GPC). These metabolites belong to the group of biomolecules called osmoprotectants, also known as osmolytes, compatible osmolytes, and/or (most precisely) counteracting osmolytes. These molecules play an essential role in the control of volumes of animal cells; they bind and keep water in the cell, but owing to their hydrophilicity they are not able to penetrate into the membranes and transport water across them.

The major organic osmoprotectants in animal cells can be divided into three groups. The first group comprises substances which contain a quaternary nitrogen moiety with three methyl groups and a positive charge. Glycerylphosphoryl-choline and betaine belong to this group. The second group consists of carbohy-drates such as sorbitol and inositol, and the third one of certain amino acids and their derivatives.

The presence of osmoprotectants in the skin is particularly important in view of the flow of ions between the inside and the outside of the skin. It is obvi-ous that a curative and/or preventive treatment of the skin with osmoprotectants can only be successful if these molecules are capable of penetration into the skin.

Phosphatidylcholine and HPC are pro-osmoprotectants that do penetrate into the skin, where they become precursors and a source of osmoprotectants. In contrast to these penetration-capable precursors, the osmoprotectants themselves are very hydrophilic and therefore are not capable of penetrating into the skin.

3.2 Phosphatidylcholine in Skin Treatment

Biological bilayers are permeation barriers which allow the formation of com-partments in a human organism. The composition of these bilayers is given by the task they have to perform. The fluid-state membranes of cells and organelles sep-arate different aqueous phases and provide means for the generation of chemical and electrical gradients. In the lung the barrier separates the aqueous and the gaseous phases, allowing an active gas exchange. In the skin it also separates the aqueous and the gaseous phases, but in addition it deals with biological, chemi-cal, and mechanical stresses.

These varying tasks are reflected in the different compositions of these bi-layers. The composition changes from the fluid-state phospholipids (mainly PC) in cell membranes to the gel-state PC in the lung and to the highly crystalline and hydrophobic structure of the skin, as imparted by ceramides. The ceramides of the latter membrane are the product of reprocessing of phospholipids and other lipids in a deeper layer of the skin, the stratum granulosum. In this specific trans-formation, the fluid, hydrophilic vesicle–forming phospholipids get converted to the hydrophobic, gel-state and sheet-forming ceramides. Such properties are nec-essary for the formation of a permeability barrier with a continuous, highly crys-talline bilayer structure.

Phosphatidylcholine is available in the form of two distinct chemical enti-ties. The first is native soybean PC, which contains approximately 70% linoleic acid, other unsaturated fatty acids, and only 15 to 16% of saturated fatty acids. Because of its fatty acid composition, this PC quality has a transition temperature of around 0°C. In water it spontaneously forms fluid-state membranes and lipo-somes. It is extensively used in skin treatment as (1) a penetration enhancer [3,4,11] and (2) as a source of linoleic acid, e.g., in the treatment of acne and greasy skin [12,13]. The second entity is PC containing saturated fatty acids only (i.e., HPC), which is used in skin treatment with the aim of strengthening or substituting the permeation barrier [14].

3.3 Phosphatidylcholine with Saturated Fatty Acids

In contrast to the fluid-state PC, the hydrogenated soybean phosphatidylcholine (HPC) contains approximately 85% stearic acid, 14% palmitic acid, and 1% other fatty acids (Fig. 2). These fatty acids have a high melting point (cf. Table 1), and the transition temperature of HPC is therefore approximately 55°C.

The INCI declaration of HPC is *hydrogenated lecithin*, a misleading term because it does not express the fact that this product is a well-defined substance. In our terminology, HPC is a chemical entity which forms bilayers with a gel-to-fluid transition temperature of 50–55°C, as compared to 50°C of the SC lipids [15]. As an excipient, HPC is used in drug formulations because it ameliorates side effects of drugs such as amphotericin B and is well tolerated by humans. It possesses thermodynamic properties similar to those of skin ceramides [2]. It is produced on an industrial scale according to the cGMP requirements. Its handling is simple and well documented. These factors suggest that for the preventive and curative treatment of dry skin, HPC could be a good industrial alternative to ceramides.

4 BIOLOGICAL FINDINGS WITH HPC

4.1 Interaction of HPC with SC Lipids

Blume et al. [16] performed differential scanning calorimetry and ^{2}H-NMR experiments on a dispersion of a SC model lipid mixture consisting of 40% ceramides, 25% cholesterol, 25% palmitic acid, and 10% cholesterol sulfate. In water at 37°C this lipid mixture formed lamellar gel-state structures which were comparable to those of the skin permeability barrier. These lamellar sheets interacted with the dispersions made of (1) a fluid-state PC fraction and (2) HPC by exchange of monomers through the water phase. For the fluid-state PC the interaction was complete in 2 hr; for HPC in 24 hr. The interaction was dependent on the lipid concentration.

These results indicate that the two PC dispersions tested have different kinetics of interaction with the skin, and also that their effect on skin homeostasis is possibly dose dependent. One can conclude that HPC does not penetrate as deeply into the skin as the fluid-state PC.

4.2 Uptake of HPC by Skin

The different kinetics of the interaction between the native skin lipids and the fluid-state PC and/or HPC was determined by several in vivo and in vitro penetration studies.

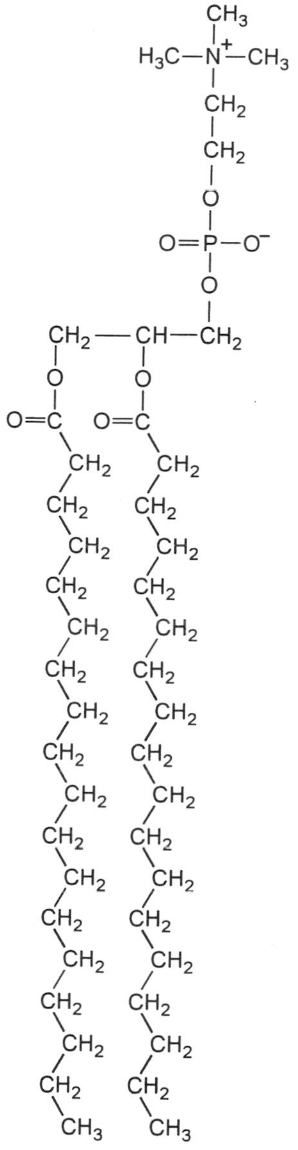

FIGURE 2 Hydrogenated phosphatidylcholine (1,2-stearoyl-phosphatidyl-choline). The molecule is shown with two stearic acids. The soybean HPC contains 85% stearic acid, 14% palmitic acid, and 1% other fatty acids.

Van Kuijk et al. [17] showed that in vivo the fluorescent-labeled liposomes made from fluid-state PC penetrate significantly deeper into the rat skin than those composed of HPC. The same results were obtained for analogous in vitro studies on human skin [18]. The uptake was higher under nonocclusive conditions, indicating the existence of an as yet unrecognized role of water in the skin penetration of the formulations containing PC.

Kirjavainen et al. [4] compared the distribution of drugs formulated with fluid-state PC and/or HPC in the skin in vitro. The HPC-based liposomes remained in the SC and were thus not able to enhance the transdermal drug penetration.

Fahr et al. [3] visualized penetration of liposomes with encapsulated fluorescent dye carboxyfluorescein into the human abdomen skin. Figure 3 shows that, compared to the liposomes made from HPC, those composed of fluid-state PC are taken up by the skin more readily, permeate it faster, and penetrate beyond the SC.

These findings suggest that HPC, and most probably also the accompanying water, is taken up by the SC but not by the deeper layers of the skin. In addition, HPC does not seem to perturb the lipid barrier to the extent that it would enhance the uptake of substances by the dermis.

4.3 Tolerance of HPC by Sensitive Skin

Damaging the permeability barrier is considered to be the first step in the process of irritation of the skin by chemical or physical noxae [19]. The consequence of this damage is the increased synthesis of cytokines and lipids as well as an increased level of TEWL [20,21]. The visual or sensory symptoms perceptible by the test persons and the investigators are scaling and erythema. These effects were used to determine and quantify the effects of different emulsifiers on the test persons as compared to those of HPC [22].

The results of this study (Fig. 4) lend themselves to the following interpretation: (1) the emulsifiers which are not related to the lipids of the permeability barrier have the highest irritation potential; (2) the sugar-containing substances which are related to the biological membranes have a lower irritation potential; and (3) HPC (substance most closely related to the permeability barrier lipids) displays no irritation potential at all.

4.4 Effect of HPC on Skin Hydration

Sodium lauryl sulfate challenge of the human skin in vivo is generally recognized as the most convincing method for imitating dry skin. We have chosen this method to evaluate the potential of HPC in the control of skin hydration. This clinical study was carried out by Gehring et al. [23] at the Dermatology Department of the University of Karlsruhe, Germany, in cooperation with the authors, and has been submitted for publication.

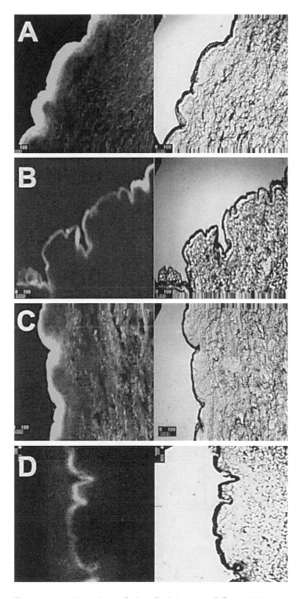

Figure 3 Uptake of the fluid-state PC and the gel-state HPC by the skin. (A) Three hours, fluid-state PC. (B) Three hours, HPC. (C) Twelve hours, fluid-state PC. (D) Twelve hours, HPC. Left side of each is a fluorescence micrograph showing the depth of penetration into the skin of the fluorescent dye carboxyfluorescein. Right side is a visible light micrograph as a reference to the fluorescence micrograph. (From Ref. 3.)

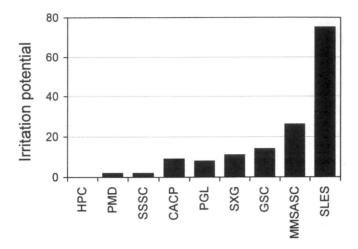

FIGURE 4 Emulsifiers and their irritation potential as assessed from the extent of erythema and scaling. HPC, hydrogenated lecithin; PMD, polyglyceryl-3 methylglucose distearate; SSSC, sorbitan stearate and sucrose cocoate; CACP, cetearyl alcohol and cetearyl polyglucose; PGL, polyglycerinlaurate; SXG, saponins–xanthan gum; GSC, glyceryl stearate citratea; MMSASC, macromolecule and stearic acid and sodium chloride; SLES, sodium laureth sulfate. (From Ref. 22.)

A total of 15 volunteers applied the dispersions to be tested on the volar side of the forearm. Sodium lauryl sulfate was applied as a 0.01 M% solution by a plastic foam roller rolled over the skin 50 times, 5 times per day; the weight of the roller ensured that a specific amount of SLS was applied on the skin surface. 200 μL of 1% HPC dispersion was distributed on the skin 30 min after the application of SLS; the 1% HPC concentration was chosen after preliminary experiments had revealed that a concentration of 0.5% showed moderate effects and that a concentration of 5% was slightly irritant. In all experiments, 1% dispersion of HPC (Phospholipon 90H) was used. The HPC dispersion was prepared by heating 495 mL distilled water to 60°C and transferring it to a high-speed mixer (Braun-Mix); 5 g HPC were added, and the mixture was homogenized at 16,000 rpm for 30 min; the product was preserved with 0.015% thiomersal and kept at 4°C before use. Skin irritation was measured by Chromameter CR 200 (Minolta), water content in the skin by Corneometer CM 820 (Courage and Khazaka), and TEWL by Tewameter TM 210 (Courage and Khazaka). The statistical evaluation was performed by a Wilcoxon pair difference test for combined random samples. The evaluation of the experimental factors took place always 12 hr after the last application.

The results are documented in Fig. 5. Figure 5A shows HPC formulated in water does not normalize the elevated TEWL. This is in agreement with the find-

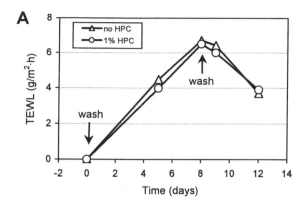

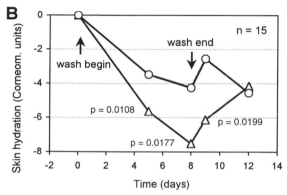

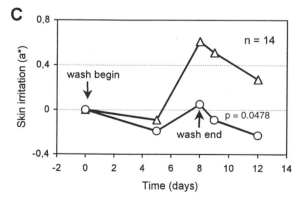

FIGURE 5 In vivo studies with human skin. Effects of (A) SLS (circles) and SLS/HPC (triangles) on TEWL; (B) skin hydration, and (C) skin irritation. Within each group the two effects were compared using Wilcoxon pair difference test for combined random samples. n indicates the size of the statistical sample; p indicates the statistical significance of the difference between the corresponding points of the two curves. (From Ref. 23.)

ings of other laboratories that the application of products containing only phospholipids [24] or only ceramides [25] to a perturbed skin is insufficient for the normalization of TEWL. Figure 5B shows that the water content of SC in the challenged skin gets significantly elevated upon the treatment with HPC. Figure 5C shows that HPC normalized the cytokine-transmitted inflammatory response of the perturbed skin.

4.5 Effect of HPC in Topical Formulations on Hydration of Healthy Skin

This cosmetic study was conducted for Kuhs GmbH by Derma Consult GmbH (Bonn, Germany). The aim of the study was to compare effects of HPC in a cosmetic formulation on healthy skin with those of three commercial oil-in-water (O/W) emulsions. The study has not been published yet, but it is available from Kuhs GmbH (Leichlingen, Germany; probiol@kuhs.com).

A total of five preparations were tested:

1. HPC-containing DMS formulation 1 (Aqua, carprylic/capric triglyceride, pentylene glycol, hydrogenated lecithin (HPC 4%), butyrospermum parkii, glycerin, squalene, 0.0066% ceramide 3)
2. HPC-containing DMS formulation 2 (Aqua, carprylic/capric triglyceride, pentylene glycol, hydrogenated lecithin (HPC 2%), butyrospermum parkii, glycerin, squalene, sodium carbomer, xantham gum, 0.0033% Ceramide 3)
3. Commercial product 1 (Aqua, caprylic/capric triglyceride, hydrogenated coco-glycerides, polyglyceryl-3 methylglucose distearate, glyceryl stearate, setyl alcohol, stearyl alcohol, phenoxyethanol, cyclomethicone, glyceryl polymethacrylate, imidazolidinyl urea, aluminum starch octenyl succinate, propylene glycol)
4. Commercial product 2 (Aqua, paraffinum liquidum, dicaprylyl ether, cyclomethicone, glyceryl stearate SE, isohexadecane, butyrospermum parkii, sodium acrylatees copolymer, phenoxyethanol, cetyl phosphate, imidazolidinyl urea, PPG-1 Trideceth-6, sodium hydroxide, PEG-8, tocopherol, ascorbyl palmitate, ascorbic acid, citric acid)
5. Commercial product 3 (Aqua, paraffinum liquidum, sorbitol, dicaprylyl ether, cyclomethicone, glyceryl stearate SE, isohexadecane, tocopheryl acetate, butryospermum parkii, sodium acrylates copolymer, panthenol, phenoxyethanol, cetyl phosphate, hexylene glycol, imidazolidinyl urea, PPG-1 Trideceth-6, retinyl palmitate, arachis hypogaea, fructose, glucose, sodium hydroxide, PEG-8, dextrin, sucrose, urea, tocopherol, alanine, ascorbyl palmitate, aspartic acid, glutamic acid, hexyl nicotinate, ascorbic acid, citric acid)

The test was performed on 20 healthy female volunteers (25 to 40 years old), who applied the formulations to be tested on the volar side of the forearm. The products were applied twice daily over a period of 28 days. The time of evaluation was 8 hr, 1 and 3 days after the last application. Skin hydration was measured with Corneometer CM 825 (Courage and Khazaka), skin roughness with Skin Visiometer (image analysis on silicon base, Courage and Khazaka) and skin firmness with Cutometer SEM 474 (Courage and Khazaka).

The results of this comparative study on healthy skin are summarized in Fig. 6. They indicate the following.

1. Both of the formulations containing HPC show similar efficacy; one can therefore presume that the highest beneficial effect is achieved at 2% HPC.

2. The superior effects of the DMS formulations, especially the longer-lasting effects after the application was terminated, are most likely based on the presence of HPC. This conclusion is supported by the penetration property of HPC as well as by the elevation of skin hydration as indicated in the case of the SLS-damaged skin. Because in healthy skin the barrier is not damaged, these findings strongly indicate that the elevated skin hydration could be a function of the intrinsic hydration force of HPC and the osmoprotectant efficacy of its metabolites, due to which HPC brings in and retains water in the permeability barrier. No other components of topical formulations possess such properties.

Because the commercial products do not include substances with the functionality of HPC outlined, the superior efficacy of the DMS formulations is understandable. This difference further indicates the relevance of HPC for the control of skin hydration also in the healthy undamaged skin.

5 DISCUSSION

The functionalities of HPC explained in this chapter support and expand our knowledge of the mechanism and the means of skin hydration control.

It was shown that SC takes up HPC. The prerequisite for this uptake is the interaction of HPC with the permeability barrier. In vitro, this interaction does not perturb the SC lipid structure. This explains the lack of any irritant capacity of HPC on healthy human skin in vivo. In contrast to the interaction of HPC with the skin, nearly all of the commercial emulsifiers dissolve the SC lipid structure in vitro, and in vivo most of them display an irritation capacity. In SLS-perturbed skin, the elevated TEWL is an indicator of the disintegration of the permeability barrier. In our experiments, HPC formulated in water does not normalize the elevated TEWL. This is in accordance with the findings of other laboratories sug-

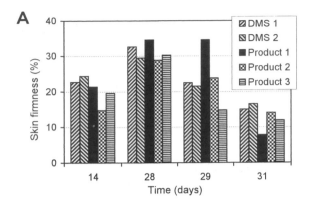

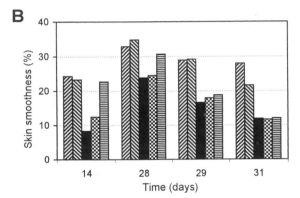

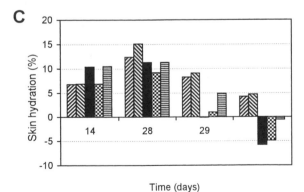

Figure 6　In vivo studies with human skin. Effects of two HPC-containing formulations (DMS 1 and DMS 2) and three commercial HPC-free products (Products 1, 2, and 3) on (A) skin firmness, (B) skin smoothness, and (C) skin hydration. (Courtesy of Kuhs GmbH, Leichlingen, Germany.)

gesting that the bilayer-forming substances, such as phospholipids [24] or ceramides [25], have to be formulated with other lipids which do not form bilayers on their own, but which will insert into existing bilayers, thus providing a form of repair to a disrupted barrier. On the other hand the water content of the SC in SLS-perturbed skin becomes significantly elevated if the skin is treated with HPC concomitantly with and after the SLS treatment. This indicates that HPC functions as a transport vehicle and storage for water, thus substituting to some degree the SLS-depleted NMF. Because of the intrinsic hydration force of HPC and the osmoprotectant properties of the HPC metabolites, such as betaine and glycerylphosphatidylcholine, and because HPC is taken up in the SC, these findings are not surprising.

The repetitive application of SLS causes not only a disruption of the permeability barrier, but also the release of cytokines, which are the indicators of inflammation. In our experiments, HPC normalized the inflammatory response of the skin to the SLS treatment. This result is supported by previous findings regarding the anti-inflammatory potential of PC in the cases of UV irritation [26] and efflorescences in acne [12]. Another supportive argument could be the proposed mode of protective effects of PC and its metabolites during a redox imbalance [5].

The finding that HPC has an anti-inflammatory efficacy but no normalizing effects on TEWL is in contrast to the common belief that the cytokine-releasing inflammatory effect of SLS is based on barrier disruption, and that a barrier repair leads to normalization of the inflamed skin [27].

Further experiments are necessary for the evaluation of the full anti-inflammatory potential of HPC because it is conceivable that due to the uptake of HPC in SC, the penetration rate of SLS through SC increases, which is a contrary effect to the amelioration of irritation by HPC.

In order to evaluate the full potential of HPC in skin hydration control we need to perform experiments with formulations containing HPC and lipids which are related to endogenous SC lipids. The positive effects of such lipid combinations on SLS-induced dry skin [24] should suggest the optimal composition of such formulations.

REFERENCES

1. Harding CR, Watkinson A, Rawlings AV, Scott IR. Dry skin, moisturization and corneodesmolysis. Int J Cosmet Sci 2000; 22:21–52.
2. Pechtold LA, Abraham W, Potts RO. Characterization of the stratum corneum lipid matrix using fluorescence spectroscopy. J Invest Dermatol Symp Proc 1998; 3:105–109.
3. Fahr A, Schäfer U, Verma DD, Blume G. Skin penetration enhancement of substances by a novel type of liposomes. SÖFW-Journal 2000; 126:49–53.

4. Kirjavainen M, Monkkonen J, Saukkosaari M, Valjakka-Koskela R, Kiesvaara J, Urtti A. Phospholipids affect stratum corneum lipid bilayer fluidity and drug partitioning into the bilayers. J Contr Release 1999; 58:207–214.

5. Ghyczy M, Boros M. Electrophilic methyl groups present in the diet ameliorate physiological states induced by reductive and oxidative stress. Hypothesis. Br J Nutr 2001; 85:409–414.

6. Rawlings AV, Scott IR, Harding CR, Bowser PA. Stratum corneum moisturization at the molecular level. J Invest Dermatol 1994; 103:731–741.

7. A Wendel. Lecithin. In: Kroschwitz JI, Howe-Grant M, eds. Encyclopedia of Chemical Technology. Vol. 15. New York: Wiley, 1995:192–210.

8. Silvius JR. Structure and nomenclature. In: Cevc G, ed. Phospholipids Handbook. New York: Marcel Dekker, 1993:1–22.

9. Israelachvili J. Intermolecular and Surface Forces. London: Academic Press, 1992:395–421.

10. Lee SH, Elias PM, Proksch E, Menon GK, Mao-Quiang M, Feingold KR. Calcium and potassium are important regulators of barrier homeostasis in murine epidermis. J Clin Invest 1992; 89:530–538.

11. Gehring W, Ghyczy M, Gareiss J, Gloor M. The influence on skin penetration by dithranol formulated in phospholipids solutions and phospholipid liposomes. Eur J Pharm Biopharm 1995; 41:140–141.

12. Ghyczy M, Nissen HP, Blitz H. The treatment of acne vulgaris by phosphatidylcholine from soybeans, with a high content of linoleic acid. J Appl Cosmetol 1996; 14:137–145.

13. Morganti P, Randazzo SD, Giardina A, Bruno C, Vincenti M, Tiberi L. Effect of phosphatidylcholine linoleic acid–rich and glycolic acid in Acne vulgaris. J Appl Cosmetol 1997; 15:21–32.

14. DMS-Concentrate: A new Hydrolipid System Similar to the Skin Lipid Structure. Langenfeld: Kuhs GmbH & Co., 1995.

15. Bonte F, Pinguet P, Saunois A, Meybeck A, Beugin S, Ollivon M, Lesieur S. Thermotropic phase behavior of in vivo extracted human stratum corneum lipids. Lipids 1997; 32:653–660.

16. Blume A, Jansen M, Ghyczy M, Gareiss J. Interaction of phospholipid liposomes with lipid model mixtures for stratum corneum lipids. Int J Pharm 1993; 99:219–228.

17. van Kuijk-Meuwissen ME, Mougin L, Junginger GE, Bouwstra JA. Application of vesicles to rat skin in vivo: a confocal laser scanning microscopy study. J Contr Release 1998; 56:189–196.

18. van Kuijk-Meuwissen ME, Junginger GE, Bouwstra JA. Interactions between liposomes and human skin in vitro, a confocal laser scanning microscopy study. Biochim Biophys Acta 1998; 1371:31–39.

19. Tsai JC, Feingold KR, Crumrine D, Wood LC, Grunfeld C, Elias PM. Permeability barrier disruption alters the localization and expression of TNF alpha/protein in the epidermis. Arch Dermatol Res 1994; 286:242–248.

20. Fartasch M. Ultrastructure of the epidermal barrier after irritation. Microsc Res Tech 1997; 37:193–199.

21. Wood LC, Jackson SM, Elias PM, Grunfeld C, Feingold KR. Cutaneous barrier per-

turbation stimulates cytokine production in the epidermis of mice. J Clin Invest 1992; 90:482–487.

22. Kutz G, Biehl P, Waldmann-Laue M, Jackwerth B. Zur Auswahl von O/W-Emulgatoren für den Einsatz in Hautpflegeprodukten bei sensibler Haut. SÖFW-Journal 1997; 123:145–149.

23. Gehring W, Ghyczy M, Vacata V, Gloor M. Effect of HPC on SLS-treated skin (submitted).

24. Summers RS, Summers B, Chandar P, Feinberg C, Gursky R, Rawlings AV. The effect of lipids, with and without humectant, on skin xerosis. J Soc Cosmet Chem 1996; 47:27–39.

25. Man MQ, Feingold KR, Elias PM. Exogenous lipids influence permeability barrier recovery in acetone-treated murine skin. Arch Dermatol 1993; 129:728–738.

26. Thiele B, Ghyczy M, Lunow C, Teichert GM, Wolff GH. Influence of phospholipid liposomes (PLL) on UVB-induced erythema formation. Arch Dermatol Res 1993; 285:428–431.

27. Nickoloff BJ, Naidu Y. Perturbation of epidermal barrier function correlates with initiation of cytokine cascade in human skin. J Am Acad Dermatol 1994; 30:535–546.

16

Hydroxyacids

Anthony W. Johnson
Unilever Home and Personal Care North America,
Trumbull, Connecticut

1 INTRODUCTION

Although there are many hydroxy acids, the focus of this chapter is on *alpha*-hydroxyacids, or AHAs as they have come to be known universally since their explosive takeover of the cosmetic facial moisturizer market in the early 1990s [1–3]. More recently, other classes of hydroxyacids have been used in skin care products [4], but at the time of writing (2001) AHAs stand alone as the only hydroxyacids supported by placebo-controlled clinical testing. In fact it is one particular AHA, glycolic acid, that was used in the first AHA facial moisturizers and remains the most common form today. As detailed herein, glycolic acid and other AHAs do more than moisturize. They are able to reduce wrinkles, eliminate fine lines, improve skin surface texture, and lessen some of the other changes associated with photodamaged skin. However, the AHA story starts long before the spectacular appearance of glycolic acid "anti-aging" skin creams in 1992. Some 25 years earlier, another alpha-hydroxyacid, lactic acid, was identified as a component of the skin's natural moisturizing factor (NMF) and introduced as a moisturizing ingredient in creams and lotions to treat and prevent dry skin, particularly winter dry skin on the hands, legs, and body [5]. At about the same time Van Scott and Yu reported that alphahydroxy acids as a class were effective for treating ichthyosis and other disorders of keratinization [6]. The new information about AHAs prompted increased interest in glycolic acid by dermatologists for chemical peel procedures. Glycolic acid solutions (50–70% concentration without neutralization) were found to be very effective as acid peels, easier to use and without side effects compared to other peeling agents [7].

The extensive use of AHAs in the last 10 years has transformed the cosmetic market place and changed consumer expectations. Women have seen that AHA moisturizers can provide skin improvements dramatically better than previous skin care creams. There has been much discussion about the biological effects and cosmetic efficacy of AHA products over the last 10 years [8–10], with the majority of publications being editorial and review articles rather than original scientific papers. This has resulted in a merging of fact and speculation relating to AHA skin actions and benefits.

Alpha-hydroxyacids have a variety of different actions on skin depending on their pH and concentration. These effects are detailed in the sections that follow. In simple terms, the salt forms of AHAs are effective humectant moisturizers, whereas the acid forms go beyond moisturizing to correct the dysfunction underlying dry skin and to enhance the normal processes of the epidermis. There is an important distinction between the strong acid solutions used as chemical peels by dermatologists and the mild buffered preparations available to consumers as everyday cosmetic creams and lotions. The former work by damaging skin, and the latter are designed to provide benefits without any adverse effect.

Alpha-hydroxyacids appear to have multiple actions on the stratum corneum and living epidermis depending on concentration and pH. But given that the primary function of the epidermis is to produce a healthy and effective outer protective layer, it is not surprising that the main benefits of AHAs are manifest as enhancements of stratum corneum quality (its look, touch, feel, and effectiveness as a protective barrier). Another property of AHAs in their buffered acid form is a tendency to induce sensory irritation (burn, sting, or tingling) in susceptible individuals, at concentrations which are not overtly irritating, i.e., do not induce an inflammatory reaction [11]. The sensory irritant effect is pH/concentration related and reduces as pH is increased (i.e., as the proportion of free acid is reduced).

Failure to take account of pH and concentration has led to a good deal of questioning and miscommunication about the benefits, safety, and effectiveness of AHA products. It is surprising how many otherwise sound scientific publications do not specify the pH of AHA preparations under study. It is therefore appropriate to start this chapter with a brief consideration of pH and some of the other basic facts about AHAs.

2 CHEMISTRY AND BIOCHEMISTRY OF ALPHA-HYDROXYACIDS

Hydroxyacids are common and essential constituents of all living cells. Simple hydroxyacids are mainly involved in the breakdown of fats and carbohydrates to produce energy. Derivatives of hydroxyacids are involved in amino acid and protein metabolism (structure and growth), neurotransmitters (brain and nerve function), and some hormones and vitamins. Lactic acid is the most important AHA involved in cellular energy metabolism.

Alpha-hydroxyacids are organic carboxylic acids having a hydroxyl group (–OH) attached to the carbon atom (–C–) next to the carboxyl group (–COOH). In the nomenclature of chemistry, this carbon atom is "alpha" to the carboxyl group. Hence the name, alpha-hydroxyacids. There are many AHAs determined by the chemical group attached to the alpha carbon atom (Figure 1).

Alpha-hydroxyacids are "weak acids," meaning that they do not completely dissociate in water. The extent of dissociation is a function of pH. The pH at which an acid is 50% dissociated (50% acid form and 50% salt form) is the pKa value for the acid. It is significant that the pKa values for glycolic acid (pH 3.83) and for lactic acid (pH 3.86) are very close [12]. Most cosmetic glycolic acid products have pH values at about this pKa value or higher, and most lactic acid hand and body moisturizers have pH values above 5. Because the slope of the dissociation curves for weak acids reaches a maximum at the pKa [13], small movements in pH make a big difference to the availability of acid versus salt, as shown in Table 1. Note that concentration does not have as much effect on acid strength, as does pH. For example, a 5% solution of fully dissociated glycolic acid has a pH of 1.7, while 10% is pH 1.6, and 50% is pH 1.2. A 10-fold difference in concentration makes a difference of only 0.5 pH unit [14].

The concentrations of glycolic acid most widely used in cosmetic face moisturizer products are from 4 to 8% glycolic acid at pH 3.8–4.0. The typical concentration of lactic acid in products for hand and body dry skin treatment is about 5%, with pH varying from pH 4–5 and above. There is one prescriptive lo-

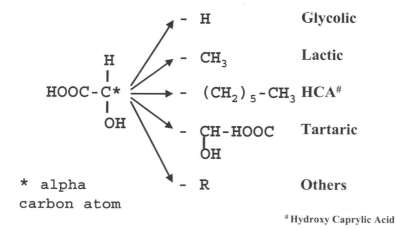

FIGURE 1 Structure of alpha hydroxyacids

TABLE 1 Free Acid Content for AHA Products (Glycolic or Lactic) Related to pH

pH	Concentration of free acid for each product concentration of AHA[a]				
	10%	8%	4%	2%	1%
2.0	9.9[b]	8.0[b]	4.0[d]	2.0[d]	1.0[e]
3.0	8.8[b]	7.0[b]	3.5[d]	1.8[e]	0.9[e]
3.5	6.8[c]	5.4[c]	2.7[d]	1.4[e]	0.7[e]
3.6	6.4[c]	5.1[c]	2.6[d]	1.3[e]	0.6[e]
3.7	5.7[c]	4.6[d]	2.3[d]	1.2[e]	0.6[e]
3.8	5.2[c]	4.2[d]	2.1[d]	1.1[e]	0.5[e]
3.9	4.6[c]	3.7[d]	1.8[d]	0.9[e]	0.5[e]
4.0	4.0[d]	3.2[d]	1.6[d]	0.8[e]	0.4[e]
4.2	3.0[d]	2.4[d]	1.2[e]	0.6[e]	0.3[e]
4.4	2.1[d]	1.2[e]	0.6[e]	0.3[e]	0.2[e]
4.6	1.5[e]	0.8[e]	0.3[e]	0.2[e]	0.1[e]
5.0	0.6[e]	0.5[e]	0.2[e]	0.1[e]	0.1[e]
6.0	0.1[e]	0.1[e]	0.0[e]	0.0[e]	0.0[e]

[a]PKa for both close to 3.8 (see text).
[b]Effective but more acid than CIR limit.
[c]Effective but more acid than most retail.
[d]Good evidence efficacy.
[e]Borderline effective/ineffective.
Note: Cells group free acid values for products according to efficacy for improving skin condition beyond simple moisturization, and superimposed on efficacy is availability/suitability for retail cosmetic moisturizer products. The cut-off for efficacy is somewhat arbitrary but based on evidence that efficacy drops off sharply below 4% AHA at pH 4.0 (1.6% free acid).

tion for dry skin that contains 12% lactic acid and is pH 5.4 [15]. It should be noted that concentrations of AHA up to 10% with pH down to 3.5 are considered safe by the U.S. Cosmetic Ingredient Review (CIR).

Glycolic acid and lactic acid appear to be similarly effective for skin moisturization and anti-aging benefits [16], and yet their biochemistry is completely different. Lactic acid is at the center of mammalian energy metabolism, whereas glycolic acid does not figure in mainstream mammalian biochemistry with only a minor pathway for processing glycolic acid coming from the diet. As we shall see later the similar effectiveness of these two metabolically different acids cannot be explained in terms of their one common feature, i.e., that they both have essentially the same pKa.

Another hydroxyacid used in facial anti-aging products is salicylic acid.

This is an aromatic hydroxyacid that has long been used as a keratolytic agent in the treatment of warts and other hyperkeratotic conditions [17] and in OTC preparations for the treatment of mild acne [18]. Unlike AHAs, salicylic acid has not been used as a moisturizing ingredient in products for treating dry skin, but it does seem to have cosmetic benefits for skin photodamage and has been promoted as an alternative to AHAs [19]. The pKa of salicylic acid is 2.97 [20], nearly 10 times more acid than the pKa of glycolic and lactic acids. Because of its potential for irritation at higher concentrations, salicylic acid is mostly used at concentrations of 1.5% or less in cosmetic skin creams. Salicylic acid has been described as a beta-hydroxyacid (BHA) by the cosmetic industry, but described correctly it is an aromatic *ortho*-hydroxyacid.

The alpha-hydroxyacids are sometimes called fruit acids because of their abundance in common fruits (citric acid in citrus fruits, malic acid in apples, tartaric acid in grapes). Ironically, the two most widely used AHAs are not major components of fruits; glycolic acid is a constituent of sugar cane juice and lactic acid occurs most abundantly in sour milk [12].

3 SKIN BENEFITS OF HYDROXYACIDS

There have been several distinct phases in the development of AHAs for cosmetic skin care products.

1. 1970 onward: use of lactic acid in products to treat and prevent dry skin (initially in the United States and Europe, extending worldwide).
2. 1992 onward: alongside lactic acid moisturizers, use of glycolic acid to treat facial photodamage (initially in the United States, extending world wide).
3. Mid-1990s onward: alongside glycolic and lactic acid products, use of other hydroxy acids including BHA, tri-hydroxyacids (THAs), poly-hydroxyacids (PHAs), combinations of these, and ascorbic acid (vitamin C), in a search for systems to improve on glycolic acid.
4. In addition to their cosmetic skin care use, AHAs, saw increasing use from the 1970s onward, specifically glycolic acid, for chemical peels. This was both as conventional peels and as combination therapies where patients use "cosmetic" AHA preparations at home and visit the dermatologist at regular intervals for supplementary glycolic acid light peels [21].

The focus for the first 20 years of AHA application was for moisturizing products to treat and prevent dry skin. The typical pH of lactate-containing dry skin creams and lotions has been above the pKa of lactic acid, usually by a pH unit or more. Therefore, the lactate in these products has been more in the salt form (ammonium, sodium, and potassium salts are most common) than as free acid. The published data suggest that lactate dry skin products vary in effectiveness and are generally only a little more effective for controlling dry skin than products based on the main alternatives, humectants such as glycerol, sorbitol, urea, and glycols. However, it is difficult to draw conclusions about the different ingredients because most of the clinical comparisons of these products have been with commercial products that contain different concentrations of humectant in different emulsion bases [22]. Over the last 30 years, most of the leading dry skin moisturizing products have been based on these alternative moisturizing ingredients more than lactic acid. [23].

The second wave of AHA products, from 1992 onward, were the facial moisturizers promoted as wrinkle reduction creams and lotions, or so-called anti-aging creams. The evidence presented here leaves little doubt that these products are effective for reducing the visible signs of photodamaged skin and that this produces a younger and healthier look to the skin. Typically, there is a marked improvement in the first week or so that can be attributed to direct effects on the stratum corneum (hydration and exfoliation). This is followed by a slow, progressive further improvement over several months with fine lines and wrinkles becoming less evident and overall complexion achieving a brighter and more even color tone. Initially, anti-aging AHA products were available in two strengths of glycolic acid, 8 and 4% glycolic acid and a pH 3.8–4.0. These products were proven effective in a placebo-controlled clinical trial (see Section 8). Their success was followed by scores of other products that were mostly highly priced items sold in prestige and specialist channels of trade. Some of these products were effective (i.e., they contained AHA, usually glycolic acid, at effective concentrations/pH), but many were probably not. The effective products have stood the test of time and remain on the market in 2001. Many of the others have disappeared or been reformulated with new ingredients and new claims.

The third phase of AHA products, which continues today, has two components. One was the extension of the original AHAs, glycolic and lactic acid, into a broader range of products addressing a wider range of everyday skin problems (see subsequent sections). The other was the introduction of "new" hydroxy acids and related ingredients, emerging from the research and exploration of cosmetic manufacturers and the raw material supply industries. The search for ingredients and combinations superior to the original AHA products for skin improvement continues.

The review in this chapter follows the chronology of AHA discovery and application in cosmetic products, a chronology that starts with research conducted in the late 1960s and published in the early 1970s.

4   BENEFITS FOR ICHTHYOSIS

The 1974 publication by Van Scott and Yu [6], indicating that hydroxyacids as a class have skin therapeutic activity beyond simple moisturization, was a major landmark in the AHA story. In a small but very elegant and revealing study, Van Scott and Yu demonstrated unequivocally that alpha-hydroxyacids have a remarkable therapeutic action on ichthyotic skin conditions. Ichthyosis describes a number of similarly appearing hereditary skin conditions in which there is abnormal keratinization, leading to an accumulation of heavy scale at the skin surface [24]. Ichthyotic skin has a characteristic fish skin–like appearance (Gr. *Ichthys,* fish). When Van Scott did his pioneering work over 25 years ago, the cause of ichthyoses, as for most skin conditions, was unknown beyond speculation based on symptoms and histological findings. Treatment of the ichthyoses was empirical, involving heavy application of moisturizing creams and ointments containing keratolytic agents such as salicylic acid and urea. These preparations provided only modest relief of symptoms. Modern molecular biology has revealed the genetic defects and associated metabolic disturbances underlying the different ichthyoses [25]. Recessive X-linked ichthyosis is caused by a deficiency of the enzyme steroid sulfatase [26,27]; epidermolytic ichthyoses are caused by defects in keratin proteins [28]; and lamellar ichthyosis is due to defects in transglutaminase cross-linking of proteins in the upper epidermis [29,30].

In their 1974 study [6], Van Scott and Yu studied the effect of some sixty or so low molecular weight organic mono- and di-acids, fatty acids, amino acids, aromatic acids including salicylic acid, urea, and analogs. These materials were applied to circular areas on the arms of patients with severe ichthyosis at concentrations of 5 or 10%. Up to six solutions were tested on each arm with twice daily application for 2 weeks. After only 4 days, some preparations cleared all the hyperkeratotic scale from the skin surface. Twelve solutions, all AHAs, were very effective for restoring normal looking skin. Forty other materials had little or no effect and the remainder, including salicylic acid (10%) and urea (5%), had a slight effect. The effective hydroxyacids were citric acid, ethyl pyruvic acid, glycolic acid, gluconic acid, 3-hydroxybutyric acid, lactic acid, malic acid, methyl pyruvic acid, 2-hydroxy-isobutyric acid, pyruvic acid, tartaric acid, and tartronic acid. Van Scott and Yu went on to show that 2% preparations of effective hydroxyacids used therapeutically could clear the visible ichthyotic condition in 2 weeks. Histological evaluation of treated and adjacent untreated sites indicated an abrupt removal of the abnormal stratum corneum rather that a slow dissolution from the surface as occurs with keratolytic agents. They also observed greatly reduce epidermal thickening, indicating a physiological effect of AHAs and not simply superficial exfoliation. Based on preliminary additional observations, Van Scott and Yu predicted AHAs would benefit other dermatological conditions involving disorders of keratinization. This has proved to be the case with clear evidence of improvement for acne [31], hyperkeratotic skin [32,33], pseudo-folliculitis barbae, i.e., ingrown hair [34], skin photodamage [35,36], and keratoses [37].

5 LACTIC ACID MOISTURIZATION, PLASTICIZATION, AND NMF

In the same year that Van Scott published his seminal paper on hydroxyacid normalization of aberrant keratinization, Middleton published results on the favorable effects of sodium lactate and more particularly lactic acid for the treatment of cutaneous dryness and flaking [5]. It had been known since the classic experiments of Blank [38] that water bound in the stratum corneum was critically important for maintaining softness and flexibility of the skin surface. Subsequent studies had shown that hygroscopic substances occurring naturally in the stratum corneum keep it hydrated. In 1968, Middleton published an insightful paper on the mechanism of water binding in the stratum corneum [39]. He showed that isolated corneum can take up and lose water by osmosis, and that powdering the corneum allows water to extract the water-soluble substances without a prior solvent extraction. He suggested that water-soluble substances are retained within the corneum by a lipid-containing semipermiable membrane system within the cell walls which allows hygroscopic substances to take up water by osmosis and protects them from washout when the intact corneum is immersed in water. He proposed that damage to the cell walls would allow water to extract the hygroscopic water-binding substances from the cells. We now know that this mechanism is the essence of water retention within the stratum corneum and the cause of dryness that arises when cells are damaged by solvents and surfactants [40]. Using his method for measuring the extensibility of isolated strips of stratum corneum, Middleton showed that water held by hygroscopic substances is responsible for most of the extensibility of stratum corneum.

In 1973, Middleton reported results of continuing work to define the water-binding properties of humectants and the relationship between stratum corneum extensibility and hydration [41]. He showed that the increase in stratum corneum extensibility after application of humectants was related to the water content of the tissue, and if the water was removed by exposure to low humidity, the increase in extensibility was lost. Sodium lactate behaved like other humectants in this respect, but lactic acid had an additional action. The increase in extensibility after application of lactic acid solution persisted after the water was removed. This effect was attributed to a direct plasticization of the stratum corneum protein by direct interaction of the lactic acid molecule. This plasticizing effect was not seen when lactic acid was applied as the sodium salt. Alderson and coworkers later showed that longer chain analogs of lactic acid had a similar plasticizing effect, which reached a maximum with the eight–carbon chain 2-hydroxy caprylic acid [42]. They also confirmed that this effect required the free acid and was reduced when pH is raised from 3 to 4 (pKa of lactic acid is pH 3.86).

Lactic acid is one of the main constituents of the natural moisturizing factor of the stratum corneum [43]. The NMF is usually considered a natural humectant system, very hygroscopic, and able to absorb and hold water even at low relative humidity. However, the direct plasticizing action of lactic acid may make a contribution to the physiological role of NMF, although at the pH of skin, approximately pH 5.5, lactic acid is mostly present as the sodium salt. Urea, another main constituent of the NMF, also has a direct plasticizing action on corneocyte protein [44] and is unaffected by pH.

6   AHA AS A TREATMENT FOR DRY SKIN

Although 1974 saw the milestone publications of Van Scott and Middleton that clearly demonstrated efficacy for alpha-hydroxyacids beyond simple hydration, it would be another 20 years before AHAs exploded on the U.S. cosmetic skin care marketplace and established a new multimillion anti-aging product category. In the intervening years, there was much development of lactic acid as a treatment for dry, flaky skin.

In his 1974 publication [5], Middleton showed that skin creams containing lactic acid were effective for reducing dry and flaky skin. In fact, these studies compared the relative effectiveness of lactic acid and sodium lactate and identified two different mechanisms for acid and salt forms. He showed that lactic acid binds to stratum corneum and has a direct plasticizing effect, and sodium lactate, which does not bind to stratum corneum but absorbs into corneocytes, acts by a hygroscopic water-holding effect. Middleton conducted two clinical studies in which 100 women used a placebo hand cream for 2 weeks, a 10% lactic acid hand cream (pH 4.0) for 2 weeks and a 10% sodium lactate hand cream for 2 weeks. Both creams were more effective than the hand cream base (an oil-in-water emulsion). In the first study, under relatively mild UK winter conditions, the lactic acid and sodium lactate creams were equally effective. In the second study, carried out under colder drier UK winter conditions, the lactic acid cream was significantly more effective (p < 0.05) than the sodium lactate cream. Middleton went on to show that a hand cream containing 5% lactic acid was as effective as 10% lactic acid cream.

There is a clear relationship between pH and primary irritation potential for lactic acid [13] with irritancy increasing rapidly below the pKa value (pH 3.86). Primary irritation potential should not be confused with the burn/sting sensory irritation that is characteristic of AHAs, and lactic acid in particular [11]. Middleton formulated his lactic acid hand creams at pH 4.0 to avoid irritation. At this pH, a little above the pKa for lactic acid, the creams would have contained a mixture of lactic acid and sodium lactate, approximately 40% acid and 60% salt. Thus, Middleton's clinical studies demonstrate that a combination of hygroscopic humectant plus protein-binding plasticizer is a more effective treatment for dry skin than humectant alone. This important insight appears to have been overlooked because dry skin lotions developed over the next 20 years (see) were almost exclusively based on hygroscopic humectants like glycerol or lactic acid used at a pH that would render it mostly the nonplasticizing humectant sodium salt.

The main humectant ingredients in over-the-counter (OTC) lotions for dry skin have been summarized [23] and these are discussed in detail elsewhere in this book. It is interesting to note that lactic acid and other hydroxyacids were little used in the main commercial products for prevention and treatment of dry skin up to the mid 1990s. One mass-market product contained 5% lactic acid, but at the product pH of 5.5 most of the lactate would be present as the sodium salt [45]. Middleton's earlier work showed that lactic acid binding to stratum corneum protein decreases as pH increases, with no detectable absorption above pH 5.0. Since 1995, presumably stimulated by the extensive use of AHAs in anti-aging creams and lotions, more dry skin products have been formulated with lactic acid, usually in addition to glycerol or other humectants.

Although there was only limited application of AHAs in commercial products in the 1980s, one notable development was a prescription lotion containing 12% ammonium lactate. This product was for treatment of dry, scaly skin (xerosis) and ichthyosis vulgaris. Several clinical studies show that this lotion is more effective than mass-market dry skin products, but not dramatically so. Dahl and Dahl reported a double-blind clinical trial where 12% ammonium lactate lotion (AML) was compared with a 5% lactic acid lotion and a nonlactate emollient lotion [22]. During the 3-week treatment phase of the study, all three products were equally effective in their ability to reduce the severity of xerosis. However, during "regression," the period after treatment was discontinued, subjects using 12% AML showed a slower return of dry skin condition than those using the other two products. Wehr et al. showed that 12% AML was a little more effective that an emollient, petrolatum-based dry skin cream in a 3-week, double-blind, paired comparison, dry skin regression study with 73 subjects [46]. After 1 week of treatment there was not a significant difference between the two products, but by weeks 2 and 3, there was a significant advantage for the 12% AML, which was even more evident during the regression period (Table 2).

Buxman et al. showed 12% AML was more effective than vehicle and petrolatum for the treatment of ichthyosis [47]. Rogers et al. compared 12% AML with a 5% lactic acid lotion and saw a small but significant benefit for 12% AML. As in the previous studies, the advantage for 12% AML was most evident during regression [48]. At the pH of 12% AML product (pH 5.4) lactate is present mostly as ammonium salt. Although the increased effectiveness of 12% AML in these studies could be attributed simply to a higher concentration of humectant than the comparator products, there is the additional evidence of a regression benefit that indicates 12% AML does more than simply enhance the water content of the stratum corneum. Others have reported effects for 12% AML which go beyond simple moisturization. Lavker et al. found that topical ammonium lactate (using 12%

TABLE 2 Comparative Effectiveness for Treating Dry Skin of a 12% Ammonium Lactate Lotion and an Emollient Lotion

| | Reduction in dry skin score versus baseline[a] | | | | |
| | Treatment period (day) | | | Regression (day) | |
	7	14	21	28	35
A (12% AML lotion)	69%	80%	86%	57%	51%
B (emollient)	63%	69%	78%	41%	31%
Significance (A versus B)	NS	SD	SD	SD	SD

[a]Initial mean dryness score for both groups was 5.1 on a 0–9 scale.
Note: Subjects with dry skin applied the products twice daily, one to left leg, the other to right leg, for 3 weeks. Leg skin condition was evaluated during the treatment period and for a further 2 weeks after treatment stopped (regression).

AML) had a sparing effect on cutaneous atrophy caused by potent topical corticosteroid [49]. This was not simply a benefit secondary to improved stratum corneum condition because there were also epidermal and dermal effects. In particular, there was a large increase in dermal glycosaminoglycans (GAGs), especially hyaluronic acid. Leyden et al. went on to show that topical application of lower concentrations of lactic acid (2–10%) also increased glycosaminoglycans content in the dermis [50].

The effects reported indicate that lactic acid and lactate salts have benefits for skin which go beyond moisturization and plasticization of dry stratum corneum. As observed by Van Scott in 1974, the hydroxyacids appear able to correct aberrant keratinization and dysfunction of normal stratum corneum maturation and turnover, making the skin more resistant to development of xerosis. The mechanism of these effects and/or most of the other biological effects of AHAs has been subject to much speculation, but so far there has been no explanation which accounts for the diversity of AHA actions (see subsequent sections).

7 STRATUM CORNEUM BARRIER IMPROVEMENT

The resistance of lactic acid–treated skin to reappearance of xerosis in the regression phase of dry skin clinical trials described indicates changes in the stratum corneum beyond simple moisturization. Leyden et al. reported dramatic difference in stratum corneum structure after 3 weeks of 12% AML treatment [50]. The thick diffuse hyperkeratotic stratum corneum characteristic of dry skin was replaced by a compact appearing stratum corneum with a normal number of cell layers. Rawlings et al. demonstrated increased stratum corneum resistance to sodium lauryl sulfate (SLS) irritation after 4 weeks of treatment with a lotion containing 4% lactic acid at pH 3.7–4.0 [51]. After twice daily application of lotion for 4 weeks, trans-epidermal water loss (TEWL) was measured on treated and vehicle control sites. These sites were then patched with 0.25% SLS for 24 hr and TEWL remeasured. The increase in TEWL caused by SLS irritation was significantly less on lactic acid–treated skin, indicating increased resistance of the stratum corneum. Lipid analysis of tape strips taken from lactic acid and control sites showed an increase in ceramide levels in lactic acid treatment sites and specifically an improvement in Ceramide 1 linoleate/oleate ratio. In follow-up studies Rawlings and his coworkers demonstrated that L-lactic acid was more effective than DL-lactic acid for improving stratum corneum barrier resistance to irritants. D-Lactic acid was ineffective [52]. They concluded that lactic acid, particularly the L isomer stimulates ceramide biosynthesis, leading to increased stratum corneum ceramide levels and a superior lipid barrier that is more resistant to irritants and development of xerosis.

8   AHA BENEFITS FOR AGED AND PHOTODAMAGED SKIN

It was a publication by Van Scott and Yu in 1989 [53] demonstrating anti-wrinkle effects of AHAs at home use concentrations that set the stage for the biggest revolution in the skin care marketplace in decades if not for all time. It was well known that acid peels would rejuvenate photodamaged skin, but here for the first time was evidence that twice-daily application of skin cream containing a potentially cosmetic concentration of glycolic acid (5–10%) for 3–10 months could reduce facial wrinkles. This was a prospective study without specific controls and with light glycolic acid peels as supplementary treatments every 1 to 6 weeks. By strict clinical criteria the evidence for anti-wrinkle effects of glycolic acid at potentially cosmetic concentrations was not conclusive. However, the evidence was compelling. The fountain of youth had been a dream of the cosmetic consumer, a hope beyond realistic expectation, and here was a rational, scientific publication showing it might be possible after all. One man in the cosmetic industry recognized the significance of this publication and took action that led to the launch of Anew Creams by Avon Products Inc. in 1992 (personal communication). Avon's Anew cream contained 8% glycolic acid at pH 4.0. The product was a huge success with consumers. They saw facial skin benefits not previously experienced with regular facial moisturizing products. Other companies followed suit and within 2 years AHAs became both a new category in the skin care marketplace and also the hottest property in town [54]. Ten years further on, AHA products continue to be the star of the cosmetic skin care marketplace. There are challengers and pretenders, but so far no other cosmetic ingredient has produced the overwhelming consumer response and the clear-cut clinical evidence seen with glycolic acid [55,56]. What then is the clinical evidence for skin anti-aging benefits of AHAs at the concentrations used in cosmetic moisturizing creams and lotions?

A publication by Nole et al. in 1994 described a new method for visual evaluation of facial "de-aging" and reported a significant improvement of skin appearance after 3 months use of AHA moisturizing creams [57]. This study compared the effects of 4 and 8% glycolic acid creams (pH 3.8) with an untreated control group over the same period. Using a variety of evaluation methods, including skin surface silicone replicas and a new clinical grading technique of complexion mapping, the study demonstrated dramatic improvements in the skin features associated with facial aging. There was a reduction in fine lines, wrinkles, enlarged pores, and uneven pigmentation and an improvement in skin texture and luminosity (radiance). The published results concentrated on the complexion mapping method and 3 months data. By 6 months, the AHA effects were more dramatic with good agreement between the subjective (complexion mapping) and objective (computer analysis of side-illuminated replica images) evaluation methods. Figures 2a and b show the complexion mapping fine line and texture results for 4% glycolic acid cream, and Figure 2c shows the skin surface replica results for the same time points.

A second clinical study of 8% glycolic acid, this time a double-blind comparison with the gelatin/glycine vehicle, was published by Morganti et al. in early 1996 [58]. This was a 3-month half-face study with 60 women aged 45–60 years with facial photodamage. There was a statistically significant reduction of fine wrinkles by the glycolic acid product after one month that was sustained through the end of the 3-month treatment period to 1-month posttreatment. The magnitude of fine wrinkle reduction in this study, 5–10%, is consistent with the earlier study where treatment beyond 3 months was required to produce larger reductions in skin signs associated with photodamage.

While the foregoing studies are good evidence for the clinical effectiveness of glycolic acid, the definitive study demonstrating efficacy of topical AHA creams was a double-blind, vehicle-controlled study done at the Massachusetts General Hospital (MGH) and published in mid-1996 [16]. This study is the only direct comparison of matched glycolic acid, lactic acid, and placebo products. Both AHAs were at 8% concentration, pH 3.8, in oil-in-water emulsion base. The base served as the vehicle (placebo) control. The creams were applied twice daily to the face and forearms using a balanced design that allowed for paired comparison of glycolic acid, lactic acid, and placebo creams on the forearms. It is interesting and maybe surprising that lactic acid cream proved at least as effective as the glycolic acid cream in this study. Both AHA products were statistically more effective than the placebo for reducing the severity of photodamage and sallowness. There were no significant differences between the glycolic and lactic acid creams. However, the lactic acid cream seemed to have a slight edge over glycol-

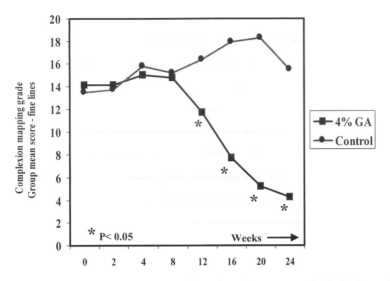

FIGURE 2A Reduction of facial fine lines in a 24-week clinical study comparing twice daily application of face cream containing 4% glycolic acid, pH 3.8,
with a control group of women continuing to use their usual facial moisturizing products. Fine lines were assessed by visual grading using the complexion mapping method.

ic acid cream for both clinical and subject self-assessed improvement from baseline photodamage.

   These studies leave no doubt that AHAs (glycolic and lactic acids) formulated as cosmetic products are effective for reducing the visible signs of aging.
However, there are no dose-response studies to establish a minimum effective
dose of AHA. The concentration of ingredients in cosmetic products is not de-
clared on the label and there is little doubt that some, perhaps many, of the hundreds of AHA creams and lotions that have come to market since 1992 contained
levels of AHA too low to provide any specific AHA benefit. These products could
be expected to provide conventional skin moisturizing benefits (soft, smooth,
healthy-looking skin) from the conventional moisturizing ingredients (oils,
humectants, occlusives) typically used in face creams and lotions.

   Other studies have been done using indirect measures that shed light on the
question of threshold concentration for AHA effectiveness. One commonly used
endpoint is "cell renewal," or stratum corneum turnover time measured by the
dansyl chloride method. This method uses a 24-hr occlusive patch of protein-
binding fluorescent dye (dansyl chloride) to stain the full depth of the stratum
corneum. The number of days for the stain to disappear is measured. Results for a

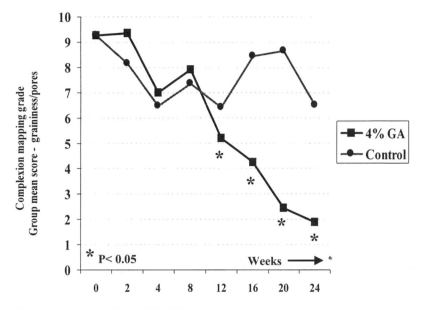

FIGURE 2B Reduction of facial texture (graininess and pores) in the same 24-week clinical study as Fig. 2a. Graininess and enlarged pores were assessed by visual grading using the complexion mapping method. These two features are the main contributors to texture, a parameter that is not assessed separately in complexion mapping. The mean values of the combined scores for graininess and enlarged pores are plotted.

series of previously unpublished studies examining a range of glycolic acid concentrations in a moisturizing cream base at pH 3.8 are shown in Figure 3. Using this test method as an indicator of AHA specific activity, there is a rapid fall in activity with decreasing concentration. Eight-percent (4% free acid) and 4% (2% free acid) Glycolic acid are effective; 2% (1% free acid) may have a slight effect; and 1% (0.5% free acid) has no effect beyond that seen with the cream base.

Using 50:50 hydroalcoholic solutions of acids, Smith observed somewhat greater increases in cell renewal values but a similar pattern related to pH [59,60]. Four percent solutions of lactic acid and glycolic acid at pH 3 (equivalent to 3.5% free acid) increased cell renewal by 35%, whereas at pH 5 (equivalent to 0.25% free acid) the increase was 25%, and at pH 7 (no free acid) the increase was 10–13%. Part of the response in these studies may have been due to a degree of irritation reported for the pH 3 and 5 solutions. Smith examined other acids at these pH values and showed that salicylic acid, trichloracetic acid, and acetic acid all increased cell renewal in the same order as glycolic and lactic acids, whereas pyruvic and citric acid had much less effect. Smith also examined cell renewal af-

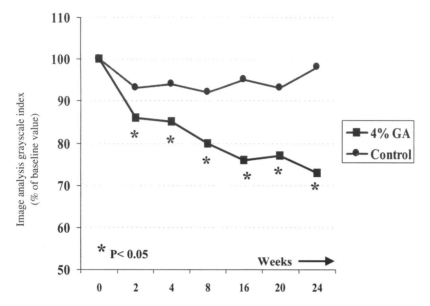

FIGURE 2c   Reduction of skin surface texture in the same 24-week clinical study as Fig. 2a, assessed by skin replica method. Silicone replicas (1 cm²) were made of the skin surface in four regions of the face (cheeks, eye crows feet, chin, and forehead) of each subject at each evaluation. Replicas were side illuminated and imaged from above using a Nikon D1 digital camera linked directly to a Pentium III processor loaded with Optima image analysis software. The gray scale variance of digital images is a measure of surface roughness. A reduction in variance corresponds to a decrease in surface roughness. Results are the group mean values of replica variance at each evaluation time. This method of replica analysis correlates well with results obtained by laser profilometery.

ter 10 weeks and 20 weeks of daily application of AHAs and found a progressive decline from initial cell renewal values, suggesting a skin accommodation response.

In another previously unpublished study, the dansyl chloride method was also used to compare glycolic acid and salicylic acid products representing the higher strengths readily available to the consumer. The marketplace standard for the "strongest" cosmetic AHA product is 8% glycolic acid at pH 3.8. Beta-hydroxyacid anti-aging creams contained 2% salicylic acid at pH 2.9 when first marketed, although this was subsequently reduced to 1.5%. In a direct comparison using the dansyl chloride method, the 8% AHA glycolic acid product was significantly more active than the 2% BHA salicylic acid product (Figure 4).

Although interpretation of the dansyl chloride test is somewhat controver-

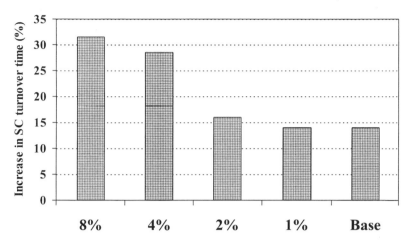

FIGURE 3 Change in stratum corneum turnover time (cell renewal) induced by glycolic acid (pH 3.8) creams of different strength applied to the upper arm. Results are the percentage increase in turnover time compared to untreated skin (measured by dansyl chloride staining method).

sial, the method will usually measure the replacement time of the stratum corneum, and this is a measure of epidermal turnover. The faster the stratum corneum is renewed from below, the quicker it will shed from the surface. The controversy arises because substances or procedures that remove superficial layers of the stratum corneum, including keratolytics, exfoliants, and acid peels, also accelerate the disappearance of dansyl chloride stain. This issue is not resolved in the literature. There are no studies that define the threshold conditions [amount, concentration, pH, frequency, and duration of contact, vehicle, skin condition (dry, hyperkeratotic, moisturized)] for AHAs to act as exfoliants or not. But the impression created by articles in the popular press, particularly women's magazines and cosmetic trade publications, that all AHA products exfoliate all skin under any conditions, is not rational and not supported by the scientific literature. Since other studies [61] have shown no reduction in stratum corneum cell layers by 8 and 4% glycolic acid creams (pH 3.8) similar to those tested here, the results presented in Figures 3 and 4 are interpreted as changes in epidermal turnover. It is of interest that the moisturizing base induces a significant increase in turnover—this is a consistent finding in dansyl chloride tests.

9 CHEMICAL PEELS

Although acid peels done in a dermatologist's office may not seem relevant to the use of AHAs in cosmetic moisturizing products, an awareness of peel procedures and results is needed to navigate the literature pertaining to skin effects of AHAs.

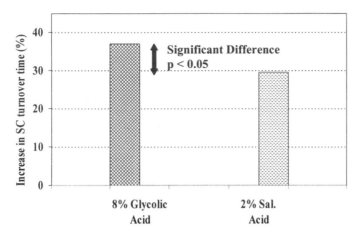

FIGURE 4 Increase in stratum corneum turnover time (cell renewal) induced by AHA cosmetic skin cream (8% glycolic acid, pH 3.8) and salicylic acid cosmetic skin cream (2% salicylic acid, pH 2.9). Test done as a paired comparison (left arm versus right arm) on a panel of 25 women. Results are the percentage increase in turnover time for each cream compared to untreated skin on the same arm (measured by dansyl chloride staining method).

In the last 10 years glycolic acid, used as a 70% acid solution or partially neutralized, has emerged as a preferred acid for chemical peels [62]. Lower concentrations (15–25% particularly neutralized) have become popular for "light peels" by estheticians in beauty salons and spas. Therefore, there are different levels of use, action, and effect for AHAs from the strongest peels through light peels and cosmetic exfoliation to simple moisturization (hydration of dry skin promotes desquamation). The AHA literature in all its forms (scientific, medical, trade journals, consumer magazines, and newspapers) covers this entire spectrum of use, but does not always make a clear distinction between the different levels when describing results and discussing mechanisms.

Chemical peeling is a procedure that has been used for many years by dermatologists to improve the condition of aged and photodamaged facial skin [63]. Related dermatological procedures are dermabrasion [64] and more recently laser resurfacing [65]. In all these procedures, damage to the epidermis (epidermolysis or tissue ablation) promotes a repair response that produces a renewed epidermis and stratum corneum. Laser resurfacing can be targeted to the underlying dermal tissues and, appropriately controlled, can provoke regeneration of collagen, elastin, and other structural elements of the dermis. The de-aging effects of lasers can be truly dramatic [66]. Chemical peels and dermabrasion can also produce very satisfactory cosmetic results. Medical skill and experience is required to control the skin contact time of concentrated glycolic acid during peels. The light peels done by estheticians also involve timed application of glycolic acid to the skin followed by a neutralizing rinse, but there is much less risk with the lower AHA concentrations used for light peels. It seems plausible that chemical peels with glycolic acid provide some element of the AHA benefit seen at nondamaging, nonirritating cosmetic concentrations and pH. However, it is less clear, and arguably unlikely, that any of the benefit of cosmetic concentrations of glycolic acid is due to an element of acid damage. But so far there have been no controlled studies to investigate these relationships. Because peel procedures and cosmetic products work in their individual fields of application, there has been no imperative to investigate the relationship of mechanisms involved, even though it has become a common practice to combine the two procedures [67].

10 OTHER BENEFITS OF AHA

Alpha-hydroxyacids are used in skin moisturizer products primarily for moisturization and skin anti-aging benefits, but as indicated these compounds have a broader range of beneficial effects for skin. Most anti-aging products for the face use glycolic acid and most hand and body moisturizer products use lactic acid. This is probably a reflection of cost. The raw material cost of glycolic acid is about four times that of lactic acid. Face care products sell at higher prices than hand and body products, and therefore glycolic acid is "affordable" for face products but too expensive for mass-market general use/hand and body products. There are other AHAs and, after the first flush of glycolic acid anti-aging creams and lotions, products containing combinations of glycolic and other AHAs appeared in the marketplace. As there is no convincing evidence for a significant performance advantage for the combinations it can be assumed that the main purpose was marketing-driven product differentiation in a crowded marketplace. Although there have been no head-to-head studies to compare AHA combinations with glycolic acid or lactic acid at equivalent acid strength, there are claims that combination products are effective for both control of dry skin and improvement of photodamaged skin (anti-aging). The Van Scott group showed that a blend of AHA and polyhydroxy acids (PHAs) was effective for improving the symptoms of xerosis, epidermolytic hyperkeratosis, and ichthyosis [68]. Another publication from Van Scott is useful for identifying and characterizing the broader range of AHAs and their effects on skin [14].

There are several publications indicating AHAs, and glycolic acid in particular, are helpful for treating acne. It may be used at high concentration (70%) as a chemical peel or daily at cosmetic strength (5–10%) where it acts to reduce cohesion of follicular corneocytes, helping to dislodge comedones and prevent their formation [37]. Glycolic acid is a less effective treatment for acne than tretinoin and acts by a different mechanism, but the combination of glycolic acid and tretinoin is more effective than either agent alone [69–71]. Alternative combination treatments using light glycolic acid peels (20–35%), daily 15% glycolic acid gel, and 4% gluconolactone cleanser, alone or in addition to prescription medications, have proved effective for dealing with recalcitrant papulopustular acne [72]. A similar mixed regimen was effective for treating rosacea, a common chronic inflammatory disorder of the face characterized by erythema and telangiectasia that is often accompanied by outbreaks of acnelike papules and pustules [73].

Cosmetic strength glycolic acid (8%, pH 4) is very effective for another follicular skin problem, razor bumps or pseudofolliculitis barbae (PFB), a foreign body inflammatory reaction to ingrown facial hair. The condition arises when shaved hairs curl and penetrate the skin near the follicle opening as they grow back after shaving. The problem afflicts over 50% of black males and a high proportion of black females who need to shave around the jaw line. Two weeks use of 8% glycolic acid cream reduces the number of papules and pustules by more than half, and continuous treatment usually provides satisfactory control of the problem [34].

Some types of sun-induced age spots, seborrheic keratoses, and actinic keratoses involve a dysfunction of normal epidermal differentiation and maturation, whereas others, the solar lentigines, reflect proliferation and hyperactivity of melanocytes. These lesions can be removed using peel concentrations of AHA, but daily application of cosmetic strength AHA is also effective and usually preferred [53]. In keeping with the ability of AHAs to correct abnormal keratinization, AHAs are more effective for reducing/eliminating keratoses than lentigines. A combination of glycolic acid with hydroquinone or kojic acid has been reported more effective than hydroquinone or kojic acid alone for treating melasma and other hyperpigmentation conditions [74]. It seems clear that AHAs do have the ability to reduce skin hyperpigmentation. However, as described subsequently, AHAs also cause a small increase in skin photosensitivity, which could be expected to promote pigmentation (tanning). A recent publication by Tsai and Maibach confirms that AHA (10% glycolic acid, pH 3.5) does promote UVB-induced skin tanning [75]. In this 3-week study, glycolic acid had no effect (did not reduce) pre-existing tan.

Although contrary to the several sunburn studies considered for the CIR review, there is a 1996 report that topical glycolic acid is photoprotective and exerts an anti-inflammatory action [76]. The anti-inflammatory conclusion is based on the finding that skin sites irradiated with 3 times the minimal erythemal dose showed a marked reduction in erythema when treated postirradiation with 12% ammonium lactate at pH 4.2. The photoprotective conclusion is based on finding an attenuation of UVB effect equivalent to SPF 2–4 on skin sites treated daily for 3 weeks with an AHA cleanser and AHA lotion both containing 8% glycolic acid at pH 3.25. Similar results were obtained in an earlier study by the same author [77].

11 SKIN COMPATIBILITY OF AHAS

There has never been any real concern about the skin compatibility of AHA products sold as dry skin moisturizers since the early 1970s. But when AHAs were first introduced in facial moisturizers in 1992 there were complaints of irritation that fueled a controversy that still continues. The reality is that AHAs induce sensory irritation (chemosensory irritability) in susceptible individuals [78]. Alpha-hydroxyacid stinging is a transient effect usually with no clinical signs of irritation, although a mild transient erythema may appear in unusually susceptible individuals. The effect is related to the susceptibility of the individual and the strength of the AHA. Some consumers regard a slight stinging as a positive sign. Those with sensitive skin often reject AHA products. Prior to the appearance of AHAs in facial products, cosmetic moisturizers were almost universally bland emollient preparations that helped to hydrate dry superficial regions of the stratum corneum. Consumers using AHA products for the first time and experiencing burning and stinging sensations were concerned. This was outside their normal experience and expectation. Some consumers assumed there was something wrong with the products. The lack of familiarity with AHA products coupled with a strong desire to try the products because of the anti-wrinkle benefits promised, encouraged widespread trial by consumers and an associated burst of complaints. This caught the attention of the media and became the issue of the week for investigative journalists for the next several months. Alpha-hydroxyacids were so new that factual information was hard to find and anecdotal comments and opinions became the currency of the day. Nearly a decade later, AHAs are far more widespread and popular than ever before. The stinging issue is recognized. There has been much work by the cosmetic industry to develop products that retain the benefits of AHAs without the sensory irritation, but so far with only modest success [79,80].

Good skin compatibility and absence of irritation is a consistent observation in all the clinical studies of cosmetic strength AHAs referenced in this chapter. Indeed, some of the studies with facial peel strength AHAs show no irritation on forearm and body parts less sensitive than the face. In Ditre's study, subjects were able to apply lotions containing 25% glycolic, lactic, and citric acid at pH 3.5 (17% free acid) to the forearm twice daily for 6 months. There was no irritation but a most dramatic improvement in the condition of the photodamaged arm skin [36]. Results of a 14-day cumulative irritation test by DiNardo provide another indication that AHAs are not primary irritants at pH values +/–0.5 pH units of the pKa value [81]. In this study, 12% ammonium lactate, pH 4.4, demonstrated an irritation score of 30 out of a possible 882 points (cumulative over 14 days). Eight percent glycolic acid, pH 4.4, demonstrated a score of 1 out of 882 points.

12   MECHANISMS OF ACTION

It will be clear from this discussion that AHAs have multiple effects on skin related to pH and concentration. It might be imagined that the popularity of AHAs for both everyday and medical skin care would have stimulated intensive research to understand the biochemical and physiological mechanisms of AHA action. In fact the few serious scientific studies that have been done have focused mostly on the end benefits of AHAs: what they do, much more than how they do it. As indicated, the published research on AHAs has significant limitations, as follows:

1.   A majority of publications do not state the pH of the preparations examined.
2.   Publications that discuss mechanisms, particularly general articles and reviews, tend not to make a distinction between cosmetic and dermatological (chemical peel) levels of action/effect.
3.   Many publications that discuss AHA mechanisms simply reiterate the 1974 suggestions of Van Scott and Yu, which these authors recognized as speculative at the time they made them.

Histological studies show that AHAs, unlike keratolytics that eliminate corneocytes from the skin surface inward, diminish corneocyte adhesion in the lower layers of the stratum corneum (stratum compactum). Van Scott and Yu speculated that this effect was due to AHA interference with intercorneocyte ionic bonding by inhibiting enzymes that add phosphate and sulfate groups to the corneocyte envelope [33]. A study by Ditre [36] provided indirect evidence that the AHA effect might be due to modification of desmosomal (protein) links between corneocytes. After 6 months of daily application to the forearm of 25% AHA (glycolic, lactic, or citric acid, all at pH 3.5), electron microscopic examination of the epidermis revealed fewer desmosomes connecting basal cells in skin sections from AHA-treated sites than from placebo-treated control sites. A more recent study by Fartasch et al. [82] applying glycolic acid cream (4%, pH 3.8) to the volar forearm twice daily for 3 weeks provides a somewhat different picture. In this study, electron microscopic examination of the stratum corneum revealed no changes or indications of reduced cohesion in the stratum compactum. In the more superficial layers of the stratum corneum (stratum disjunctum), where desmosome degradation is initiated as part of the normal process of desquamation, there was enhanced degradation of desmosomes (corneosomes) in AHA-treated sites compared to control sites. Also, in contrast to the Ditre study, there was no change detected in the epidermis. Comparing the Ditre and Fartasch results, it appears that AHAs may exert actions at different levels of the stratum corneum depending on the strength of AHA applied to skin. The strength used by Fartasch is a cosmetic strength that is effective. The strength used by Ditre, although apparently not irritating when applied daily to the forearm for several months, is a much higher concentration than used in cosmetic products.

Research in the 1990s revealed some of the biochemical mechanisms involved in cellular adhesions and degradation of these adhesions during desquamation [83,84]. At points of adhesion, including desmosomes, cells are connected by transmembrane proteins called cadherins. Calcium bound to cadherins protects the structures from enzymic proteolysis. Combining these insights with clinical and experimental data published for AHAs, Wang proposed "a theory for the mechanism of action of AHAs applied to the skin" [85]. The essence of this theory is that AHAs remove calcium from cadherins by chelation, resulting in proteolysis and enhanced desquamation. Wang also suggested that lowering epidermal calcium levels promotes cell proliferation and retards differentiation of keratinocytes. Wang's theory appears to be a possible explanation for effects of AHAs on the stratum corneum, but it does not explain the specific enhancement of corneocyte adhesion by alpha-acetoxyacids acids [86]. Nor does it explain the metabolic effects of AHAs, such as the sparing effect on steroid-induced cutaneous atrophy [49], increased epidermal ceramide synthesis [52], increased transglutaminase expression in dermal dendrocytes [87], increased dermal and epidermal hyaluronic acid [88], and increased collagen deposition in the papillary dermis [81]. Like any theory, Wang's proposed mechanism of AHA action must be put to the test by appropriate experimentation, particularly as the theory relies in part on calcium-induced changes observed using in vitro systems.

The diversity of metabolic changes induced by AHAs could reflect multiple mechanisms of action or, as most would argue, an effect on a fundamental cellular target that initiates a procession of consequential actions and reactions. It is established that perturbation of the stratum corneum barrier produces a cascade of stimulatory and inhibitory cytokines [89] that would be expected to migrate to the epidermis and dermis and exert a host of effects, either directly or by impacting other cell regulatory pathways. Is cytokine activation and release the mechanism of the AHA effect on skin? I don't know and the literature to date (2001) does not provide the answer.

13 AHA SAFETY: THE COSMETIC INGREDIENT REVIEW

Because of escalating use of AHAs in cosmetic skin care products in the early 1990s and the U.S. Food and Drug Administration (FDA) concern to ensure consumer safety was thoroughly evaluated, the Cosmetics, Toiletries and Fragrance Association (CTFA) asked the Cosmetic Ingredient Review to review AHAs, principally glycolic and lactic acids, their salts, and simple esters. The CIR is a comprehensive program for independent review of the safety of cosmetic ingredients in the United States. Although CIR is supported by industry funding it is staffed and operated independently. All decisions regarding safety of cosmetic ingredients are made by the CIR Expert Panel, a panel composed of seven physicians and scientists with expertise in dermatology, toxicology, pathology, carcinogenicity, and biochemistry. In addition, there are three nonvoting members of the CIR panel representing industry (CTFA), consumers (the Consumer Federation of America), and government (FDA Office of Cosmetics and Colors).

The CIR compiled a scientific literature review of published data on AHAs plus unpublished industry data made available to CIR via CTFA. There were over 350 studies covering all aspects of safety of glycolic acid and lactic acid [90]. The CIR Expert Panel discussed the safety data and their particular areas of concern at CIR public meetings in 1995 and again in 1996. The CIR acknowledged that in most respects there were no concerns about the safety of AHAs [91]. There was much data from which to conclude that AHAs are not mutagenic or carcinogenic, are not reproductive or developmental toxins, and are not skin sensitizers. The areas CIR identified for particular consideration were (1) the irritation potential of AHAs and (2) the exfoliating effect of AHAs that could potentially enhance penetration of other ingredients and/or increase the sensitivity of skin to solar UVR.

With respect to irritation, the CIR Expert Panel concluded that there were data indicating acceptable limits for concentration/pH of AHAs for leave-on skin products. The panel also concluded that there were studies indicating no need for concern about use of AHA enhancing the penetration of other chemicals. They noted that AHAs themselves do penetrate skin readily, but because of low systemic toxicity this was not a concern. However, the expert panel stated that the evidence did point to a small and variable increase in sun sensitivity after use of AHA products. They noted that there were studies providing contradictory evidence on the effect of AHA on minimal erythemal dose. One study suggested MED was increased (reduced UV sensitivity) after use of AHAs, but a second study showed a reduction in UVR dose required to produce skin reddening. The average reduction in MED (increased UV sensitivity) was 13%, but some individuals showed greater than 50% reduction. Additional studies were carried out using sunburn cell (SBC) production as the endpoint for indicating UVR penetration of skin. After 4 days of application of standard AHA preparation (10% glycolic acid at pH 3.5) there was no significant increase in SBC production following UVR challenge. However, after 12 weeks of AHA treatment there was a small but significant increase in SBC formation after UVR challenge. The increase in number of SBCs after a 12-week AHA pretreatment was equivalent to increasing UV exposure of untreated skin by the equivalent of 1.6 MED. Therefore, addition of a sunscreen with an SPF 2 to an AHA product containing 10% glycolic acid at pH 3.5 would be sufficient to eliminate the AHA-induced increase in UVR sensitivity. In fact, the most widely available commercial AHA products have a concentration of 8% glycolic acid and a pH of 3.8. This product strength provides less than half the free acid contained in the standard AHA preparation used in the SBC studies (approximately 4% free acid for 8% glycolic acid, pH 3.8, compared to 8.7% free acid for 10% glycolic acid, pH 3.5). The 1996 recommendations of the CIR Expert Panel were based on the SBC results showing a relatively small AHA-induced increase in sun sensitivity that could be eliminated by addition of low SPF to AHA creams and lotions. The Expert Panel concluded that AHAs are safe for use in cosmetic products at concentrations equal or less than 10%, at a final formulation pH equal to or greater than 3.5, when formulated to avoid increasing sun sensitivity or when directions for use include the daily use of sun protection. A recent publication [61] confirms that commercial AHA products (8 and 4% glycolic acid at pH 3.8) containing SPF 4 sunscreen do not increase sun sensitivity over 6 months of twice daily application to forearms. More recent studies by the FDA add further support for the 1996 CIR recommendation. The FDA did additional studies to examine AHA effect on the sensitivity of skin to UVR, using MED, SBCs, and thiamine dimer formation as endpoints for indicating UVR penetration of skin [92]. The first study used a 10%, pH 3.5, glycolic acid solution applied 6 days per week for 4 weeks followed by UVR challenge, and a second UVR challenge 1 week after the last AHA application. Results indicated a small AHA-induced reduction in MED and small increase in SBC formation after 4 weeks of treatment. One week after AHA treatment was stopped, AHA-induced changes were no longer evident. In a second study, there was no significant increase in thiamine dimer formation after 4 weeks treatment with the same AHA solution. The CIR Expert Panel reviewed the FDA results and reported at the February 2000 CIR meeting their conclusion that the new results supported the 1996 panel conclusion [93].

14 FUTURE TRENDS

Research over 30 years has revealed that AHAs, most particularly lactic acid and glycolic acid, have many mostly beneficial actions on skin. The mechanisms of action are less clear. Explanations for some actions are more a statement of effect on a process (e.g., AHAs reduce corneocyte adhesion) than true mechanistic descriptions of the physiological, biochemical, and molecular biological causes for the observed effects. In the future, with accelerating advances in diagnostic and analytical techniques, such as DNA arrays to probe subtle changes in gene expression and cellular biochemistry, we can expect the actual mechanisms of AHA effects on skin will be worked out. It seems unlikely that the future will see discoveries of major new effects of AHAs on skin. Instead, clarification of mechanisms of action should enable more effective targeting and optimal use of AHAs for the indications of skin benefit already identified.

REFERENCES

1. Jackson EM. AHA-type products proliferate in 1993. Cosmet Dermatol 1993; 6(12):22–26.
2. Branna T. The skin care market. Happi 1991; 29(5):49–64.
3. Jackson EM. Update on AHA-containing products. Cosmet Dermatol 1994; 7(1):29–30.
4. Draelos ZD. Sorting out all your hydroxy acid options. Skin Aging 1998; 6(4):45–47.
5. Middleton JD. Development of a skin cream designed to reduce dry and flaky skin. J Soc Cosmet Chem 1974; 25:519–534.
6. Van Scott EJ, Yu RJ. Control of keratinization with α-hydroxy acids and related compounds. Arch Dermatol 1974; 110:586–590.
7. Elson ML. The utilization of glycolic acid in photoaging. Cosmet Dermatol 1992; 5(1):12–15.
8. Jackson EM. Supporting advertising claims for AHA products. Cosmet Dermatol 1996; 9(5):40–47.
9. Jackson EM. AHAs: what's wrong with this picture? J Toxicol Cut Ocular Toxicol 1997; 16(4):203–205.
10. Jackson EM. Do AHA products really work? Cosmet Dermatol October 1994; (suppl):21–22.
11. Frosch PJ, Kligman AM. A method for appraising the stinging capacity of topically applied substances. J Soc Cosmet Chem 1977; 28:197–209.
12. Rosan AM. The chemistry of alpha-hydroxy acids. Cosmet Dermatol October 1994; (suppl):4–9.
13. Johnson AW, Nole GE, Rozen MG, DiNardo JC. Skin tolerance of AHAs: a comparison of lactic and glycolic acids and the role of pH. Cosmet Dermatol 1997; 10(2):38–45.
14. Yu RJ, Van Scott EJ. Alpha-hydroxy acids: science and therapeutic use. Cosmet Dermatol October 1994; (suppl):12–20.
15. Greaves MW. Alpha hydroxy acid derivative for relieving dry itching skin. Cosmet Toil 1990; 105(10):61–64.
16. Stiller MJ, Bartolone J, Stern R, Smith S, Kollias N, Gillies R, Drake LA. Topical 8% glycolic acid and 8% L-lactic acid creams for the treatment of photodamaged skin. Arch Dermatol 1996; 132:631–636.
17. Nook TH. In vivo measurement of the keratolytic effect of salicylic acid in three ointment formulations. Br J Dermatol 1987; 117:243–247.
18. Leyden JJ, Shalita AR. Rational therapy for acne vulgaris: an update on topical treatment. J Am Acad Dermatol 1986; 4:507–515.
19. Kligman AM. Salicylic acid: an alternative to alpha hydroxy acids. J Geriatr Dermatol 1997; 5(3):128–131.
20. Draelos ZD. Hydroxy acids for the treatment of aging skin. J Geriatr Dermatol 1997; 5(5):236–240.
21. Bergfeld W, Tung R, Vidimos A, Vellanki L, Remzi B, Stanton-Hicks U. Improving the cosmetic appearance of photoaged skin with glycolic acid. J Am Acad Dermatol 1977; 36:1011–1013.

22. Dahl MV, Dahl AC. 12% lactate lotion for the treatment of xerosis. Arch Dermatol 1983; 119:27–30.
23. Johnson AW. Dry skin: recent advances in research and therapy. J Retail Pharmacy 1994; 4(suppl):S1–S8.
24. Hanifin JM, Rajka G. Diagnostic features of atopic dermatitis. Acta Derm Verereol (Stockholm) 1980; 92(suppl):44–47.
25. Roop D. Defects in the barrier. Science 1995; 267:474–475.
26. Williams ML. Lipids in normal and pathological desquamation. Adv Lipid Res 1991; 24:211–262.
27. Morita E, Katoh O, Shinoda S, Hiragun T, Tanada T, Kameyoshi Y, Yamamoto S. A novel point mutation in the steroid sulphatase gene in X-linked ichthyosis. J Invest Dermatol 1997; 109:244–245.
28. Rothnagel JA, Roop DR. Analysis, diagnosis, and molecular genetics of keratin disorders. Curr Opin Dermatol 1995; 2:211–218.
29. Huber M, Rettler I, Bernasconi K, Frenk E, Lavrijsen SPM, Ponec M, Bon A, Lautenschlager S, Schorderet DF, Hohl D. Mutations of keratinocyte transglutaminase in lamellar ichthyosis. Science 1995; 267:525–528.
30. Bale SJ, Compton JG, Russell LJ, DiGiovanna JJ. Genetic heterogeneity in lamellar ichthyosis. J Invest Dermatol 1996; 107 (Letters to the Editor):140–141.
31. Petratos MA. Drug therapies and adjunctive uses of alphahydroxy and polyhydroxy acids. Cutis 2000; 66:107–111.
32. Siskin 3B, Quinlan PJ, Finkelstein MS, Marlucci M, Maglietta TG, Gibson JR. The effects of ammonium lactate 12% lotion versus no therapy in the treatment of dry skin of the heels. Int J Dermatol 1993; 32:905–907.
33. Van Scott EJ, Yu RJ. Hyperkeratinization, corneocyte cohesion, and alpha hydroxy acids. J Am Acad Dermatol 1984; 11:867–879.
34. Perricone NV. Treatment of pseudofolliculitis barbae with topical glycolic acid: a report of two studies. Cutis 1993; 52:233–235.
35. Smith WP. Epidermal and dermal effects of topical lactic acid. J Am Acad Dermatol 1996; 35:388–391.
36. Ditre CM, Griffin TD, Murphy GF, Sueki II, Telegan B, Johnson WC, Yu R, Van Scott EJ. Effects of alpha-hydroxy acids on photoaged skin: a pilot clinical, histologic, and ultrastructural study. J Am Acad Dermatol 1996; 34:187–195.
37. Van Scott EJ, Yu RJ. Alpha hydroxyacids: therapeutic potentials. Can J Dermatol 1989; 1(5):108–112.
38. Blank IH. Factors which influence the water content of the stratum corneum. J Invest Dermatol 1952; 18:433–440.
39. Middleton JD. The mechanism of water binding in stratum corneum. Br J Dermatol 1968; 80:437.
40. Harding CR, Watkinson A, Rawlings AV. Dry skin, moisturization and corneodesmolysis. Int J Cosmet Sci 2000; 22:21–52.
41. Middleton JD. The influence of temperature and humidity on stratum corneum and its relation to skin chapping. J Soc Cosmet Chem 1973; 24:239.
42. Alderson SG, Barratt MD, Black JG. Effect of 2-hydroxyacids on guinea-pig footpad stratum corneum: mechanical properties and binding studies. Int J Cosm Sci 1984; 6:91–100.

43. Harding CR, Bartolone J, Rawlings AV. Effects of natural moisturizing factor and lactic acid isomers on skin function. In: Loden M, Maibach HI, eds. Dry skin and Moisturizers: Chemistry and Function. Boca Raton: CRC Press, 2000:229–241.

44. Takahashi M, Kawasaki K, Tanaka M, Ohra S, Tsuda Y. The mechanism of stratum corneum plasticization with water. In: Marks R, Pine PA, eds. Bioengineering and the Skin. Lancaster: MTP Press, 1981:67–73.

45. Yu RJ, Van Scott EJ. Bioavilability of alpha-hydroxy acids in topical formulations. Cosmet Dermatol 1996; 9:54–62.

46. Wehr R, Krochmal L, Bagatell F, Radsdale W. A controlled two-center study of lactate 12 percent lotion and a petrolatum-based cream in patients with xerosis. Cutis 1986; 37:205–209.

47. Buxman M, Hickman H, Ragsdale W, et al. Therapeutic activity of lactate 12% lotion in the treatment of ichthyosis: active versus vehicle and active versus a petrolatum cream. J Am Acad Dermatol 1986; 15:1253–1258.

48. Rogers RS III, Callen J, Wehr R, Krochmal L. Comparative efficacy of 12% ammonium lactate lotion and 5% lactic acid lotion in the treatment of moderate to severe xerosis. J Am Acad Dermatol 1989; 21:714–716.

49. Lavker RM, Kaidbey K, Leyden J. Effects of topical ammonium lactate on cutaneous atrophy from a potent topical corticosteroid. J Am Acad Dermatol 1992; 26:535–544.

50. Leyden JJ, Lavker RM, Grove G, Kaidbey K. Alpha hydroxy acids are more than moisturizers. J Geriatr Dermatol 1995; 3(suppl):33A–37A.

51. Rawlings AV, Conti A, Feinberg C, Van Dyk K, Nicoll G. Improvements in stratum corneum ceramide level and barrier function following treatment with alpha hydroxy acids. Poster exhibit, American Academy of Dermatology, San Francisco, 1994.

52. Rawlings AV, Davies A, Carlomusto M, Pillai S, Zhang K, Kosturko R, Verdejo P, Feinberg C, Nguyen L, Chandar P. Effect of lactic acid isomers on keratinocyte ceramide synthesis, stratum corneum lipid levels and stratum corneum barrier function. Arch Dermatol Res 1996; 288:383–390.

53. Van Scott EJ, Yu RJ. Alpha hydroxy acids: procedures for use in clinical practice. Cutis 1989; 43:222–228.

54. Smith W. AHAs or Retin A—the dermatological view of actives. Proceedings Advanced Technology Conference, Paris, 1995:3–45.

55. Draelos ZD. Therapeutic moisturizers. Dermatol Clinics 2000; 18:597–606.

56. Ghadially R. Do anti-aging creams really work? Cosmet Dermatol 2000; 13(12):13–17.

57. Nole G, Edgerly S, Johnson A, Znaiden A. Global face assessment—a clinical evaluation method. Cosmet Toil 1994; 109(7):69–72.

58. Morganti P, Randazzo SD, Bruno C. Alpha hydroxy acids in the cosmetic treatment of photo-induced skin aging. J Appl Cosmetol 1996; 14:1–8.

59. Smith WP. Hydroxy acids and skin aging. Soap Cosmet Chem Specialities 1993; 69(9):54–76.

60. Smith WP. Hydroxy acids and skin aging. Cosmet Toil 1994; 109(9):41–48.

61. Johnson AW, Stoudermayer TS, Kligman AM. Application of 4% and 8% glycolic acid to human skin in commercial skin creams formulated to CIR guidelines does not

thin the stratum corneum or increase sensitivity to UVR. J Cosmet Sci 2000; 51:343–349.

62. Ditre CM, Nini KT, Vagley RT. Practical use of glycolic acid as a chemical peeling agent. J Geriatr Dermatol 1996; 4(suppl):2B–7B.

63. Elson ML. The Art of chemical peeling. Cosmet Dermatol, October 1994; (suppl):24–28.

64. Benedetto AV, Griffin TD, Benedetto EA, Humeniuk HM. Dermabrasion: therapy and prophylaxis of the photoaged face. J Am Acad Dermatol 1963; 27:439–447.

65. Ratner D, Tse Y, Marchell N, Goldman MP, Fitzpatrick RE, Fader DJ. Cutaneous laser resurfacing. J Am Acad Dermatol 1999; 41:365–389.

66. Guttman C. Branching into cosmetic procedures no stretch. Dermatol Times 1999; 20(2):1.

67. Murad H, Shamban AT. Various combinations of peeling agents improve results. Cosmet Dermatol, 1994; (suppl):29–32.

68. Kempers S, Katz HI, Wildnauer R, Green B. An evaluation of the effect of an alpha hydroxy acid-blend skin cream in the cosmetic improvement of symptoms of moderate to severe xerosis, epidermolytic hyperkeratosis, and ichthyosis. Cutis 1998; 61:347–350.

69. Hermitte R. Aged skin, retinoids and alpha hydroxy acids. Cosmet Toil 1992; 107(7):63–66.

70. Kligman A. Results of a pilot study evaluating the compatibility of topical tretinoin in combination with glycolic acid. Cosmet Dermatol 1993; 6(10):28–32.

71. Elson ML. Differential effects of glycolic acid and tretinoin in acne vulgaris. Cosmet Dermatol 1992; 5(12):36–40.

72. Briden ME, Kakita LS, Petratos MA, Rendon-Pellerano MI. Treatment of acne with glycolic acid. J Geriatr Dermatol 1996; 4(suppl):22B–27B.

73. Briden ME, Rendon-Pellerano MI. Treatment of rosacea with glycolic acid. J Geriatr Dermatol 1996; 4(suppl):17B–21B.

74. Garcia A, Fulton JE Jr. The combination of glycolic acid and hydroquinone or kojic acid for the treatment of melasma and related conditions. Dermatol Surg 1996; 22:443–447.

75. Tsai T, Paul BH, Jee S, Maibach HI. Effects of glycolic acid on light-induced skin pigmentation in Asian and Caucasian subjects. J Am Acad Dermatol 2000; 43:238–243.

76. Perricone NV, DiNardo JC. Photoprotective and anti-inflammatory effects of topical glycolic acid. Dermatol Surg 1996; 22:435–437.

77. Perricone NV. An alpha hydroxy acid acts as an antioxidant. J Geriatr Dermatol 1993; 1(2):101–104.

78. Christensen M, Kligman AM. An improved procedure for conducting lactic acid stinging tests on facial skin J Soc Cosmet Chem 1996; 47:1–11.

79. Cosmederm-7 anti-irritant "substantially reduces" AHA irritation. The Rose Sheet. F-D-C Reports, Washington, D.C., June 16, 1997.

80. Morganti P, Randazzo SD, Fabrizl G, Bruno. C. Decreasing the stinging capacity and improving the antiaging activity of AHAs. J Appl Cosmetol 1996; 14:79–91.

81. DiNardo JC, Grove GL, Moy LS. 12% ammonium lactate versus 8% glycolic acid. J Geriatr Dermatol 1995; 3(5):144–147.

82. Fartasch M, Teal J, Menon GK. Mode of action of glycolic acid on human stratum corneum: ultrastructural and functional evaluation of the epidermal barrier. Arch Dermatol Res 1997; 289:404–409.
83. Burge S. Cohesion in the epidermis. Br J Dermatol 1994;131:153–159.
84. Harding CR, Watkinson A, Rawlings AV, Scott IR. Dry skin, moisturization and corneodesmolysis. Int J Cosmet Sci 2000; 22:21–52.
85. Wang X. A theory for the mechanism of action of the alpha-hydroxy acids applied to the skin. Medical Hypotheses 1999; 53:380–382.
86. Van Scott EJ, Yu RJ. Actions of alpha hydroxy acids on skin compartments. J Geriatr Dermatol 1995; 3(suppl):19A–24A.
87. Griffin TD, Murphy GF, Sueki H, Telegan B, Johnson WC, Ditre CM, Yu RJ, Van Scott EJ. Increased factor XIIIa transglutaminase expression in dermal dendrocytes after treatment with alpha hydroxy acids: potential physiological significance. J Am Acad Dermatol 1996; 34:196–203.
88. Bernstein EF, Uitto J. Connective tissue alterations in photoaged skin and the effects of alpha hydroxy acids. J Geriatr Dermatol 1995; 3(suppl):7A–18A.
89. Nickoloff BJ, Naider Y. Perturbation of epidermal barrier function correlates with initiation of cytokine cascade in human skin. J Am Acad Dermatol 1994; 30:535–546.
90. Cosmetic Ingredient Review. Scientific Literature Review on Glycolic and Lactic Acids, Their Common Salts, and Their Simple Esters. Washington, D.C.: Cosmetic Ingredient Review, April 7, 1995.
91. Cosmetic Ingredient Review. Final report on the safety assessment of glycolic acid, ammonium, calcium, potassium, and sodium glycolates, methyl, ethyl, propyl, and butyl glycolates, and lactic acid, ammonium, calcium, potassium, sodium, and TEA-lactates, methyl, ethyl, isopropyl, and butyl lactates, and lauryl, myristyl, and ceryl lactates. Int J Toxicol 1998; 17(suppl 1):1–242.
92. The Rose Sheet. F-D-C Reports, Washington, D.C., September 13, 1999, p. 3.
93. The Rose Sheet. F-D-C Reports, Washington, D.C., February 28, 2000, p. 3.

17

Salicylic Acid and Derivatives

**Jean Luc Lévêque and
Didier Saint-Léger**
L'Oréal, Clichy, France

To the trees from the Salix and Spiraea spp, for so many vanished pains . . .

1 INTRODUCTION

From the bark of trees to the human stratum corneum, salicylic acid (SA) has followed a unique, now legendary, trajectory. Early and pragmatically recognized by dermatological masters as a valuable help in disorders of hyperkeratinization, SA progressively became a standard. As a russian doll, from therapy to research, SA offered successive and intricate developments, being both a therapeutic agent and a tool of research as well. More recently, since it is well tolerated by the human skin, SA logically entered the cosmetic field as a major skin care agent. The rationale of its introduction in this application, with other molecules such as α-hydroxyacids (AHAs), retinoic acid, etc., is mostly grounded in their so-called keratolytic action, a property that leads to skin softening which, in turn, improve the aspect (hue, color) of the consumer's skin.

Within this domain, new and recent findings have shown that by itself and as a mother molecule SA still shows promise with regard to its derived products.

The aim of this chapter is, through its properties and those of one of its derivatives, to illustrate how such an ancient product may be "self-rejuvenating."

353

2 SALICYLIC ACID—FROM TRADITION TO RATIONALE

From the most ancient human memories, the willow tree (Salix spp.) has brought a precious offering to both human and animal well being [1]. The salicylate-rich extract from the bark, later shown to contain salicin and salicylic acid, was as early as 1763 recognized to be efficient as both an antipyretic and pain reliever in various forms of rheumatic diseases [2–4]. Later on, the adverse side effects of SA (irritation of mucosa, gastrointestinal intolerance, etc.) were partly encompassed by acetylation of the hydroxyl group (OH), leading to the fascinating saga of Aspirin® [5,6], commercialized in 1899, as science, politics, World War I, and commercial conflicts admixed.

Although aspirin, a century old product, has proven anti-inflammatory properties (inhibition of prostaglandin synthesis) [7], its interest as a prophylactic drug in thrombosis and myocardial infarction has been emerging during the last decades. This old multifaceted compound likely deserves its designation as a miracle drug [6], although, ironically enough, if present standards of toxicological safety were applied, its development would definitely be banned.

Chemically, SA is 2-hydroxybenzoic acid and may possibly be viewed as a β-hydroxyacid, (Fig. 1), although such denomination does not strictly apply to cyclic radicals such as its benzene ring:

With regard to skin, the rationale for its topical use, back to the early 20th century, is sparsely documented. It is reasonable to assume that it arose from two main factors:

1. Reported to have antibacterial activities, it was commercialised, too, as food preservative. In those times, the crucial need for skin disinfectants was obvious, and its topical use as a phenol alternative dates back to 1874 [8].
2. Its well-known (and early detected) side effects on oral mucosa likely induced some to see SA as a potential help in hyperkeratotic disorders (ichthyosis, pityriasis, etc.) and later to dyskeratinization disorders, such as acne, where its early use originated in the 1950s.

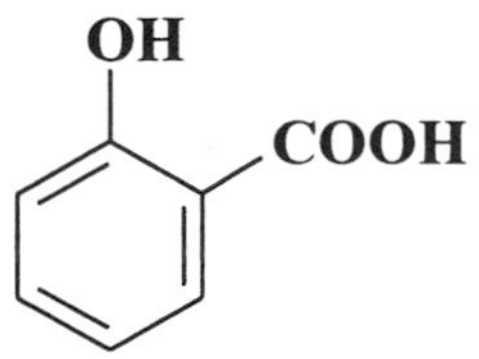

FIGURE 1 Chemical structure of salicylic acid.

2.1 Dermatological and Cosmetical Properties

For decades, SA has certainly been one of the most commonly used compounds among both dermatological and cosmetical arsenals. A 1975 review [9] conferred to topical SA a mosaic of actions according to dosages (0.3 to 5% and above), i.e., germistatic, acidogenic, photoprotective, anti-eczematous, and the so-called keratolytic effect. Presently, both scientific works and routine practice have, in fact, largely focused interest on the latter action [10–13] for three main reasons:

1. The first four actions were of a very modest amplitude as compared to other candidates (true germicides, powerful sunscreens, etc.).
2. Clinically, its progressive (and empirical) use in common hyperkeratotic conditions showed clear benefits, coupled with an acceptable tolerance.
3. The intense development of bioengineering methods during the last three decades allowed a precise quantification of its "keratolytic" property when applied to skin. Salicylic acid rapidly became, too, an important tool for researchers involved in exfoliative cytology or transcutaneous penetration studies [14,15].

It is now a common statement that keratolytic and derived effects are unjustified. Neither SA nor AHA lead to breakage of keratin chains as this invented term suggested [16].

In fact, SA appears to be a clear disrupter agent of the horny cell junctions. Desmosome or Corneodesmosome attachments between adjacent cells mostly ensure the latter, maintaining stratum corneum cohesion. These cellular "snap fasteners" of glycoprotein structures are progressively degraded through (endogenic) enzymatic attacks, leading to a loosening of the cell junctions and consequent monocellular desquamation, in the normal situation. Our group has recently shown that desmosomes-like organizations are the precise privileged sites of action of SA, leading to their degradation [17]. As suggested, "desmolysis" would be a much better term for such action.

In hyperkeratotic conditions (xerosis, acne, warts), where the SC appears thick, cracking, fluffy, or badly organized, topical SA restores within a few weeks a normalized and thinner horny organization [18,19]. This action is coupled to the following criteria:

Form. Salicylic acid is sparingly hydrosoluble. It is, most of the time, introduced in lipophilic ointments or alcoholic lotions. In most cases, SA is introduced as a free form, i.e., at a spontaneous acid pH, the free states of both OH and COOH groups seemingly a prerequisite for desmolytic action.

Dose dependence. Desmolysis is dose dependent, ranging from 2 to 3% in the minor cases of xerosis, to 17% (coupled to lactic acid) for wart treatment [20]. Above that (50%), it has been shown to exert a peeling effect of the hands, helping to treat actinic damage and pigmented lesions [21].

Specificity. Topical SA which penetrates the SC modifies its properties and acts as plasticizer [22,23] It may cause irritation in a dose-related manner. However, according to the vehicle, daily applications of 2 to 3% SA appear safe, well tolerated, and rarely irritating [24]. Desmolysis seems directly induced by the presence of SA within the SC, rather than by an indirect action onto the living (basal) epidermis. Previous studies dealing with its effect on epidermopoeisis are conflicting [16,25,26].

It is only recently that one study [27] has shed new light on a possible moisturizing action of SA. As compared to "classic" references of SC hydrating compounds, SA leads to an appreciable amplitude of moisturizing effect, although the latter seems reached at high concentration (10%) of SA. This work was, however, carried out on the skin of miniature swines. It remains uncertain whether SA per se directly acts as a moisturizing agent on human skin. In fact, such effect if really proven might well be a secondary event following the SA-induced normalization of the SC barrier.

3 SA DERIVATIVES

Studies from our group dealing with lipophilic derivatives of SA led us to select the C8 derivative (herein referred to as LSA), among many, as the best candidate in terms of both keratolytic and microbiological effects (Fig. 2). The screening procedures were the following:

Keratolysis. This property was assessed in vivo in man through trans-epidermal water loss (TEWL) since it clearly increases following repeated topical applications of SA [28]. When used to record the effects of SA derivatives of varying chain lengths, TEWL variation with baseline pro-

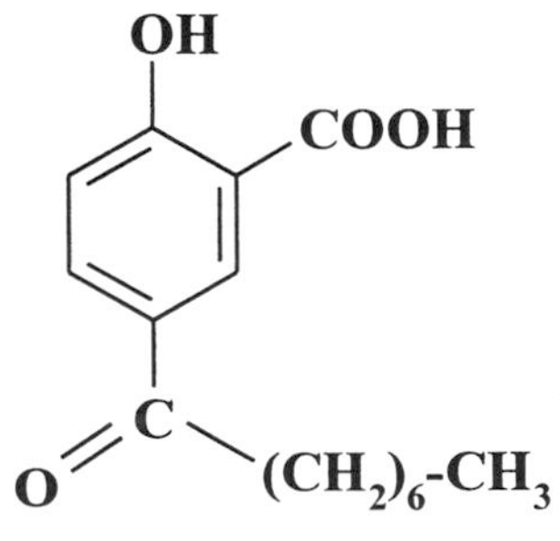

FIGURE 2   Chemical structure of LSA (n-octanoyl-5 salicylic acid).

gressively increases with increasing length (from C4 to C8), peaks at C8, and declines afterward. As compared to SA, LSA leads to comparable variation in TEWL for a reduced concentration (w/w), about three times lower than that of SA [26]. Expressed as molar ratios, this increased activity is even more in favor of LSA since it has a much higher molecular weight (264 versus 138). According to these expressions, LSA therefore shows for a "keratolytic" property an intrinsic potency of three to six times that of SA.

Microbiological data. MIC's of the various derivatives on different strains of the resident human skin flora appear lower with longer chains (C8, C10, and above) as compared to shorter ones (C2, C4, and C6) [29]. Based on such in vitro findings, a better efficacy is therefore given privilege to chains greater than C8.

These two citeria, coupled to safety data profiles, led us to investigate further the cosmetological interest of LSA, by comparing it to previously well-recognized keratolytic agents such as SA, glycolic acid (GA), lactic acid (LA), and retinoic acid (RA).

3.1 Comparative Effects of the Keratolytic Compounds on Human Epidermis

3.1.1 Effects on Stratum Corneum in Vitro

Samples from either strippings or biopsies from healthy human volunteers were submitted to the actions of LSA (1 and 5%), LA, and SA (3 and 15%), all introduced in the same propylene glycol vehicle and further processed by transmission electronic microscopy (TEM) coupled to freeze fracture (FF) according to classical technical procedures [17].

The results clearly show that corneodesmosomes (CDs) are the main targets of these three agents. Keratin filaments remain intact in all samples.

However, some differences between the respective effects of these compounds may be outlined. Salicylic and lactic acid seem to act uniformly into the overall thickness of the stratum corneum, whereas LSA appears to limit its action to the superior third, a location of the SC where corneodesmosomes have previously been modified/degraded by proteolytic enzymes. The nature of the modifications of the CDs seems different, too; LSA appears to act on their whole structure, completely detaching them from one full side, while LA and SA seem to fractionate these CDs. With regard to SA, the glycoproteins, which cross the membrane, appear strongly denatured. These changes are illustrated in Figs. 3 and 4.

According to the authors of these works, the different modes of actions of these agents are closely related to their intrinsic lipophilic property. The latter

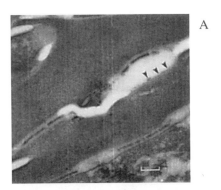

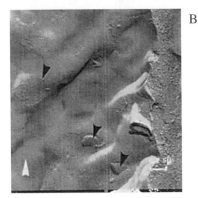

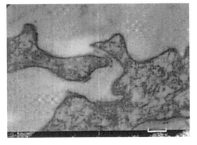

Figure 3 Corneosome degradation by SA. (A) The corneosomes are fragmented. When the plug detaches from one of the corneocytes, the opposite lipid envelope is still visible (arrow heads). Biopsy—OsO4 fixation. Scale bar: 150 nm. (B) Freeze-fracture replica showing affected corneosomes in the stratum compactum. The P fracture face of corneosomes appears as loosely spaced particles. Protusions of plug fragments (black arrow heads) occur on the P face of corneosomes. The direction of shadowing is shown by the white arrow head. The bar represents 250 nm. (C) Like central corneosomes, peripheral corneosomes are fragmented, some fragments remaining attached to one corneocyte and others to the opposite corneocyte. Biopsy—OsO4. Scale bar: 250 nm. (From Ref. 17.)

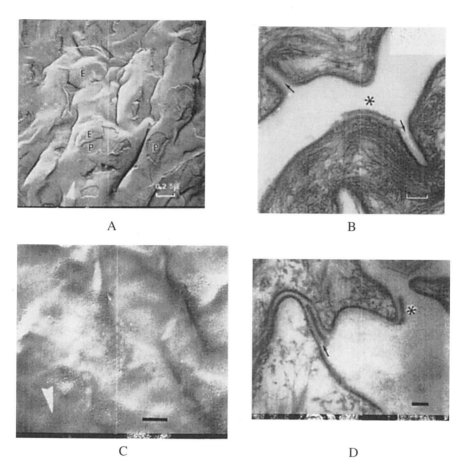

FIGURE 4 Corneosome rupture by LSA. (A) In the stratum compactum, the corneocyte membranes are sinouos. The plane of fracture jumps from P to E face in the same corneosome, suggesting slight altered fracture behavior of the junctional areas. The direction of shadowing is shown by the white arrow head. The bar represents 250 nm. (B) The plub has detached from the upper corneocyte (asterisk). The corneocytes membranes are sinuous (arrows). Biopsy—OsO4 fixation. Scale bar: 90 nm. (C) At the compactum/disjunctum interface, fractured corneosomes display abnormal particle distribution, delineating the corneosomes edge. The number of membrane-associated particles of corneosomes is clearly decreased. The direction of shadowing is shown by the white arrow head. Scale bar 250nm. (D) Neqar the skin surface, the peripheral corneosomes undergo a clean rupture (arrow) and remain attached to one of the corneocytes (asterisk). Biopsy—OsO4 fixation. Scale bar: 90 nm. (From Ref. 17.)

would, in turn, "orientate" their action either on the membrane (LSA) of the CDs or on their proteins/glycoproteins for the least lipophilic agents (SA, LA).

3.1.2 Effects on Epidermal Renewal in Vivo

It has been shown that on human photoaged skin repeated topical applications of retinoic acid lead to clear changes in the epidermal turnover, even for as short a period as 4 weeks [23]. Following a similar protocol, Pierard et al. compared in vivo on man the respective activities of SA (5%) and LSA (1.5%) versus RA (0.025%) [30]. The study was carried out for 4 weeks in a double-blind procedure, and the three agents were compared to their respective vehicles. On biopsies, automated histometry measurements, immunohistology allowed the recording of changes in cell proliferation (Ki67), cell differentiation (K), and activity of the papillary dermis as well.

The skin sites treated by vehicle and SA do not differ from a nontreated control site in any aspect. However, both sites treated by RA and LSA revealed significant increases in the thickness of the viable epidermis and its renewal rate. In the papillary dermis, dendrocytes FXIII positive were shown significantly activated and of higher amplitude in the RA-treated site than that of the LSA.

Another study of a comparable methodology (double-blind, vehicle-controlled) compared on three groups of human volunteers (eight per group) the effects of RA (0.05%), LSA (2%), and GA (10%, pH 3.5), each product being applied onto one forearm for two months, the other receiving the vehicle (common to the three agents) alone [31].

In addition to standard histometric and immunohistologic measurements, classical histology (H&E, Luna, Hale, Fontana–Masson, and PAS-Giemsa stains) was undertaken.

This study, in conflict with previously published data, failed to detect any modification brought by GA. This study confirms, however, the RA and LSA effects that were initially found in the Pierard study [23]. Additionally, classical histology revealed a partial correction of epidermal atrophy, atypia, and dysplasia. Again, this study noted higher amplitude of effect brought by RA than by LSA.

As far as melanins are concerned, both products show comparable activity; the large and dense melanosome conglomerates present on the basal layer become dispersed into small units.

These studies illustrate the effectiveness of this lipophilic derivative of SA in the skin care of photoaged skins and its superiority vis a vis SA, LA, and GA in these precise experimental conditions.

3.2 LSA-Treated Skin and Cosmetic Implications

The usual cosmetic concepts (skin smoothness, firmness, hue, glow) can hardly be reduced to the measurements of one or two objective cutaneous parameters.

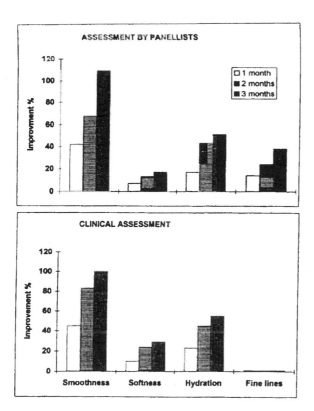

FIGURE 5 Improvement of the skin after 1, 2, and 3 months of treatment with an excipient containing 1% LSA. Assessment by the panelists and dermatologists.

The need to describe the overall effect of a given treatment requires either the help of a well-trained clinician and/or comments by the consumer, who in fact is the ultimate judge of the benefits brought to the skin by this treatment.

In a first experiment, an oil-in-water (O/W) emulsion containing 1% LSA was given to 35 subjects [26]. They were asked to judge, each month, for a 3-month period, the improvement of their facial skin through four predetermined criteria: smoothness, suppleness, hydration, and fine wrinkles). A trained clinician recorded his own appreciation during each monthly visit. Results given by Fig. 5 illustrate the close agreement between the subjects and the clinician for three of the four criteria under study. The discrepancy noticed in the fourth parameter (fine wrinkles) likely lies in the personal and subjective interpretation/ definition of fine wrinkle.

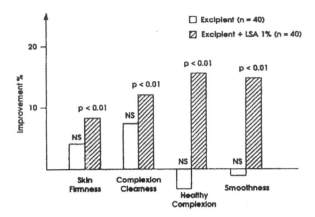

Figure 6 Improvement of the skin of 80 volunteers after 6 months of treatment. Half of the volunteers were treated with an excipient containing 5% glycerol and the other half with the same excipient containing 1% LSA.

In this study, skin smoothness, likely resulting from an induced descaling effect, highly increased (more than twofold on a nonparametric range).

A second study was carried out with the same emulsion (containing 5% glycerol and 1% LSA) and was compared to the vehicle alone (an emulsion containing glycerol but without LSA) on two groups of 40 subjects each. They applied the products (active or vehicle) for a 6-month period. Results, shown in Fig. 6, illustrate for months 1, 4, and 6 the significant improvements brought by LSA to four cutaneous parameters (firmness, hue, glow, and smoothness). With regard to dry skin, both treatments (active and vehicle) led to comparable improvement, likely due to the common presence of 5% glycerol among the two preparations.

4 CONCLUSIONS

The so-called keratolytic agents bring an appreciable contribution to skin care. They clearly improve the overall aspect of the skin and its smoothness as well, probably by eliminating clusters of corneocytes resulting from slight dysfunction in the desquamative process. As discussed, the main targets of these compounds are, in fact, the corneodesmosomes that link adjacent horny cells and not on keratin filaments as their name suggests.

Among this category of compounds, α-hydroxyacids, used in cosmetic/skin care for years, should be distinguished from the salicylate family. The efficacy of AHA to help with squama removal or epidermal renewal appears highly dependent to their formulation (pH, concentration). Such does not seem to be the case with salicylates, especially the C8 lipophilic derivative which combines both the effects of a slight boost of cell renewal and a dispersing of the basal melanin aggregates, leading to a more uniform and clearer aspect to the skin. The results reviewed here highlight the LSA as a promising active agent for skin care where a slight stimulation of the epidermal turnover is desirable.

REFERENCES

1. Stone E. An account of the success of the bark of the willow in the cure of agues. Philos Trans R Soc Lond (Biol) 1763; 53:195–200.
2. Stricker F. Aus der Traubschen Klinik. Über die Resultate der behandlung der polyarthritis rhumatica mit salicylsäure. Berl Klin Woschr 1876;13:1–15.
3. Gross M, Greenberg LA. The salicylates: a critical bibliographic review. New Haven, CT: Hillhouse Press, 1948:8.
4. Hedner T, Everts B. The early clinical history of salicylates in rheumatology and pain. Clin Rheumatol 1998; 17:17–25.
5. Kubnert N. Hundert Jahre Aspirin. Chemie 1999; 3364:213–220.
6. Jourdier S. A miracle drug. Chemistry in Britain 1999; Feb:33–35.
7. Vane JR. Inhibition of prostaglandin synthesis as a mechanism of action for aspirin-like drugs. Nature 1971; 231:232–235.
8. Kolbe H. Ueber eine neue Darstellungmethode und einige bemerkenswerte Eigenschaften der Salicylsäure. Arch Pharm 1874, 5–45.
9. Weirich EG. Dermatopharmacology of salicylic acid. Dermatologica 1975; 151:268–273.
10. Huber C, Christophers E. "Keratolytic" effect of salicylic acid. Arch Derm Res 1977; 257:293–297.
11. Kligman LH, Kligman AM. The effect on rhino mouse skin of agents which influence keratinization and exfoliation. J Invest Dermatol 1979; 73:354–358.
12. Roberts DL, Marshall R, Marks R. Detection of the action of salicylic acid on the normal sratum corneum. Br J Dermatol 1980; 103:191–196.
13. Loden M, Boström P, Kneczke M. Distribution and keratolytic effect of salicylic acid and urea in human skin. Skin Pharmacol 1995; 8:173–178.
14. Elias PM, Cooper ER, Korc A, Brown BE. Percutaneous transport in relation to stratum corneum structure and lipid composition. J Invest Dermatol 1981; 76:297–301.
15. Harada K, Murakami T, Yata N, Yamamoto S. Role of intercellular lipids in stratum corneum in the percutaneous permeation of drugs. J Invest Dermatol 1992; 99:278–282.
16. Davies M, Marks R. Studies on the effect of salicylic acid on normal skin. Br J Dermatol 1976; 95:187–192.
17. Corcuff P, Fiat F, Gracia AM, Lévêque JL. Hydroxyacid induced desquamation of the human stratum corneum: a comparative ultrastructural study. Proc 19th IFSCC Congress 1996; 3:85–94.
18. Mark R, Davies M, Cattel A. An explanation for the keratolytic effect of salicylic acid. J Invest Dermamol Abstracts 1975; April:283.
19. Nook TH. In vivo measurement of the keratolytic effect of salicylic acid in three ointment formulations. Br J Dermatol 1987; 117:243–245.

20. Lawson EE, Edwards H, Barry BW, Williams AC. Interaction of salicylic acid with verrucae assessed by FT raman spectroscopy. Journal of Drug Targeting 1998; 5(5):343–351.

21. Swineheart JM. Salicylic acid ointment peeling of the hands and forearms. J Dermatol Surg Oncol 1992; 18:495–498.

22. Rasseneur L, De Rigal J, Lévêque JL. Influence des différents constituants de la couche cornée sur la mesure de son élasticité. Int J Cosmet Sci 1982; 4:247–260.

23. Pierard-Franchimont C, Goffin V, Pierard GE. Modulation of human stratum corneum properties by salicylic and all-*trans* retinoic acid. Skin Pharmacol 1998; 11:266–272.

24. Davis DA, Krasu AL, Thomson GA, Olerich M, Odio MR. Percutaneous absorption of salicylic acid after repeated (14 days) in vivo administration to normal, acnegenic or aged human skin. J Pharmaceut Sci 1997; 86(8):896–899.

25. Weirich EG, Longauer JK, Kirkwod AH. Effect of topical salicylic acid on animal epidermopoiesis. Dermatologica 1978; 156:89–96.

26. Lévêque JL, Corcuff P, Gonnord G, Montastier C, Renault B, Bazin R, Pierard GE, Poelman MC. Mechanism of action of a lipophilic derivative of salicylic acid on normal skin. Skin Res Technol 1995; 1:115–122.

27. Goshi KI, Tabata N, Sato Y. Comparative study of the efficacy of various moisturizers on the skin of the ASR miniature swine. Skin Pharmacol Appl Skin Physiol 2000; 13:120–127.

28. Guillaume JC, De Rigal J, Lévêque JL, Dubertret L, Touraine L. Etude comparée de la perte insensible d'eau et de la pénétration cutanée des corticoides. Dermatologica 1981; 162:380–390.

29. International patent L'Oreal no. 850.69.53.

30. Pierard GE, Nikkels-Tassoudji N, Arrese JE, et al. Dermo-epidermal stimulation elicited by a lipohydroxyacid: a comparison with salicylic acid and all-*trans* retinoic acid. Dermatology 1997; 194:398–401.

31. Pierard GE, Kligman AM, Stoudemayer TJ, et al. Comparative effects of retinoic acid, glycolic acid and a lipophilic derivative of salicylic acid on photoaged epidermis. Dermatology 1999; 199:50–53.

18

The Efficacy, Stability, and Safety of Topically Applied Protease in Treating Xerotic Skin

David J. Pocalyko and Prem Chandar

Unilever Research, Edgewater Laboratory, Edgewater, New Jersey

Clive R. Harding, Lynn Blaikie, and Allan Watkinson

Unilever Research, Colworth Laboratory, Sharnbrook, Bedford, United Kingdom

Anthony V. Rawlings

Unilever Research, Port Sunlight Laboratory, Bebington, Wirral, United Kingdom

1 INTRODUCTION

Abnormal desquamation arises from an inability to effectively degrade the molecular components that provide cohesive force and thereby maintain tissue integrity. In such conditions corneocytes do not detach as single cells, but are shed in large clusters forming visible scales. The degree of scaling varies from severe in genetically determined disorders such as ichthyoses (which are also associated with increased thickness of the stratum corneum) to "cosmetic" dry skin. The appearance of the latter form of dry skin is a common feature in the population and is usually associated with extrinsic damage (e.g., surfactants, UV irradiation) and

365

following seasonal changes in the weather (cold winter conditions with a low relative humidity). Dry skin associated with the steady decline into old age (senile xerosis) reflects an increased susceptibility of the skin to extrinsic damage due to a decreased intrinsic ability to respond to challenges from the environment.

Abnormal desmosomal retention [1] into the most superficial layers is a characteristic of dry, flaky skin conditions. The inability to degrade desmosomes may result from a number of changes within the corneum. The reduction of active SCCE and possibly other desquamatory hydrolases, either through leaching out from the stratum corneum [2,3] or insufficient conversion from pro-enzyme, may contribute to the condition. In acute dryness this may reflect damage/inactivation of the enzyme, especially if the condition is exacerbated by surfactant use. Alterations to the extracellular environment surrounding the desmosomes (essentially the organization/composition of the lipids) may influence the intrinsic ability of the enzymes to work effectively. Ultimately, the alteration in stratum corneum lipid organization will affect the levels of free water available to both hydrate the desquamatory enzymes and to participate in their catalytic reactions. This will result in these water-requiring desquamatory enzymes having reduced activity in the outermost layers of the stratum corneum [4].

Thus the water distribution and content of the stratum corneum, and the interaction of SCCE and other enzymes with the lipid environment in the intracellular space, have become targets for modulating desquamation in an effort to improve the texture and appearance of skin. Figure 1 depicts the current understanding surrounding the formation of cosmetic dry skin. In normal skin, the de novo production of keratinocytes at the basal layer is balanced by the loss of cells at the surface of the skin due to desquamation. External factors such as surfactants and low humidity environments lead to barrier damage and reduced water-holding capacity, resulting in a loss of desquamatory enzyme activity and retention of desmosomes in the upper layers of the stratum corneum. The increased cohesiveness of cells at the surface prevents the loss of single cells and results in the formation of visible flakes.

Conventional treatment involves moisturization, which by attempting to boost the water content of the stratum corneum aims to enhance desquamation. Indeed, glycerol, a highly effective agent for treating xerotic skin, has been shown to increase dsg1 hydrolysis resulting in increased cell dissociation, probably working by a combination of occlusivity, humectancy, and modulation of lipid phase behavior [3,5,6]. Although moisturization is an effective treatment for alleviating dry skin, there is room for improvement in the effiicacy of these agents. Because one potential cause of the perturbation in the desquamation process is a decrease in the activity of the protease SCCE, supplementation with topically applied proteolytic enzymes therefore represents a novel potential treatment for alleviation of xerotic skin scaling.

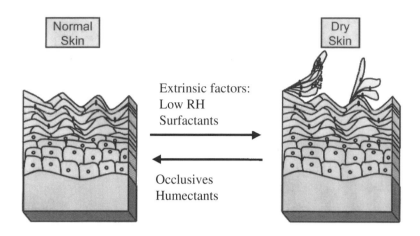

- Intact barrier
- Active SCCE
- Completely degraded desmosomes in upper stratum corneum
- Imperceptible loss of corneocytes

- Disrupted barrier
- Loss of SCCE activity
- Intact desmosomes retained in upper stratum corneum
- Visible scales formed

FIGURE 1 Conceptual model describing the role of desmosome degradation in dry skin formation.

2 EFFICACY OF TOPICAL PROTEASES

2.1 Clinical Effect of Protease on Visual Scaling

The effect of topically applied protease on visual scaling has been assessed clinically as described by El-Kadi et al. [7]. Briefly, subjects wash their lower legs for 20 s two times a day for one week. Enzyme is then applied and after a period of time the enzyme is washed off, and the site is evaluated visually using a scale ranging from zero (no dryness) to four (severe scaling and severe fissuring). Using this protocol, the ability of bovine pancreatic chymotrypsin to augment this loss in proteolytic activity is demonstrated in Fig. 2. Occluded treatment of dry skin with 0.5% (43 GU/mg, where a GU, or glycine unit, is the amount of enzyme that at pH 8.0 and 50°C produces an amount of amino terminal groups from acetylated casein equivalent to 1 μg/mL of glycine) of chymotrypsin resulted in a rapid decrease in visual scaling within 3 hr. The effect of this treatment is shown in Fig. 3. Visual scaling began to return after 24 hr, however, after 72 hr a significant difference in the level of visual scaling observed relative to vehicle treatment remained. Inactivation of the enzyme by heat prior to application resulted in no

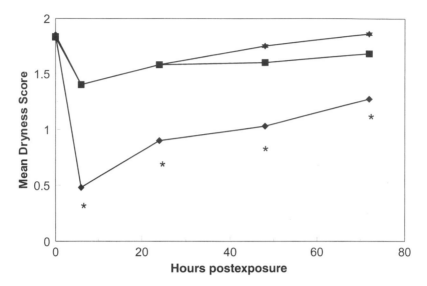

FIGURE 2 Effect of bovine pancreatic chymotrypsin on visual scaling after 3 hr occluded application. Vehicle (100μM Tris-HCl, pH 8, 5 μM Na₂EDTA) (square), 0.5% chymotrypsin (43 GU/mg) (diamond), heat inactivated chymotrypsin (star). *p < 0.05 for chymotrypsin versus vehicle and chymotrypsin versus inactivated enzyme.

effect beyond that observed by the vehicle, indicating that the reduction in visual scaling was due to proteolytic activity of the enzyme and was not due to a simple emollient effect of the protein itself.

The effect of chymotrypsin is both time and dose dependent. A steady increase in mean dryness reduction is observed as exposure time is increased from 30 to 180 min, suggesting that the enzyme is still catalytically active after this extended exposure time [7]. A dose-dependent effect is observed at both 0.1 and 0.5% chymotrypsin after 3 hr of occlusion (Fig. 4). The reduction in dryness achieved with 0.1% chymotrypsin is reduced to the level of the vehicle after 24 hr postexposure, while the reduction achieved with 0.5% is still evident at this time.

The ability to induce desquamation does not appear to be unique to chymotrypsin. Several enzymes from plant sources induce desquamation, although due to their lower specific activity, significantly more enzyme is required than in the case of chymotrypsin (Fig. 5). Some bacterial proteases are particularly efficient at inducing desquamation [7]. Serine proteases derived from *Bacillus licheniformus* sold commercially under the trade names Alcalase or Optimase contain both endo- and exopeptidase activity. The enzymes have broad substrate

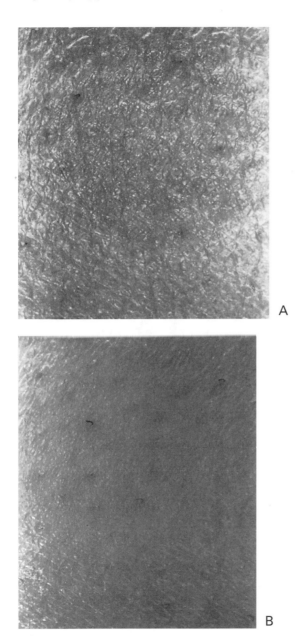

Figure 3 Effect of bovine pancreatic chymotrypsin in 100 μM Tris-HCl, pH 8, 5 μM Na₂EDTA after 3 hr occluded application. (A) Before treatment. (B) After treatment.

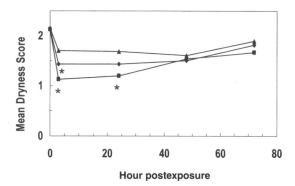

FIGURE 4 Effect of bovine pancreatic chymotrypsin on visual scaling after 3 hr occluded application. Vehicle (100 μM Tris-HCl, pH 8, 5 μM Na$_2$EDTA) (triangle), 0.01% chymotrypsin (1.1 GU/mg) (diamond), and 0.5% chymotrypsin (59 GU/mg) (square). *$p < 0.05$ for chymotrypsin versus vehicle.

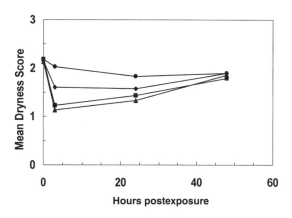

FIGURE 5 Visual scaling reduction achieved using various plant derived proteases under occluded application for 3 hr. All enzymes dosed at 5% by weight. Vehicle (100 μM sodium acetate, pH 6, 5 μM Na$_2$EDTA) (circle), bromelain (diamond), ficin (square), papain (triangle). $p < 0.05$ for all enzymes versus vehicle at 3 and 24 hr.

specificity and have pH optimum at neutral to alkaline pH. In part due to these properties, the enzymes are highly efficient, on a weight basis, at degrading large proteins. Their efficiency at inducing desquamation suggests that the cleavage of desmosomes required for cell shedding does not require a high degree of specificity.

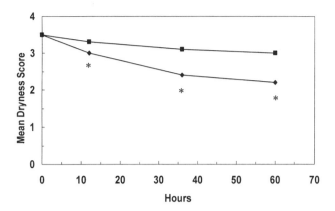

FIGURE 6 Reduction in visual dryness achieved using Optimase. Aqueous enzyme was applied unoccluded followed by the application of a commercial moisturizer. Vehicle (100 µM Tris-HCl, pH 8, 5 µM Na$_2$EDTA) (square) and Optimase at 50 GU/cm^2 (diamond). *$p < 0.05$ for Optimase versus vehicle.

Topical application of protease can be used to improve the efficacy of commercially available moisturizers. As seen in Fig. 6, the application of Optimase followed by the application of a commercial moisturizer resulted in a greater visual dryness reduction than the application of the aqueous vehicle and moisturizer. The reduction in dryness does not occur as quickly as when the enzyme is occluded. The effect is measurable after 12 hr and continues to increase over the next 48 hr. The stability of protease in typical oil-in-water emulsion–based moisturizes is low, primarily due to autolysis and denaturation. Thus a two-step application method was developed to circumvent the stability problem. The half-life of Optimase in a oil-in-water base moisturizer is long enough to conduct a clinical study provided that the samples are stored at 4°C during the course of the study. Using the procedure, a moisturizer containing Optimase was tested in a single-step application, applying the product once a day. Optimase improved the efficacy of the moisturizer in a manner similar to that achieved in a dual application (Fig. 7).

2.2 Mechanism of Protease-Induced Desquamation

The role of SCCE, a chymotrypsin-like protease, in degrading the corneodesmosome suggested that chymotrypsin enzymes would be the most effective when topically applied. However, as described, the action of topically applied proteolytic enzymes showed no such specificity; indeed the broader specificity enzymes proved to be the most effective. This suggested that the highly effective amelioration of xerotic skin scaling may have been due simply to generalized

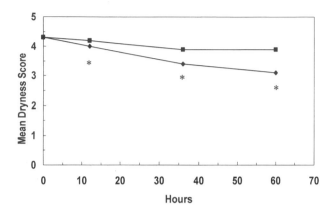

FIGURE 7 Reduction in visual dryness achieved using Optimase in a comercial moisturizer. Vehicle (commercial moisturizer) (square) and Optimase at 50 GU/cm² (diamond). *p < 0.05 for Optimase versus vehicle.

proteolysis, rather than emulating desquamation by causing the degradation of the corneodesmosomal linkages. To assess the mechanism of action of topically applied proteases on stratum corneum, an in vitro desquamation model was devised [7].

The model involved placing dermatomed skin on a bed of agar, to prevent tissue desiccation, applying Optimase to the skin, and incubating at a constant RH of 80%. Subsequent measurement of corneocyte release demonstrated that Optimase aided in enhancing cellular detachment, rather than by completely degrading the stratum corneum (Fig. 8a). Furthermore, indirect immunofluorescence, using an antiserum raised against extracellular regions of dsc1, revealed decreased levels of dsc1 epitopes on the surface of corneocytes in Optimase-treated skin (Figure 8b). This result indicated that at least one target of topically applied Optimase was the binding proteins of the corneodesmosome and supports the view that these enzymes work by an increased level of desmolysis. To confirm that the bacterial protease was indeed inducing desmosomal degradation, the morphology of desmosomes in enzyme-treated plantar stratum corneum was investigated.

In brief, pieces of plantar stratum corneum were incubated in buffer, with and without enzyme, and electron-microscope analysis was used to investigate the effect upon corneodesmosomes. This analysis revealed an increased incidence of degraded or degrading desmosomes in treated tissue compared to controls. Moreover, there was no evidence that Optimase had any effect upon the cornified envelope or the intermediate filaments within the corneocytes, except where the cornified envelope was obviously damaged, allowing enzyme entry (Fig. 9). This

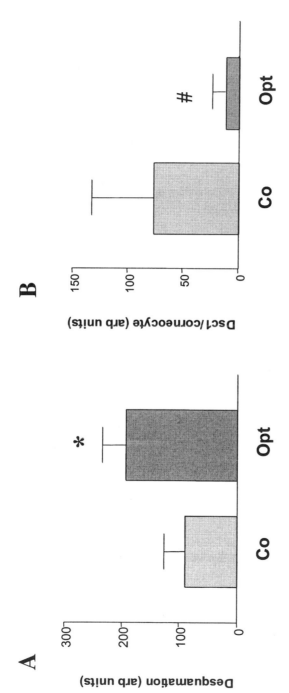

FIGURE 8 Effect of topically applied Optimase upon desquamation and desmolysis in vitro. Optimase (Opt) (100 μg/mL) was topically applied to pig skin in 100 mM Tris-HCl pH 8 at 50 μL/cm² and incubated for 24 hr at 37°C in 80% RH. Enzyme treatment was compared to the buffer control (Co). Panel A shows corneocyte release (n = 8) and panel B the levels of dsc 1 immunoreactivity per corneocyte (n = 15). Statistical analysis was by Whitney-Mann Rank Sum test; *p < 0.0002; #p < 0.0001.

A   B

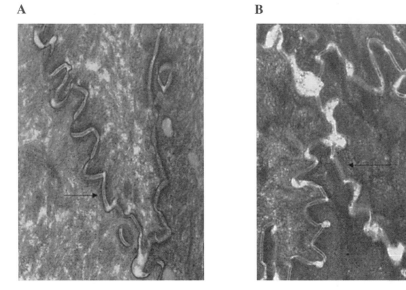

Figure 9 Typical electron micrograph images of control- and Optimase-treated plantar startum corneum. Optimase-treated stratum corneum (B) shows more degraded and degrading corneodesmosomes (arrow) compared to the control tissue (A), where intact corneodesmosomes predominate (arrow). (×32,000.)

indicates that as long as the cornified envelope remains intact, protease treatment of stratum corneum results in proteolysis of extracellular elements such as the desmosomal proteins.

The in vitro methodology strongly supports a mode of action of Optimase treatment that involves desmolysis. To confirm that this was happening in vivo under clinical conditions, corneocytes were collected using tape strips and analyzed by indirect immunofluorescence using dsc1 antiserum [7]. A 3-day unoccluded treatment with Optimase resulted in reduced levels of desmosomal protein on the corneocyte surface supporting the hypothesis that bacterial proteases rapidly improved the visual symptoms of xerosis by degrading the aberrantly retained desmosomes in scaling skin.

3 STABILITY OF PROTEASES IN CREAMS AND LOTIONS

From the previous sections, it is clear that topical application of proteolytic enzymes results is the rapid alleviation of the rough, flaky skin condition associated with soap-induced xerosis. However, proteases incorporated into cosmetic lotions containing high concentrations of water are unstable due to autolysis and denaturation. Typically an aqueous solution of Optimase is completely inactive after one day of storage at room temperature due primarily to autolysis. Thus, storage stability of enzymes in skin care cosmetics represents an inherently difficult challenge. Techniques to achieve storage stability have been developed for laundry detergents where the use of proteases has been widespread [8]. These include methods such as encapsulation, coacervation, precipitation, use of anhydrous (low water activity) vehicles, and the addition of stabilizers or enzyme inhibitors. However, these techniques are not immediately applicable for topical skin care products. In addition to safety and cosmetic acceptability considerations, a key difference is that such methods of stabilization rely on dilution in the laundry wash water to release or activate the enzyme from its stable storage condition and thus trigger its activity in use; in skin care products the reverse situation persists. The evaporation of volatile ingredients, primarily water, tends to concentrate the enzyme keeping it in the stable, inactive form. An obvious approach to circumvent this problem is through the use of dual compartment packages, which serve to physically separate a stable enzyme formula from a cosmetic emulsion. Formulations designed to effectively trigger the activation of enzyme through dilution or another mechanism upon mixing of these separate parts during application to skin can be conceived and developed. However, the complexity and cost of the packaging is often a prohibitive limitation.

The limitations associated with many of the stated approaches suggest that encapsulation routes which serve to isolate the enzyme into a hydrophobic, anhydrous matrix within the microstructure of the cosmetic lotion and subsequently release the enzyme through the shear and abrasion during topical application to

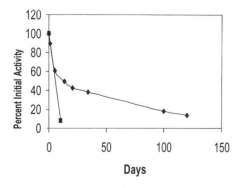

FIGURE 10 Comparison of the stability of encapsulated (diamond) versus unencapsulated (square) protease in a commercial oil-in-water cosmetic lotion.

the skin would offer significant advantages. Figure 10 compares the relative storage stability of Optimase AP 45 in a typical cosmetic skin lotion with and without encapsulation. The details of the encapsulation and analysis of protease activity are described elsewhere [9]. Briefly, the anhydrous enzyme powder is dispersed into petrolatum and emulsified in a concentrated aqueous solution to produce 100- to 500-µm droplets. The emulsion is blended into the skin lotion using low shear mixing to prevent breakage of the droplets.

Encapsulation clearly provides a considerable enhancement in stability compared to the direct incorporation of the enzyme into the lotion. Following this proof of principle we next considered factors that affect the rate of decomposition. As shown in Fig. 10, the shape of the decay curve is biphasic. The initial rapid loss can be attributed to the dissolution of poorly encapsulated enzyme into the aqueous solution and the consequential loss of activity due to autolysis. The slower loss of activity reflects the inactivation of encapsulated material. Overall the kinetics of decay can be described by Eq. (1):

$$[E] = ([E_t] - [E_{enc}]) \exp(-k_1 t) + [E_{enc}] \exp(-k_2 t) \tag{1}$$

where E is the active enzyme remaining at time t, E_t is the total enzyme, E_{enc} represents encapsulated enzyme, and k_1 and k_2 are the first-order rate constants for degradation of unprotected and protected enzyme, respectively: E_{enc} and k_2 can be obtained from fitting the data from more than 10 days.

A second consideration for the stability of encapsulated enzyme is water diffusion into the hydrophobic matrix and subsequent dissolution of the anhydrous enzyme within the capsule. With respect to this, it important to note that the anhydrous enzyme granules used in Fig. 10 (Optimase AP45) are spray-dried on

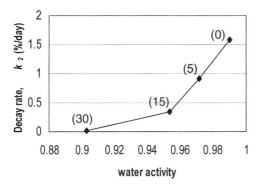

FIGURE 11 Effect of water activity reduction in the aqueous phase of an oil-in-water lotion on the degradation rate of encapsulated protease. Glycerol levels in aqueous phase corresponding to the water activity are shown in parantheses.

a lactose matrix. The consequence of this is a considerable osmotic driving force for water penetration into the capsule resulting from the water solubility of lactose. Figure 11 shows clearly that controlling this osmotic imbalance by reducing the water activity of the external aqueous phase through the addition of glycerol leads to a considerable enhancement in stability. Indeed, the data indicate that k_2 significantly decreases below water activity of ~0.94, which is approximately equal to the water activity of a saturated solution of lactose. Thus, the implication is that when the water activity in the external phase is equal or less than that of saturated lactose, water penetration into the capsule is greatly retarded, enabling the enzyme to remain in a mostly anhydrous form and thereby greatly enhancing storage stability.

A final consideration in the use of encapsulated enzyme is ensuring the enzyme is released upon application to skin. In this context petrolatum forms an ideal matrix for encapsulation because it is sufficiently hydrophobic and viscous to immobilize the anhydrous enzyme, but is sufficiently friable under shear forces associated with rubbing to release the enzyme. In clinical studies, encapsulated enzymes have been shown to be as effective as direct incorporation of the enzyme into the vehicle (Fig. 12). Overall these studies indicate that with further optimization, encapsulation methods offer a viable method to deliver stable, effective levels of proteases in skin care products.

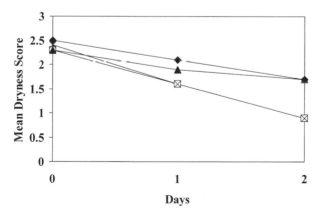

FIGURE 12 Comparison of clinical effectiveness of encapsulated protease systems (cross) versus unencapsulated systems (open square). Also shown is the effectiveness of the base moisturizer alone (diamond) as well as the base moisturizer containing placebo capsules (triangle). The improvement in dryness of both enzyme-containing products is significant at p < 0.01 compared to the nonenzyme-containing controls at Day 1 and Day 2 timepoints.

4 SAFETY ISSUES ASSOCIATED WITH THE USE OF ENZYMES IN SKIN CARE PRODUCTS

4.1 Potential Health Effects Associated with the Use of Enzymes

The primary toxicological hazard presented by the use of enzymes in any application is that they are potentially allergenic. The capacity of proteins, including enzymes, to cause sensitisation of the respiratory tract and thus to have the potential to induce asthma is well known [10–13], and enzymes are recognized occupational allergens [14]. Respiratory sensitization is an immediate IgE antibody–mediated Type I hypersensitivity response regulated by T_H2 lymphocytes and associated cytokines [15,16]. The principal safety concern for the use of enzymes in any application is therefore the potential for the induction of Type I sensitization and most particularly respiratory sensitization.

Another concern with the use of enzymes is the possibility of direct reactions when enzymes are topically applied to the skin. Skin sensitization, referred to clinically as allergic contact dermatitis, is a cell-mediated Type IV delayed hypersensitivity reaction. The delayed contact hypersensitivity reaction is immunologically based and is dependent on T_H1 lymphocytes [15,16]. To behave as a skin sensitizer a substance must first penetrate the stratum corneum, partition into the epidermis, and react with endogenous proteins to form a hapten–carrier conjugate. Such substances will therefore normally be of low molecular weight (normally <400 D), e.g., metals (nickel), plant extracts [the poison ivy/oak family (pentadecyl catechols)], dyes [17–19]. Proteins (and thus enzymes) are not implicated as a cause of delayed contact hypersensitivity and this is supported by the experience in the detergent industry where there have been no reported cases of delayed contact hypersensitivity due to enzymes. However, there are other types of dermatitis in man, including irritant contact dermatitis (ICD) [20]. While proteins are not commonly associated with ICD, this can occur with proteolytic enzymes, presumably as a direct consequence of barrier damage [21], and this may be a factor in the accommodation of skin barrier penetration in the much less common protein contact dermatitis. Protein contact dermatitis is a type of contact urticaria [22]. Although the majority of contact urticaria is nonimmunological, a small proportion is caused by a Type I hypersensitivity reaction mediated by specific IgE antibody [23]. Typically immunological protein contact urticaria is expressed on skin where the barrier function has been compromised through wet work and contact with surfactants. This condition was recognized largely in the occupational context of food preparation—common causes are (shell) fish and vegetables—and has a substantial skin irritation component [24]. However, it is not known whether repeated contact of foreign protein with intact skin will lead to the formation of specific IgE antibody. Although occupational protein contact dermatitis is not uncommon, the frequency of reported cases caused by enzymes is limited relative to exposure [25,26]. While in these cases the reaction is elicited via the skin, it is not possible to exclude the possibility that sensitization was induced via another route. Exposure to foreign proteins (enzymes) can occur via several routes: respiratory, mucosal, and skin (particularly if damaged/compromised, e.g., in eczema) and although the role of dermal contact in the induction of Type I sensitization is unclear, immunological protein contact urticaria can occur in a sensitized individual after skin exposure. The route of exposure which induces the production of specific IgE antibody may not be the same as that by which a clinical response is elicited. In the case of enzymes the most likely route of primary sensitization is via the respiratory tract.

Although enzymes are recognized as potential occupational respiratory allergens [10,14], consumers have used them safely in laundry detergent products for many years. With the exception of a few isolated cases of allergic reactions in the consumer population when enzymes were first introduced into products and were extremely dusty, there have to date been no reported cases of the induction of Type I hypersensitivity. This is most probably due to the extremely low levels of enzyme exposure during consumer use of enzyme-containing laundry detergent products (estimated as <0.067 ng/m^3) [27,28]. However, there have been reported incidences in the consumer population of allergic reactions to enzymes when used in other applications. Allergic reactions to papain have been reported due to its use in contact lens cleaning solution [29,30] and cosmetics [31]. The history of the safe use of enzymes in laundry products has prompted the consideration of the use of these enzymes in other applications, including personal products. Given the recognized potential of enzymes as occupational respiratory allergens and the reported cases of allergy from other consumer uses of enzyme-containing products, a careful risk assessment of any new use scenario is vital. The main concern is possibility inducing Type I hypersensitivity, primarily respiratory sensitization, because the fate of the enzyme following use in topical or personal cleansing applications is uncertain. The potential for inhalation of airborne or deposited enzyme in the home of the consumer, due to loss from the skin surface following desquamation or by aerosolization during washing as well as absorption via mucosal and dermal exposure, is therefore a major concern. The possible risks of the induction of Type I hypersensitivity reactions associated with the use of enzymes in leave-on products have therefore been assessed in several studies.

4.2 Safety Studies on the Use of Enzymes in Personal Care Products

A study to assess the levels of aerosolized enzyme generated during showering using an enzyme-containing personal cleansing product was carried out and this was followed by a 6-month pilot use test with concurrent monitoring for the development of specific IgE antibody [32]. Levels of airborne enzyme were monitored during showering using prototype soap bars containing different concentrations (0.2, 0.4, and 2.8%) of a *Bacillus subtilis*–derived protease. The levels of enzyme measured in the shower cubicle increased proportionately with the concentration of enzyme in the product (mean values 11.4, 15.7, and 183 ng/m^3). Repeated experiments using the 0.2% level confirmed the measurements (mean values 5.7–11.8 ng/m^3). The enzyme levels in the room outside the shower cubicle were also measured and found to be approximately 2.5-fold less than the level in the shower cubicle itself. In the follow-up 6-month use test, volunteers with a reported history of seasonal allergic rhinitis substituted test (with 0.2% enzyme) or control soap bars for their normal products. Prior to the start of the test and at two monthly intervals, skin prick tests (SPT) using the enzyme and appropriate controls were carried out on the volunteers. All SPT analysis was negative up to the 4-month assessment point. However, after 6 months 4 out of the 61 individuals in the test group gave a positive SPT response to the enzyme, and all four positive results were confirmed by the identification of specific IgE antibody using serological analysis. Although none of these individuals reported clinical symptoms, the potential to develop symptoms with extended use cannot be ruled out.

When used in the manufacture of laundry detergent products, occupational airborne exposure levels for the *Bacillus subtilis*–derived protease used in the soap bar study (and other enzymes of similar antigenic potency) have been limited to 15–20 ng/m^3. In this controlled occupational environment, data show that clinical symptoms are prevented and the rate of sensitization is minimized [33,34]. The assumption was therefore that because the frequency, duration, and magnitude of the exposure to enzyme from the soap bar application was much less than that observed in the occupational environment, the use would be safe. However, the induction of specific IgE antibody in several of the study participants emphasizes the need for caution when developing a risk assessment for any proposed new enzyme use application. The possibility that Type I hypersensitivity can be induced through routes other than via inhalation, e.g., dermal or mucosal, is uncertain. As discussed previously, it is known that dermal contact with proteins (e.g., latex proteins) [35] can elicit IgE antibody–mediated allergic reactions thus confirming the ability of proteins to penetrate the skin barrier under certain conditions. Although the primary route of induction is thought to be via the respiratory tract, the mechanisms are not fully understood, and the dermal and mucosal routes may be contributory. Other studies, including the assessment of enzyme-containing laundry bars for hand laundry and personal cleansing over a 6- to 18-month period with no induction of IgE antibody [36,37], indicate that it is unlikely that the dermal route alone was responsible for the sensitizations observed in the soap bar study.

Further studies have investigated the use of enzymes in topically applied leave-on products and have confirmed the potential for the generation of inhalable enzyme. The important consideration here was not skin penetration, but rather the fate of the enzyme lost from the skin surface. In a study to assess the airborne levels of enzyme generated following the use of a topically applied skin cream, groups of five volunteers applied a skin cream with (~0.03%) or without a *Bacillus*-derived proteolytic enzyme twice daily for 12 weeks [38]. At 2- to 4-week intervals during the 12-week use phase and for 6 weeks after use, the panellists' bedroom air was sampled before and after vacuuming and changing the bed linen. No airborne enzyme was detected before vacuuming and changing of linen in any of the groups. No enzyme was detected in the control group following vacuuming and changing the bed linen; however, enzyme was detected on a number of occasions in the low-dose (0.5 g cream/application) group but with no obvious pattern. In the high-dose group (3 g cream/application) there was with continued exposure clear evidence of a trend to increasing airborne enzyme levels (up to 29 ng/m^3) that dropped back to nondetectable levels 6 weeks after the applications were discontinued. Although no specific IgE antibody was detected in any of the small number of individuals participating in this study, this is most probably due to the relatively short duration of the exposure period. Specific IgE antibody is usually induced after 6–12 months of exposure, as illustrated in the soap bar study [32], the papain in contact lens solution case [29], and the extensive experience from occupational exposure to enzymes within the detergent industry. The possibility of the induction of a specific IgE antibody response with prolonged exposure should not be ignored.

The potential for the deposition of enzyme on the skin and aerosolization after showering following the use of an enzyme-containing leave-on product were investigated in another study [39]. This study demonstrated that immuno-reactive enzyme could remain on the skin (100–400 ng/cm^2) for at least 24 hr following application of a leave-on vehicle containing less than 0.02% of a proteolytic enzyme. The study also showed that the "reservoir" of residual enzyme on the skin could become aerosolized during showering. The leave-on vehicle containing <0.02% enzyme was applied by six volunteers to the whole body and after 12 hr the levels of airborne enzyme were measured during showering, and levels of up to 1.13 ng/m^3 were detected.

4.3 Potential for the Future Use of Enzymes in Personal Care Products

While the exposure patterns to enzymes in the occupational environment are very different to those arising from the consumer use of enzyme-containing personal products, the levels of airborne enzyme demonstrated in various studies [32,38,39] are orders of magnitude greater than estimated in the consumer use of laundry detergent products [28]. This gives cause for concern and means that a risk assessment for topically applied or personal wash products containing enzyme must include as a primary consideration the potential for respiratory sensitization arising from the inhalation route of exposure. In all the cases presented here, the risk assessment conclusion would be that the proposed use of the enzyme would be unacceptable in the absence of further detailed evaluation.

The conduct of thorough risk assessments, including detailed evaluation of potential sources and routes of exposure, when developing safety evaluations for enzymes in new applications is paramount. As part of this process, it is important to understand the levels of exposure which might induce an immunological (specific IgE antibody) response under normal use conditions, i.e., it is necessary to understand something of the dose response relationship for the enzyme/application in question. Although evidence indicates clinical skin problems associated with the use of enzymes are limited, any risk assessment should also include an assessment of the possible effects of repeated skin exposure to enzyme on changes in skin structure and function. Enzymes are implicated in irritant dermatitis, and compromised skin is recognized as a critical factor in protein contact urticaria and may also be a factor in the induction of specific IgE antibody and thus potentially respiratory sensitization. Appropriately designed clinical evaluations are therefore required. The duration of the clinical study is critical, with the potential development of an IgE antibody response requiring 6–24 months. Proper statistical analysis must be carried out to ensure the calculation of any risk in the consumer population. Postmarket surveillance should also be considered following any introduction of a new enzyme-containing product, and all complaints should be carefully evaluated, including a medical assessment if required.

5 SUMMARY

Considerable evidence has been presented in this chapter that supports the hypothesis that a reduction in proteolytic activity within the stratum corneum and a subsequent retention of desmosomes in the upper layers of stratum corneum contribute to the visible scaling associated with xerotic skin. Topical application of protease has been shown to rapidly reduce this scaling leading to a significant reduction in the visible signs of dryness. From our research, broad specificity proteases appear to be most efficient at producing this effect. The benefit of protease can be achieved from a conventional moisturizer, and routes to stabilize the enzyme using encapsulation can be envisioned. Concerns regarding the safety of such products have been investigated and indicate that until the technologies exist to address the safety of enzymes, for example, modification to reduce the inherent allergenicity, they are probably not appropriate for use in topical or personal cleansing products. Consequently, further research will be required to commercialize this promising technology.

REFERENCES

1. Rawlings AV, Watkinson A, Rogers J, Mayo A, Scott IR. Abnormalities in stratum corneum structure, lipid composition and desmosome degradation in soap-induced winter xerosis. J Soc Cosmet Chem 1994; 45:203–220.

2. Watkinson A, Smith C, Coan P, Wiedow O. The role of pro-SCCE and SCCE in desquamation. 21st IFSCC Congress, Berlin, 2000.
3. Harding CR, Watkinson A, Rawlings AV, Scott IR. Dry skin, moisturization and corneodesmolysis. Int J Cosmet Sci 2000; 22:21–52.
4. Watkinson A, Rogers JS, Harding CR. Water activity: the critical factor controlling SCCE and desquamation J Invest Dermatol 1999; 112:573.
5. Froebe CL, Simion FA, Ohlemeyer H, Rhein LD, Mattai J, Cagan RH, Friberg SE. Prevention of stratum corneum lipid phase transition by glycerol—an alternative mechanism for skin moisturisation. J Soc Cosmet Chem 1990; 41:51–65.
6. Long S, Banks J, Watkinson A, Harding C, Rawlings AV. Desmocollin 1: a key marker for desmosome processing in the stratum corneum. J Invest Dermatol 1996; 106:397.
7. El-Kadi KN, Rawlings AV, Feinberg C, Watkinson A, Nunn CC, Battaglia A, Chandar P, Richardson N, Pocalyko DJ. Broad specificity alkaline proteases efficiently reduce the visual scaling associated with soap-induced winter xerosis. Arch Dermatol Res (in press).
8. Hawkins J, Chadwick P, Messenger ET. Method for preparing stabilized enzyme dispersion. US patent 5,198,353.
9. Chandar P, Richardson NK, Battaglia A, Cicciari KJ, El-Kadi KN. Oil-in-water cosmetic emulsions containing stabilized protease. US patent 5,811,112.
10. Flindt MLH. Pulmonary disease due to inhalation of derivatives of *Bacillus subtilis* containing enzyme. Lancet 1969; 1:1177–1181.
11. Venables KM, Tee RD, Hawkins ER, Gordon DJ, Wale CJ, Farrer NM Lam TH, Baxter PJ, Taylor AJN. Laboratory animal allergy in a pharmaceutical company. Br J Industr Med 1988; 45:660–666.
12. Douglas JDM, McSharry C, Blaikie L, Morrow T, Miles S, Franklin D. Occupational asthma caused by automated salmon processing. Lancet 1995; 346:737–740.
13. Quirce S, Diéz-Goméz ML, Eiras P, Cuevas M, Baz G, Losada E. Inhalant allergy to egg yolk and egg white proteins. Clin Exper Allergy 1998; 28:478–485.
14. Pepys J, Haregreave FE, Longbottom JL, Faux JA. Allergic reactions of the lungs to enzymes of *Bacillus subtilis*. Lancet 1969; 1:1181–1184.
15. Dearman RJ, Basketter DA, Coleman JW, Kimber I. The cellular and molecular basis for divergent allergic responses to chemicals. Chem-Biol Interactions 1992; 84:1–10.
16. Kimber I. Cytokines and regulation of allergic sensitisation to chemicals. Toxicology 1994; 93:1–11.
17. Cronin E. Contact Dermatitis. New York: Churchill Livingstone, 1980.
18. Fisher AA. Contact Dermatitis. Philidelphia: Lea and Febiger, 1986.
19. Rycroft RJG, Menne T, Frosch PJ, Benezra C. Textbook of Contact Dermatitis. Berlin: Springer-Verlag, 1992.
20. van der Valk PGM, Maibach HI. The Irritant Contact Dermatitis Syndrome. Boca Raton: CRC Press, 1996.
21. Zachariae H, Thomsen K, Rasmussen OG. Occupational contact dermatitis. Acta Dermatovener 1973; 53:145–148.
22. Hjorth N, Roed-Petersen J. Occupational contact dermatitis in food handlers. Contact Dermatitis 1976; 2:28–42.

23. Shafer T, Ring J. Epidemiology of contact urticaria. In: Burr ML, ed. Epidemiology of Contact Allergy. Vol. 31. Basal: Karger Press, 1993:49.

24. Cronin E. Dermatitis of the hands in caterers. Contact Dermatitis 1987; 17:265–269.

25. Kanerva L, Vanhanen M, Tupasela O. Occupational contact urticaria from cellulase enzyme. Contact Dermatitis 1998; 38:176–177.

26. Kanerva L, Vanhanen M. Occupational protein contact dermatitis from glucosamylase. Contact Dermatitis 1999; 41:171–173.

27. Belin L, Hoborn J, Falsen E, Andre J. Enzyme sensitisation in consumers of enzyme-containing washing powder. Lancet 1970; 2:1153–1157.

28. Hendricks MH. Measurement of laundry product dust levels and characteristics in consumer use. J Am Oil Chem Soc 1970; 47:207–211.

29. Berbstein DI, Gallagher JS, Grad M, Bernstein IL. Local ocular anaphylaxis to papain enzyme contained in a contact lens cleansing solution. J Allergy Clin Immunol 1984; 74:258–260.

30. Fisher AA. Allergic reactions to contact lens solutions. Cutis 1985; 36:209–211.

31. Niinimaki A, Reijula K, Pirila T, Koistinen AM. Papain-induced rhinoconjunctivitis in a cosmetologist. J Allergy Clin Immunol 1993; 92:492–493.

32. Kelling CK, Bartolo RG, Ertel KD, Smith LA, Watson DD, Sarlo K. Safety assessment of enzyme-containing personal cleansing products: exposure characterisation and development of IgE antibody to enzymes after a 6-month use test. J Allergy Clin Immunol 1998; 101:179–187.

33. Juniper CP, Roberts DM. Enzyme asthma: fourteen years clinical experience of a recently prescribed disease. J Soc Occup Med 1984; 34:127–132.

34. Gaines WG. Occupational health experience manufacturing multiple enzymes detergents and methods to control enzyme exposures. The Toxicology Forum 1994; 143–147.

35. Hamann CP. Natural rubber latex protein sensitivity in review. Am J Contact Derm 1993; 4:4–21.

36. Sarlo K., Cormier E, MacKenzie D, Scott L. Lack of Type-I sensitisation to laundry enzymes among consumers in the Phillipines: results of an 18-month clinical study. J Allergy Clin Immunol 1996; 97(1):749.

37. Cormier E, Sarlo K, Scott L, Vasunia K, Smith M, Payne N, MacKenzie D. Lack of sensitisation to laundry enzymes among consumers in the Phillipines. J Allergy Clin Immunol 1997; 99(1):321.

38. Blaikie L, Richold M, Whittle E, Lawrence RS, Keech S, Basketter DA. Airborne exposure from topically applied protein (proteolytic enzyme). Hum Exp Toxicol 1999; 18:528.

39. Johnson G, Innis JD, Mills KJ, Bielen F, Date RF, Weisgerber D, Sarlo K. Safety assessment for a leave-on personal care product containing a protease enzyme. Hum Exp Toxicol 1999; 18:527.

19

Enzymes in Cleansers

Takuji Masunaga

Kosé Corporation, Tokyo, Japan

1 INTRODUCTION

The essential function of skin care cosmetics is to maintain beautiful and healthy skin. Skin care cosmetics, including creams, lotions, facial packs, cleansers, and astringents, have specific purposes and effects. The main purpose of a skin cleanser is to clean the skin surface by removing dirt to promote beautiful and healthy skin. Any dirt remaining on the skin surface or plugged in the pilosebaceous orifices is easily oxidized or degraded by oxygen and microorganisms, leading to skin trouble, including inflammation and acne vulgaris.

Dirt on the skin surface consists of sloughed corneocytes, sebum, sweat remnants, products from bacteria on the skin surface, and environmental pollutants. Keratin is a main component of corneocytes, which are continually sloughed from the skin surface. Stratum corneum is formed by terminal differentiation of epidermal keratinocytes, and both epidermal proliferation and keratinization increase in response to daily life ultraviolet exposure [1] and dry environmental conditions [2]. As a result of inappropriate keratinization, the skin tends to become rough or dry and can lead to scarring. Sebum is excreted from pilosebaceous orifices and spreads on the skin surface. The lipid on the skin surface is easily oxidized and converted to lipid peroxidation. Such peroxidized lipid can cause skin irritation, leading to skin damage. Acne vulgaris can result from sebum becoming plugged in the pilosebaceous orifices. Certain kinds of bacterial product are believed to generate singlet oxygen [3]. Reactive oxygen species are generated even under daily life conditions, and can oxidize materials on the skin surface to form skin irritants. Removing the dirt is an essential requirement for healthy skin and personal hygiene.

Enzymes can be used as a cosmetic ingredient in skin cleansers due to their unique characteristics as a biocatalist which effectively catalyzes the specific reaction under mild conditions, although the main component of cleaning product is detergents. Because protease and lipase can degrade high molecular weight materials into smaller fragments, their incorporation into skin cleansers is helpful in removing dirt on the skin surface. Bell reported that application of suitable protease could remove the adherent corneocytes and produce softer skin [4]. Because an enzyme is a kind of protein and exhibits less stability of three-dimensional structure, incorporation of an enzyme generally results in short shelf-life of the products. Therefore, stabilization of enzymes is important for cosmetic applications.

In this chapter, we mainly focus on the application of protease in a skin cleanser, and describe the evaluation of its function and improvement of its stabilization.

2 PROTEASE

Proteins in skin dirt are generally high molecular weight materials. To facilitate their removal by detergents, it is preferable to degrade them into smaller fragments. Protease is often used in skin cleansers to catalyze such a reaction. Protease showing low specificity is preferable for a skin cleanser because there are many kinds of proteins in dirt. Commonly used proteases in skin cleanser are Bioprase® (Nagase Biochemicals, Japan) and papain.

Bioprase is an extracellular protease from *Bacillus subtilis* with molecular weight of 31 kD (Fig. 1). Bioprase is inhibited by di-isopropyl fluorophosphate (DFP) and phenylmethylsulfonyl fluoride (PMSF), but not by EDTA, mono-iodoacetic acid (MIA), and N-ethylmaleimide (NEM), and is not activated by cysteine, which indicates that Bioprase is a serine protease.

Papain is a thiol protease obtained from papaya [5]. This protease is inhibited by NEM and MIA, but not by DFP and PMSF, and is activated by cysteine and EDTA, which confirms that papain is a thiol protease.

In general, oxidation of cysteine residue in the active center in thiol protease results in reduction of its activity. Therefore, oxidizing agents would affect Bioprase less than papain because Bioprase has no cysteine residues in its active center, a benefit of Bioprase as a cosmetic raw material.

3 EVALUATION OF PROTEASE FUNCTION

Proteases in skin cleansers are expected to degrade protein in dirt on the skin surface so that they may be easily removed by detergents, as mentioned. The main

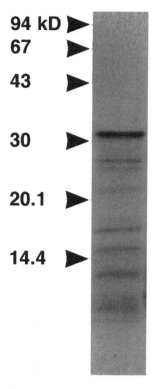

FIGURE 1 Sodium dodecyl sulfate–polyacrylamide gel electrophorograms of Bioprase. Molecular weight markers are indicated on the left. (From Ref. 10.)

protein included in dirt on skin surface is thought to be keratin, which is a main component of sloughed corneocytes. Sweat protein is thought to be another component of protein in dirt. Therefore, the proteolytic activity toward keratin and sweat protein can be employed as a marker of protease function in a skin cleanser.

3.1 Keratin Hydrolytic Activity

Keratin is an intermediate filament expressed in keratinocyte [6]. Normal epidermal keratinocytes express four major keratins. Epidermal keratinocyte in basal layer expresses basal type keratins, keratin 5 and 14. On the other hand, differentiated keratinocyte in suprabasal layer expresses keratin 1 and 10, markers for skin type differentiation.

To investigate the hydrolytic action of protease toward keratin, we used a commercial keratin preparation extracted from human epidermis as a substrate. The keratin preparations used in this evaluation have four main polypeptides with molecular weights of 73, 56, 51, and 45 kD. Keratin hydrolytic activity was evaluated by analyzing the degraded polypeptide fragments by sodium dodecyl sulfate–polyacrylamide gel electrophoresis after mixing keratin substrate solution with protease.

In the case of Bioprase (Fig. 2A), original keratin bands began to degrade into the fragments of 28–35 kD within the first 5 min. After 20 min incubation, no intact keratin bands were observed, and the smaller fragments less than 20 kD were generated. By 60 min, almost all keratins and their fragments had disappeared. When keratins were incubated for 60 min without Bioprase as a negative control, no degradation was observed. These results clearly show that Bioprase hydrolyzed the keratins.

Since papain was found to have lower hydrolytic activity on keratin than Bioprase (Fig. 2B), the latter is a more effective ingredient for skin cleansers.

3.2 Sweat Protein Hydrolytic Activity

The major components of sweat are water and salts. However, some proteins are known to be included in sweat [7] although the amount is considered to be less than in sloughed keratin. Marshall analyzed sweat proteins by two-dimensional electrophoresis followed by methylamine incorporating silver stain [8], and Rubin and Penneys analyzed ^{125}I-labeled sweat proteins by two-dimensional electrophoresis [9]. Sodium dodecyl sulfate–polyacrylamide gel electrophoresis com-

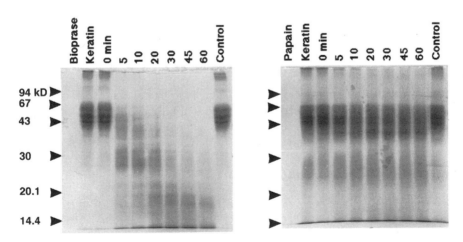

FIGURE 2 Keratin hydrolytic activity of Bioprase (left) and papain (right). Keratin solution was incubated with respective protease for various periods indicated. The fragments were analyzed by sodium dodecyl sulfate–polyacrylamide gel electrophoresis. No protease was incubated with keratin in control. Nearly the same amount of proteases on a molar basis was used in respective experiment. (From Ref. 10.)

bined with ordinary silver staining technique is a convenient and highly sensitive way to analyze sweat proteins as a substrate for proteases in skin cleansers. The sweat proteins can be collected from the facial skin after exercise by using gauze. The details are described elsewhere [10].

As shown in Fig. 3, Bioprase can hydrolyze the sweat proteins of ranges 21–26 and 32–41 kD within 60 min. The results indicate that enzyme in skin cleanser is effective in removing the dirt originating from sweat proteins.

3.3 Experimental Conditions

In the assay of keratin and sweat protein hydrolytic activity described, the employed incubation time of 60 min is very long compared with the time typically spent washing the face. It is not clear how much protein is degraded in actual face washing. However, complete degradation of the protein in dirt is not necessary because detergent, but not protease, is the main component in removing dirt. The amount of protease in the formula should be decided by considering not only functionality, but also safety, cost, and so on.

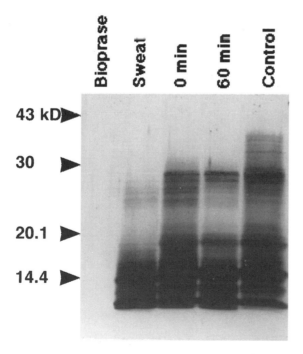

FIGURE 3 Sweat protein hydrolytic activity of Bioprase. Sweat protein was incubated with Bioprase for 60 min. The fragments were analyzed by sodium dodecyl sulfate–polyacrylamide gel electrophoresis. The bands were revealed by silver staining. (From Ref. 10.)

4 STABILIZATION

Bioprase, a protein hydrolytic enzyme, is a useful ingredient in skin cleansers, as shown. However, the shelf-life of Bioprase is known to be short, especially in water-containing products. No reduction of the activity of Bioprase in a powder-type preparation was observed in the first 4 weeks, whereas its activity in an aqueous solution was drastically reduced and completely lost within 1 day (Fig. 4). Even with the addition of glycerin, which is a well-known protein stabilizer [11,12], half of the Bioprase activity was lost in 1 week, and no activity was observed after 4 weeks. This short shelf-life would be a barrier to widespread application. To develop various types of cleansing preparations containing protein hydrolytic enzymes, improvement of the shelf-life is required.

Several approaches are possible to improve the stability of enzymes. The simplest approach is to use heat-stable enzymes [13]. Some thermophilic microorganisms are known to produce heat-stable proteases, such as thermolysin [14], aqualysin I and II [15,16], caldolysin [17], and thermitase [18]. Thermophilic enzymes generally show high stability not only against heat, but also against protein denatures induced by urea, detergents, and organic solvents. These characteristics are also advantageous in cosmetic ingredients. Of course, safety and functional efficacy must be established before incorporation into a skin cleanser.

The second approach is a gene engineering method. Site-directed mutagenesis is one such technique, enabling the substitution, deletion, and insertion of specific amino acids in protein by changing the nucleotide sequence of the encod-

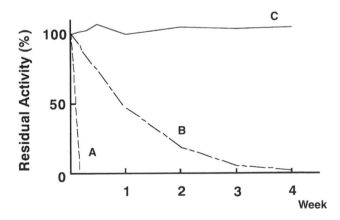

Figure 4 Stabilities of native Bioprase in an aqueous solution without (A) or with (B) glycerin and as dried powder (C). The samples were stored at 40°C. (From Ref. 10.)

ing gene. This technique enables us to freely design an enzyme protein molecule to obtain heat-stable protein molecules. Because safety and cost concerns remain to be solved, this technique can be applied only to laboratory level experiments, not to manufacturing level production.

The third approach is chemical modification, whereby a modifier is bound to protein molecules by covalent bonds. Polyethylene glycol and its derivatives, polysaccharide and its derivatives, maleic acid–styrene copolymer, and so on, are used as modifiers. This approach is one of the best ways to improve the stability of protease used as cosmetic ingredients, because many of the modifiers are used as cosmetic ingredients or its derivatives or analogs. Furthermore, chemically modified protein with a high molecular weight modifier generally shows low antigenicity, which is desirable from the standpoint of ingredients safety.

5 CHEMICAL MODIFICATION OF BIOPRASE

Here, I would like to single out the chemical modification of Bioprase with copolymers of α-allyl-ω-methoxy polyoxyethylene and maleic anhydride to show how Bioprase can improve heat stability.

5.1 Chemical Modifier

Modifiers were synthesized according to the method of Yoshimoto et al. [19]. The synthesis procedure is briefly summarized in Fig. 5. The modifier shows various lengths of a polyoxyethylene (POE) group (n) and the various degree of polymerization of a monomer unit (k). This modifier was designated as PEG-MA(n, k).

5.2 Determination of Procedure for Chemical Modification

The chemical modification of Bioprase with PEG-MA copolymer is carried out to form covalent bonds between amino groups located on the surface of the Bioprase molecule and anhydride group of the copolymer (Fig. 5). The reaction is performed by mixing both materials, followed by drying the mixture.

Selection of the modification procedure was carried out using PEG-MA(33, 8) as a modifier. First, the method for adding the modifier was investigated. When the modifier was dissolved in acetone, the recovery of activity of the modified Bioprase was 16%, whereas a 78% recovery was obtained by adding it as a fine powder to a Bioprase aqueous solution (Fig. 6). Consequently, the modifier should be added in the form of a fine powder. The difference in recovery of activity is probably due to denaturation of Bioprase by acetone.

Second, the solvent for Bioprase was selected by analysis of the modified Bioprase preparations by gel permeation chromatography. As shown in Fig. 7A, only a small amount of Bioprase was modified when distilled water was used as a

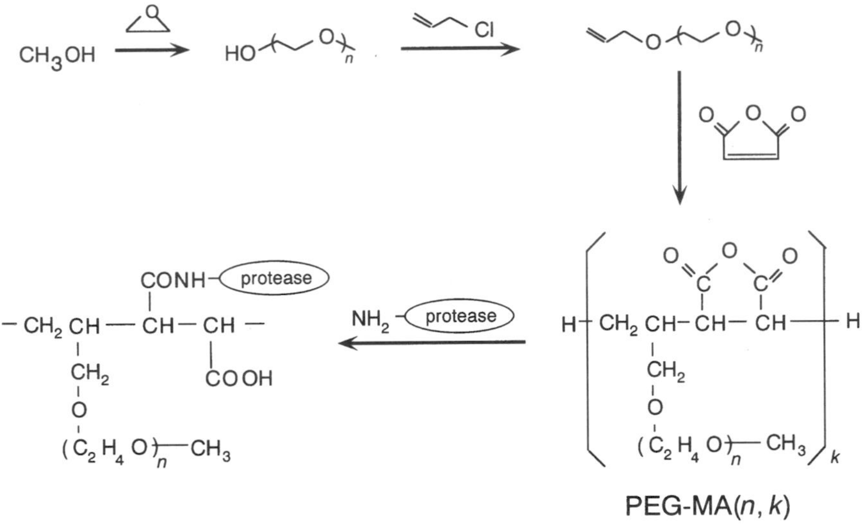

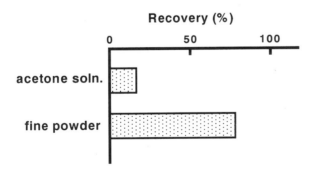

FIGURE 5 Synthesis of copolymer of α-allyl-ω-methoxy polyoxyethylene and maleic anhydride [PEG-MA(n, k)], and chemical modification of Bioprase. (From Ref. 10.)

Recovery (%)

acetone soln.

fine powder

FIGURE 6 Yield of activity of modified Bioprases prepared by two procedures for addition of modifier.

solvent for Bioprase. On the other hand, the yield of the modified Bioprase was increased when Bioprase was dissolved in 0.25M borate buffer, pH 8.8 (Fig. 7B). Because a high pH increases the number of free amino groups in the Bioprase molecule, Bioprase effectively reacted with anhydride groups of the modifier. Consequently, a borate buffer was used as a solvent for Bioprase in the following experiments.

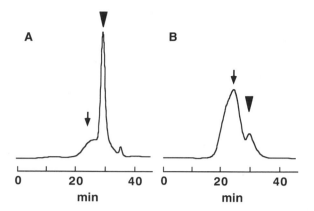

Figure 7 Gel permeation chromatograms of modified Bioprases. (A) Bioprase dissolved in water: (B) Bioprase dissolved in 0.25M borate buffer, pH 8.8. Arrowhead and arrow indicate elution point of modified Bioprase and native Bioprase, respectively. (From Ref. 10.)

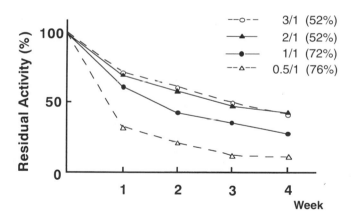

Figure 8 Determination of modifier/Bioprase ratio. The values in parentheses were the recovery of activity. All samples were stored at 40°C. (From Ref. 10.)

Finally, the modifier/Bioprase ratio was determined. The ratio based on weight in the reaction mixture was changed from 0.5 to 3, and the stabilities of respective modified Bioprases were evaluated (Fig. 8). The modified Bioprase conjugated with the smaller amount of the modifier showed lower stability and higher recovery. In contrast, when the ratio was 2 or 3, the modified Bioprases showed higher stability, but their recoveries of activity were lower. These results can be explained as follows. When the amount of the modifier was increased, the degree of modification also increased, which means that the surface of Bioprase molecule was covered more completely with the modifier. Because the structure of the protease was protected in this modified Bioprase, the stability also improved. However, enzyme activity was decreased because the approach of Bioprase to substrate was inhibited by the presence of the surface modifier. The modifier/Bioprase ratio was set at 2 because our main purpose was to improve the stability of Bioprase, not to obtain high recovery of activity.

From the results described, the modification procedure was determined as follows: All modification procedures were carried out at 4°C. The fine powdered modifier was added incrementally (2.5 g, 4 times) to 5 grams of Bioprase in 100 mL of 0.25M borate buffer, pH 8.8. The mixture was stirred for 30 min after each addition of the modifier, and 50 mL of the buffer was added each time to maintain the pH. Then the mixture was dried to obtain the modified Bioprase.

5.3 Characterization of Chemically Modified Bioprase

Chemically modified Bioprase with other modifiers having various numbers of n and k in their structures were synthesized, and their stability and activity recovery rate were evaluated (Fig. 9). The results show that modified Bioprase with low re-

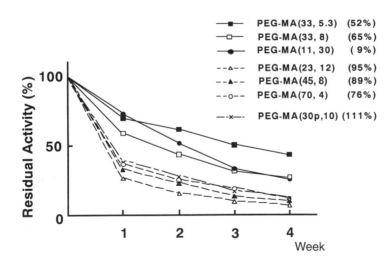

FIGURE 9 Stability of modified Bioprases with various modifiers. The values in parentheses were the recovery of activity. The stability was evaluated at 40°C. (From Ref. 10.)

covery rate tended to exhibit high stability, and the one showing high recovery rate tended to be less stable.

To clarify the reason for this, the modified Bioprase preparations were analyzed by gel filtration chromatography (Fig. 10). There was no native Bioprase in the modified Bioprase preparation with PEG-MA(33, 8) and (33, 5.3), which showed low recovery rate and high stability. In contrast, some unreacted Bioprase remained in samples modified with PEG-MA(23, 12), (45, 8), and (70, 4), which

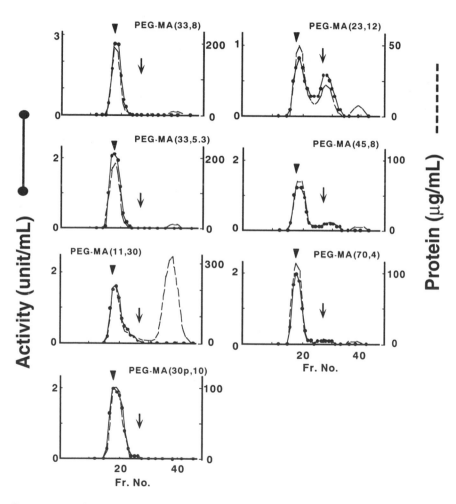

FIGURE 10 Sephadex G-75 gel filtration chromatograms of modified Bioprases. Arrowhead and arrow indicate void volume and elution volume of native Bioprase, respectively. (From Ref. 10.)

showed high recovery rate and low stability. Higher recovery rate and lower stability of the latter three preparations are attributed to the unreacted Bioprase. In the chromatogram of the modified Bioprase preparation with PEG-MA(11, 30), a large amount of low molecular weight peptide fragments was detected, probably due to degradation of Bioprase into fragments, and this caused the low recovery rate seen in Fig. 9.

A PEG-MA(30p, 10) is the modifier with 15 moles of propylene oxide group and 15 moles of ethylene oxide group in its polyoxyalkylene moiety. The modified Bioprase with this modifier displayed lower stability than that of the one modified with PEG-MA(33, 8), indicating that ethylene oxide group is more effective on stabilization than propylene oxide group.

Thus, we found that the characteristics of Bioprase modified with various modifiers are different, and appropriate modifier should be chosen to fit the purpose. From the viewpoint of stability, two Bioprases modified with PEG-MA (33, 5.3) and (33, 8) are most useful, and the latter was used in the following experiments.

5.4 Effect of Ingredients on Stability of Modified Bioprase

To prepare the formula in which the protease can be further stabilized, the effects of other ingredients on the stability of modified Bioprase were investigated as follows.

It is well known that polyol increases the stability of protein [11,12]. Therefore, to further stabilize the modified Bioprase, the stabilizing effects of four polyols which are commonly used in cosmetics were investigated by evaluating the stabilities of the modified Bioprase dissolved in 50% polyol solutions (Fig. 11). The results were that more than 80% of activity remained in glycerin, 1,3-butylene glycol, and propylene glycol. These three polyols increased the stability of modified Bioprase more effectively, but dipropylene glycol had a little stabilizing effect. Accordingly, glycerin, 1,3-butylene glycol, or propylene glycol should be added to further stabilize the modified Bioprase.

Surfactant is an essential component in skin care cosmetics, especially in a skin cleanser, although it is well known to be a denaturing reagent against protein [20]. Thus, it is also important to investigate the effect of surfactants on the stability of the modified protease. As shown in Fig. 12, nonionic surfactants did not affect the stability of the modified Bioprase, while anionic surfactants reduced the stability. Accordingly, nonionic surfactants are preferable to anionic surfactants for this purpose.

Finally, based on the results of the experiments carried out with the simple buffer system, two cleansers, a cleansing cream and a cleansing lotion, were prepared, and the stabilities of modified Bioprase in those products were tested. The

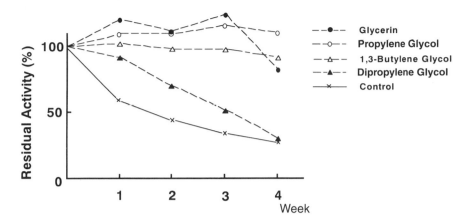

FIGURE 11 Increase of the stability of modified Bioprase by addition of polyols. Stability of modified Bioprase with PEG-MA(33, 8) was evaluated at 40°C. Control experiment was carried out in the absence of any polyols (From Ref. 10.)

residual activities of modified Bioprase in these products were over 50% in 1 week, while almost all activities of the native Bioprase in both preparations were lost within 1 week. This result is consistent with the results obtained with a simple buffer system, and shows that the modified Bioprase is more stable than the native Bioprase in a product preparation as well as in a simple buffer system.

5.5 Activity of Modified Bioprase

To confirm whether the modified Bioprase with improved stability also maintained the protein hydrolytic function, the keratin and sweat protein hydrolytic activities were measured (Fig. 13). Modified Bioprase could degrade the keratins, although it displayed a slightly lower keratin hydrolytic activity than the native one, due to steric hindrance by the modifier located on the surface of Bioprase molecule. However, the activity displayed is sufficient for a skin cleanser because almost all of the main keratin bands disappeared. In contrast to the slightly reduced keratin hydrolytic activity, almost no reduction in the hydrolytic activity toward sweat proteins was observed, as shown in Fig. 13B. It was presumed that the surface modifier did not hinder the approach of the modified Bioprase to sweat proteins, which were lower molecular weight proteins than keratins. These experiments confirm that the modified Bioprase possesses sufficient hydrolytic activity toward protein in dirt on the skin surface, confirming the usefulness of modified Bioprase as an ingredient in skin cleansers.

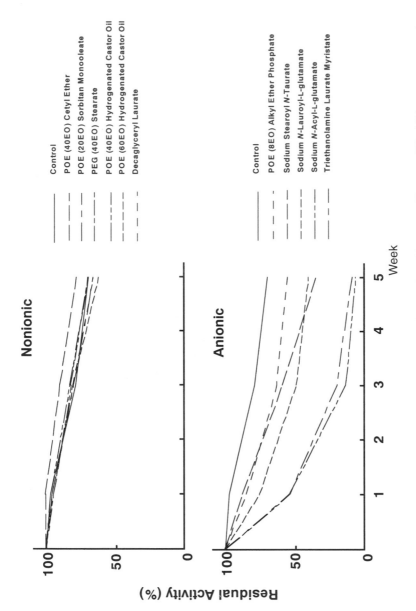

FIGURE 12 Influence of surfactants on stability of modified Bioprase. The modified Bioprase was subjected to evaluate the stability at 40°C. Control experiment was carried out in the absence of any surfactants. (From Ref. 10.)

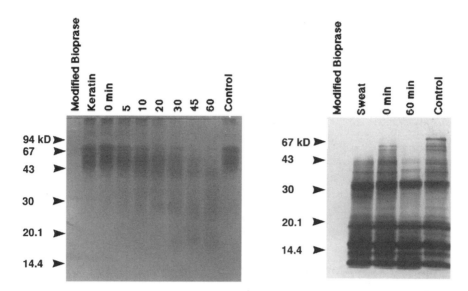

FIGURE 13 Hydrolytic activity of modified Bioprase toward keratins (left) and sweat proteins (right). Modified Bioprase with PEG-MA(33, 8) was used. (From Ref. 10.)

5.6 Safety Test

In general, chemical modification of protein molecules enables reduction of the antigenicity of native ones. Indeed, in the field of pharmaceuticals, chemical modification of protein has been investigated for the purpose of avoiding immunological adverse reactions [21]. This characteristic is also desirable for cosmetic ingredients from the standpoint of safety, a benefit of chemical modification of protease.

Regarding the modified Bioprase, primary and cumulative skin irritation tests were carried out (Table 1). The modified Bioprase shows no primary and slight cumulative irritations, although the native one had mild primary and cumulative irritations. Namely, the irritation of Bioprase was reduced by chemical modification with the modifier, which has no irritation. The modified Bioprase is quite useful from the safety viewpoint.

5.7 Use Test

Finally, we investigated the cosmetic effect of continual use of a skin cleanser containing the modified Bioprase. The results showed that coarse skin became fine in skin texture after using the skin cleanser containing the modified Bioprase. The modified Bioprase removed protein in dirt, especially adherent corneocytes

TABLE 1 Irritation Tests of Native and Modified Bioprases and the Modifier

	Modifier[a]	Modified Bioprase	Bioprase
Primary (n = 3)	No	No	Mild
Cumulative (n = 5)	No	Slight	Mild

Note: Primary irritation was measured by a closed patch test, and cumulative irritation was evaluated after continual application for 14 days.
[a]PEG-MA(33, 8).
Source: Ref. 10.

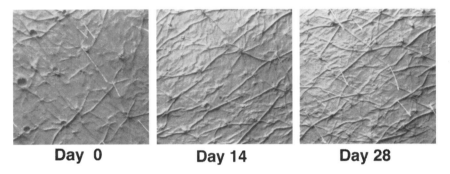

Day 0   **Day 14**   **Day 28**

FIGURE 14 Cheek skin replicas before (day 0) and after (days 14 and 28) continual use of skin cleanser. It contained 0.04% of the modified Bioprase and 24% of polyol. Volunteers washed their face every day with the skin cleanser containing the modified Bioprase. (From Ref. 10.)

on the top of stratum corneum, and then the rate of epidermal turnover could be normalized as suggested by Bidmead and Rodger [22]. Normalization of epidermal turnover rate allowed recovery of fine skin texture. Again, it is important to confirm the cosmetic usefulness of product preparation by actual use.

5.8 Summary

In this section, chemical modification of Bioprase was singled out as an example. The stability of Bioprase was improved by chemical modification with PEG-MA modifier, and the effect of other ingredients on stability was investigated as well. Simultaneously, hydrolytic activity, improvement of safety, and cosmetic usefulness by actual use were also investigated. Our investigations enable us to develop new skin cleanser containing enzymes.

Ohta et al. reported on the chemical modification of esperase, a kind of protease [23]. Esperase was chemically modified with dextran to improve stability and to reduce skin sensitization potential. They successfully obtained the dextran–esperase conjugate, investigated the influence of cosmetic ingredients for further stabilization in cosmetic formulations, and finally prepared the commercial product. Their strategy and the results obtained were similar to those described in this paper.

6 OTHER ENZYMES

In this chapter, we have focused on the protease as an enzyme in skin cleanser. However, besides protease, some other enzymes are proposed as an effective ingredient of skin cleanser.

Lipase is one such useful enzyme. This enzyme hydrolyzes triglyceride to diglyceride, monoglyceride, and finally to free fatty acids. On the skin surface, especially on the face, sebum is one of the main components of the dirt, and lipid is oxidized, generating lipid peroxidation which can lead to skin trouble. The major component of sebum is triglyceride, which is not easily washed out by detergent compared with diglyceride, monoglyceride, or free fatty acid. The incorporation of lipase into skin cleanser can improve its efficacy in washing out fatty dirt on the skin surface.

Lysozyme, usually extracted from egg white, is a bacteriolyzing enzyme through the cleavage of polysaccharide of plasma membrane of bacteria. Its activity can be measured by the tubidimetric assay of *Micrococcus lysodeikticus*. In a skin cleanser, this enzyme could impart antibacterial and anti-inflammatory effects.

Superoxide dismutase (SOD) is an enzyme quenching the reactive oxygen species; SOD catalyzes the dismutation of superoxide anion (O_2^-) into oxygen and hydrogen peroxide to protect cells against toxic reactive oxygen species. Because superoxide anion can react with various materials, including protein and lipid, and such an oxidized material may act as a skin irritant, it is important to prevent the oxidation of the dirt on skin surface and to maintain personal skin hygiene.

7 FUTURE

Enzymes are protein, which means that they have low stability but unique action. Therefore, stabilization of enzymes is key to their incorporation into skin cleansers or other cosmetic products. In the near future, it will be possible to include the various enzymes into a skin cleanser due to the progress in enzyme stabilization itself, pharmaceutical technology, formulation of cleansers, and manufacturing methods. The development of new cosmetic products, including skin cleansers containing enzymes, will depend on the progress of all these aspects of cosmetic science.

REFERENCES

1. Asano H, Masunaga T, Takemoto Y, Kawada A, Kominami E. Influence of consecutive irradiation of low dose UVB on the mice epidermis. Proceedings of the 20th Annual Meeting of the Japanese Society of Photomedicine and Photobiology, Kumamoto, Japan, 1999, pp. 89–90.
2. Denda M, Sato J, Tsuchiya T, Elias PM, Feingold KR. Low humidity stimulates epidermal DNA synthesis and amplifies the hyperproliferative response to barrier disruption: implication for seasonal exacerbations of inflammatory dermatoses. J Invest Dermatol 1998; 111:873–878.
3. Arakane K, Ryu A, Hayashi C, Masunaga T, Shinmoto K, Mashiko S, Nagano T, Hirobe M. Singlet oxygen ($^1\Delta g$) generation from coproporphyrin in *Propionibacterium acnes* on irradiation. Biochem Biophys Res Commun 1996; 223:578–582.
4. Bell KW. Enzymes in cosmetics. Am Cosmet Perf 1972; 87:39–44.
5. Arnon R. Papain. In: Perlmann GE, Lorand L, eds. Methods in Enzymology. New York: Academic Press, 1970:226–244.
6. Sun T-T, Tseng SCG, Huang AJ-W, Cooper D, Schermer A, Lynch MH, Weiss R, Eichner R. Monoclonal antibody studies of mammalian epithelial keratins: a review. Ann NY Acad Sci 1985; 455:307–329.
7. Jenkinson DM, Mabon RM, Manson W. Sweat proteins. Br J Dermatol 1974; 90:175–181.
8. Marshall T. Analysis of human sweat proteins by two-dimensional electrophoresis and ultrasensitive silver staining. Anal Biochem 1984; 139:506–509.
9. Rubin RW, Penneys NS. Subpicogram analysis of sweat proteins using two-dimensional polyacrylamide gel electrophoresis. Anal Biochem 1983; 131:520–524.
10. Masunaga T, Yasukohchi T, Hirobe M, Arakane K, Adachi K. The protease as a cleansing agent and its stabilization by chemical modification. J Soc Cosmet Chem Jpn 1993; 27:276–288.
11. Gekko K, Ito H. Competing solvent effects of polyols and guanidine hydrochloride on protein stability. J Biochem 1990; 107:572–577.
12. Arakawa T, Kita Y, Carpenter JF. Protein–solvent interactions in pharmaceutical formulations. Pharm Res 1991; 8:285–291.
13. Cowan D, Daniel R, Morgan H. Thermophilic proteases: properties and potential applications. Trends Biotech 1985; 3:68–72.
14. Matsubara H. Purification and assay of thermolysin. In: Perlmann GE, Lorand L, eds. Methods in Enzymology. New York: Academic Press, 1970:642–651.
15. Matsuzawa H, Hamaoki M, Ohta T. Production of thermophilic extracellular proteases (aqualysins I and II) by *Thermus aquticus* YT-1, an extreme thermophile. Agric Biol Chem 1983; 47:25–28.
16. Matsuzawa H, Tokugawa K, Hamaoki M, Mizoguchi M, Taguchi H, Terada I, Kwon S-T, Ohta T. Purification and characterization of aqualysin I (a thermophilic alkaline

serine protease) produced by *Thermus aquaticus* YT-1. Eur J Biochem 1988; 171:441–447.

17. Cowan DA, Daniel RM. Purification and some properties of an extracellular protease (caldolysin) from an extreme thermophile. Biochim Biophys Acta 1982; 705:293–305.

18. Frömmel C, Höhne WE. Influence of calcium binding on the thermal stability of 'thermitase', a serine protease from *Thermoactinomyces vulgaris*. Biochim Biophys Acta 1981; 670:25–31.

19. Yoshimoto T, Ritani A, Ohwada K, Takahashi K, Kodera Y, Matsushima A, Saito Y, Inada Y. Polyethylene glycol derivative-modified cholesterol oxidase soluble and active in benzene. Biochem Biophys Res Commun 1987; 148:876–882.

20. Schomaecker R, Robinson BH, Fletcher PDI. Interaction of enzymes with surfactants in aqueous solution and in water-in-oil microemulsions. J Chem Soc Faraday Trans I 1988; 84:4203–4212.

21. Yoshimoto T, Nishimura H, Saito Y, Sakurai K, Kamisaki Y, Wada H, Sako M, Tsujino G, Inada Y. Characterization of polyethylene glycol–modified L-asparaginase from *Escherichia coli* and its application to therapy of leukemia. Jpn J Cancer Res (Gann) 1986; 77:1264–1270.

22. Bidmead MC, Rodger MN. The effect of enzymes on stratum corneum. J Soc Cosmet Chem 1973; 24:493–500.

23. Ohta M, Goto A, Mori K, Fukunaga S, Nakayama H, Fujino Y. A dextran–protease conjugate for cosmetic use. A stabilized dextran–protease conjugate leads to cleaner, smoother, more attractive skin. Cosmet Toil 1996; 111(6):79–88.

20

Moisturizing Cleansers

**Kavssery P. Ananthapadmanabhan,
Kumar Subramanyan, and
Gail B. Rattinger**
Unilever Research, Edgewater Laboratory, Edgewater, New Jersey

1 INTRODUCTION

Historically, the primary purpose of cleansing has been to achieve cleanliness and freshness by removing oily soils from face and body. Hygienic benefits of cleansing have also been recognized for a very long time. While soap-like materials for cleansing have been around as early as 2500 BC [1], soap itself is believed to have been invented sometime around 600–300 BC [2]. The first industrial type manufacturing of soap in an individually wrapped and branded bar form was in 1884 in England [2]. The desire for cleanliness and freshness coupled with the sensory pleasures and health benefits has driven the growth of soap in the 20th century [3]. Thus, deodorant soaps grew from a desire for health and hygiene benefits. The beauty segment, on the other hand, grew from a desire for beautiful skin coupled with the sensory pleasures of cleansing using cleansing bars of different colors, fragrances, and shapes [3].

With increasing use of soaps, awareness of soap-induced skin irritation, itching, dry skin, and other potential effects also increased. This led to an increased desire on the part of the consumer to have mild cleansing bars. Introduction of synthetic detergents into the cleansing arena in 1948 made it possible to develop cleansing bars that were demonstrably milder than soaps [3]. These bars provided superior skin care benefits as well as unique sensory cues. This was the first step toward providing skin care benefit from cleansing systems.

The mild cleanser segment has grown over the years with increasing interest in achieving skin functional benefits, especially moisturization, from wash-off systems. Availability of novel chemicals such as milder surfactants and polymers coupled with an understanding of cleanser-induced changes in skin have led to novel approaches in delivering skin care benefits from cleansers. Introduction of new product forms such as liquid cleansers and nonwoven fabrics have made it easier to deliver skin care benefits from wash-off systems.

The focus of this chapter is on moisturization from cleansers. Specifically, the focus will be on how cleansers affect skin moisturization, how critical it is to prevent/minimize cleanser-induced damage as a first step toward achieving moisturization from cleansers, and finally how to deliver moisturization benefit from cleansers.

A schematic of the evolution of the skin-cleansing technology from the basic soap to syndet bars with moisturizing creams and shower gels that provide positive skin care benefits is given in Fig. 1.

2 SKIN MOISTURIZATION

In a simplistic sense, skin moisturization implies maintaining a certain level of hydration in skin that will allow it to retain its normal viscoelastic properties [4]. This will ensure adequate extensibility and flexibility for the movement of skin.

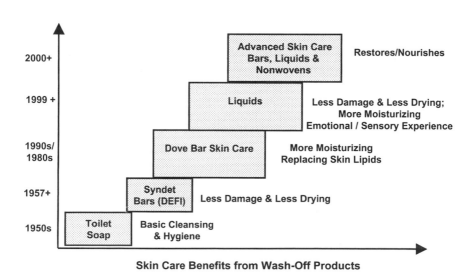

FIGURE 1 Schematic of the evolution of personal cleansing technology.

Absence of moisturization, on the other hand, is a state of skin that can manifest in a variety of forms including a sensation of after-wash tightness (AWT), lack of flexibility/extensibility, visible dryness (skin whitening), skin roughness, scaling, cracking, and ultimately irritation in the form of visible erythema, and itching. Thus there are emotional, tactile, and visual manifestations of absence of skin moisturization.

Stratum corneum upper layers contain about 15% water, 65–75% proteins, and 10–15% lipids [5]. Most of the water in the corneum is present as water bound to the proteins. Water level changes markedly with depth in the corneum, increasing to levels as much as 40% at the innermost level [6]. Water content of the corneum can vary markedly with changes in the relative humidity [6], water binding capacity of corneum proteins, concentration of natural moisturizing factors (NMFs), and the integrity of the barrier lipids [7]. The NMFs in the corneum include short chain amino acids (40%), pyrrolidone carboxylic acid (12%), lactate (12%), urea, (7%), and Na/Ca/K/Mg phosphate/chloride (18.5%) [8]. Stratum corneum lipids, in addition to being a water barrier, also play an important role in maintaining its elasticity. Moisturization technology in the leave-on skin care area usually involves a combination of actives such as humectants that increase water-holding capacity of the corneum, emollients that form a light lubricant coating, and occlusives that provide an external water barrier film on skin. Thus, a moisuturizer provides several positive benefits to improve the skin hydration and alter the unpleasant tactile and visual manifestations of skin dryness.

Cleansers are designed to remove oily soils, dirt, sweat, and sebum from skin. This is achieved through the use of surfactants that aid in the uplifting of dirt and solubilization of oily soils including sebum. In addition to removal of unwanted materials from skin, the cleansing process also helps the normal exfoliation process by removing the dead skin cells, leading to rejuvenation of the skin. These beneficial effects can, however, be accompanied with other interactions with the corneum that can be deleterious to skin. For example, cleanser surfactants can bind to stratum corneum proteins leading to a reduction in their ability to bind and hold water [9,10]. Surfactants can also cause dissolution of fluid skin lipids during cleansing [11] or alterations to the lipid layers by adsorption and intercalation into lipid layers [12–14]. In addition, washing with cleansers can also lead to a reduction in the level of NMFs in skin [15,16]. All these factors that reduce the water content of skin can lead to changes in the viscoelastic properties of skin and this in turn can manifest as after-wash tightening of skin [17]. Continued use of such cleansers can lead to dry skin, barrier damage, and erythema. Thus, in a simplistic sense, while cleansers have the potential to negatively impact the hydration and viscoelastic properties of skin, a moisturizer is expected to improve such conditions. In the case of cleansers, minimizing the damaging/deleterious effects leading to dry skin and erythema is the first step toward moisturization.

Most cleansers currently available in the marketplace make claims of moisturization based on minimizing damage. Limited ones have begun to combine the minimizing damage concept with positive skin benefits by depositing moisturizing agents on skin. This is clearly in the direction of positive skin moisturization. Several excellent reviews have appeared recently on mechanistic aspects of cleanser-induced damage to stratum corneum [4,18–22] and therefore this chapter will have a limited discussion on the damage itself and focus more on current approaches to minimizing the deleterious effects of cleansers and providing moisturization benefits.

3 EFFECTS OF CLEANSERS ON STRATUM CORNEUM

3.1 Stratum Corneum Structure

Stratum corneum, the upper most layer of the skin, is a nonliving layer consisting of proteins, lipids, and water. The proteins and lipids in the corneum are organized in a brick and mortar–like structure with protein (corneocyte) bricks embedded in a lipid mortar phase [23]. Available data seem to support the notion of two types of lipids, specifically, relatively fluid lipids as well as covalently bonded relatively rigid lipids in the matrix [24,25]. Available ESR and DSC data seem to support the presence of complex lipid domains in the stratum corneum [26]. Corneocytes with a keratin envelope and NMFs (e.g., pyrrolidone carboxylic acid, urea, lactic acid, short chain amino acids) within them have the potential to bind water molecules to keep the skin moisturized [27]. Corneocytes in different layers are also linked to each other through membrane protein links referred to as desmosomes [28]. As a part of the normal desquamation process, desmosomes are degraded by protease enzymes present in the upper layers of skin [29]. In healthy skin, the corneum is renewed about every two weeks and this process of desquamation requires a certain level of hydration of the skin.

3.2 Surfactant Interactions with Stratum Corneum Proteins

Interactions of cleanser surfactants with stratum corneum proteins and model proteins have been studied extensively in the past [30–38]. Typically, anionic surfactants, because of their excellent foam and lather characteristics, find use as primary surfactants in cleansers. Liquid cleansers often have a combination of anionic and amphoteric surfactants. Nonionic surfactants also find limited application, mostly in combination with anionic or amphoteric surfactants. In general, the tendency of surfactants to interact with proteins follow the following order: anionic surfactants > amphoteric surfactants > nonionic surfactants. Typical anionic surfactants used in cleansers include soaps (salts of fatty acids), synthetic surfactants such as alkyl ether sulfates, alkyl acyl isethionates, alkyl phosphates, and alkyl sulfonates. The binding tendency of anionic surfactants to proteins follow the order sodium lauryl sulfate (SLS) = sodium laurate $\gg$ monoalkyl phosphate (MAP) > sodium cocoyl isethionate [19,37]. Recently, Imokawa has shown that in studies using Yucatan microswine in vivo, the binding of surfactants upon exposure at 100 mM level for 30 min at 30°C follow the order soap > SLS $\gg$ MAP > sodium cocoyl isethionate (SCI) > triethanolamine N-lauroyl β-aminopropionate (LBA) [19]. In general, for a given chain length surfactant, the larger the headgroup size, the lower is its binding to proteins. Thus, ethoxylated alkyl sulfates tend to have lower binding to keratin compared to the corresponding alkyl sulfates [31]. For a given surfactant headgroup, there is an optimum chain length for maximum binding, and this governed by a balance between surfactant solubility in the aqueous phase and its surface activity [30,38]. This optimum for most surfactants at room temperature is around C_{12}. Even though the higher chain length surfactants have higher surface activity, because of their limited solubility their binding is limited. At higher temperature, increased solubility of higher chain length surfactants can increase their binding.

Surfactants that tend to bind strongly to corneum proteins, in general, have a higher potential to cause significant protein denaturation leading to barrier damage, erythema, and itching. Some of the common approaches to lowering the tendency of anionic surfactants to bind to proteins are (1) increase in the size of head/polar group of the surfactant [31,39] and (2) use anionic surfactants with amphoteric or nonionic surfactants [40]. A typical example of modulating the activity of sodium lauryl ether sulfate (SLES) by adding an amphoteric surfactant, cocoamido propylbetaine (CAPB) is shown in Fig. 2 in terms of the solubility of a corn protein, zein. The ability of a surfactant to dissolve zein has been used as a measure of its irritation potential [41]. Thus, in this example, there exists a certain ratio of SLES to CAPB where the dissolution of zein is minimum and this coincides with the minimum in the critical micelle concentration (CMC) of these mixed surfactants. The commonly accepted hypothesis for the reduced binding of the anionic surfactant in the presence of amphoteric or nonionic co-surfactant is the competition between binding and co-micellization for monomers that tend to favor co-micellization in the presence of lower CMC surfactants. Thus, at a given level of anionic surfactant, addition of lower CMC surfactant whether it is nonionic, amphoteric, or even anionic can result in reduced irritation [18]. These effects can often be synergistic since co-micellization is often synergistic, resulting in CMC values that are lower than the CMC of either surfactant.

Surfactant binding to protein can significantly affect the water-binding and -holding capacity of proteins. Several studies show that surfactant solutions cause swelling of the corneum [42] and this effect saturates at about the CMC of the surfactant, suggesting that the swelling is controlled by surfactant monomers [42]. The swelling itself is due to increased water uptake resulting from an increase in the net negative charge of the protein because of surfactant binding.

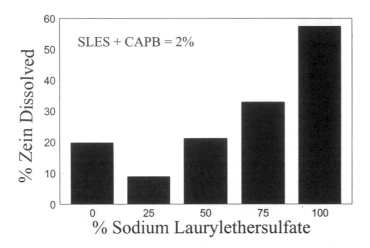

FIGURE 2 Solubility of zein, a corn protein, showing a minimum as a function of composition of anionic-amphoteric (sodium lauryl ether sulfate-cocoamidopropyl betaine) surfactant mixtures. Past work [41] has shown that the tendency to dissolve zein is a reflection of the irritation potential of surfactants.

This increased water uptake may appear to be rather contrary to the intuitive notion that harsh surfactants tend to reduce the water-binding capacity of the corneum. Note that this hyperhydration effect is rather transient occurring immediately after exposure to surfactant solution. As the water evaporates with time after wash, re-equilibration of the skin to hydration levels that are actually below the surfactant pre-exposure levels takes place [10,43]. The latter is thought to be due to the reduced water-binding capacity of the proteins because of surfactant adsorption to protein hydration sites as well as loss of water-holding NMFs during wash. The effect of this on after-wash tightness is examined in a later section.

3.3 Surfactant Interactions with Stratum Corneum Lipids

Similar to the case of proteins, surfactant interactions with skin lipids has also been a subject of extensive study [5,11,18,19,44–48]. While the binding of cleanser surfactants to proteins is well recognized as a potential problem that can lead to skin irritation and barrier damage, the role of surfactant interactions with lipids and their effects on skin condition has been a rather controversial one [19,44–49]. It has been suggested that surfactants above their CMC cause some delipidation of the corneum by solubilization of the lipids in surfactant micelles [11,19]. Selective removal of certain components such as cholesterol, ceramides, or fatty acids can alter the optimum levels of various lipids required to maintain a healthy corneum. Subramanyan et al. have shown that washing skin with a cleanser base (anionic/amphoteric surfactant mix without any moisturizing ingredients) can cause reduction in levels of fatty acids and cholesterol in skin even after a single wash [50]. Rawlings et al. showed that in the case of soap-induced winter xerotic dry skin, ceramides decreased with severity of xerosis grades [47]. The latter may have a biochemical origin rather than be due to removal of lipids since ceramides are not likely to be extracted from skin under wash conditions [51]. An alternative view is that surfactants, especially anionic surfactants, adsorb and intercalate into the lipid structure leading to increase in bilayer permeability and destabilization of the bilayer structure [12–14,52]. It has been shown that the tendency of surfactants to intercalate into a model lipid bilayer structure is very much governed by the hydrophobicity of the surfactant [14]. Surfactant charge also can play an important role in the destabilization of the bilayer structure. Yet another view is that the surfactants alter the biological lipid biosynthetic process leading to changes in the relative levels of various lipids. [18].

Relative tendencies of surfactants to interact with proteins and lipids are not necessarily the same. For example, in general, anionic surfactants tend to interact strongly with proteins as well as cause some delipidation. Nonionic surfactants, on the other hand, exhibit minimal interactions with proteins, but have the potential to cause delipidation. Relative tendencies of SLES, CAPB, dodecyl dimethyl amine oxide (DMAO), and a sugar-based nonionic surfactant, APG, to solubilized stearic acid under controlled conditions is shown in Fig. 3. Clearly, nonionic surfactants have a higher tendency to dissolve fatty acids than anionic surfactants and this may translate to higher delipidation of skin if nonionic surfactants are incorporated into a cleanser. In a mixed surfactant system, however, such effects can be modulated by choosing appropriate co-surfactants.

In vitro experiments by Froebe et al. determined the amount of lipid removed by anionic surfactants such as sodium lauryl sulfate and linear alkyl benzene sulfonate at levels in the range of 0.01 to 2% [51]. The results obtained showed that the surfactants removed lipids only above the surfactant CMC and that the amount of lipid removed as a fraction of the total lipid in the corneum was relatively low even at 2% level of the surfactant. Froebe et al. also showed that SLS and LAS can induce erythema at levels well below the surfactant CMC. Based on these results the authors have argued that lipid removal does not play a role in the induction of erythema [51]. Imokawa et al. in in-vivo studies showed that SLS at 5% level can cause significant lipid depletion even at contact times as short as 1 min [11]. Lipid analysis showed that SLS treatment led to selective removal of cholesterol, cholesterol ester, free fatty acid, and sphingolipids. Transmission electron microscopy pictures of skin biopsy samples showed the absence of intercellular lamellae after the SLS treatment. According to Imokawa, there is a close relationship between the potential for removing intercellular lipids and the

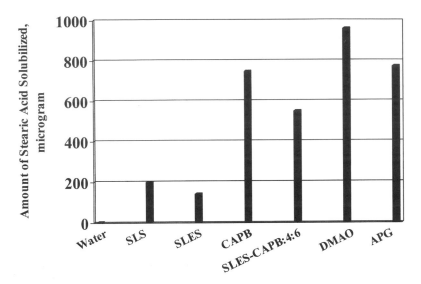

FIGURE 3 Lipid dissolution tendency of various surfactants as indicated by their ability to dissolved stearic acid. Total surfactant = 2%; stearic acid = 1 mg. Contact time, 5 minutes. Clearly nonionic surfactants seem to dissolve more fatty acid than anionic surfactants reflecting their high defatting tendency. SLS, sodium lauryl sulfate; SLES, sodium lauryl ether sulfate; CAPB, cocoamido propyl betaine; DMAO, dodecyl dimethyl amine oxide; APG, alkyl poly glucoside.

potential to induce skin roughness for several anionic surfactants. Imokawa also investigated the effect of two daily topical applications of four chromatographically separated fractions from the stratum corneum lipids (cholesterol ester, free fatty acids, cholesterol, and sphingolipids) from the stratum corneum lipids on SLS-damaged skin [11]. The results showed that cholesterol ester and sphingolipids induced a significant increase in conductance, whereas treatments with cholesterol and fatty acids did not effect a significant increase in conductance value. Abraham [20] has argued that the increased water retention is possibly due to glycolipids rather than stratum corneum lipids since endogeneous lipids of stratum corneum are not capable of holding water. While the latter comment is a valid one, it is not clear if the observed effects are necessarily due to the water-holding capacity of the lipids or because of the improved barrier repair properties of the applied lipids.

While the importance of lipid removal by surfactants and its role in cleanser-induced changes in skin condition may be a matter of debate, the role of lipids in maintaining the barrier function is better established [53]. For example, Grubauer et al. using acetone- and petroleum ether-extraction procedures for removing lipids from hairless mice skin showed that there exists a linear relationship between total lipid content of the corneum and the stratum barrier function [53]. Based on the trans-epidermal water loss (TEWL) differences between acetone- and petroleum ether–extracted sites, the authors have hypothesized that while the total lipid content is important, removal of sphingolipids and free sterols lead to a more pronounced level of barrier breakdown.

3.4 Clinical Manifestations of Cleanser-Induced Effects on Skin

It is clear from the preceding discussion that several factors contribute to cleanser-induced skin damage. In addition to cleansers, factors such as age, genetic conditions, nutrition, weather, and other environmental factors also influence skin condition. A schematic diagram of factors that can lead to skin damage is shown in Fig. 4. In general, a combination of these factors can lead to increased damage, and the use of harsh cleansers will aggravate the situation even further. The emphasis here will be on cleanser-induced damage.

3.4.1 After-Wash Tightness

Harsh cleansers such as soaps induce perceivable skin tightness compared to mild syndet surfactant-based cleansers [54]. Factors that cause skin tightness, a sensa-

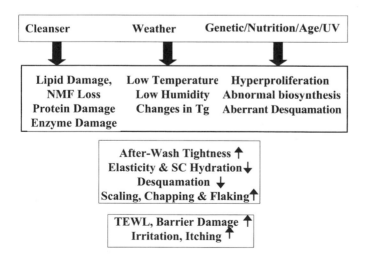

Figure 4 Schematic diagram of factors that contribute to skin dryness, irritation, and itching. While any one of the factors such as cleanser, weather, poor nutrition, genetic factors, or UV damage can lead to skin problems, a combination can significantly increase the potential for skin problems.

tion that manifests about 5 to 10 min after wash with a cleanser, have been linked to stresses created in skin because of rapid evaporation of water from surface layers. As mentioned earlier, treatment with harsh surfactants can actually lead to hyperhydration immediately after wash, followed by rapid evaporation of water to equilibrium values that are below the presurfactant treatment levels [19]. This hyperhydration coupled with lower equilibrium hydration levels sets up a higher rate of evaporation, and this creates a differential stress in the upper layers leading to AWT. The hyperhydration itself is possibly due to surfactant-induced corneocyte swelling, which in turn is linked to surfactant binding to proteins. The reduction in equilibrium levels of water in skin, on the other hand, is possibly due to loss of NMFs as well as reduction in water-binding capacity of keratinous proteins. Results reported in the literature seem to indicate that the tendency to cause skin tightness parallels both lipid removal as well as binding to proteins [19]. The correlation between tightness and NMF removal appears to be rather weak compared to surfactant binding to proteins [19]. According to Imokawa, skin lipid removal enhances the tightness but is not essential for tightness [19].

3.4.2 Skin Dryness, Scaling, and Roughness

It is well recognized that harsh cleansers such as soaps can induce dry skin leading to scaly rough skin. Note, however, that irritation is not a prerequisite for skin dryness [22]. In fact, some of the lipid solvents such as alcohols, acetone, [55] and even some nonionic surfactants that cause minimal or no irritation can cause significant dry skin. Thus there may be a link between lipid removal and dry skin. These effects may be much more acute during winter months and low humidity conditions. This is not unreasonable since changes in skin elasticity at temperatures below the glass transition temperature of skin lipids make the corneum more vulnerable to chapping/cracking, leading to barrier breakdown. Similarly, water being an excellent plasticizer of skin, under low humidity conditions, glass transition temperature of skin decreases markedly, making the corneum more susceptible to cracking. Thus a combination of harsh cleanser use, cold temperatures, and low humidity make the conditions ideal for dry skin.

Increase in visible skin dryness has been found to exhibit a positive correlation with surface hydration, but not necessarily with an increase in TEWL. This clearly suggests that significant barrier breakdown is not a requirement for skin dryness. Continued increase in dryness to values above a certain level may, however, lead to cracking and chapping leading to a barrier breakdown and eventually to irritation.

3.4.3 Skin Irritation

Harsh surfactants that can cause significant barrier damage have the potential to cause skin irritation, erythema, and itching. Erythema and itching are basically inflammatory responses to penetration of a foreign substance such as surfactant.

It is not necessary that surfactant has to penetrate into dermal layers to elicit a response. Communication via production of cytokines can also elicit a response from the dermis.

Harsh soaps and soap-based liquids have the potential to cause skin irritation and itching. Most of the currently available syndet surfactant-based cleansers are formulated to be significantly milder than soap and cause considerably less irritation and itching under normal use conditions.

Irrespective of the exact mechanisms involved in AWT, skin dryness/roughness, and irritation—a moisturizing cleanser would be expected to prevent/minimize/eliminate these effects. Thus in the case of cleansers, preventing and/or minimizing damage is clearly the first step toward providing moisturization benefits from a cleanser.

4 MOISTURIZING SYNDET BARS VERSUS SOAP

It is clear from the analysis so far that a mild moisturizing cleanser should have relatively mild surfactants that exhibit minimal or no interaction with skin proteins and lipids. In the evolution of cleansers, syndet bars clearly represented a distinctly different class of mildness in the cleansing arena [56]. Syndet bars utilized sodium cocoyl isethionate, a milder surfactant compared to soap with carboxylate functionality. As mentioned earlier, soaps bind much more strongly to skin proteins than SCI [19,37]. Syndet bars are also formulated at a neutral pH, which can cause only minimal damage to skin lipids [57]. Furthermore, moisturizers in the syndet bar help enhance their mildness.

Mildness benefits of syndet bars over conventional soap have been demonstrated by a variety of in vivo methodologies under different degrees of exaggerated washing conditions. These frequently used tests include soap chamber [56], flex wash [58], arm wash [59], and forearm controlled application technique (FCAT) [60,61]. In several of the examples of comparisons of syndet bar and soap in the following sections of this chapter have been generated using bar compositions shown in Table 1. Results demonstrating superiority of a syndet bar versus a soap bar in such controlled use tests are also shown in Table 1.

Mildness of syndet bars is also reflected in improved viscoelastic properties of skin compared to those achieved by soap bars. For example, using a newly developed instrument, the Linear Skin Rheometer, that is considered to be more sensitive to upper layers of the corneum [62], our recent in vivo results (Fig. 5) show that the syndet bar leaves the skin in a softer and less stiff state compared to soap bars [63]. Extensibility of human corneum after exposure to bar slurries and a delipidating solvent (acetone) measured using a Miniature Mechanical Tester (Fig. 6) also show that the syndet bar–treated corneum behaves similar to water treatment, whereas the soap treatment leads to cracking of the corneum.

TABLE 1 Irritation and Dryness Potential of Syndet and Soap Bars as Measured by Soap Chamber Test, Flex Wash, Arm Wash, and FCAT Tests

	Soap chamber test (irritation score)	Flex wash (mean total erythema score)[c]	Arm wash[d]		FCAT		
			Erythema	Dryness	Erythema	Dryness	SKICON (conductance)
Syndet bar[a]	0.5	5.7 +/- 1.2	0.3	0.7	0.11	0.57	-60.5
Soap bar[b]	2.8	27.7 +/- 2.0	2.6	1.7	0.33	1.04	-148.9
Ref.	56	58	59	59	61	61	61

[a]Syndet bar: sodium cocoyl isethionate, stearic acid, sodium tallowate, water, sodium isethionate, coconut acid, sodium stearate.
[b]Soap bar: sodium Tallowate, potassium soap, water.
[c]$p < 0.05$.
[d]$p < 0.0001$.

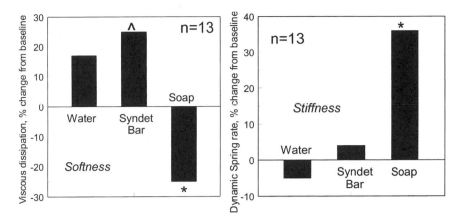

Figure 5 Linear Skin Rheometer measurements of changes in skin after a single wash with water, soap bar, or syndet bar showing that the syndet bar enhances skin softness and reduces stiffness. *p < 0.05; ^directionally different from baseline (p = 0.06).

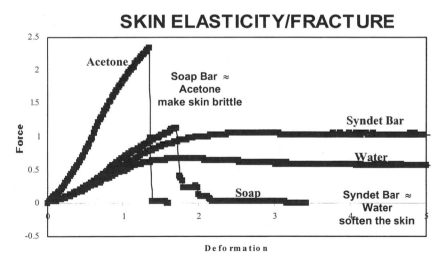

Figure 6 Force–deformation plots for human stratum corneum samples treated with water, acetone, soap bar, or syndet bar tested using a miniature mechanical tester. Samples soaked in the respective slurries/solutions for 1 hr and rinsed thoroughly prior to testing. Soap makes stratum corneum more brittle, a behavior similar in pattern to that of acetone. In contrast, syndet bar–treated corneum samples appear to be closer to water-treated samples.

4.1 Skin Ultrastructural Changes Induced by Soap Versus Syndet Bars

As stated earlier, common soaps consist of surfactants having carboxylate head-groups, and these are somewhat analogous to the harsh SLS and therefore have the potential to cause significant damage to proteins and lipids leading to irritation and itching. Cleanser-induced changes in the ultrastructure of the corneum is a powerful method to assess the nature and extent of damage that a cleanser can impart [11,64]. Recently, using an ex vivo arm wash methodology (Fig. 7) [64,65] in combination with TEWL measurements, environmental scanning microscopy (ESEM) and TEM have been used to compare the ultrastructure of human skin after multiple washes with a soap bar and a syndet bar. Results reproduced in Fig. 8 from Misra et al. [65,66] show changes in TEWL after 15 washes with soap and syndet bars. Corresponding changes in the surface morphology of skin obtained using ESEM is shown in Fig. 9. Clearly, these results show the significant increase in TEWL and uplifting of cells in the soap-washed sample. In

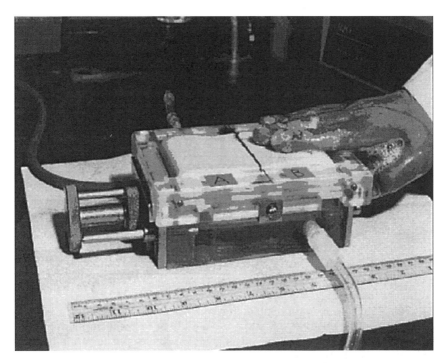

FIGURE 7 An ex vivo arm wash set-up. Wash protocol: wash cadaver skin with lather for 2 min; rinse for 15 s (rinse water temperature 38°C); measure TEWL using evaporimeter; punch biopsy samples for TEM and ESEM analyses. (From Ref. 64.)

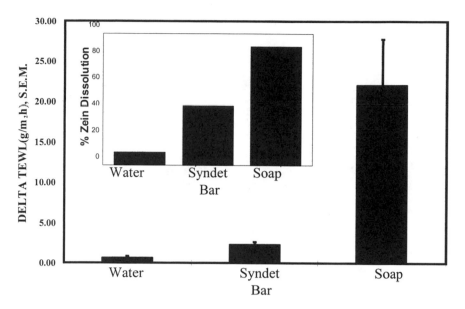

FIGURE 8 Change in TEWL of human skin after 15 washes with water, syndet bar, and soap bar. Inset shows the zein dissolution by the same products illustrating how protein dissolution correlates with the changes in TEWL. n = 9; 15 2-min washes; 25°C and 30% RH; rinse temperature 40°C. (From Ref. 65.)

contrast, syndet-washed samples showed much less increase in TEWL with no signs of uplifting of cells. The TEM results given in Fig. 10 showed significant damage to both lipid and protein regions after the soap wash. In contrast, under the same conditions the syndet bar–washed skin showed well-preserved lipid and protein regions. These results also show a good correlation between high TEWL and damage to corneum ultrastructure. Interestingly, a nonionic surfactant-based cleanser wash resulted in disrupted lipid region with much less damage to proteins [65]. Even though these represent rather exaggerated conditions, they clearly demonstrate the potential for damage from soap systems. These results are consistent with well-accepted mildness of syndet bars over soap bars.

4.2 Deposition of Skin Lipids from Syndet Bars

One of the reasons for the mildness of syndet bars has been the incorporation of moisturizing cream in the bar. A key component of the moisturizing cream is long chain fatty acids similar to the fatty acids present in skin. Presence of fatty acids can minimize the lipid damage by two different mechanisms. Fatty acids can actively deposit onto skin during wash to replenish the fatty acids that are lost dur-

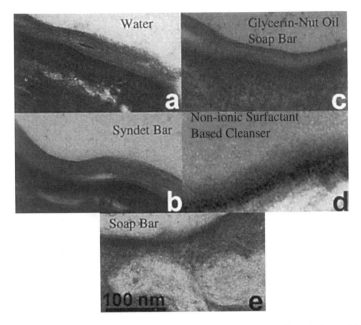

FIGURE 9 TEM pictures of stratum corneum of cadaver skin that has been washed 15 times with (a) water, (b) synder bar, (c) Glycerin-Nut Oil Bar, (d) nonionic surfactant–based liquid cleanser, and (e) soap bar. Soap shows maximum damage to both proteins and lipids; nonionic surfactants shows significant damage to lipids; syndet bar shows well-preserved lipids; glycerin bar shows some damage to lipids. (From Refs. 65 and 66.)

ing the wash process. Fatty acids also can minimize the lipid depletion by the surfactant micelles by acting as sacrificial lipids to saturate the micelles. While the relative roles of these two mechanisms are not fully established, it has been shown that these mild syndet bars do deposit fatty acids during wash conditions [67]. In this study, deuterated fatty acids were used to distinguish the deposited fatty acids from those present in skin. Specifically, 11 subjects rubbed a wet bar on their forearm for 10 s and the lather was allowed to remain on the skin for another 10 s. This was followed by a 15-s rinse under running water at a temperature of 95–100°F. The forearm was patted dry using a soft disposable towel. After an hour, 20 sequential tape-strip samples were taken and analyzed using a GC-MS procedure. Results obtained showed that fatty acids from the syndet bar deposits at a level of about 1 to 2 micrograms/cm^2 during wash. Importantly, deuterated fatty acid was detected even at a depth of 20 tape strips. Results for the first 10 tape strips are given in Fig. 11. It is not clear if the deposited lipids actually got incorporated into skin lipids or they remained as deposits that simply fill the crevices and cracks, thus preventing the water loss and allowing skin to maintain

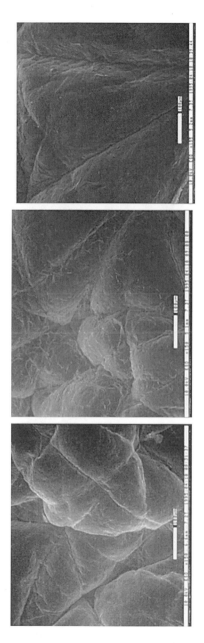

FIGURE 10 ESEM of stratum corneum of cadaver skin that has been washed 15 times, using the set-up and procedure shown in Fig. 7. Left, water; middle, soap bar; right, synder bar. Soap-washed sample shows onset of uplifting and scale formation. (From Ref. 65.)

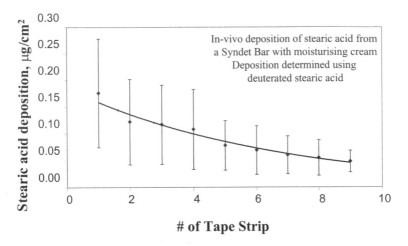

FIGURE 11 In vivo deposition of stearic acid after wash with a syndet bar containing fatty acids as beneficial lipids. n = 11. Study using deuterated stearic acid. Wash protocol: 15 s rubbing of the bar on forearm, 15 s lather retention on skin, 15 s rinse under running water, pat dry. Tape strip extraction after 1 h. Analysis using GC-MS technique. (From Ref. 67.)

its moisture levels. In any case, the cleanser induced changes of skin ultrastructure discussed earlier using this moisturizing syndet bar versus soap suggest that the lipids are well preserved in the case of the syndet bar even after exaggerated wash conditions.

An attempt to determine if the lipids that can be deposited from a syndet bar can alter the state of skin lipids was tested using ESR spectroscopy [68]. In this study, human stratum corneum was first exposed to a nitroxide spin probe that mimics fatty acids (doxyl 5-stearic acid) and a spectrum was obtained. This was followed by immersion of the corneum in a syndet or soap bar slurry for 1 min. This was followed by a rinse to mimic regular wash and then the ESR spectrum was obtained. Results given in Fig. 12 show that the untreated corneum has two lipid regions, one corresponding to relatively fluid lipids and the second to a rigid lipid region. This is consistent with the DSC results, which also showed two lipid transitions in the corneum. Importantly, the syndet bar slurry–treated corneum appears to have a more fluid lipid region compared to the soap-treated corneum (see Fig. 13). Even though this does not represent actual wash conditions, the results indicate that the cleansers with moisturizing lipids have the potential to fluidize the skin lipids. These types of studies to understand the molecular level interaction of deposited lipids on skin are important to establish the fate of beneficial agents deposited on skin.

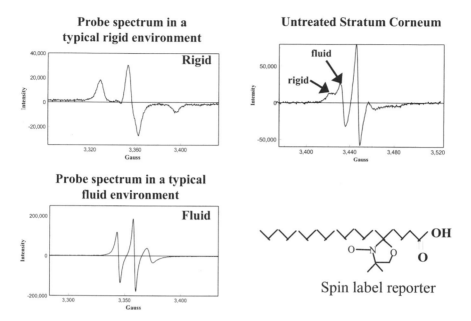

FIGURE 12   ESR probe, doxyl stearic acid, shows a sharp spectrum in a fluid lipid environment and an uneven spectrum in rigid environment; Stratum corneum shows presence of two types of lipid regions, rigid and fluid. (From Ref. 68.)

4.3   Liquid Cleansers

The introduction of liquid cleansers in the 1990s clearly offered new opportunities for formulators to make the systems significantly milder than bars. Since Liquid systems have significantly less processing problems, it was possible to select surfactants and surfactant mixtures from a much wider choice of surfactants to provide enhanced mildness benefits. Liquids technology also allowed deposition and delivery of beneficial agents to skin from a wash-off system. Thus, borrowing technology from shampoo systems that allow deposition of conditioning materials such as silicone oils onto hair, deposition and delivery of emollients and occlusive from wash-off systems using polymeric deposition aids have become a reality. Liquids technology allow deposition of beneficial agents at a much higher efficiency than the current bar technology. This advancement has made it possible to consider deposition/delivery of moisturizing ingredients from wash-off systems. Specifically, deposition of emollients, occlusives, and humectants under wash-off conditions can lead to delivery of moisturization benefits from cleansers. Some of the leading liquid cleansers in the market contain skin lipids,

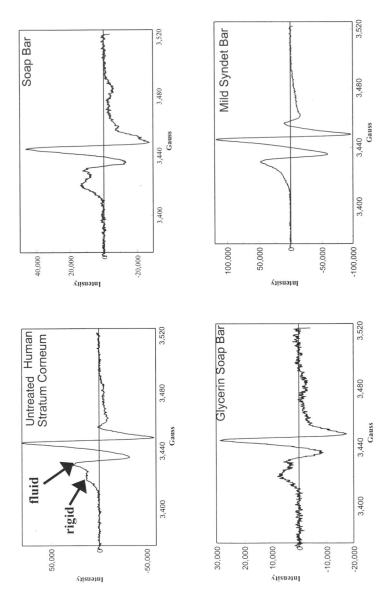

Figure 13 ESR probe, doxyl stearic acid, shows a rigid and a fluid spectrum in human stratum corneum. Stratum corneum samples were soaked in bar slurries for 1 minute followed by water wash in excess water. Rigid regions appear to be enhanced for stratum corneum samples that have been soaked in slurries of a regular soap bar and a glycerin soap bar. Soaking stratum corneum in the syndet bar slurry, however, appears to leave the lipids in a more fluid state as indicated by the sharp spectrum. (From Ref. 68.)

vegetable oils, petrolatum, emollient alcohols, and glycerol as beneficial agents for skin. The market is continuing to explode with activity with a variety of novel combinations of ingredients and novel skin care claims from wash-off systems.

Liquid cleansers can be designed to deposit beneficial lipids such as cholesterol and fatty acids during wash. Recently, Subramanyan et al. conducted a clinical study to determine the deposition of fatty acids and cholesterol deposited from a liquid shower gel during a single wash [50]. Main ingredients in the body wash were sodium cocoyl isethionate, sodium laureth sulfate, cocamidopropyl betaine, glycerin, stearic acid, and lanolin alcohol. The lipids in the product were tracked on skin by deuterium labeling to distinguish them from the lipids that naturally occur in skin. Results indicated that during cleansing with the base cleanser without the beneficial active ingredients (stearic acid and lanolin alcohol), significant amounts of endogenous cholesterol and stearic acid were removed from the stratum corneum, and the marketed cleansing product containing the beneficial

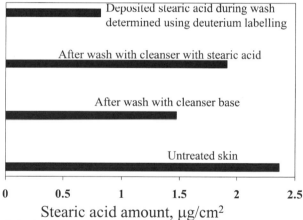

N=16, Arm wash, 2 min wash,
15 second rinse

Figure 14 Stearic acid extracted from skin using 1:1 IPA/methanol mixture after wash with various shower gels. Baseline shows the level of extractable stearic acid in the corneum. A comparison of the control wash with baseline shows a reduction in extractable stearic acid indicating that the cleanser has removed a certain level of stearic acid from the corneum. Comparison of product with stearic acid and the baseline shows a higher level of extractable stearic acid after the product wash. Since this was done using deuterated stearic acid, active deposition could be estimated and this is also shown in the figure. (From Ref. 50.)

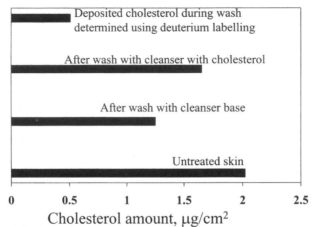

Deposited cholesterol during wash
determined using deuterium labelling

After wash with cleanser with cholesterol

After wash with cleanser base

Untreated skin

Cholesterol amount, $\mu g/cm^2$

N=16, Arm wash, 2 min wash,
15 second rinse

FIGURE 15 Cholesterol extracted from skin using 1:1 IPA/methanol mixture after wash with various shower gels. Baseline shows the level of extractable cholesterol in the corneum. Comparison of control wash with baseline shows a reduction in extractable cholesterol showing that the cleanser has removed a certain level of cholesterol from the corneum. Comparison of product wash with the control wash shows a higher level of extractable cholesterol after the product wash. Since this was done using deuterated cholesterol, active deposition could be estimated and this is also shown in the figure. (From Ref. 50.)

agents actively replaced about 50–60% of the cholesterol and stearic acid (see Fig. 14 and 15).

Recently a dual formula body wash was introduced with skin nourishing claims. This shower gel with a unique dual chamber packaging has been shown in in vivo studies to deposit about 10 $\mu g/cm^2$ of triglycerides and 0.6 $\mu g/cm^2$ of cholesterol onto skin during wash [69]. Clearly the level of deposition of triglycerides from this system is significantly higher than that from bars, demonstrating that liquid cleanser technology allows deposition of materials at much higher levels than bars. In separate autoradiography experiments using cadaver skin, it has also been shown that the deposited triglycerides penetrate several layers into skin (Fig. 16) [70].

Progress in liquid cleanser technology will continue to occur in the coming years. The success of the technology will depend upon how effectively the deposition and delivery of beneficial agents can be balanced against the ability of the

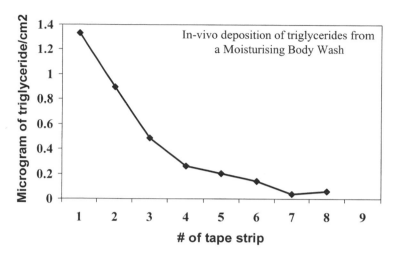

FIGURE 16 In vivo deposition of triglycerides from a commercial dual chamber shower gel. Penetration profile of triglyceride determined using cadaver skin. (From Ref. 70.)

cleanser to provide freshness and cleanliness with the desired in-use sensory and lather properties.

5 SUMMARY

Cleanser technology has come a long way from their primary purpose of removing oily soil, dirt, and bacteria from skin to providing skin mildness and moisturization benefits. Soap-based cleansers have the potential to interact with skin proteins and lipids leading to dry skin and irritation. The first step toward providing skin care benefits from wash-off systems is to minimize damage to skin by cleansers. A clear understanding of the potential damage that can be induced by cleansers provides a road map to minimize damage and begin to examine opportunities to deliver moisturization benefits from cleansers. The introduction of syndet bars about half a century ago was a major breakthrough in the direction of minimizing damage to skin from cleansers. Delivering moisturization benefits from cleansers is a real technical challenge since this involves actually depositing and delivering skin care materials under wash-off conditions that are normally designed to remove materials from skin. New product forms such as liquid cleansers introduced in the 1990s and nonwoven product technology introduced recently offer exciting opportunities for delivering moisturization benefits from wash-off systems. Skin cleansing products that contain emollients, occlusives, humectants, and skin nutrients have begun to appear in the marketplace already. This trend of providing skin care benefits from wash-off systems will continue to be an area of active research resulting in novel product forms and technologies in the coming years.

Acknowledgments

The authors would like to thank Drs. S. Mukherjee, X. Lei, and N.J. Turro for granting permission to use their unpublished data on ESR spectroscopy of corneum treated with cleanser solutions. We would also like to thank Drs. M. Misra and M. Aronson for their helpful discussions and Unilever Research for allowing us to publish this work.

REFERENCES

1. Spitz L. In: Spitz L, ed. Soap Technology for the 1990's. Champaign, IL: Am Oil Chem Soc 1990:1–47.
2. Stanislaus IVS, Meerbott PB. In: American Soap Makers Guide. New York: Henry Carey Baird, 1928:914–919.
3. Murahata RI, Aronson MP, Sharko PT, Greene AP. In: Rieger MM, Rhein LD, eds. Surfactants in Cosmetics. New York: Marcel Dekker, 1997:307–330.
4. Matthies W. Dermatological observations. In: Gloxhuber C, Kunstler K, eds. Anionic Surfactants. New York: Marcel Dekker, 1992:291–329.
5. Warner RR, Lilly NA. Correlation of water content with ultrastructure in the stratum corneum. In: Elsner P, Berardesca E, Maibach HI, eds. Bioengineering of the Skin: Water and the Stratum Corneum. Boca Raton: CRC Press, 1994:3–12.
6. Leveque J. Water–keratin interactions. In: Elsner P, Berardesca E, Maibach HI, eds. Bioengineering of the Skin: Water and the Stratum Corneum. Boca Raton: CRC Press, 1994:13–22.
7. Yamamura T, Tezuka T. The water holding capacity of the stratum corneum measured by ^{1}H-NMR. J Invest Dermatol 1989; 93(1):160–164.
8. Loden M, Lindberg M. Product testing—testing moisturizers. In: Elsner P, Berardesca E, Maibach HI, eds. Bioengineering of the Skin: Water and the Stratum Corneum. Boca Raton: CRC Press, 1994:275–289.
9. Imokawa G, Sumura K, Katsumi M. Study on skin roughness caused by surfactants. II. Correlation between protein denaturation and skin roughness. J Am Oil Chem Soc 1975; 52:484.
10. Wihelm KP, Wolff HH, Maibach HI. Effects of surfactants on skin hydration. In: Elsner P, Berardesca E, Maibach HI, eds. Bioengineering of the Skin: Water and the Stratum Corneum. Boca Raton: CRC Press, 1994:257–274.
11. Imokawa G, Akasaki S, Minematsu Y, Kawai M. Importance of intercellular lipids in water-retention properties of the stratum corneum: induction and recovery study of surfactant dry skin. Arch Dermatol Res 1989; 281:45–51.
12. Inoue I, Miyakawa K, Shimozawa K. Interaction of surfactants with vesicle mem-

brane of dipalmitoylphosphatidylcholine—effect on gel-to-liquid crystalline phase transition of lipid bilayer. Chem Phys Lipids 1986; 42:261–270.

13. Lichtenberg D, Robson J, Dennis EA. Characterization of the lipid bilayers by surfactants. Biochim Biophys Acta 1985; 821(3):470–478.

14. de la Maza A, Coderch L, Lopez O, Baucells J, Parra JL. Permeability changes caused by surfactants in liposomes that model the stratum corneum lipid composition. J Am Oil Chem Soc 1997; 74(1):1–8.

15. Middleton JD. The mechanism of action of surfactants on the water binding properties of isolated stratum corneum. J Soc Cosmet Chem 1969; 20:399–412.

16. Prottey C, Ferguson T. Factors which determine the skin irritation potential of soaps and detergents. J Soc Cosmet Chem 1975; 26:29–46.

17. Kawai M, Imokawa G. The induction of skin tightness by surfactants. J Soc Cosmet Chem 1984; 35:147–156.

18. Rhein LD. In vitro interactions: biochemical and biophysical effects of surfactants on skin. In: Rieger MM, Rhein LD, eds. Surfactants in Cosmetics. New York: Marcel Dekker, 1997:397–425.

19. Imokawa G. Surfactant mildness. In: Rieger MM, Rhein LD, eds. Surfactants in Cosmetics. New York: Marcel Dekker, 1997:427–471.

20. Abraham W. Surfactant effects on skin repair. In: Rieger MM, Rhein LD, eds. Surfactants in Cosmetics. New York: Marcel Dekker, 1997:473–487.

21. Rizvi PY, Morrison BM. Bioengineering techniques for investigating the effects of surfactants on skin. In: Rieger MM, Rhein LD, eds. Surfactants in Cosmetics. New York: Marcel Dekker, 1997:489–499.

22. Simion FA. Human in vivo methods for assessing the irritation potential of cleansing systems. In: Rieger MM, Rhein LD, eds. Surfactants in Cosmetics. New York: Marcel Dekker, 1997:519–532.

23. Elias PM. Epidermal lipids, barrier function, and desquamation. J Invest Dermatol 1983; 80:44S–49S.

24. Swartzendruber DC, Wertz PW, Madison KC, Downing DT. Evidence that the corneocyte has a chemically bound lipid envelope. J Invest Dermatol 1987; 88(6):709–713.

25. Madison KC, Swartzendruber DC, Wertz PW, Elias PM. Presence of intact intercellular lipid lamellae in the upper layers of the stratum corneum. J Invest Dermatol 1987; 88(6):714–718.

26. Rehfeld SJ, Plachy WZ, Williams ML, Elias PM. Calorimetric and electron spin resonance examination of lipid phase transition in human stratum corneum: molecular basis for normal cohesion and abnormal desquamation in recessive X-linked ichthyosis. J Invest Dermatol 1988; 91:499–505.

27. Middleton JD. The mechanism of action of surfactants on the water binding properties of isolated stratum corneum. J Soc Cosmet Chem 1969; 20:399–412.

28. Chapman SJ, Walsh A. Desquamation, corneosomes and desquamation. An ultrastructural study of adult pig epidermis. Arch Dermatol Res 1990; 282:304–310.

29. Egelrud T, Lundstrom A. The dependence of detergent induced cell dissociation in non-palmo-plantar stratum corneum on endogenous proteolysis. J Invest Dermatol 1992; 90:456–459.

30. Imokawa G, Mishima J. Cumulative effects of surfactants on cutaneous horny layers—adsorption onto human keratin layers in vivo. Contact Dermatitis 1979; 5(6):357–366.

31. Faucher JA, Goddard ED. Interaction of keratinous proteins with sodium lauryl sulfate: sorption. J Soc Cosmet Chem 1978; 29:323–338.

32. Breuer MM. The interaction between surfactants and keratinous tissues. J Soc Cosmet Chem 1979; 30:41–64.

33. Dominguez JG, Parra JL, Infante RM, Pelejero F, Balaguer F, Sastre TA. New approach to the theory of adsorption and permeability of surfactants on keratinic proteins: specific behavior of certain hydrophobic chains. J Soc Cosmet Chem 1977; 28:165–182.

34. Conrads A, Zahn H. A study of interaction of sodium dodecyl sulfate with proteins of human stratum corneum. Int J Cosmet Sci 1976; 9:29–46.

35. Schwuger MJ, Bartnik FG. Interaction of anionic surfactants with proteins, enzymes, and membranes. In: Gloxhuber C, ed. Anionic Surfactants, Surfactant Science Series, Vol. 10. New York: Marcel Dekker, 1980:1–49.

36. Ananthapadmanabhan KP. Protein–surfactant interactions. In: Goddard ED, Ananthapadmanabhan KP, eds. Interaction of Surfactants with Polymers and Proteins. Boca Raton: CRC Press, 1993:319–366.

37. Ananthapadmanabhan KP. Binding of surfactants to stratum corneum. J Soc Cosmet Chem 1996; 47:185–200.

38. Rhein LD, Simion FA. Surfactant interactions with skin. In: Bender M, ed. Interfacial Phenomena in Biological Systems. Surfactant Science Series. Vol. 39. New York: Marcel Dekker, 1991:33–49.

39. Pierard GE, Goffin V, Pierard-Franchimont C. Corneosufametry: a predictive assessment of the interaction of personal care cleansing products with human stratum corneum. Dermatology 1994; 189:152–156.

40. Dominguez JG, Balaguer F, Parra JL, Pelejero CM. The inhibitory effect of some amphoteric surfactants on the irritation potential of alkyl sulfates. Int J Cosmet Soc 1981; 3(2):57–68.

41. Gotte E. Skin compatibility of tensides measured by their capacity for dissolving zein In: Proceedings of the 4th International Congress on Surface Active Substances, Brussels; 1964, pp. 83–90.

42. Rhein LD, Robbins CR, Kernee K, Cantore R. Surfactant structure effects on swelling of isolated human stratum corneum. J Soc Cosmet Chem 1986; 37:125–139.

43. Wilhelm KP, Cua AB, Wolff HH, Maibach HI. Predicting surfactant induced stratum corneum hydration in vivo: prediction of the irritation potential of anionic surfactants. J Invest Dermatol 1994; 101:310–315.

44. Fulmer AW, Kramer GJ. Stratum corneum lipid abnormalities in surfactant-induced dry scaly skin. J Invest Dermatol 1986; 86:598–602.

45. Fartasch M, Diepgen TL, Hornstein OP. Morphological changes of epidermal lipid layers of stratum corneum in sodium lauryl sulfate induced dry skin: a functional and ultrastructural study. J Invest Dermatol 1991; 96(4):617.

46. Rieger M. Skin lipids and their importance to cosmetic science. Cosmet Toil 1987; 102(7):36–49.

47. Rawlings AW, Watkinson A, Rogers J, Mayo HJ, Scott IR. Abnormalities in stratum corneum structure, lipid composition, and desmosome degradationin soap-induced winter zerosis. J Soc Cosmet Chem 1994; 45:203–220.

48. Imokawa G, Akasaki S, Hattori M, Yoshizuka N. Selective recovery of deranged water-holding properties by stratum corneum lipids. J Invest Dermatol 1986; 187:758–761.

49. Leveque JL, DeRigal J, Legere DS, Billy D. How does sodium lauryl sulfate alter the skin barrier function in man—a multiparametric approach. Skin Pharmacol 1993; 6(2):111–115.

50. Subramanyan K, Wong J, Ananthapadmanabhan K, Pereira A. Deposition of lipids from personal wash cleansers. Poster presentation at the IFSCC conference, Berlin, Sep 2000.

51. Froebe CL, Simion FA, Rhein LD, Cagan RH, Kligman A. Stratum corneum lipid removal by surfactants: relation to in vivo irritation. Dermatologica 1990; 181:277–283.

52. Downing DT, Abraham W, Wegner KK, Willman KW, Marshal JL. Partition of sodium dodecyl sulfate into stratum corneum lipid liposomes. Arch Dermatol Res 1993; 285(3):151–157.

53. Grubauer G, Feingold KR, Harris RM, Elias PM. Lipid content and lipid type as determinants of the epidermal permeability barrier. J Lipid Res 1989; 30:89–96.

54. Simion FA, Rhein LD, Morrison BM, Scala DD, Salko DM, Kligman AM, Grove GL. Self-perceived sensory responses to soap and synthetic detergent bars correlate with clinical signs of irritation. J Am Acad Dermatol 1995; 32:205–211.

55. Imokawa G, Hattori M. A possible function of structural lipids in the water-holding properties of the stratum corneum. J Invest Dermatol 1985; 84(4):282–284.

56. Frosch PJ, Kligman AM. The soap chamber test. J Am Acad Dermatol 1979; 1(1):35–41.

57. Murahata RI, Aronson MP. The relationship between solution pH and clinical irritancy for carboxylic acid-based personal washing products. J Soc Cosmet Chem 1994; 45:239–246.

58. Strube DA, Koontz SW, Murahata RI, Theiler RI, The flex wash test: a method for evaluating the mildness of personal washing products. J Soc Cosmet Chem 1989; 40:297–306.

59. Sharko PT, Murahata RI, Leyden JL, Grove GL. Arm wash with instrumental evaluation—a sensitive technique for differentiating the irritation potential of personal washing products. J Dermoclinical Eval Soc 1991; 2:19–27.

60. Ertel KD, Keswick BH, Bryant PB. A forearm controlled application technique for estimating the relative mildness of personal cleansing products. J Soc Cosmet Chem 1995; 46:67–76.

61. Azri-Meehan S, Edison B, Borowski D. Clinical evaluation of soap bars. Unilever Research US, Nov 1998.

62. Matts PJ, Goodyer E. A new instrument to measure the mechanical properties of human stratum corneum in vivo. J Cosmet Sci 1998; 49:321–333.

63. Subramanyan K, Bautista B, Mok W, Meyers L. Unpublished results, Unilever Research, Sep 2000.

64. Ananthapadmanabhan KP, Prowell S, Hoyberg K, Misra M, Spaltro S, Mukherjee S,

Aronson MP. Cleanser induced structural changes in human stratum corneum. Proc 4th Congr Eur Acad Dermatol Venereol, Brussels, 1995, p. 143.

65. Misra M, Ananthapadmanabhan KP, Hoyberg K, Gursky RP, Prowell S, Aronson MP. Correlation between surfactant-induced ultrastructural changes in epidermis and transepidermal water loss. J Soc Cosmet Chem 1997; 48:219–234.

66. Misra M, Ananthapadmanabhan KP. Quantitative analysis of surfactant induced ultrastructural changes in skin lipids. In: Lal M, Lillford PJ, Naik VM, Prakash V, eds. Supramolecular and Colloidal Structures in Biomaterials and Biosubstrates. Proc. 5th Royal Soc Unilever-Indo-UK Forum in Materials Science and Engineering, Jan 10–14, 1999, pp. 183–196.

67. Yu K, Hargiss L, Wong JK, Anathapadmanabhan KP. In-vivo deposition of stearic acid from syndet bars: a clinical study using deuterated stearic acid. Unpublished results, Unilever Research US, 1995.

68. Mukherjee S, Lei X, Turro NJ, ESR study of cleanser induced changes in human stratum corneum. Unpublished results, Unilever Research US, 1995.

69. Naser M, Atlas J, Chang E, Meyers L, Morgan L, Velez S, In-vivo deposition of cholesterol and triglycerides from dual chamber body wash. Unpublished results, Unilever Research US, 1998.

70. Subramanyan K, Prowell S, Ananthapadmanabhan KP. Unpublished results, Unilever Research US, 1998.

21

Consumer Testing Methods

**Steven S. Braddon and
Gwendolyn S. Jarrett**
Unilever Home and Personal Care North America,
Trumbull, Connecticut

Alejandra M. Muñoz
International Resources for Insights and Solutions,
Mountainside, New Jersey

1 INTRODUCTION

Moisturizers are big business. Consumers spend millions of dollars each year in search of efficacious products. All one needs to do is scan the monthly "women's magazines" to understand that moisturizers of all types—hand and body lotions, facial moisturizers, and body washes—are being advertised in record numbers. Approximately 80% of women in the United States use a hand and body lotion regularly. Products offer benefits ranging from dry skin relief to youthful, less wrinkled, and firmer skin. Formulations include such ingredients as α- and β-hydroxyacids (AHA and BHA), retinols, and seaweed extract. Vitamins are added as antioxidants and firming agents. It is common knowledge that herbs, long used for healing purposes, are finding new life in skin preparations [1]. Herbal extracts, considered by some as good for the inside, are now being used on the outside as well. Foods have also found their way into moisturizers—soya, whey protein, oats, sugar, cucumbers, and green tea are but a few of these ingredients. It is possible to purchase moisturizers that are fragranced or unfragranced in every color imaginable.

Products are sold not only in the more traditional locales of supermarkets and drug, discount, and department stores, but also in mall specialty shops which provide an endless supply of moisturizing lotions, creams, and body washes offering exotic fragrances in expensive packaging. The internet, the latest shopping medium, is another source of supply for the consumer's insatiable quest for new and different products. To understand more about what will entice the consumer to actually buy a product, it is up to the testing professional to ascertain their likes and dislikes.

In the fast-paced environment of the personal care industry, who to test, what to test, and how to test are conundrums posed daily by many marketing brand managers. Start-up operations and smaller businesses, some with limited or no research dollars, may rely on the intuition of a company's president, marketing team member, or development chemist as the deciding factor in selecting product formulas, colors, or fragrances. At more established companies those types of questions are normally directed to the in-house experts: market research and research guidance testing departments.

Market research is traditionally conducted within a marketing department which, in turn, usually operates within the corporate headquarters. It explores such areas as brand awareness, trial and repeat purchase, category segmentation, habits and attitude studies, advertising effectiveness, and large-scale performance and acceptance tests for current brands and potential new products. Within the research and development department (R&D), with which the authors are most familiar, research guidance testing seeks insight into products and prototypes through the analysis of early-in consumer evaluations and the assessments of trained descriptive panels. Their main responsibility is to help guide the development chemist's efforts to "build" products that will delight consumers and induce them to become loyal brand users. Some companies rely more heavily on the insights derived from trained panels because their judgments are free of bias. Others lean toward tests with naive consumers because they are the ultimate purchasers of a product and because the cost of trained panels can be prohibitive.

This chapter provides a comprehensive overview of moisturizer testing methodologies currently utilized in the personal care industry for the reader with little or no experience in the field as well as a review for the professional. On the following pages the authors first provide a brief history of moisturizer use. Although commercially sold product is a relatively new invention of the 20th century, there is evidence that moisturizer-like products were in use from the earliest times [2]. While no testing was conducted on those early products, there exists today a number of options for extensive consumer, sensory, and expert testing of moisturizers.

Before testing can begin it is crucial to identify meaningful terms for both the consumer and expert to evaluate a product. Terminology is important because it provides the professional with a common lexicon for deciphering consumer feedback. It is important to clearly understand the objectives of a study, for without explicitly defined goals it is impossible to choose appropriate test methods. The various methodologies discussed will comprise discrimination tests, descriptive panels conducted by expert evaluators, and naive consumer testing. Data analysis is then examined as a way of understanding consumer responses. The chapter ends with a discussion of irritation issues and a number of testing applications such as claim substantiations.

2 HISTORY OF MOISTURIZERS

Concern about the appearance of skin predates modern society. Just how far back in time cosmetics originated is somewhat surprising. Cosmetics and perfumes have been found at ancient burial sites in Egypt [3], and the use of homemade mixtures to moisturize and rejuvenate dry and aging skin have been documented in early Greece and Rome [4,5].

2.1 Egypt

Viewing the powerful art that remains on the walls of ancient Egyptian burial sites presents a picture of a highly refined, painted culture. The early Egyptians were not only interested in color cosmetics; home-worked products for skin moisturizing and anti-aging also abounded. Stylish Egyptian women applied a product called Coan Quince Cream for silky complexions [6], and anthropological literature shows that women in Greece and Rome were doing much the same thing.

2.2 Greece and Rome

Some Greek women followed a routine of spreading a poultice of bread and milk on their faces before retiring at night "to repair the effects of time as a cause of cutaneous aging" [4]. Often referred to as the father of medicine, the Greek physician Hippocrates, in his discourse on "Considerations of treatment of wounds," speaks of using honey on the face, arguing that it "assures a fresh and jovial look" [4]. Roman women were doing likewise. Masks prepared from "breadcrumbs soaked in milk, or rye flour with honey" [7] were used at night and usually removed in the morning. Some women wore them all day, cleansing their faces only to run an important errand [7]. Also, some Roman women applied the dregs from the bottom of wine vats looking for the same results that moisturizing products claim today: soft and smooth skin [7]. Still others attempted to maintain their skin with milk baths [7]. Thomas Spelios, writing in a historical review of cosmetics, states that Galen of Pergamon, the renowned physician, is credited with developing cold cream sometime around 200 AD and that "the product was used widely by Roman women as a beauty aid for aged and dry skin . . ." [8].

Times have not changed much despite the passage of several thousand years. Women of today might be surprised to learn that while their face products are touted as new and revolutionary, some of the concoctions used so long ago by their Greek and Roman sisters are similar to the currently popular moisturizing creams and lotions formulated with AHA. What a surprise to find the roots of our expensive moisturizers in the mixtures of Roman and Greek housewives!

2.3 Anglo-Saxons and the English

Hundreds of years later, the Anglo-Saxons developed moisturizing products they used specifically for their hands [5]. A recipe remains for a "hand cream" that included lily of the valley, old lard, and wine. The lily of the valley and lard were pounded together, heated with the wine, and worked into a mixture. Living in the damp and cold apparently caused many cases of dry, chapped hands.

During Elizabethan times lotions and ointments were prepared with "ass's milk, hog lard, honey and beeswax with added embellishments of cherries, rose petals and herbs" [5]. Elizabeth I is purported to have made many of her own cosmetics including a forehead cream with "a compound of posset curd" to remove wrinkles and a skin lotion from a concoction of "egg white, powdered egg shells, alum, borax and white poppy seeds" [5].

For the next several hundred years the majority of moisturizer-like preparations were made at home for personal use. During the 1800s, there was no cosmetic industry as we know it today. Some of the following account of the industry's growth comes from a recent excellent book entitled, *Hope In a Jar: The Making of America's Beauty Culture* [9]. During the 19th century cosmetics referred to creams and lotions that protected the face. These were the precursors of modern day facial moisturizers. Women basically had three choices during this period: home preparation, local druggist, and, somewhat less common, overseas sources and larger wholesale drug suppliers.

2.4 Twentieth Century

By the turn of the century "the era of soap and water, and the modest application of home-made face creams, was certainly at an end" [5]. At the same time, one of the first hand lotions to be introduced was Jergens Benzoin and Almond Lotion Compound, later to be known as Jergens Lotion. Initially the only mass-produced moisturizers were cold cream and vanishing cream [5]. Cold cream was used as a cleanser and moisturizer to restore dry, flaky skin. Vanishing cream, an emollient, served as a make-up base and also protected facial skin against moisture loss. The now legendary figure Helena Rubinstein opened her first beauty salon in London in 1908 selling a wide array of creams and lotions. She was followed by Elizabeth Arden, who in 1910 also opened a salon in New York. Both sold products claiming to provide the same benefits that today's women desire and will pay so dearly for—youthful complexions. It was at this stage that women were less interested in what could be purchased from their pharmacist than from beauty salons. As products became more effective an increased demand arose for better products; coupled with this, women were exerting a growing independence. By the end of World War I, cosmetics were readily available in Woolworths and other large department stores. The transition from "class to mass" took little time. By the 1930s the beauty industry was in full swing. Advertisements in the popular ladies magazines of the times such as *Ladies Home Journal* and *Good Housekeeping* promoted face products that offered smooth, soft skin. The introduction of television provided yet another opportunity for industry to reach the masses by promoting the latest skin care preparations. Manufacturers spent millions of dollars each year extolling the benefits of their latest moisturizing products.

Moisturizers of all types are literally used by millions of people around the globe every day. They are looking for many of the same benefits our ancestors did thousands of years ago. Only now, they have an endless array of choices with products that have been tested and retested among the correct user groups. As we enter the 21st century the buzzword is innovation. The keys to the new products of tomorrow are ingredients that work better and faster to provide healthy looking, moisturized skin.

3   MOISTURIZING TERMINOLOGY

3.1   Naive Consumers and Trained Sensory Panelists

To provide direction for product development, moisturizer terms or attributes must have actionable meanings. In other words, a pattern of ratings or scores must be convertible into one or more courses of action for the moisturizer formulation. When consumers rate products on attributes such as "silky" or "greasy" their definitions are culture dependent and are also affected by the product set with which they are familiar. The terms are fuzzy. There are core meanings plus many shadings or nuances radiating out from the center of the definition. Product development formulators learn with experience that certain changes in a moisturizer systematically move consumer ratings, even though no two participants in a large study may define the attributes identically.

In contrast, moisturizer terms when used by descriptive sensory panels have meanings defined through lengthy training with reference standards and rating scales [10,11]. "Spreadibility" has a technical and precise meaning that is not combined with other terms in the mind of the expert. Panelists strive to perform ratings as human machines, generating replicable sensory "signatures" for products, as well as providing detailed information in order for chemists to know the subtle differences that changes in a formula can make. The descriptive results are nonhedonic, that is, without reference to liking or skin benefit. A more detailed treatment of descriptive sensory panels and their unique terminology can be found in Sec. 4.2.2.

3.2 Hedonic Terminology

Like foods, moisturizers have a dual identity. They are experienced as functional as well as hedonic/"pleasure-giving" substances. It is clear that some lotions are positioned as more functional or therapeutic than others. Terminology or descriptors should then in turn emphasize the nuances of efficacy and skin healing. Conversely, the more hedonically focused or experiential lotions require a more detailed treatment of pleasure or emotive qualities. Traditionally, hedonic survey items such as overall liking or purchase intent are not seen as the purview of the trained sensory professional because of the "possibility of bias and resultant error in predicting consumer preferences" [12]. Enjoying a product and functioning as a dispassionate sensory machine are incompatible. As a result, sensory language related to experiential qualities is not nearly as developed as, say, texture or skin-feel properties. Fortunately, a new research discipline called hedonic psychology may in time rectify this by bringing attention to the experiential and improving our understanding of what makes some moisturizers pleasurable. In their edited collection launching the field, Kahnemann et al. [13] target psychology in general. They argue that pleasure and well-being are ignored topics. Consumer behavior is not addressed specifically. But they present some provocative findings that may in time find their way into consumer psychology to expand our understanding of the dimensions of liking and preference. One important inference from their work is that retrospective assessments of one's state of happiness or unhappiness (as measured by the standard post-product use questionnaire) are not as accurate as the moment-by-moment feelings experienced in real time as a product is used. This suggests a greater use of diaries or handheld microcassette recorders to capture what consumers feel. In the same volume, Stone et al. [14] argue for the use of "ecological momentary assessment," which entails the frequent probing of a consumer's feelings and mood states during the day as a product is used. They suggest data entry into portable computers but note that the feasibility depends upon a generous research budget.

4 TESTING

4.1 Study Objectives

Requests for consumer and sensory studies are made every day by marketing and formulation chemists in research and development eager to learn what consumers think of their latest products. In today's work environment, deadlines and budgets are invariably tight. A common reaction by many testing professionals is to conduct a test as quickly as possible, presumably meeting client needs without asking what the goal or objective is. However, the first reaction to any request should be to review the available information concerning all aspects of the test product so that the appropriate test can be designed. In today's fast-paced, cooperative business environment, it is important for the testing professional to be included as early as possible in discussions on development projects to create clearly defined objectives before consumer testing begins. Cooperation, good communication among team members, and the determination of correct methodology to meet test objectives are critical to achieve success. To think of consumer testing as a service group only to be involved when executing studies is a critical error because it does not allow for a program of systematic testing to be developed. It encourages a scattershot approach that is not an efficient testing strategy. The days of working in a vacuum are long gone. Snap judgments and general assumptions are a waste of time and may prove costly if studies are fielded without the total understanding and agreement of team members. Product testing has become a very expensive business. Budgets necessary to conduct the myriad studies required to support business goals have increased dramatically from the early days of solely going desk to desk asking for employee opinions. Budgets are wisely used when objectives are tailored to the phase of the development cycle.

Objectives for studies in the early development phase tend to be more broadly defined and focused on general product assessments such as overall acceptability and presence/absence of gross negatives (irritation). Later studies require more specific details about product characteristics and user groups. For example, "does product x produce a lower stinging (irritation) rate than product y" among women, 35–59 years old. Later studies may also address other important issues including performance relative to concept or a competitive product, or claim substantiations.

4.2 Methodology

Product testing methodologies used in the evaluation of skin moisturizers are built on a foundation established by decades of research in the food industry, about which so much has been written, especially in the area of sensory evaluation (see Ref. 15 for a historical review). Some texts now focus exclusively on the application of these well-established principles to cosmetics [16,17]. The selection of the appropriate test method for the evaluation of moisturizers depends on the development process phase. Generally speaking, discrimination testing precedes expert panels and naive consumer assessments.

4.2.1 Discrimination Testing

Discrimination testing is a sensory method used to determine if two products are distinguishable or not. In general, there are two types of discrimination tests: overall and attribute tests. In the overall discrimination tests, panelists consider all sensory characteristics in making a judgment. Therefore, the response reflects overall differences and similarities between products. In contrast, the more focused attribute discrimination tests zero in on a person's ability to detect differences between products on a particular attribute, for instance, the difference between two products in speed of rub-in. In most projects, the overall discrimination tests are used to determine if, overall, two products are similar or different. Attribute tests are used only when there is a specific interest in an attribute. Caution must be taken when designing and interpreting attribute tests. The researcher has to be careful in choosing the attribute, since panelists will be asked to concentrate on only that one attribute. In addition, results have to be analyzed carefully. If two products are not found to be different in one attribute test (e.g., greasiness), it should not be implied that they are not different overall. There may be other attributes (e.g., fragrance intensity, shininess) that may differentiate the two products.

The two most popular discrimination methods are the triangle and duo-trio tests. In the standard triangle test, two of the samples are the same and one is different. The task is to select the odd product. In a duo-trio test, one product is identified as the reference. The participant is asked to pick which of the remaining two samples is the same as the reference. Other methods include the two-out-of-five test, A–not A test, difference from control test, etc. [18]. The selection of the test depends on the desired type of response [nominal data (yes/no) or degree of difference], limitations on the number of product applications/evaluations to reach a judgment, etc.

When designing and interpreting discrimination tests, the researcher needs to assess if the interest is in finding a difference or similarity between products. In the past, all discrimination tests were handled as difference tests. One has to be aware that in projects such as ingredient and process substitution, discrimination tests should be handled as similarity tests (i.e., to protect against committing Type II error—incorrectly declaring that samples are indistinguishable when in fact they are different) [18].

Discrimination tests are classified as analytical/laboratory tests. Traditionally, panelists/discriminators are used to participate in these tests [11,18]. A screening process should be followed either prior to participation or once panelists have participated in series of tests to insure that panelists participating in these tests are discriminators [11]. There are some companies that have used naive consumers as judges for discrimination tests. However, there are many criticisms within the sensory community as to the use of consumers in discrimination tests. This debate will continue until research proves that consumers can reliably participate in these tests.

4.2.2 Descriptive Panels

Definitions and Importance. Moisturizers are frequently tested by descriptive/attribute panels to characterize their appearance, fragrance, and skin-feel characteristics. Descriptive analysis is one of the most complex and involved sensory tests used in the evaluation of personal care products. This technique is used by a trained panel to qualitatively and quantitatively characterize the perceived sensory attributes of a product (i.e., evaluate the intensity of perceived attributes in the product) [11,19]. In the case of moisturizers, the evaluated sensory dimensions include appearance, fragrance, and skin-feel characteristics. Descriptive analysis results provide information not obtained though other methods. For example, descriptive tests provide technical and specific information on perceived attributes and their intensities, free of (or minimally influenced by) psychological errors (halo effect, stimulus error, etc.) and personal preferences.

History and Current Skin-feel Descriptive Methods. All current skin-feel descriptive evaluations of moisturizers and other personal care products are based on the modified texture profile method [20]. In this method, the concepts of the food texture profile method [21,22] were adapted to the evaluation of skin care products. Schwartz [20] classified the main stages of evaluation of skin care products as pick-up (the removal of the product from the container), rub-out (the application of the products to the skin), and after-feel (the evaluation of the effect of the product on the skin). This pioneering work was adapted by all professionals working in skin-feel evaluations for their specific applications. A milestone in descriptive skin-feel evaluation occurred when the standard practice for descriptive skin-feel analysis of creams and lotions was published by the ASTM committee E18 on sensory evaluation [23]. The techniques published in the ASTM standard are also based on the modified texture profile method for skin care product evaluations [20]. Currently most personal care products companies base their descriptive skin-feel evaluations on this methodology. Table 1 details many of the sensory attributes that should be considered in moisturizer evaluation.

Panels. The evaluation of product attributes and intensities requires the use of a panel, or group of trained individuals. Names given to panels involved in descriptive/attribute evaluations include descriptive, expert, attribute, and experienced panels.

Descriptive and expert panels. Used interchangeably by some professionals to describe the same panel type, a descriptive or expert panel is a group of individuals who have undergone a formal and rigorous training [24–27]. This panel evaluates products following common established procedures. The term "descriptive panel" is preferred over "expert panel." The latter often connotes those professionals who are experts on specific products who have acquired their expertise through their continuous exposure to products and product evaluations. Frequently these experts work alone/independently and have not participated in a group training.

Table 1 Appearance and Skin-Feel Descriptive Attributes for Lotions and Creams, Including Moisturizers

Product Delivery	After 6, 9, 12, and 15 rubs:
Immediate:	Thermal melting
Ease of dispensing	Spreadability
Amount of spread	Whitening (when applicable)
Integrity of shape (thickness)	When applicable:
After 10 s:	Chemical warm
Integrity of shape (thickness)	Thermal cool
Amount of spread	Chemical cool
Smoothness (appearance of surface)	Tingle
Gloss	Absorbency
Pick-up evaluation	*After-feel evaluation*
Amount of peaking	Gloss
Firmness	Slipperiness
Stickiness	Film residue (waxy, greasy, oily)
Stringiness	Moisture
Denseness	Stickiness/tackiness
Rub-out evaluation	When applicable:
After 3 rubs:	Cool
Thermal melting	Warm
Spreadability	Burn
Wetness	Tingle
Thickness	Tautness
Denseness	
Thermal cooling	

Source: Ref. 23.

> *Attribute panel.* This is a group of individuals who have only been trained on specific product attributes. That is, this panel is not trained to evaluate all attributes that characterize the product category, but only a few attributes of interest. Attribute panels are trained for specific applications when the complete product characterization is not needed. These applications may be for shelf-life/stability, quality control, or claim support evaluations.
>
> *Experienced/semi-trained panel.* This is a group of individuals who either have not participated in a training program but are experienced in product evaluations or a group that has undergone a very general training program. When no training is involved, the panelists have become experienced through their frequent participation in product evaluations. This often occurs when consumers have participated in frequent consumer

product evaluations and become experienced through this frequent product assessment. Experienced/semi-trained panels should only be used for product screening purposes, not for formal and important product evaluations. Frequently, experienced panels participate in a formal training program and become trained descriptive panels. This training is generally shorter and simpler than a training with naive panelists, since the experienced panelists have acquired considerable product experience.

4.2.3 Descriptive Characterization of Moisturizers

Appearance and Skin-Feel Attributes.   When experts evaluate moisturizers, they divide the characteristics into four categories that depend on the time course of the lotion application event. Table 1 shows these categories, which are

Product delivery (e.g., ease of dispensing, amount of spread)
Pick-up evaluation (e.g., firmness, stickiness, denseness)
Rub-out evaluation (e.g., wetness, spreadability)
After-feel characteristics (e.g., gloss, residual film, tautness)

See ASTM Standard Practice E 1490–92 [23] for a detailed description of procedures and attributes.

Fragrance Attributes.   The fragrance evaluations for moisturizers are completed in two ways. The fragrance submissions are evaluated by themselves (i.e., not in the product) or in the product. When evaluated by themselves, the fragrances are evaluated in glass containers. When the fragrance is evaluated in the product, it is applied and the fragrance is sniffed on the skin. The panel can be trained to evaluate basic fragrance/odor attributes or complete fragrance profiles. When a panel is trained on basic fragrance notes, the attributes may include overall fragrance, overall base odors, and off-odors. Panelists may be asked to describe the character of the fragrance. This information is only qualitative.

A panel can be trained to recognize and score specific fragrance characters. The evaluations can be general and address main fragrance components (e.g., floral, fruity) or address specific notes within each category (e.g., rose, carnation, white flower, violet). Table 2 shows an example of fragrance/odor categories that a panel can be trained on [28].

Establishing a Descriptive Panel.   The establishment of a descriptive capability for the evaluation of moisturizers requires management support, the building or procurement of testing facilities, and the recruitment/selection and training of the panel. Many sources [10,11,24–27] provide thorough coverage of how to set up and train a descriptive panel.

Applications and Uses of Descriptive/Attribute Data.   The main applications of this type of data are

TABLE 2 Examples of Fragrance/Odor Categories

Citrus	Nutty
Coconut, almond	Leather
Non-citrus fruit	Rubber
Cool	Green
Minty	Burnt
Caraway	Brown
Anise	Sulfidic
Floral	Spicy
Woody	Animal/foul
Fishy	Solvent

Source: Adapted from Ref. 28.

Documentation of sensory properties. The data provide a product "finger-print" of the sensory properties of moisturizers. This is crucial in the characterization of controls, prototypes, and competitor products.

Screening of moisturizers. Products may be screened based on specific sensory attributes (i.e., spreadability, absorbency).

Product maintenance. Descriptive/attribute data are used to track product characteristics of moisturizers in shelf-life studies and during production (quality control) and to assess differences from and similarities to controls in ingredient/process substitution and cost reduction projects.

Product guidance/optimization. Descriptive/attribute data are used to guide developers in the development, reformulation, and optimization of moisturizers. Descriptive/attribute analysis provides information on the perceived attributes of moisturizers, which are developed and/or modified in the formulation/reformulation of products.

Consumer test design. Descriptive/attribute analysis provides attribute information on the moisturizers to be evaluated. This information is used to determine the best test design (e.g., product presentation/rotation) and for questionnaire development.

Identification of drivers of liking. Descriptive/attribute data allow the identification of attributes that drive/affect the acceptance of moisturizers when coordinated with consumer hedonic data.

Interpretation of consumer information. Descriptive/attribute data provide information on the product attributes that are considered by consumers in rating attributes, thus allowing the interpretation of consumer responses.

Supportive information for claim support. Data support a claim on specific perceived product attributes and product performance.

Upon completion of the experts' efforts the next step is evaluation using naive consumers.

4.2.4 Naive Consumer Tests

Testing with consumers falls into two categories: qualitative and quantitative. In qualitative studies, inferences are drawn from patterns in the ideas or opinions offered by consumers. In quantitative evaluation, recommendations are based on statistical inferences from product ratings. Results from consumer testing of moisturizers are only as good as the recruitment and screening process used to select study participants.

For naive consumer testing, the counterpart to expert training is the careful screening for the appropriate moisturizer user. The complete set of questions used to qualify or disqualify a study participant is termed a screener. Typically, a screener probes demographics, habits, and attitudes; personality or cognitive characteristics; lifestyle; and routine background items such as whether one works for a market research firm or has taken part in a consumer study in the past six months.

When consumers qualify for a study, it is a good practice to reconfirm that they qualify by asking key screening questions at the time products are picked up. It is disconcerting but common for the question "what is your one most frequently used brand of facial moisturizer" to be answered inconsistently from one week to the next.

Qualitative Testing. Qualitative research provides a forum for people to express in their own words what moisturizers mean to them as well as what effect they have on dry skin. All the emotion, logic, free association, and irrational thought that may be behind the checkmark in the answer box is revealed by qualitative research.

Focus Groups Principles. The focus group is the best known technique for gaining qualitative insight into consumer attitudes. It can be used to generate product ideas, new product benefits, weaknesses in current products, as well as to understand how people think about brand categories, advertising, product usage habits, product concepts, and much more. There is no substitute for real discussions with people. Qualitative research typically precedes quantitative especially when the project is about new products. However, an effective project often winds back and forth between the two types of research, each benefiting the other. Focus groups confirm and expand on the statistically derived conclusions of survey research. They also help to sharpen surveys by highlighting the terminology actually used by people discussing products.

Focus group leaders should reconfirm the qualifications of participants on key criteria before the sessions begin. Some people should be kept on-hand as "alternates" by over-recruiting the group. That is, invite more people than the number of available seats in case some potential participants need to be disqualified at the last minute.

Guidelines for the conduct of effective qualitative research are readily found [29–31]. Many are basic rules of civil conduct. Examples are talk in turns, listen to what it said by others, allow people to hold their own opinions.

Focus groups are conducted with 8–10 participants per group. Sessions last 90–120 minutes. The moderator follows a discussion guide preapproved by the project team. Discussions that are even more focused can be achieved with one-on-ones, so-called because only a moderator and one participant are present. One-on-ones can remove the influence of a dominating or bullying focus group member. Other variations that fall between full focus groups and one-on-ones are possible and have unique benefits. For example, two-on-ones (two participants, one moderator) might enable a panelist and a friend to discuss their differences in shopping strategy or how they hear about interesting new products from one another.

When properly conducted, qualitative research can provide a wealth of information to help guide a project. It can be used to clarify and understand the terms that people actually use to describe moisturizers and their effects on the skin, to understand how people categorize products in a given segment, and, most typically for the r&d environment, to learn what people think of one or more prototypes. On this last point, since prototypes often go through several phases of refinement before launch, focus groups can be a powerful tool when they include an iterative component. Inviting the same people back to evaluate and discuss successive improvements can show what it takes, in microcosm, to win over an audience. Caution though should be exercised here. Generalizing to the population from a small sample of people in a qualitative setting is not appropriate.

INNOVATIVE TECHNIQUES. The insight and creativity derived from a focus group is a joint product of the participants and the techniques the moderator uses to engage the imagination. To recruit qualified research participants requires more than screening for the appropriate category users. Personality and cognitive skills factor in also. There are screening tools for finding people who like to think [32] or who are open to novel products [33,34]. Less formal methods are also possible. Lists of creative people can be compiled by a nomination process, that is, regularly asking study participants to identify friends who they view as creative, trend-setting, off-beat, etc. The use of projective techniques and metaphor [35] are tools the moderator should employ to make the two hours enjoyable and entertaining to the participants as well as productive for the project team. An example of such a technique is "brainwriting" [36]. The moderator asks people to write down a new product idea or improvement. The piece of paper gets passed to the next person who builds on the idea and so on around the room.

OBSERVATIONAL STUDIES. While focus groups and one-on-one interviews free people from the constraints of a product survey, they still have limitations. The focus group or testing facility, as comfortable as it may be, extracts people away from the natural context in which products are used. The consumer researcher is thus cut off from seeing how and where the product fits in with other products and routines. The solution is to talk to people in their home and observe them as they use health and beauty products such as moisturizers. This option fits within the growing movement in consumer research to utilize ethnographic techniques to more fully understand people and their products. Most associated with the field of anthropology, ethnography involves "participating, overtly or covertly, in people's daily lives for an extended period of time, watching what happens, listening to what is said, asking questions—in fact, collecting whatever data are available to throw light on the issues that are the focus of the research" [37]. The resultant account, which can be captured on video, may be as realistic as a straightforward documentary or quite impressionistic and personal [38]. Either way, the ethnographic approach endeavors to create "thick descriptions" [39] which capture the particulars of the habit or product regimen in all its richness. The application of moisturizers may be embedded in a series of personal care and cleansing events which give it deeper meaning. As well, the physical product itself may be stored in ways that illuminate the range of cognitive categories it falls within. It is hard to glean this information without the ethnographic tools.

PHOTOGRAPHIC TECHNIQUES.   Unfortunately for the consumer researcher on a tight budget or timetable, observational research may not often be feasible. Luckily, the advent of inexpensive disposable cameras has been a boon. Moisturizer users can be given the cameras and asked to photograph the physical layout of their products on the shelf or vanity as well as to document product usage with the help of a willing family member stationed behind the lens. These pictures can be brought to a focus group, photocopied, discussed, and organized. While there is a risk that the photographs may be "posed" or self-selected, the consumer should be encouraged to "flesh out" the story behind the image to reveal what was left out, if anything. These photographs could also be circulated around the focus group in brainwriting fashion [36].

THE INTERNET.   Various projections put U.S. on-line consumer spending in 2000 at $38–61 billion [40]. As a tool for both quantitative and qualitative investigations of consumer behavior, the internet is having a similarly enormous impact though the field is still in its infancy, and there have been difficulties assimilating on-line research into traditional market research organizations [41]. Regardless, it is clear how the internet is being harnessed to consumer research objectives. Some of the uses include

> Consumers are being encouraged to visit a company or product website. There, they register, complete a personal profile, and agree to participate in future testing/surveys. A database can thus be created from which a test sample can be drawn for the testing of moisturizer products or concepts.
>
> Personal care companies contract with an outside agency that can create an

on-line chat about product or concepts between a moderator and registered consumers who fit the relevant screening criteria.

Consumer researchers create and post a survey to be completed on-line by
registered members.

There are many clear plusses for internet research: feedback is immediate; nar-
rowly defined niche markets can be more easily tapped; and it offers participants
the freedom to complete surveys when they want—at 3 am if they desire! Negatives are the lingering uncertainty about who exactly is completing the survey,
whether it is being completed independently, and the projectability of the opinions of the on-line audience to the target of, say, mass market hand and body lotion users. Clearly, the growth of on-line accounts points to a time when internet
users will more closely reflect national demographics, rather than a limited, more
educated, upscale audience. Once qualitative investigations are complete, projects normally progress to quantitative research.

Quantitative Test Methods. One of the advantages of the quantitative
study is the completion of a standardized product questionnaire by all respon-
dents to reach statistically based conclusions. Aside from an open-ended question
such as "what did you like or dislike about the product?" the questionnaire contains primarily closed-ended items using terminology and rating scales selected
by the researcher.

Table 3 shows some quantitative designs and several variants on the sequential option. These are defined by how many surveys are used, when they are
given, and what sorts of questions they contain. For example, in the paired preference procedure, two products are used but there is no survey until after the second usage period. The questions are entirely about preference for one product or
the other.

The choice of a monadic or sequential test design is more than just a decision about how products are assigned to consumers. Each design actually mirrors
a real-world encounter with products. The compatibility of the test objective with
that encounter should be considered when selecting a design. The monadic design
is more reflective of normal product use. People rarely use two different brands
simultaneously, in alternation, or in quick succession for purposes of comparison.
Monadic presentation is also aligned with an encounter with a dramatic "breakthrough" type product. There is no regular brand on the shelf and none is provided as context in the study. The sequential design, in contrast, is aligned with a
product substitution, upgrade, or brand switching experience. For example, sup-
pose a company plans to substitute a new, improved, or less expensive moisturizer for a currently marketed product. The shopping experience of the loyal consumer of that brand will, at some point, be the use of the current variant followed
by its replacement when the new variant is purchased. The sequential monadic
design reflects or recreates that shopping experience. Half the participants use the

TABLE 3 Research Designs for the Quantitative Assessment
of Moisturizers

Design name	Characteristics
Monadic	One product per person
	Survey after product use
Sequential monadic	Two (or more) products used in sequence for equal amounts of time
	Balanced order of presentation
	Complete survey for all products, including attribute and overall preference
Proto-monadic	Two products used in sequence for equal amounts of time
	Balanced order of presentation
	Complete survey for first product
	Preference questions in second survey
	May also include acceptance questions
Paired preference (sequential presentation)	Two products in sequence for equal amounts of time
	Balanced order of presentation
	No survey after completion of first product, only after both products are used
Paired preference (simultaneous presentation)	Two products used simultaneously on half the body or face
	Product presentation balanced for side of application
	Preference questions after both products are used; additional diagnostic items may be included

current control followed by the new prototype. Of course, in a balanced design, half the people get the products in reverse order: new followed by current. This does not correspond to reality, as mentioned earlier (except, for example, when an old familiar product like Coke Classic is brought back after the introduction of New Coke). It is included to tease apart product from order effects. One alternative to the balanced sequential design is to employ a two-cell monadic design in which all study participants are screened to be current users of the brand of moisturizer in question. The monadic assessments of the new formula will now implicitly be with reference to that regular brand. In addition, a direct question "how does the product you used compare with your regular brand?" may also be included.

TESTING LOCATIONS. Generally speaking, quantitative testing is conducted either in the consumers' homes or at a testing facility, called a central location. In-home testing most approximates real life extended use. In contrast, the central location test evaluates a product often used only once, but most importantly allows the investigator the opportunity to observe product use. Frequently, the research question does not require extended use by the consumer. In these circumstances, the central location test is all that is needed to answer the research question.

QUESTIONNAIRE DESIGN. Regardless of where the test is conducted, the quality of the information collected hinges on the development of a suitable questionnaire. Much has been written on this topic (see, for example, Ref. 42), but a good questionnaire should comprise the following kinds of questions:

> *Hedonic*. Overall, how much do you like this product? How much do you like this product for _____ (attribute)?
>
> *Open ended*. What, if anything, is there about this product that you like?
>
> *Attributes*. Ratings of attributes on a 5- or 7-point "excellent-to-poor" scale, for example, rub-in, silkiness, greasiness, softness, smoothness.
>
> *Agree/disagree items*. Is a fragrance for someone just like me? Is a moisturizer for a contemporary woman?
>
> *Directional/intensity*. Using a "just about right" scale, for example, "too thin," "just about right," "too thick"; or a unipolar intensity scale such as "not at all greasy" to "much too greasy."
>
> *Comparison to regular brand*. A scale that typically includes "much better" and "much worse" at the extremes and "equal to" in the middle.
>
> *Uniqueness*. A scale anchored by "similar to all others" at one end and "similar to no others" at the other end.
>
> *Preference* Which product did you prefer overall? (Only appropriate if more than one product is being tested.)

When developing the questionnaire the researcher has to be careful to include terms that consumers understand and scale rating points that make sense intuitively to the average consumer. Questionnaires should also be formatted for clarity and ease of use by the consumer.

IMPROVING TEST SENSITIVITY. One factor in the decision to select one research design over another is the test's ability to detect product differences. For example, when a cost reduction is being considered, the happy outcome is that consumers not notice the difference in esthetics, efficacy, fragrance, etc. It is easier to "prove" product parity if people are not given sufficient opportunity to detect the difference, as when the product usage period is too short. In contrast, when difference detection is desired, extending the usage period or employing the half-body procedure is recommended. The half-body technique improves sensitivity because both products are experienced nearly simultaneously. Product A is applied to the left side and product B to the right for half the sample, and the other half receive the reverse order. Whatever differences there are can be perceived without the distorting effects of the passage of time or the presence of intervening events that are part of a sequential design by definition.

COMPLIANCE. The chances of obtaining reliable data are enhanced when measures are taken to check that participants follow procedures and understand directions. For example, the half-body procedure places some added compliance burdens on the research participant, especially in a home-use test. Participants must be instructed to keep the products separate or not to mix the products. Yet people may not easily comply with a cross-handed product application instruction (put product A in right hand and apply to left side of body; do reverse for product B) when using products at home. The technique should be demonstrated before products are taken home or the first application occasion should be in the testing facility under the observation of a project team member. Such controls are typical of a central location test (CLT), where the entire study takes place at an independent test facility rather than at home (home-use test; HUT). A CLT is monitored by a member of the project team or a briefed employee of the CLT agency. They ensure that the participant is attending to the products as instructed by being present during product usage.

Compliance in another sense is somewhat easier to monitor. This is use-up compliance which is accomplished by a product weight check. Did the consumer use the moisturizer twice a day for four weeks? The product should be weighed before and after a home usage period to ascertain that the samples were actually used sufficiently. This requires that product developers provide to consumer researchers a "reasonable" dose value. Calculations will then establish a lower bound for product use-up. People who used less than that amount should be discarded from the data analysis.

SEASONALITY. The time of year and regional climate affects the efficacy of moisturizers. If the usage and purchase frequency of hand lotions drops in the summer, tests relating to therapeutic benefits, such as relief of dry, chapped skin, should be delayed until the winter months or perhaps relocated to a dry climate. Testing in the wrong season limits the ability to see product differences.

4.3 Data Analysis

Sensory and consumer responses collected in moisturizer studies are analyzed statistically to enable separation of random from real treatment effects.

4.3.1 Summary Statistics and Graphical Representation

Prior to applying any statistical tests, it is advisable to summarize data and complete some simple diagnostic and/or graphical analyses to assess the nature of the data [43]. Basic summary statistics for continuous data may include sample size, average, ranges, standard deviation and other deviation measures, skewness measures, interquartile range, etc. Graphical representations are used to observe certain data characteristics of interest. The researcher may choose graphs such as stem leaf, boxplot, data distributions (number or percent of observations/scores), bar, radar/spiderplot, and other charts to display data.

These summary statistics and graphs provide simple and revealing information of the data to be analyzed. The outcome of some statistical tests may be anticipated through this assessment. In addition, these simple summaries and graphs provide preliminary information on the data to help decide on the statistical analysis to apply. For example, a simple distribution graph displaying the percentage of observations across a scale indicates if the data distribution is uni- or multimodal. Data that are not unimodal should not be analyzed through parametric statistics.

4.3.2 Common Statistical Analyses for Sensory and Consumer Data

This topic is covered extensively in the literature. The books describe the characteristics of the basic statistical tests used to analyze sensory and consumer data [44,45]. Sensory/consumer research publications cover the topic specifically for the data collected in sensory/consumer studies of consumer products, including moisturizers [11,18,46,47].

Analysis for Treatment Effects and Panelist Performance. The analysis completed on the sensory and consumer data from moisturizers and other consumer products may have two objectives: to study treatment effects or to study panelist performance. Routinely, upon completion of a consumer, descriptive/attribute, or discrimination test, data analyses are completed to reach conclusions about product or sample treatment effects [11]. For example, analyses on treatment effects may address questions such as Are two moisturizers, control and product A, equally liked? or Is one significantly better liked over the other? or Does one moisturizer spread significantly easier than another? or Is the competitor's moisturizer and product X perceived significantly differently when applied on the skin? All these questions deal with product or attribute differences/similarities. The statistical tests for each data type [18,19,48–50] address these questions related to treatment effects (or product attributes).

Practitioners who work with trained or semi-trained panelists to evaluate attributes and attribute intensities do need to analyze the data with an additional objective. This objective is to learn about panelist performance. These analyses are conducted on a routine basis to monitor panelists, assure that their responses are valid and reliable, and ensure that sound product conclusions are obtained. Panelist monitoring analyses investigate ability of panelists to (1) find significant differences if differences exist, (2) replicate their own judgments, (3) agree with the rest of the panel as far as the direction of product differences, and (4) match intensity references (if used). Different statistical procedures for panel monitoring have been and continue to be developed [51–54].

5 APPLICATIONS

Sensory and consumer testing methods have many applications. It would be impossible to cover all applications and with the detail each application deserves. A summary of the main applications are discussed.

5.1 Product Matching

Product matching projects are very common in any industry. Testing conducted for these projects assesses if a prototype matches a control. This control can be the competition, the "gold standard," or the current product. Product matching projects can be completed either through discrimination or descriptive tests. Discrimination tests indicate if, overall, products are sufficiently similar or different. Descriptive tests will, in addition, provide information on the attributes that differentiate products, if they are found to be different.

Discrimination tests are conducted if the interest is only in overall difference/similarity (as the first step), when there are a few products to test, and when enough panelists are available. Similarity tests should be conducted for matching projects, which require a large number of panelists [55]. The testing of fragrances in moisturizers is commonly completed using discrimination tests.

The testing of a match for skin-feel characteristics of moisturizers is most commonly conducted using descriptive tests. Since skin-feel properties require time intensity or assessment at different stages (e.g., immediate and 5- and 10-minute evaluations, etc.), discrimination tests may not be as useful.

5.2 Assessment of Differences and Similarities

There are many projects where the differences and similarities among moisturizers need to be determined. These evaluations are conducted when comparing the company's current product to competition, a new formula, different prototypes that encompass new packaging materials, ingredients, process variables, etc.

Ultimately, companies are interested in determining the differences (or lack thereof) in liking between and among products. Frequently, a company may conduct a consumer study to test the differences and similarities between the control and test samples/prototypes as perceived by consumers without completing any other tests. Although this test strategy is sound and followed by many companies, it may not be the most efficient approach.

The use of sensory tests (e.g., discrimination and descriptive tests) prior to a consumer test represents a more efficient testing strategy, since the former are usually less expensive and can have a faster turnaround time. The rationale in using such tests first is to assess the differences and similarities in perception, then make a decision if an ensuing consumer test is needed. In addition, the discriminative or descriptive tests provide information on the products to be tested and thus aid in designing a better consumer study (e.g., in guiding decisions on sample presentation strategy, attributes in the consumer questionnaire, etc.).

For example, a descriptive test is conducted first if the objective is to confirm that a perceivable difference exists between a new formula and the control (or a new formula and the competition) and to characterize the difference(s). If the descriptive tests show that there are no differences or not large enough difference(s), a recommendation is given to reformulate the product before conducting a more expensive and involved consumer test. If a trained panel does not find a difference, a consumer will not find the difference nor indicate a difference in liking or preference. If the descriptive panel finds a difference, the consumer test can be conducted to explore how consumers react to the perceived difference(s). This sequence of testing represents an effective test strategy. In addition, the complete data set—the descriptive information and the consumer reaction to the differences—can then be put together to interpret data, make decisions, and provide recommendations.

5.3 Research Guidance and Optimization

Sensory and consumer test methods are widely used for research guidance in the development of new products. Formulators/researchers are interested in studying the effect of certain variables (e.g., ingredients, technologies, packaging, and processes) on the product's perceived properties and consumer responses. Ultimately, the goal is to develop the best liked product in the category or within the limits of the raw materials and technologies used. Formulators/researchers need to obtain guidance in case products need to be reformulated. This guidance is provided either using the consumer diagnostic information or the descriptive/attribute information linked with the consumer information (see Sec. 5.5).

Research guidance can be provided in two ways: (1) through individual sample evaluation (one-at-a-time approach) or (2) through designed experiments, where a set of products is produced to represent variables and ranges of interest. From the experimental point of view the first type of study is called a nondesigned experiment or one-way treatment structure study; the latter is called a design experiment, treatment structure, or optimization study [56,57].

5.3.1 Nondesigned Experiments

Nondesigned experiments are very common in industry and are used to test a series of products either in a sensory or consumer study. The products are a set of qualitatively distinct objects, having no particular association among themselves. In such tests, the products tested may include the company's products, a few commercial products, and one or more prototypes. There is no association among themselves in the formula, package, performance, etc.

These experiments are favored by those companies that require the testing of a series of products with fast turnaround and do not want to or cannot invest the time, effort, and funds to systematically produce samples following an experimental design and do not want to or cannot test the larger number of products generated by designed experimental plans. The design and execution of these tests is relatively simple, since samples are produced, purchased, or collected and then tested.

Once the test is completed, results are analyzed through statistical procedures which indicate if the products are different and how they are different in the response measured (e.g., liking, oiliness, glossiness). No inferences can be made on the effect of one variable or concentration on the response measured. Often, if analytical data (e.g., sensory or any instrumental measure) are collected, they are related to liking or any other consumer response (e.g., greasiness). A relationship can be build between the consumer response (e.g., liking or greasiness) and the descriptively perceived attributes (e.g., greasy, oily, waxy) or the concentration of a certain variable (if measured or known for all samples). Even though these relationships can be built, the interpretation of results may not be clear, since variables may be confounded and not cover the complete intensity ranges [58].

5.3.2 Designed Experiments

A most effective way to study the effect of variables (or factors) on a response is to use experimental designs to produce the set of samples/prototypes that represent specific variables and levels. These prototypes are then tested (e.g., in a descriptive or consumer study), and the results can be analyzed to accurately infer the effect of such variables on the response (e.g., liking), on the way the response varies as a function of the variable studied (if and how the response increases or decreases with increasing concentrations/levels of the variables), and on an optimal (if any) combination of variables to achieve the lowest or highest response [57].

For example, an optimization study for moisturizers may include two variables such as the amount of aloe and sunflower seed oil. An experimental plan is then used to determine the samples that need to be produced to represent specific combinations and concentrations of these variables. The prototypes are then tested (e.g., in a consumer study). Results (e.g., liking) are analyzed statistically vis-a-vis the nature of the experimental design. Models can be developed and results can be displayed in graphs or plots that show the relationship of the response variable (e.g., liking) as a function of the concentration and combination of the two variables studied.

Common plans or treatment structures used in consumer product tests are factorial treatment structures and response surface structures (RSM) [56]. Many designed approaches and optimization studies have been predominantly published in the food industry [56–61]

5.4   Claim Support

Clinical claims are addressed in the next chapter. Here, the focus is on consumer-based claims. The application of sensory and consumer methods is essential in claim support projects. Advertising claims most often address perceived product attributes and/or differences as perceived by consumers or trained panelists. Therefore, no sensory related claim can be substantiated without the use of these methods. This area is of particular importance to a company not only because proper claim support testing provides the basis for sound advertising claims, but also for the legal implication that may result from unsupported claims. Being such a critical application of sensory/consumer methods, the ASTM committee E18 on sensory evaluation formed a task group to document the design and implementation of sound sensory and consumer testing practices geared to validate claims addressing sensory properties [62]. The most important step in a claim support study is to delineate an explicit statement of what the claim will be. This statement will in fact dictate the type of testing strategy to follow. Most claim support studies are completed with consumers, even if they deal with perceived attributes (e.g., "our product leaves your skin feeling softer than brand X"). However, much claims support testing is completed using discriminative/laboratory tests. When these tests are used, they are intended to provide more objective data regarding perceived attributes without regard for personal preference.

5.4.1   Consumer-Based Claim Support Testing

Consumer-Based Claims.   Consumer-based claims can be tested stating a hedonic/liking or a perceived attribute responses. These claims can be comparative and noncomparative. In addition, comparative claims can be parity or superiority claims [62]. Examples of each of these claims follow:

> *Comparative/parity.* Our product is as well liked as product A. Our product is as moisturizing as product C.
> *Comparative/superiority.* Our product is preferred over any other product. Our product leaves your skin looking more radiant than product D.
> *Noncomparative.* Our product leaves your skin feeling soft. Our product is gentle to your skin.

Consumer Studies for Claim Support.   Consumer studies designed to support claims need to be carefully designed and executed. Special attention needs to be paid to sample size [57], product selection, and questionnaire design.

5.4.2 Discriminative/Laboratory-Based Claim Support Testing

The two discriminative/laboratory tests used in claim support are discrimination (e.g., duo-trio, attribute difference tests) and descriptive tests [62]. Discrimination tests are used when information needs to be collected regarding the overall (or attribute) difference/similarity between products. Usually, claim support studies use discrimination tests to obtain additional back-up information, but not exclusively to support a claim. Descriptive tests are more commonly used, since they address attribute perception.

Descriptive-Based Claims. Descriptive-based claims have the following characteristics compared to consumer-based claims: (1) they do not address preference and acceptance/liking and (2) they address attribute perception by a highly trained panel. The attributes are not consumer terms (gentle, silky, moisturizing, radiant), but technical and descriptive, as described in Sec. 3.1 (oily, greasy, spreadable, sticky, dense, taut). Frequently, descriptive information is collected in claim support studies only as supportive information for the claim. The concurrent consumer study may address the advertisement claim per se. However, the claim becomes much stronger if the consumer results are supported by the descriptive information.

Examples of comparative and noncomparative claims based on descriptive information include

Comparative/parity. Our product is as absorbent as product C.
Comparative/superiority. Our product is less greasy than product D.
Noncomparative. Our product leaves a cool sensation on your skin.

Descriptive Studies for Claim Support. As with consumer tests, special attention has to be paid to the test design and test parameters of a descriptive study for claim support. The product selection and acquisition needs to be carefully completed. Unique aspects of descriptive studies to be controlled are

Trained panel. Descriptive evaluations for claim support have to be completed by a highly trained and calibrated panel.
Test design and ballot development. The attributes evaluated only have to address those attributes related to the claim. All descriptive attributes do not need to be measured. The sample preparation and presentation needs to be carefully controlled.
Test execution and replications. The evaluations are completed following strict and controlled protocols. If appropriate, references are reviewed prior to the study to calibrate the panel. No claim support evaluation should be conducted without an assurance that the panel is well trained and calibrated. In addition, the study needs to be replicated to be able to confirm adequate panelist performance.

5.5   Category Appraisals

A category appraisal or review is one of the most fascinating projects conducted by a consumer products company. In these projects, a product category is evaluated to assess differences and similarities among products in the category. The study usually includes the main commercial products within the category, the company's products, and sometimes prototypes.

Category appraisals are conducted (1) only with consumer data (traditional category reviews) or (2) both with consumer and analytical data (e.g., descriptive and instrumental) as in multifaceted category research studies [53]. In general, the main benefit of the individual category studies is the documentation of the differences and similarities among products which yield an understanding of the category. The consumer category study provides information on the differences and similarities among products in liking and consumer-perceived attributes [63]. The laboratory category study provides information on the differences and similarities among products in the properties measured. If the laboratory data are descriptive, these results show the differences and similarities in perceived attributes by a trained panel. There are many benefits and applications when studies in both categories are completed. The most important applications are [64]

1. The determination of drivers for liking (in descriptive terms) to provide actionable and clear direction to researchers in the formulation and reformulation of acceptable products within the category.
2. The interpretation and understanding of consumer responses.
3. The establishment of a system in which laboratory data can be used to infer consumer responses.

5.6   Irritation

Some facial moisturizers, especially those containing AHA, produce skin irritation or an "adverse reaction." Typical descriptive terminology includes tingling, stinging, burning, rashing, pulling, tightness, and itchiness. Consumer research projects are frequently motivated by a need to know whether the obtained irritation rate is below a pre-established action standard level or whether an ingredient change is effective at reducing irritation levels.

5.6.1   Measurement Issues

Asking about and accurately measuring irritation is a delicate issue. On the one hand, simply raising the issue by including irritation items on a survey may clue the consumer into certain expectations of the project and create an inflated rate of such comments via a self-fulfilling prophecy type effect. On the other hand, including relevant questions or warning of possible irritation reactions provides a context for understanding the product. A respondent is told that some level of ir-

Q.1. Did you experience any pleasant or unpleasant skin sensations from the product?

>Yes ( ) Continue
>No ( ) Skip to next question

Q.1A What did you experience? _____

Q.1B Where did you experience it? _____

Q.1C Would you say the sensations were...

>Strong ( )
>Moderate ( )
>Mild ( )
>Slight ( )

Q.1D When did it start?

>Immediately after application ( )
>Within 5-10 minutes ( )
>Within 15-30 minutes ( )
>After 30 minutes ( )
>Other ( )

Q.1E How long did it last? _____

Q.1F Did it eventually stop?

>Yes ( )
>No ( )

Q.1G Would you say this influenced your opinion of the product...

>Very much ( )
>Somewhat ( )
>Slightly ( )
>Not at all ( )

Q.1H Was the influence positive or negative?

>Positive ( )
>Negative ( )

FIGURE 1 Irritation questions for a facial moisturizer normally appear near the end of a survey so as not to influence product judgments.

ritation is part and parcel of the moisturizer's mode of action. The level of reported irritation may, in this case, be under-reported because, given a rationale for it, the consumer discounts the experience. To create a perfectly balanced position between these concerns may not be possible. In practice, the consumer's cognitive machinery is activated in complex ways by the presentation of a product concept, by the naming of the product (e.g., "age-defying" or "pore-refining"), and even by the courtesy instructions and warnings that ethically accompany moisturizers that may irritate the skin, for instance, "You may experience a brief burning or tingling. Discontinue use, if severe." All one should ask of the questionnaire is that it be probing and free of bias. One option is to have balanced wording in the questionnaire so that specific product expectations are not divulged. For example, asking Did you experience any pleasant or unpleasant sensations after using the product for two weeks? is balanced and nonbiasing, whereas Did you experience any unpleasant sensations after using the product for two weeks? suggests that this sort of reaction is expected. One full set of possible irritation questions is presented in Fig. 1.

It is important to realize that unpleasant sensory stimulation does not necessarily correlate with disliking for a product. Questions Q.1G and H in Fig. 1 look at this possibility. Brief stinging may be a signal of a product's efficacy, i.e., that it is working to smooth or exfoliate the skin. As such, the unpleasantness may not negatively influence purchase intent.

6 CONCLUSION

The authors have attempted to present a selective overview of current methods and issues. Moisturizers can no longer be formulated in a laboratory vacuum. Companies large and small can not afford to dismiss or ignore the voice of the consumer in the product development process. More and more emphasis is being placed on understanding the consumer as a person and not as a marketing object (J. Kastenholz, personal communication, 2000). The evaluation of moisturizers has come a long way since the early days of informal product appraisals. Emphasis should be placed on studying the consumer in their normal environment. While more traditional methods (e.g., trained panels, home-use tests, mall intercept) will continue to be effective, new approaches should be explored.

Acknowledgment

We would like to thank M. Davis and C. Wesolowski for their research assistance.

REFERENCES

1. Grievson M, Barber J, Hunting A. Natural Ingredients in Cosmetics: Based on a Symposium Organized by the Society of Cosmetic Scientists. Weymouth, England: Michelle Press, 1989.

2. DeNavarre MG. Oils and fats: the historical cosmetics. J Am Oil Chem Soc 1978; 55.
3. McDonough EG. Truth About Cosmetics. New York: The Drug and Cosmetics Industry, 1937:12.
4. Fernandez Rodriguez MC, Selles Flores E. The splendour of the cosmetology in the ancient Greece. Cosmetic News 1998; XXI.
5. Gunn F. The Artificial Face: A History of Cosmetics. New York: Hippocrene Books, 1983.
6. Angeloglou M. A History of Make Up. London: Macmillian, 1970:22.
7. Fernandez Rodriguez MC. The beginnings of esthetic and cosmetological care in ancient Rome. Cosmetic News 1999; XXII.
8. Spelios T. An Informal History Of Cosmetics II. Drug Cosmet Ind 1983; 133:42.
9. Peiss K. Hope In A Jar: The Making of America's Beauty Culture. New York: Henry Holt and Company, 1998.
10. American Society for Testing and Materials. Guidelines for the Selection and Training of Sensory Panel Members. ASTM Special Technical Publication 758. Philadelphia: ASTM, 1981.
11. Stone H, Sidel JL. Sensory Evaluation Practices. 2nd ed. New York: Academic Press, 1993.
12. American Society for Testing and Materials. Manual on Sensory Testing Methods. ASTM Special Technical Publication 434. Philadelphia: ASTM, 1981:6.
13. Kahneman D, Diener E, Schwarz N, eds. Well-Being: The Foundations of Hedonic Psychology. New York: Russell Sage Foundation, 1999.
14. Stone AA, Shiffman SS, DeVries MW. Ecological Momentary Assessment. In: Kahneman D, Diener E, Schwarz N, eds. Well-Being: The Foundations of Hedonic Psychology. New York: Russell Sage Foundation, 1999.
15. Schutz HG. Evolution of the sensory science discipline. Food Technol 1998; 52(8):42–46.
16. Moskowitz HR. Cosmetic Product Testing: A Modern Psychophysical Approach. New York: Marcel Dekker, 1984.
17. Moskowitz HR. Cosmetic Testing and Evaluation of Personal Care Products. New York: Marcel Dekker, 1996.
18. Meilgaard M, Civille GV, Carr BT. Sensory Evaluation Techniques. 2d ed. Boca Raton: CRC Press, 1991.
19. Lawless HT, Heymann H. Sensory Evaluation of Food. New York: Chapman and Hall/International Thomson Publishing, 1998.
20. Schwartz NO. Adaptation of the sensory texture profile method to skin care products. J Texture Studies 1975; 6:33–42.
21. Brandt MA, Skinner EZ, Coleman JA. The texture profile method. J Food Sci 1963; 28:404–409.
22. Szczesniak AS. Classification of textural characteristics. J Food Sci 1963; 28:385–389.
23. American Society for Testing and Materials. ASTM practice for descriptive skinfeel analysis of cream and lotions (E 1490–92). In: Annual Book of ASTM Standards. Philadelphia: ASTM, 1999.
24. Keane P. The flavor profile. In: ASTM Manual Series MNL 13. Manual on Descriptive Analysis Testing. Philadelphia: ASTM, 1992.

25. Stone H. Quantitative descriptive analysis (QDA). In: ASTM Manual Series MNL 13. Manual on Descriptive Analysis Testing. Philadelphia: ASTM, 1992.
26. Muñoz M, Civille GV. The spectrum descriptive analysis method. In: ASTM Manual Series MNL 13. Manual on Descriptive Analysis Testing. Philadelphia: ASTM, 1992.
27. Muñoz AM, Szczesniak AS, Einstein MA, Schwartz NO. The texture profile. In: ASTM Manual Series MNL 13. Manual on Descriptive Analysis Testing. Philadelphia: ASTM, 1992.
28. Jeltema MA, Southwick EW. Evaluation and applications of odor profiling. J Sensory Studies 1986; 1:123–136.
29. Hayes TJ. The flexible focus group: designing and implementing effective and creative research. In: Wu LS, ed. Product Testing with Consumers for Research Guidance. Philadelphia: ASTM, 1989:77–84.
30. Hawkins DI, Best RJ, Coney KA. Consumer Behavior: Building Market Strategy. 7th ed. Boston: Irwin/McGraw-Hill, 1998.
31. Morgan DL, Krueger RA. The Focus Group Kit. Thousand Oaks, CA: Sage Publications, 1998.
32. Cacioppo JT, Petty RE. The need for cognition. J Personality Social Psychol 1982; 42:116–131.
33. Lynn M, Harris J. The desire for unique consumer products: a new individual difference scale. Psychology and Marketing 1997; 14:601–616.
34. Goldsmith RE, Hofacker CF. Measuring consumer innovativeness. J Acad Marketing Sci 1991; 19:209–221.
35. Coulter RH, Zaltman G. Using the Zaltman metaphor technique to understand brand image. In: Allen CT, John DR, eds. Advances in Consumer Research XXI. Provo, UT: Association for Consumer Research, 1994:501–507.
36. Mattimore BW. 99% Inspiration: Tips, Tales, and Techniques for Liberating Your Business Creativity. New York: American Management Association, 1994.
37. Hammersley M, Atkinson P. Ethnography: Principles in Practice. 2d ed. London: Routledge, 1995:1.
38. Joy A. Interpretations of ethnographic writing in consumer behavior. In: Belk RW, ed. Highways and Buyways: Naturalistic Research from the Consumer Behavior Odyssey. Provo, UT: Association for Consumer Research, 1991:216–233.
39. Geertz C. The Interpretation of Cultures. New York: Basic Books, 1973.
40. Weber N. E-commerce projections: which to believe? Home Furnishing Network 2000; 74(21):15.
41. Gonier DE. Factionalization imperils market research groups. Advertising Age 2000; 71(25):40.
42. Sudman S, Bradburn NM. Asking Questions. San Francisco: Jossey-Bass Publishers, 1982.
43. Richmond SB. Statistical Analysis. New York: The Ronald Press Company, 1964.
44. Dixon WJ, Massey FJ Jr. Introduction to Statistical Analysis. New York: McGraw-Hill, 1969.
45. Snedecor GW, Cochran WG. Statistical Methods. 7th ed. Iowa State University Press, 1980.
46. Gacula MC, Singh J. Statistical Methods in Food and Consumer Research. Florida: Academic Press, 1984.

47. Powers JJ. Descriptive methods of analysis. In: Sensory Analysis of Foods. Piggott JR, ed. Essex, England: Elsevier Science, 1988.
48. Neter J, Wasserman W. Applied Linear Statistical Models. Illinois: Richard D. Irwin 1974.
49. Hollander M, Wolfe D. Nonparametric Statistical Methods. New York: John Willey & Sons, 1973.
50. American Society for Testing and Materials. ASTM standard test method for unipolar magnitude estimation of sensory attributes (E 1697–95). In: Annual Book of ASTM Standards. Philadelphia: ASTM, 1999.
51. Sinesio F, Risvik E, Rodbotten M. Evaluation of panelist performance in descriptive profiling of rancid sausage: a multivariate study. J Sensory Studies 1990; 5:33–52.
52. Lundahl DS, McDaniel MR. Use of contrasts for the evaluation of panel consistency. J Sensory Studies 1990; 5:265–277.
53. Naes T, Solheim R. Detection and interpretation of variation within and between assessors in sensory profiling. J Sensory Studies 1991; 6:159–177.
54. Schlich P. GRAPES: a method and a SAS® program for graphical representations of assessor performances. J Sensory Studies 1994; 9:157–169.
55. American Society for Testing and Materials. ASTM standard test method for sensory analysis—triangle test (E 1885–97). In: Annual Book of ASTM Standards. Philadelphia: ASTM, 1999.
56. Montgomery DC. Design and Analysis of Experiments. New York: John Willey & Sons, 1976.
57. Gacula MC. Design and Analysis of Sensory Optimization. Trumbull, CT: Food and Nutrition Press, 1993.
58. Muñoz AM, Chambers E IV. Relating sensory measurements to consumer acceptance of meat products. Food Technol 1993; 47(11):128–131.
59. Giovanni M. Response surface methodology and product optimization. Food Technol 1983; 37(11):41–45.
60. Henika RG. Use of response surface methodology in sensory evaluation. Food Technol 1982; 36(11):96–101.
61. Galvez FCF, Resurreccion AVA. Optimization of processing of peanut beverages. J Sensory Studies 1990; 5:1–17.
62. American Society for Testing and Materials. ASTM standard guide for sensory claim substantiation (E 1958–98). In: Annual Book of ASTM Standards. Philadelphia: ASTM, 1999.
63. Moskowitz H. Food Concepts and Products. Just in Time Development. Trumbull, CT: Food and Nutrition Press, 1994.
64. Muñoz AM, Chambers E IV, Hummer S. A multifaceted category research study: how to understand a product category and its consumer responses. J Sensory Studies 1996; 11:261–294.

22

Clinical Testing of Moisturizers

Gregory Nole
Unilever Home and Personal Care North America,
Trumbull, Connecticut

"A moisturizer is a topically applied substance that overcomes the signs and symptoms of dry skin" [1]. When Dr. Kligman wrote that definition in 1978, moisturizers were generally either emulsions or oleaginous mixtures. As a result, products were generally designed around two primary mechanisms of action, humectancy and/or occlusion. In both cases, as Dr. Kligman's definition shows, moisturizing products of that time focused on treatment of symptoms, that is, the appearance and feel of dry skin.

Today, the amelioration of symptoms is still the primary benefit to the consumer, however, many if not most products attempt to go beyond simple humectancy and occlusion to treat the underlying causes of dryness. Products today often deliver skin lipids, natural moisturizing factors (NMF), essential fatty acids (EFA), or other components of healthy skin that are deficient in dry skin. Moreover, who would have predicted 20 years ago that even some cleansers would begin to move toward delivering low level moisturization benefits.

These changes in product technology have had significant impact on the role and means of clinical testing of moisturizing products. No longer can product investigators be content with measuring the end benefit to the skin, they must now follow the example of researchers in trying to understand what the product is doing to skin. With a wide array of clinical tools and techniques at their disposal, the choice of measurement and interpretation of the measurements is of course critical to good experimental design. But bioinstruments and skin assays are just the tools. Equally important in good clinical design is the protocol, that is, the complete description of the experiment in robust scientific terms.

1 HISTORY OF DRY SKIN TESTING

1.1 Early Method for Describing Skin Barrier Properties

Clinical testing is conducted for the purposes of research, technology evaluation, or product claim support. In the earliest days the work was principally for research. The origins of modern dry skin understanding rightly belong to Dr. Irwin Blank when he described the mechanism of water content in skin [2,3]. He demonstrated that water, not oils, were necessary for maintaining skin plasticity. He described the problem in terms of regulating the barrier function. Dryness was viewed as a function of water loss rate from the surface to the environment versus replacement rate from the lower layers. In this early research, Blank was the first to describe barrier integrity by measuring the transpiration rate of water through excised human skin in a diffusion cell. He measured the water loss rate of normal, damaged, and treated skin and demonstrated that this rate was a function and direct measure of skin barrier quality.

Since that time, trans-epidermal water loss (TEWL) has been an accepted means of describing skin condition. Where Blank's experiments were conducted in vitro, methods to measure water loss in vivo were later being devised [4,5]. Before the development of the modern evaporimeter, TEWL was measured by passing a stream of dry nitrogen over skin through a closed cup that was in contact with the skin surface and measuring moisture pick-up with a dew point hygrometer. For the product investigator, evaporimetry not only described skin barrier quality, but could be used objectively to compare the performance of emollient lotions and creams [6]. However, TEWL alone says little about the momentary hydration state and is not appropriate for comparing product humectancy. Even with modern instrumentation, TEWL measurements can be confounded by the presence of surface moisture or an alteration in skin condition [7]. For example, an increase in TEWL could indicate an increase in surface moisture levels or could be the result of skin damage. Unless testing conditions are well controlled, TEWL alone could lead to ambiguous results which call for further investigation.

1.2 Biomechanical Developments

The 1960s brought further understanding of the relationship of water content in skin and its effect on physical skin properties. This led to development of in vitro analytical and biomechanical methods for describing skin conditions beyond vapor transpiration rate [8–11]. Gravemetric approaches measured the amount of water loosely held in the skin that could be feely lost to the atmosphere under low humidity. Differential scanning calorimetry (DSC) was used to describe the water that was tightly bound within the cellular matrix in an attempt to better describe the underlying hydration state. Tensile testing was used to describe elastic properties of skin in order to relate skin plasticity to hydration state. All of these approaches provided opportunity for the product investigator to further understand product efficacy, but as in vitro methods, they could not demonstrate the end benefit of products in actual usage.

1.3 Regression Testing

Through most of the 1970s the underlying principle of lotion product testing was that there is a correlation between skin mechanical properties and the effects of moisturizer treatment. In 1978, Dr. Kligman challenged this assumption. He pointed out that while physical properties of skin can vary, their true relationship to dry skin is unclear. The lack of real understanding of dry skin is summarized in his assertion (or more likely frustration) that "we cannot even say that dry skin is dry; that is, lacks water" [1]. For the clinician, this raises a serious question of what to measure. Kligman's proposal, in this seminal paper, was the dry skin regression test.

The thinking behind the regression method was derived from an understanding of "cosmetic dry skin." Kligman recognized that classical signs of dryness such as skin flaking can be effectively masked with emollient lotions that give the appearance of moisturized skin but do not provide a fundamental improvement in skin quality. He observed that while treatments continued, dry skin may look and even feel better, but as soon as treatment was stopped, the skin quickly reverted or regressed back to its original state. Kligman's view was that it was this rate of regression that was the true measure of moisturizer efficacy.

The original regression method was a 4- to 6-week process separated into distinct treatment and regression phases. The studies were conducted on legs in a paired comparison design. Treatments were applied twice daily, Monday through Friday for 3 weeks with no treatments occurring over the weekends. Because visual assessments were made on Monday mornings (three days after the last treatment) they better reflected the true condition of the skin. After 3 weeks, treatments were discontinued altogether, and during this regression phase the skin was assessed on Mondays and Thursdays until baseline was reached, which could take 2 weeks or longer. Assessments involved visual grading of the test sites on a four-point scale for the overall appearance (or lack) of dryness. A quarter century later, with the many advances in our knowledge of dry skin and instrumental analysis, the principles of the regression method remain sound and continue to be the backbone of modern dry skin testing programs.

1.4 Bioinstrumental Methods

The original regression method used visual observation of skin as the primary measurement. About the time this method was proposed numerous bioinstrumental methods were just beginning to emerge [13–18]. These various techniques, many described elsewhere in this volume, were developed to quantify skin hydration (electrical hygromety), texture (profilometry), elasticity (dynamometry and ballistometry), optical properties (spectroscopy and photography), and other physical states (squamometry), just to name a few. These methods were often developed for research into the fundamental properties of skin, and the emphasis in the literature was on what these measurements told about skin. For the product investigator they provided new opportunities for describing product effects; however, there was insufficient guidance in how the instrument should be used in the context of a consumer product clinical trial. While these instruments are excellent tools, there is an ever-present danger of seeing them as the test method rather than as tools within a test method.

1.5 Regression Testing Revisited

Following publication of the regression method there was a growing body of literature on instrumental methods but a lack of writings on clinical evaluation. Yet there was evidence that researchers were using the principles of the regression method as framework for bioinstrumental evaluations [19]. Bioinstruments provided finer resolution than a four-point visual scale, and this improved the ability to clearly separate the strictly visual (cosmetic) effects from fundamental changes to skin condition.

　　For product investigation, the need for a well-structured test design in which to use these new measurement techniques became clear. Because skin moisturization can be achieved through various routes (occlusion, humectancy, dryness prevention, and healthy skin repair), study details and the selection of the measurement tools must be made appropriately. Further, as measurements became more sophisticated and the demands for product discrimination increased, some refinements (but not changes!) to the original regression method were needed to meet the increased requirements [20]. These refinements proposed basic parameters such as weather and panelist recruitment criteria as well as defining procedures such as for product assignment and application to ensure unambiguous results for evaluating consumer products. The robustness of the regression method remains evident in clinical testing where it is almost no longer a consideration but simply treated as a de facto approach for product evaluation [21,22].

1.6 The Miniregression Test

For the product investigator, bioinstrumental measures within a well-structured test provided a sensitive measurement of product performance. Within these multiweek trials, it was recognized that methods such as hygrometery had potential to predict after one week the overall product performance seen after three weeks. This led to the development of a more rapid predictive product evaluation test called the Miniregression [23]. In this test, all of the principles of the original regression method test are retained, just shortened. Treatment is for 5 days, followed by a treatment-free weekend and then a 7-day regression period. Using instrumental measures instead of visual, the miniregression method focuses on predicting the functional benefit (increased hydration state) rather than visual (cosmetic) benefit of treatment. This method provides value to the investigator not just for quickly screening products, but also for demonstrating the early treatment benefits of products on skin.

1.7 "Nutrition Protocol" Regression Test

A novel approach took the standard regression test and turned it inside-out in order to better evaluate the quality of skin following treatment [24]. Referred to as the nutrition protocol, it starts with a 4-week pretreatment phase which allows full stratum corneum turnover of the treated skin site. With fully treated skin and no further product use, the test phase focuses principally on a 3-week regression. The healthier the skin quality, as a result of pretreatment, the greater should be the persistence of "good" skin during the regression period.

1.8 Short-Term Alternative to Regression Testing

While a well- and widely established test, the regression method and its variations are by no means the only acceptable approaches to product evaluation. Regression testing in all its forms always involves the use of multiple product applications over time. However, rapid and sensitive bioinstrumental measures such as hygrometry have allowed the development of methods to look at the immediate hydrating effects of even a single lotion application. These immediate hydration tests are typically used to discriminate product performance within 4 hr of application though they can be extended [25,26]. With controlled application and restrictions on subject activities, the tests almost always involve a multiple product design, typically evaluating up to six sites simultaneously, usually on lower legs, which allows for highly sensitive, direct within-subject interproduct comparisons.

Note that while appropriate for showing moisturization effects, short-term protocols involving moisturemeters are not appropriate for predicting longer-term behavior. For example, occlusive materials such as petrolatum show no immediate benefit based on a moisturemeter yet are highly effective in the longer term.

Short-term testing is best limited to describing the immediate effect of a treatment. Bioinstruments to look at elasticity, surface roughness, and other skin properties can also be used in a single-use test to understand how quickly and effectively a particular treatment delivers relief to the user. In fact, a thorough understanding of immediate effects can be as important to the product investigator as determining the long-term benefit because when consumers begin to feel their skin getting dry and tight, they want immediate relief.

1.9 Testing Moisturizers Today and Tomorrow

Today the product investigator has a wide array of tools, both visual and instrumental measurement methods, and well-designed long- and short-term protocols to fully understand the effects of moisturizer treatment on skin. These techniques have been used by researchers and product manufacturers to develop a solid understanding of lotion technology. While the growing array of bioinstrumental tools complements the more traditional visual evaluation methods, the need for a well-designed, structured framework for using any measurement technique is fundamental.

We are already seeing today that the delivery of moisture is beginning to come from a most unlikely source, body cleansers. As the range of moisturizing products expands, it creates a need for a broader range of clinical methods [27]. As we look forward, the future in leave-on products bodes new delivery mechanisms, biomimemics, and new forms [28]. However, in the end, to be accepted as a true moisturizer, new technologies will still need to deliver immediate and sustained relief and the well-developed methods for measuring short- and long-term effects will still apply.

2 BASIC ELEMENTS OF CLINICAL DESIGN

The more objective and controlled the clinical trial, the more detached it becomes from the normal-use consumer experience. The competing interests of clinical control and consumer relevance cannot be easily reconciled. No single method is all-encompassing. Taking a broad view of testing, one finds a spectrum of methods, from loosely controlled panel tests to the rigorously controlled clinical trials. Moreover, dry skin has many aspects, from how it looks to how it feels to how it functions, all of which further complicate the testing choices. Determining the ideal course for testing is not always easy. Clearly the variety of available bioinstrumental methods can play an important role in dry skin testing; however, instruments tend to give a unidimensional picture for a multidimensional problem. Thus the answer is often a stepwise approach to product evaluation [29,30].

In developing a clinical testing plan, the product investigator must balance the requirements of each experiment against the objectives and conclusions to be drawn from the results. Before the details of a clinical trial can be determined, the broad requirements of the trial must first be established. Discussed herein are three basic questions that underlie the study design. Only once the fundamentals are established can then the details of the protocol can be considered, and these are discussed in the next section.

2.1 Setting the Size and Scope of the Trial

Depending on the stage of the research or product development program, trials of different size and scope are entirely appropriate. In the early stages of a program, preliminary or pilot trials are often used as a cost-effective and rapid means of getting indicative information as a guide toward further study and full clinical trials. Sometimes referred to as preclinicals, these trials tend to be short with a minimal number of subjects and are typically used as screening tools or as predictors of product effects.

In preparing a study proposal, it is necessary to understand the value and limitations of pilot trials but also to approach such trials with the same thoughtful diligence as larger clinical trials. A danger in labeling trials as preliminary is that they can be perceived as informal, resulting in an unacceptable degree of laxity. Preliminary trials should never be approached as "quick and dirty," but must receive the same detailed consideration as large-scale trials. When done properly, preliminary trials provide scientifically valid supporting evidence and incrementally add to the knowledge base. The data may not necessarily be sufficient to stand entirely on their own, but should constitute a solid first step.

Pilot trials must not be confused with small trials. The mere fact that a test is small does not mean that it is preliminary. Pilot tests should be defined on the basis of statistical risk, not just complexity. All studies carry with them some risk of error, and preliminary studies carry higher levels of this risk. To illustrate the difference between a pilot trial and small trial, consider two proposals: a 6-week regression test with only six subjects per cell versus a 1-hr hygrometer trial on 100 subjects. The regression trial would likely be set up as a pilot trial because expectations for the statistical power is low (i.e., high risk of error due to small sample size) despite the complexity of conducting a 6-week trial. Depending on objectives, the simpler hygrometer study may or may not be approached as a pilot trial. If the objective were to record the before/after effects of a lotion, it can pass as a definitive clinical study. But if the same trial were being used surrogate for a 3-week home-use test, then it would be considered preliminary because it was being used to make predictions well beyond the scope of its data.

So the first element in designing a clinical trial is to establish the size and scope. How much risk can you accept in order to save time, money, or other resources? How comfortable will you be making a decision based on the outcome? How does this trial fit in with next steps? How does this trial fit in with the timeline of your research program? With the study objectives in mind, the trial must be developed appropriately, but to do so consideration must first be given to specifically determining what is appropriate and necessary to meet those objectives.

2.2 Selecting the Measurements

Closely linked with setting the scope of the trial is selection of test methods. The choice of measurement method is ultimately what will define the study. After all is done, it is the output of these measurements, the numeric data, that is compiled, analyzed, and pored over in order to describe the effects of skin treatment.

Based on a review of product claims, it has been shown that moisturizer benefits can be divided into three categories: what moisturizers do for the skin, how the skin looks, and how the skin feels [31]. Clinical tests can follow this path using a three-prong approach. This multimeasurement approach offers strong advantages as each method has its own strengths and weaknesses (Table 1). More importantly, the multiprong approach allows the conclusions based on one method to be corroborated and reinforced by the others. These three classes of evaluation methods are discussed below and further in Sec. 3.

Instrumental methods are ideal at providing objective data to individual aspects of what the product does for skin. They can provide quantification of invisible aspects such as moisture content within the skin, and a battery of instrumental measurements helps draw a detailed picture of physiological changes in skin. They are, nevertheless, unidimensional, which can lead to an incomplete view of product performance. Instruments also can be highly sensitive to small differences suggesting skin benefits that are neither consumer relevant nor perceivable.

With expert assessment, a qualified human judge integrates many aspects into a measurement of the visual appearance of skin. Normal healthy skin is visually apparent, and this is the ultimate goal of a dry skin treatment. Any deviation from normal/healthy appearance can be captured in the evaluation. Visual grading is traditionally the cornerstone of dry skin measurement.

Subject self-assessment within the context of the clinical trial gives quantitative measure to the perception of skin look and feel. Self-assessment measurements have two roles: they provide a means of measuring sensory attributes that cannot be measured instrumentally and they demonstrate whether the instrumentally measured changes are resulting in meaningful and perceivable benefits to the user.

Clearly, the selection of measurement(s) must be made appropriately for the products being evaluated. Moreover, it is axiomatic that they are made in the context of the study objectives. No measurement is perfect; all have cost and resource requirements associated with them, and all have certain limitations. Choice of measurement must balance the different study needs, and compromise

TABLE 1 Comparison of Three Classes of Skin Measurement

	Strengths	Weaknesses
Instrumental	Rapid, objective quantification of skin condition	Unidimensional, takes individual aspects out of context of entire skin condition
	Unidimensional, provides clear measure of singular aspects of skin condition	Capable of measuring parameters that are imperceptible or consumer irrelevant
	Uniform measurement; lower operator dependency than other methods	Not always able to detect confounding influences
	Wide variety of instruments for various skin attributes	
Expert visual	Holistic, integrates numerous aspects of condition into measurements	Requires rigorous training and experience
	Can make judgmental comparisons of different skin types or sites	Dependent upon individual grader for consistency
	Measurement capability continually improves with additional experience	Limited to superficial (i.e., visible at the surface) conditions
Subject self-assessment	Direct measure of user perceptions	No frames of reference; no consistency in grading between subjects
	Can quantify visual and sensory attributes	Perceptions can be highly influenced by unrelated external stimuli
	Can be done almost any time, anywhere, and under a variety of usage conditions	

may be necessary. Careful consideration must be given to what information is needed and what methods are best suited to provide it.

2.3 Establishing the Protocol

While measurements may be the defining aspect of the trial, they are nevertheless only tools. It is the protocol for the trial that provides the framework in which the measurements are made. In line with the choice of measurements, the protocol must be defined appropriately for the objectives of the trial. Dry skin has a wide range of etiologies, and dry skin treatment can be achieved through a variety of routes such as occlusion, humectancy, preventing dryness, and healthy skin repair [29,32]. Thus, the difficulty facing the product investigator is that there is no single all-encompassing clinical approach that addresses all of the aspects of product performance.

For the evaluation of leave-on moisturizing lotions, common clinical testing approaches can be divided into two groups: single application trials and multiple application trials, each of which can be further divided into trials for short- or long-term effects (Table 2). Each has its own distinct purpose, which must be considered in developing a clinical testing program.

> Single application tests assess the physical changes in skin due to the product and predict the physiological changes with repeated use. In short-term moisturemeter hydration tests, measurements can be made within seconds of applying lotion. This is appropriate for determining the immediate, even instantaneous effect of a lotion on skin but is extremely weak for predicting long-term repeat use benefits. The entire study usually takes place under controlled indoor conditions to eliminate environment effects. This test can be used to compare the overall moisture delivery of competing products.
> The longer-term moisturemeter hydration test measures the persistence of the immediate physical changes to skin. It is often used to demonstrate "all-day" or "24-hour" effects. Due to the length of time involved, accommodation for panelist comfort must be considered; however, panelist activities can add variability to the measurement. This test can be used to compare the long-lasting moisturization ability of competing products.

Multiple application tests assess the true physiological changes in skin over time. The advantage of tests with a 3-week or longer treatment phase is that it allows time for complete stratum corneum turnover.

> A test of 1 to 2 weeks with no regression shows the rate of benefit, that is, the rate of healing of dry skin. Traced over time, it is a strong predictor of overall benefit, though the skin may not achieve a level of complete recovery. This test can be used to compare speed of benefit between competing products.
> The miniregression test shows the rate of healing and better predicts the overall benefit by also showing the persistence in regression. This test can be used to compare speed of benefit and predict the quality of that benefit between competing products.
> The Kligman regression test shows the speed of benefit as well as the overall benefit of treating skin through a complete cycle of stratum corneum turnover. Further, it separates the cosmetic (superficial) benefit from

TABLE 2 Common Clinical Testing Approaches for Leave-On Skin Moisturizers

Product application	Study duration	Regression or retreatment	Uses	Study name
Single application	Short duration (<4 hr)		Immediate hydration effects	Moisturemeter hydration test
	Long duration (8–24 hr)		"long lasting" moisturization	
Multiple application	Short term (1–2 weeks)	No regression	Rate of benefit	
		With regression	Predict overall moisturizer performance	Miniregression test
	Long term (3–6 weeks or more) with regression	No retreatment	Demonstrate overall moisturizer performance	Kligman regression test
		With retreatment	Measure of underlying healthy condition	Nutrition study

substantive benefits by measuring how well the fully treated skin persists in regression. This test can be used to directly compare the overall effectiveness of competing products to treat dry skin and improve skin quality.

The nutrition protocol ignores speed of benefit to focus on the quality of the skin due to product use. More than just measuring persistence of benefit in regression, it measures the resistance of skin to external assault as indicator of the underlying skin health condition. This test can be used to compare the overall effectiveness of competing products to restore skin health.

The selection of measurement tools and general framework for the study provide the necessary structure for a well-designed protocol. But regardless of the approach taken, numerous aspects must still be considered which not only define what must be done, but ensure that the results are scientifically sound. There is no single right way to conduct a clinical trial, though there are always opportunities for improvements. (It is the nature of scientists to provide critical review and identify what could be done better.) General protocols such as the regression test provide well-established principles, but the specifics of the trial must be given individual consideration in the detailed protocol. The product investigator actually has wide latitude to tailor a study to particular needs and must demonstrate sound rationale for decisions.

3 DETAILED CONSIDERATIONS OF CLINICAL DESIGN

To fully elucidate the effects of a moisturizer on skin requires careful planning, and every aspect of the study must be considered. These considerations go far beyond the mechanics of the test and measurement tools. Some considerations that can impact on a study's outcome have been well described in the literature, such as the effect of weather, environment, temperature, and humidity on skin measurements [32–37]. General descriptions of how to design and conduct trials are harder to come by, although some excellent references can be found[38–41]. However, the real details of how a study is conducted are often the result of years of experience by the investigating lab. These details become part of the operating routine and are often taken for granted as their standard, good practice. While some of these details may not be formally documented in the study protocol, they are extremely important for a well-designed and well-conducted trial.

Following is a reference list of points to consider when developing a protocol or conducting a clinical trial. This list is not nearly exhaustive, but is fairly extensive. Thinking through these points will place detail on the general protocol framework and help create an unimpeachable study design. The points are discussed with respect to the clinical evaluation of dry skin and are relevant to all manner of dry skin trials from the 2-hr hydration trial to the 6-week full regression trial.

3.1 General Factors

The first level of detail is to define the structure of the trial. Following are some operational parameters that define the framework for the protocol.

3.1.1 Statement of the Test Objective

An obvious and necessary part of any study, a well-written objective will clearly articulate what is to be achieved from the trial in a just few words. This objective statement is the first stake in the ground and every aspect of trial must be measured against this statement. Therefore it must be the first consideration for the detailed protocol and should be written specifically to the desired test. Broad or generically written objectives should be avoided.

3.1.2 Body Site

Where on the body to focus treatment is not a trivial question. Legs, forearms, hands, and face are the most commonly used sites and each has its strengths and weaknesses. Site selection must balance the study objectives with the practicalities of the clinical method. Most dry skin clinical trials are conducted on legs, hands, and forearms and to a lesser extent on faces. Table 3 provides a comparison of strengths and weaknesses of each site. Other areas such as feet, knees, and elbows are occasionally used when there is specific interest.

3.1.3 Number of Cells and Cell Size

Statistical analysis can predict the minimum panel size required to show an expected level of change where the level of variability is known. However, data variability are not always known. Moreover, very large samples can sometimes be used to demonstrate statistical significance on small differences that are neither consumer perceivable nor relevant. Another chapter in this book provides thorough discussion of statistics and relevant cell size.

The product investigator who operates in the real world must think beyond just the theoretical considerations and must also consider the practical aspects of panel logistics. For example, how long each measurement takes will limit how many panelists can be assessed in a given period of time. Equally important is clinician fatigue that will occur with repetitive measurements. Both of these issues have direct bearing on sample size and the number of cells that can be run by exerting very real practical constraints. For reference, regression tests have typically ranged from 10 to 20 subjects per cell, while hydration tests typically range

TABLE 3   Comparison of Body Sites in Dry Skin Testing

	Strengths	Weaknesses
Lower legs	Excellent display of dryness/flaking Ideal for a two-product direct comparison test Suitable for treatment by the subjects at home With clinician application, suitable for testing up to six products simultaneously	Awkward to evaluate Not highly exposed to the environment Shaving may be restricted to prevent interactions Does not exhibit erythema
Hands	Wide range of dry skin symptoms Receives the greatest amount of environmental exposure Highly relevant to consumers Excellent for treatment by the subjects at home	Not appropriate for two-product direct comparison due to potential for cross-contamination Wide variability in symptoms between subjects; may be difficult to assemble homogeneous test cells Not suitable for some instrumental evaluations
Forearms	Easily accessible; ideal for two-product direct comparison test With clinician applications, suitable for testing up to four products simultaneously Ideal for most instrumental measurements	Not highly exposed to the environment Does not exhibit erythema Lacks range of dryness symptoms of hands or legs
Face	Most appropriate for testing facial products Unique skin type cannot be perfectly modeled elsewhere on the body High level of environmental exposure Wide range of dry skin symptoms	Not well suited to two-product direct comparison tests Not suitable for some instrumental evaluations Subject compliance is constant issue Limits to degree of dryness many subjects will allow Limits to extent of what many subjects will apply

from 20 to 30 per cell. In the end, actual study size must be established within the context of what can effectively be handled by the lab.

3.1.4 Control Products

Control cells generally come in three varieties:

> Positive or benchmark product: a product with a known effect against which other products can be compared.
> Negative or placebo product: a nonperforming product or a vehicle product (test product minus "active" ingredients) to monitor background "noise" which can be factored out of the test results
> Untreated: baseline skin left on its own.

Typically a hydration test will include an untreated cell as the baseline reference. Base vehicles are often used in a two-product direct comparative leg regression. In a regression test, benchmark products are often included as a common point of comparison across trials.

3.1.5 Number of Products per Subject

Hand trials are usually limited to one product per subject due to the propensity for cross-contamination. In multiple application tests where home applications are performed, no more than two products per person should be considered in a leg test (left leg/right leg) and only with great effort made to insure there is no potential for cross-over or left/right confusion. Clinician controlled application tests can comfortably accommodate up to six sites on the legs (three on each leg) or four on the forearm (two on each arm).

3.1.6 Test Duration

Study duration depends first on the study objective. Measuring the "immediate moisturization" can be accomplished in under 2 hr, but demonstrating persistence of the moisture will require a longer time. Skin hydration tests are commonly conducted over a 4-hr period. However, if a specific claim such as "lasts all day" is sought, then test duration must be extended appropriately. To see beyond hydration effects, the first indications of physiological improvement usually require multiple applications over a few days and full recovery may require up to several weeks.

While scientific requirements should be the primary factor in deciding how long to run a study, environmental issues, panelist concerns, and logistics must also all be considered. As discussed next, unpredictable weather conditions are a significant risk in multiweek trials. Longer studies also have more difficulties in maintaining panelist interest/compliance and are inherently more complex to organize and more costly to complete. Even with single-day trials, the logistics of organizing panelists for a 4-hr study is much different than for an 8- or 12-hr study. The requirements for test duration must be considered in context of real world constraints.

3.1.7 Test Period/Environment: Weather, Season, and Location

Weather plays a significant role in the induction and maintenance of dry skin and therefore is an overarching force in dry skin evaluation. The relative effectiveness of moisturizing products can appear very different when evaluated in the dead of winter versus early spring. For a regression test, it is not possible to evaluate dry skin under anything other than dry skin conditions; however, depending on the product, very harsh conditions are not always required. For example, a hot dry desert condition (such as 90+°F with average RH consistently under 40%) can induce skin dryness, albeit without the severe cracking and chapping of cold dry conditions. This may be ideal for testing a light, everyday moisturizer, but for that heavy occlusive skin protectant more severe cold winter conditions may be preferable, where average temperatures are consistently below freezing.

In trials of a few hours duration, weather and season are less of a factor. As a model for predicting lotion performance, dry skin can be induced with soap for 2–7 days before the test, and on the day of the trial subjects can be maintained indoors in a controlled dry environment (such as 70°F, 40% RH) for the duration of the test.

In selecting the location and the time of the year, consider what type of benefit your product will deliver, how much dryness is needed at baseline, and how weather conditions will affect performance. If the available conditions do not make sense for your study objectives, be prepared to wait for appropriate conditions or seek an alternative location where conditions are favorable.

For multiweek studies, consistency of weather conditions can be as important as the average temperature and humidity. A sudden shift in weather, such as a period of warm rainy weather, can completely overwhelm product effects falsifying conclusions about product benefits. It is a good practice to define the acceptable range of weather criteria and be prepared to discontinue a study if the criteria are adversely exceeded.

3.2 Subject Recruitment

The practical issues around subject recruitment are often overlooked. An adequate supply of bodies is not enough. The following points will help insure the right panelists are available and that there is no misunderstanding with them over requirements.

3.2.1 Panelist Criteria

Good clinical practice requires that characteristics of test subject are clearly defined both in terms of what to seek (inclusion) and what to avoid (exclusion). The goal is to assemble a group of potential subjects from which homogenous subsets can be assembled for testing. General inclusion criteria to consider may include sex, age, and skin type as well as availability to participate. Exclusion criteria may cover skin diseases and use of medications, known sensitivities, and participation by pregnant or nursing women.

In addition to these, criteria for the acceptable type and quality of skin necessary for dry skin testing should be established. For dry skin testing, it is self-evident that you need dry skin. Valid comparisons across test cells require that homogenous groups are established at baseline. Therefore, to insure adequate dryness is available, set specific criteria for acceptable dryness and be prepared to dismiss panelists who fail to achieve it. If necessary, a pretrial dry-down or preconditioning period can be used to induce dryness.

In studies involving contralateral sites on arms or legs, panelists should additionally show bilateral consistency at baseline, that is, both legs (or arms) within each subject should be similar. Likewise, for a multiproduct trial, the entire test area on each leg (or arm) should be uniform. Inconsistencies at baseline immediately create variability and can set up for inequitable and unfair comparison after treatment.

Some typical criteria to be considered in dry skin clinical testing on legs are listed in Table 4.

3.2.2   Over-Recruitment Factor

After initial telephone recruitment, it is not uncommon to for some studies to experience 10 20% no-shows at the start of the trial. Moreover, if a dryness or skin

TABLE 4   Typical Basic Dry Skin Panelist Criteria

Inclusion	Exclusion
Females, 30–60 years old	Pregnant or nursing females
Willing and freely able to participate, agreeable to all directions, and available to attend all scheduled appointments	Visible skin disorder at or near treatment site
Exhibiting moderate to marked visible dry skin on test site (grade 2–3 on 0–4 point scale) at baseline	Under the care of a dermatologist and/or using topical prescriptive or OTC treatment
Exhibiting uniformity of dryness across contralateral test sites on legs	Use or prescriptive medications that can increase skin sensitivity or reactivity (e.g., retin A or tetracycline)
	Known history of sensitivity to cosmetic products or ingredients

condition criteria is established, losing a certain percentage of panelists at base-line must be expected. To prepare for this, studies should be over-recruited by an appropriate factor, perhaps as much as 50% if criteria are very restrictive. It is al-ways better to start a panel with an excess of acceptable panelist than to have to consider changing criteria because insufficient panelists are available.

3.2.3 Panelist Restrictions

During recruitment, well in advance of the start of the trial, it is important that subjects fully understand the personal restrictions to be placed on them, that is, the products that they cannot use and activities they must stop. The restrictions should also be fully spelled out in the panelist paperwork. This will help insure compliance and avoid misunderstandings later. Similarly, in multivisit trials, pan-elist must commit to the observation schedule and understand the penalties for not following it.

3.3 Grading/Measurements

As discussed earlier, the three-prong approach of expert assessment, instrumental assessment, and self-assessment allows the results of one method to be corrobo-rated and reinforced by the others. Within these three categories, the choice of techniques must be rational and appropriate to the objectives. More measurement is not always better. Data from measurements that are irrelevant to the objective or, worse, inappropriate to the objective can be a distraction and waste resources. Quality data will flow from a well-conceived set of measurements.

3.3.1 Expert Visual Grading

Dry skin condition is typically graded in terms of its main symptoms, flakiness (scaling), roughness, and erythema, though it is also common to use a single as-sessment of overall dryness. Because expert grading is only as good as the expert grader, experience and training is critical. The use of photographic reference stan-dards and/or descriptive texts to define grading levels is strongly recommended [42,43]. Because visual grading is subjective, all expert grading scales should be described in the protocol with the precise language used to delineate scale points. It is the ability to discriminate each point unambiguously that defines the limits of sensitivity.

Even the most experienced graders are not free from potential bias. To en-sure complete objectivity of the visual grading procedures, visual assessors must be completely independent of all other aspects of the trial and must be blind to the products being tested and the allocation of cells. Grading must also be performed absolutely, that is, how it appears at that moment. There should be no reference to prior data for comparison.

3.3.2 Bioinstruments

The many instruments which are available to quantify a wide range of physical attribute are discussed in detail elsewhere in this volume. For the study designer, the selection of instrumental measures must be relevant to the objectives and should be aligned with expert grading. Procedures for bioinstrumental readings must be defined in the protocol, for example, that three replicate readings are being taken and averaged for each measurement. Also, in that skin can be influenced by transient environmental conditions, the protocol should specify the acceptable test conditions for instruments.

3.3.3 Self assessment

In clinical testing, self-assessment is not the same as in consumer panels. Where consumer panels are interested in likes and dislikes of product attributes, self-assessment clinical grading is concerned with how skin looks and feels to the user. Clinical self-assessment demonstrates whether the changes in skin condition are resulting in meaningful and perceivable benefits to the subject. It also allows measurement of a much richer set of attributes than can be achieved with either visual or instrumental evaluations both in terms of descriptive attributes (such as roughness, redness, chapping, and cracking) and in terms of sensory attributes that cannot be otherwise measured (such as soreness, itching, tight feel).

Self-assessment scales are commonly of two types. The first is analog, or line scale, where subjects place a mark anywhere along a continuous line between two endpoints. With this type of scale the relative distance from the end point is simply measured and recorded. The alternative is a fixed interval scale, where subjects select a relative grade of increasing severity, usually a series of bubble dots. In either case, the language used to define the anchor points must be clear and unambiguous (Table 5).

Self-assessment within a clinical trial can not replace consumer testing. The relatively small sample size and controlled structure of the clinical trial are inappropriate for measuring consumer habits and attitudes. Within a clinical trial, self-assessment should remain focused on the perception of skin condition (physical and sensory) and the changes in condition due to product use.

3.3.4 Order of Measurements

Instrumental probes that contact the skin can alter the test sites. It is also difficult to keep the subjects from having an awareness of the various evaluations, even if they are not fully understood, and this can bias their own perceptions of skin condition. Therefore the order of measurements should be thought through in terms of how each could affect the next. It is generally good to allow subjects to complete their self-evaluation first, with visual expert assessments next, followed by any instrumental measures in order of increasing invasiveness.

TABLE 5 Example of Two Types of Self-Assessment Scales for Skin Dryness

Analog scale	Panelists mark X on the line relative to where they feel their skin is. Measure the distance from left edge. *Advantage:* fine resolution and ability to separate small differences *Disadvantage:* poor reproducibility Not dry ⊢————————————————————⊣ Very dry
Fixed interval scale	Panelists mark bubble which they feel best describes their skin. *Advantage:* good consistency within panelists for measuring changes over time *Disadvantage:* less sensitive to small differences O O O O O O O Not dry Slight dryness Moderate dryness Marked dryness Extremely dry

3.4 Observation Events

Observation is the essence of a clinical trial. When all is done, the output of the study is the collection of observation data. Exactly how, when, and under what conditions the measurements are taken must be well documented in the protocol.

3.4.1 Equilibration Period

Transient activities and environmental conditions can temporarily affect the physical properties of skin. For example, the face can become flushed coming inside on a brisk day or perspiration can increase with nervousness. Subjects need to accommodate to the testing environment prior to measurements being made. A quiet period of 15–30 min is generally accepted as sufficient to equilibrate to the testing conditions and allow the subject to reach a relaxed physiological state.

3.4.2 Blinding Procedures

Double-blind procedures are necessary to prevent product knowledge by subjects and evaluators that could bias study results. Because they are such an important part of good clinical practice, the specific blinding procedures should be defined in the protocol. A double-blind trial includes both product and assignment blindness, that is, all products are in coded plain white containers and evaluators are unaware of which subjects are using which products.

3.4.3 Frequency of Observations

A study with only two observations, baseline and end point, leaves much to be desired. A schedule of interim observations provides valuable insight into how the skin reacts to the product over time, which allows a time course of improvement to be plotted. A sensible time response profile is a very good indication of a valid study. For a multiweek test, a schedule of Monday/Thursday or Monday/Wednesday/Friday is typical. Daily observations over several weeks are not usually necessary, except perhaps at the very start of the treatment or regression phases. In single application trials, readings at 30- to 90-min intervals are common, with at least two interim observations between baseline and the end point.

3.4.4 Observation Schedule

Diurnal rhythms can have a significant physiological effect with potential implications for clinical measurements. In addition to natural cycles, the time gap since morning shower or last product application should be consistent among subjects. If it is not possible to ensure uniformity, having each subject evaluated at the same time at each observation and having subjects from each study cell uniformly distributed throughout the observation day can at least minimize the diurnal effects.

3.4.5   Condition of Skin Immediately Prior to Measurement

Skin reflects not just the effect of treatment, but the transient effect of any activity prior to measurement. For example, baseline hygrometer measurements can be depressed immediately following a wash cycle or the visual appearance of dryness can be affected by the presence of residual product still on the skin. Because activities immediately prior to measurement can affect the measurement, the protocol should describe how skin is to be prepared. For example, in hygrometer studies, a standard mild wash procedure can be implemented across all subjects 30 min prior to the baseline observations. For regression studies, daily treatment on observation days can be delayed until after observations are complete.

3.4.6   Number of Independent Judges

Despite all efforts to ensure any two judges work similarly, there is always potential for inconsistencies between them to occur. It is more important that judges remain consistent within themselves (intrajudge consistency) than between other judges (interjudge consistency). A practice to avoid is one judge being responsible for half of the study and another judge being responsible for the balance, or some other such configuration. In any trial, a single primary judge responsible for all observations throughout the study is ideal.

3.4.7   Observation Schedule: Timing and Traffic Flow

Machines never tire, but people certainly do. It is difficult to maintain the same mental acuity for assessing the 99th panelist as the 9th panelist. A rule of thumb would be to determine the typical amount of time it takes to complete an observation, then allow 50% more time. This will prevent the pace from becoming too hectic. Short breaks should also be scheduled every hour to prevent fatigue. Panelists too will become fatigued if they are endlessly probed by a succession of instruments. When setting up a schedule, consider what is reasonable for subjects as well. The pace and break schedule will define the throughput, that is, the number of panelists per hour, that can be evaluated; the throughput in turn defines the total number of subjects that can be evaluated in a day. The total subjects that can be evaluated is often the maximum limit for participants in your trial.

The daily observation schedule should be described in the protocol. In a regression test, throughput of 10–20 subjects per hour is reasonable, depending on experience and efficiency of the clinicians. In a hydration test, throughput of 30 subjects per hour can be achieved.

In a trial where multiple measurements are being collected by different clinicians, a panelist checklist is recommended. The panelist follows the list in sequence to be sure the correct order is maintained, and as each measurement is completed it is initialed by the clinician. Before the subject is dismissed, a checklist is reviewed to make sure everything has been completed.

3.4.8 Lighting and Environmental Conditions

For all observations—visual, self-assessment or instrumental—consistency of conditions is very important both from one observation to the next and from one panelist to the next. Visual evaluations are best done under fixed lights and away from windows where sunlight changes throughout the day. A 2x magnifying ring-lamp is commonly used for dry skin visual evaluation. Instrumental measures benefit from having subjects equilibrate to a standard indoor temperature and humidity. For single-use tests, an air conditioned lab with good control is generally acceptable; for more rigorous control, a humidity/temperature control room is recommended.

3.4.9 Bathing and Shaving Restrictions

In studies over several weeks, it is recommended to standardize the bathing habits of subjects, for example, by issuing a standard mild soap bar and requiring all bathing be done in the morning, within 30 min of product application. Shaving during leg trials poses a particular challenge as shaving can exacerbate the appearance of dryness. A uniform schedule of how and when to shave should be included in the panelist instruction.

3.5 Sample Administration

In any trial, the product is usually the only thing subjects are concerned with. In clinician applied studies, subject interaction with the product is minimal. But in trials with home applications, the product is the most prominent source of information disclosed to subjects. In such trials, products must be presented without bias and should be adequately blinded. Label contents and product handling should be defined in the protocol. The following points are relevant only to clinical studies involving at-home application.

3.5.1 Uniform Packaging

Ideally all products would be presented in identical plain, coded containers. If product forms are different (creams versus lotions) the different packaging should be nondescript. Pump packages are preferred as they insure a more uniform dosage.

3.5.2 Descriptive Label Contents

Labels should contain absolute minimal descriptive information about the product. Three pieces of information are sufficient: study number, a cryptic product code, and a unique bottle number or subject identification. Good product codes are randomly assigned letter/number combinations. Bottle numbers can be sequentially assigned independently of product codes to aid in traceability of the products.

3.5.3 Warnings/Restrictions

If necessary, warning and caution statements must be included on the package. It is good practice to include a contact phone number in case of emergency on the label. Additional information may be provided in an accompanying sheet.

3.5.4 Weight Record and Sample Disposition

It is good practice to preweigh all bottles and reweigh at each observation. Using the bottle numbers, products can be traced to the individual panelists, and non-compliance (subjects applying too little or too much product) can be identified. Clinical test products must always be returned by the end of the trial, even if returned empty.

3.5.5 Retained Samples

It is always a good practice to retain one to three additional samples of each test material in the test package for reference during and after the study.

3.6 Pretreatment Phase

To evaluate the effectiveness of a dry skin treatment requires some degree of dry skin at baseline. The greater the initial level of dryness, the greater the potential for demonstrating effects. In the real world, few people allow their skin to reach marked or severe levels of dryness without taking action, therefore some type of pretreatment may be needed. In designing the dry skin protocol it is necessary to define the acceptability criteria for dryness, and if a pretreatment phase is needed, then the means for achieving baseline dyrness must likewise be defined.

3.6.1 Product Use/Exclusion

The generally accepted means of achieving sufficient baseline dryness is with a moisturizer weaning period, that is, where all cream/lotion use is stopped. For leg studies, the use of moisturizing cleansers or moisturizing leg shaving products must likewise be discontinued. During this phase subjects should be supplied with a commercial mild cleansing bar (such as Dove) for general bathing.

3.6.2 Length of Preconditioning Phase

Inducing dryness too harshly can lead to irritation. Superficial dryness for single application studies can usually be achieved in 24–72 hr even under moderate dry skin weather. Moderate to marked dryness for regression tests typically requires 3–7 days under more severe dry skin conditions.

3.6.3 Soap Washing Procedure

If weather conditions are severe, adequate dryness will occur naturally with lotion weaning. To enhance the drying process when necessary, a routine of two or three times daily washing can be included. A dry-down wash procedure is more stringent than an ordinary wash. For example;

> Lather bar in wet hand 10 rotations in 10 seconds.
> Apply lather to wet leg (or arm) and lather test site for 30 seconds.
> Rinse site thoroughly with water.
> Lightly pat dry.

Note that overwashing, especially with plain soap, must be avoided as it can go beyond flaky dry to a condition where surface squames are removed and skin lipids are hyperdepleted.

3.7 Product Treatment Phase

Whether the product is applied once or repeatedly, by clinician or by subjects at home, questions of how the products are applied, how much is used, where it is used, when it is used, and when it is to be avoided must all be answered. In a controlled clinical trial, the goal is to eliminate the variability of consumer use by defining every aspect of the treatment phase so that all subjects across all product groups are doing the exact same thing. Only by ensuring consistency across the groups can valid comparison of the groups be made.

3.7.1 Usage Rate

The rule set down by the FDA in the 1970s for sunscreen testing was to apply a uniform film of lotion at a rate of 2 mg/cm^2 [44]. This standard has been widely accepted for any lotion treatment, as it is in fact a reasonable amount. Higher application levels lead to excess on the skin which is unpleasant to the subject and will likely get rubbed off anyway.

For clinician-applied studies, test sites of $15–30 \text{ cm}^2$ are typically marked on the arm or leg. Treatment amounts are precisely dispensed using a pipette and rubbed in uniformly within the demarcated area with a gloved finger.

Because trials with home application cannot achieve this level of precision, detailed instructions to the panelists are required. For example, a pump which dispenses 0.5 g per press can be used as a convenient means of dispensing a standard dose. An instruction to apply one pump of product to the lower outer leg and rubbing in thoroughly is acceptably close to the desired application rate and, at the very least, is a uniform application procedure across test groups. In general, 0.5 g of a facial product is adequate for treating the entire face, while 1 g of a hand lotion is needed to treat both hands.

3.7.2 Frequency of Application

The original regression method called for twice daily application. At this rate, skin generally improves slowly over a week or two. While more frequent application would appear to allow skin to improve more quickly, much of the additional "benefit" would be cosmetic only and it could obscure the differences in real performance between products. Moreover, twice daily is a very easy routine for home-based panelists to follow: once when subjects get up in the morning and again before going to bed at night.

3.7.3 How Long to Use Product

For regression testing, 1 week is minimum to begin to see true physiological effects (i.e., discernable from mere cosmetic effects). In 3 weeks the skin has achieved full stratum corneum turnover so the entire skin layer at that point is the result of the treatment product. Two weeks is a middling approach that gives a performance prediction very near the 3-week results.

3.7.4 Weekend Treatments

The original regression test discontinued product over the weekends in order to strip away the cosmetic benefits and view more clearly the substantive benefits to dry skin. This procedure has its merit particularly where daily applications are conducted by a clinician. However, for home-use trials, simplicity of routine is key and it may be better to continue the same daily regimen over the weekends.

3.7.5 Observation Day Treatments

During regression tests, to avoid the cosmetic effect of residual lotion on skin, there should never be a product application prior to observations. The recommendation is to apply (as usual) the night before, then shower as normal on the day of the observation to wash away residual product. The daily treatment resumes immediately after the observation session is completed.

3.7.6 Panelist Instructions

Panelist instructions can never be clear enough or simple enough. The treatment procedure should be described as plainly as possible. On the first day of the trial, subjects must read these instructions and review them with the clinician. If possible, the first application should take place at the test center under supervision. A brief review of the instructions at each observations is recommended.

3.8 Regression

The regression phase is the signature component of the regression test. To properly evaluate the rate of return of dry skin, as much consideration must be given to what panelists do not do during this phase as was given to what they did during treatment phase.

3.8.1   What Products to Allow/Exclude

All treatment during this phase is discontinued. Panelists continue to refrain from using their normal lotion products and must continue to use only the prescribed wash products in the prescribed manner.

3.8.2   Length of Regression

Generally the regression phase is set up as a fixed term of 1–2 weeks after the final treatment. Seven days is sufficient to establish a rate of dry skin return though skin may not reach baseline. A 2-week regression allows skin to approach the original baseline level of dryness. In the nutrition protocol, regression can be extended to 3 weeks.

3.8.3   Observation Schedule

The difference between a cosmetic and substantive product should show up immediately after treatment is discontinued, where the healthier skin shows greater persistence. Therefore, a daily or every-other-day observation schedule is used during the first half of the regression phase.

4   EXAMPLE PROTOCOLS

From this discussion of points to consider when developing a protocol, it is evident that there is no single right way to conduct a trial. It is a generally poor practice to take a standard protocol and use it without thinking through the listed points to insure that the proposed study design is appropriate for your products and objectives.

Having said that, some guidance can be helpful. Table 6 provides a side-by-side listing of typical protocol specifications for four common approaches to dry skin. This table provides quick reference for some details of procedures and provides easy comparison of the size and scope of each procedure. Keep in mind that these should only be used for guidance; the fine points of your own final protocol must flow from your objectives and your consideration of the study details.

TABLE 6 Example Specifications for Four Clinical Study Protocols

	4-hr hydration	Mini regression	Kligman regression	Skin nutrition
General Requirements				
Objective	Compare the effect of 5 lotions to impart and maintain moisture in dry skin.	Predict the comparative effectiveness of 3 novel moisturizing ingredients in a cream base.	Directly compare the effectiveness of a prototype lotion versus 3 leading products on summer dry skin.	Compare the ability of 4 lotions to make severe winter dry skin healthy.
Test period	September	November	May	February
Location	New Jersey	Pennsylvania	Arizona	Montana
Weather Criteria	<70°F, <75% RH	<40°F, <60% RH	<95°F, <40% RH	<30°F, any RH
Test Duration	4 hours	2 weeks	5 weeks	4 weeks
Site	Lower legs	Volar forearms	Lower legs	Hands and lower legs
Size (n)	30	15	20	15
Number of test cells	6	4	3	4
Product/cells per subject	6 sites: 5 product and 1 untreated per subject	4 sites: 3 test products and 1 vehicle product per subject	2 sites: one on each leg; each subject directly compares a prototype against the standard lotion	1 product per subject applied to both hands
Total subjects	30	15	60	60
Control products	Untreated	Vehicle	Benchmark product	None

Subject recruitment				
Number recruited	35	20 at dry down	90 at dry down	75
Inclusion/exclusion	See Table 4	See Table 4	See Table 4	See Table 4
Dry skin requirement	<20 Skicon hydration index units	<45 corneometer hydration units	Grade 2–3 (0–4 point scale) visual dryness on both legs	None
Grading				
Visual	0–4 overall dryness	0–4 scaling; 0–4 erythema	0–4 overall leg dryness	0–6 overall hand dryness; 0–4 overall leg dryness
Instrumental	Hygrometer	Hygrometer	Hygrometer; squame adhesive	TEWL (legs); hygrometer (legs); tape biopsy for lipid and NMF analysis
Self-assessment	No	No	Yes	Yes
Observations				
Equilibration period	Wash legs with mild soap. Equilibrate 30 min. Panelists remain in room for duration of test.	20 min at room conditions prior to measurement.	20 min at room conditions prior to measurement.	20 min at room conditions prior to measurement.
Blinding procedure	Coded samples; clinician applied independently from evaluations.	Coded samples; clinician applied independently from evaluations.	Coded samples in plain white tubes. Random product assignment. Product assignment independent from evaluations.	Coded samples in plain white tubes. Random product assignment. Product assignment independent from evaluations.

Table 6 Continued

	4-hr hydration	Mini regression	Kligman regression	Skin nutrition
Observations (cont.)				
Frequency of observations	Baseline, 1, 2.5, and 4 hr	Treatment phase: Day 0, 1, 2, 4, 7. Regression phase: Day 8, 9, 11, 14.	Treatment phase: Day 0, 3, 7, 10, 14, 17, 21. Regression phase: Day 24, 28, 31, 35.	Regression phase: Day 0, 3, 7, 10, 14. Retreatment phase: Day 27, 21, 24, 28.
Viewing schedule	8:00 am to 1:00 pm	All observations in am	All observations in am	All observations in am
Preparing skin before visit	None.	Shower in am minimum 1 hr prior to visit.	Shower in am minimum 1 hr prior to visit. Do not apply lotion.	Shower in am minimum 1 hr prior to visit.
Observation test environment	Controlled for duration of test: 70°F, 50% RH.	Controlled for hygrometer. Visual under 2x ring-lamp.	Controlled for hygrometer. Visual under 2x ring-lamp.	Controlled for instruments. Visual under 2x ring-lamp.
Bathing/shaving restrictions	Shave legs 48 hr prior to study.	Shower in am. Use only provided cleanser.	Shower in am. Use only provided cleanser. Shave legs on day 4, 11, 18, 25, 32 only.	Shower in am. Use only provided cleanser. Avoid solvents and harsh detergent cleaners.
Pretreatment phase				
Product use	Discontinue lotion on legs	Wash arms twice daily with provided mild cleanser. Discontinue lotion use on arms	Wash legs daily with provided soap bar. Discontinue lotion use on legs.	Treat hands ad libitum, minimum 3 times per day. Recommend to apply whenever hands are washed.
Duration	3 days prior to baseline	7 days prior to baseline	7 days prior to baseline	28 days prior to baseline

				Retreatment phase[a]
Treatment phase				
Treatment procedure and product use rate	Three 25-cm^2 sites marked on each lower outer leg. Clinician applies 50 mg to each site. Five product and one untreated sites are rotated across panelists.	50 mg to 5-cm^2 sites.	Wash legs 15 s with provided soap bar. Pat dry and follow with 1 pump (0.5 g per pump) to each leg.	2 pumps (1 g) to hands.
Frequency of application	Once	Twice daily, am (between 8:00 and 10:00) and pm (between 6:00 and 8:00)	Twice daily, am and pm before going to bed	Twice Daily, am and pm before going to bed
Duration	4 hours	5 days	3 weeks	2 weeks
Weekend treatment	Clinician applied	No treatment	Regular schedule	Regular schedule
Observation day schedule		Clinician applied	Applied at home after am observation	Applied at home after am observation
Regression phase				
Product	No lotion on arms. Wash arms once daily with provided mild cleanser.		No lotion on legs. Wash legs twice daily for 15 s with provided soap bar.	No lotion on hands. Wash hands as normal using only the provided mild cleansing bar.
Duration	1 week		2 weeks	2 weeks

[a] For the nutrition protocol, the retreatment phase occurs *after* the regression phase.

REFERENCES

1. Kligman A. Regression method for assessing the efficacy of moisturizers. Cosmet Toil 1978; 93:27–35.
2. Blank I. Factors which influence the water content of the stratum corneum. J Invest Dermatol 1952; 18:433–440.
3. Blank I. Further observatons on factors which influence the water content of the stratum corneum; J Invest Dermatol 1953; 21:259–271.
4. Spruit D, Malten KE. Epidermal water barrier formation after stripping of normal skin. J Invest Dermatol 1965; 45(1):6–14.
5. Berube G, Messinger M, Burdick M. Measurement in vivo of transepidermal moisture loss. J Soc Cosmet Chem 1971; 22:361–368.
6. Berube G, Burdick M. Transepidermal water loss. II. The significance of the use thickness of topical substances. J Soc Cosmet Chem 1973; 25:397–406.
7. Rietschel R. A method to evaluate skin moisturizers in vivo. J Invest Dermatol 1978; 70:152–155.
8. Wildauer R, Bathwell J, Douglass A. Stratum corneum biomechanical properties. J Invest Dermatol 1971; 56:72–78.
9. Rieger M, Deem D. Skin moisturizers. I. Methods for measuring water regain, mechanical properties and transepidermal moisture loss of stratum corneum. J Soc Cosmet Chem 1974; 25:239–253.
10. Rieger M, Deem D. Skin moisturizers. II. The effects of cosmetic ingredients on human stratum corneum. J Soc Cosmet Chem 1974; 25:253–262.
11. Quattrone A, Laden K. Physical techniques for assessing skin moisturization. J Soc Cosmet Chem 1976; 27:607–623.
12. Christenson M, Hargens C, Nacht S, Gans E. Viscoelastic properties of intact human skin: instrumentation hydration effects and the contribution of the stratum corneum. J Invest Dermatol 1977; 69:282–286.
13. Cook T. Profilometry of skin: a useful tool for the substantiation of cosmetic efficacy. J Soc Cosmet Chem 1980; 31:339–358.
14. Tagami H. Electrical measurement of the water content of the skin surface. Cosmet Toil 1982; 97:39–47.
15. Leveque J. Physical methods for skin investigation. Int J Dermatol 1983; 22:368.
16. Nole G, Boisits E, Thaman L. The Salter complex impedance device as an instrument to measure the hydration level of the stratum corneum in vivo. Bioeng Skin 1988; 4(4):285–296.
17. Grove G, Grove M. Objective methods for assessing skin surface topography noninvasively. In: Leveque J, ed. Cutaneous Investigation in Health and Disease. New York: Marcel Dekker, 1988:1–32.
18. Grove G. Noninvasive methods for assessing moisturizers. In: Waggoner W, ed. Clinical Safety and Efficacy Testing of Cosmetics. New York: Marcel Dekker, 1990:121–147.
19. Prall J, Theiler R, Bowser P, Walsh M. The effectiveness of cosmetic products in alleviating a range of skin dryness conditions as determined by clinical and instrumental techniques. Int J Cosmet Sci 1986; 8:159–174.
20. Boisits E, Nole G, Cheney M; The refined regression method; J Cutan Aging Cosmet Dermatol 1989; Vol 1(3):155–163.

21. Moss J. The effect of 3 moisturizers on skin surface hydration. Skin Res Technol 1996; 2:32–36.

22. Loden M. Biophysical methods of providing objective documentation of the effects of moisturizing creams. Skin Res Technol 1995; 1:101–108.

23. Grove G. Skin surface hydration changes during a mini-regression test as measured in vivo by electrical conductivity. Current Therap Res 1992; 52(4):556–561.

24. Rawlings A. Effect of lactic acid isomers on keratinocyte ceramide synthesis. Arch Derm Res 1996; 288:383–390.

25. Batt M, Davis W, Fairhurst E, Gerrard W. Changes in the physical properties of the stratum corneum following treatment with glycerol. J Soc Cosmet Chem 1988; 39:367–381.

26. Grove G. The effect of moisturizers on skin surface hydration as measured in vivo by electrical conductivity; Current Therap Res; Vol 50:712–718.

27. Ertel K, Neumann P, Hartwig P, Rains G, Keswick B. Leg wash protocol to assess the skin moisturization potential of personal cleansing products. Int J Cosmet Sci 1999; 21:383–397.

28. Barker M. Moisturizers of tomorrow. Toxicol Cutan Ocular Toxicol 1992; 11(3):257–262.

29. McCook J, Berube G. Evaluation of hand and body lotions: correlation of objective and subjective responses. J Soc Cosmet Chem 1982; 33:372.

30. Boisits E. The evaluation of moisturizing products. Cosmet Toil 1986; 101:31–39.

31. Jackson E. Moisturizers of today. Toxicol Cutan Ocular Toxicol 1992; 11(3):173–184.

32. Hannon W, Maibach H. Efficacy of moisturizers assessed through bioengineering techniques. In: Cosmetology for Special Locations. pp. 246–269.

33. Rogiers V, Derde M, Verleye G, Roseeuw D. Standardized conditions needed for skin surface hydration measurements. Cosmet Toil 1990; 105:73–82.

34. Black D, DelPoza A, Lagarde J, Gall Y. Seasonal variability in the biophysical properties of stratum corneum from different anatomical sites. Skin Res Technol 2000; 5:70–76.

35. Goh C. Seasonal variations and environmental influences on the skin. In: Serup J, Jemec G, eds. Handbook of Non-Invasive Methods and the Skin. Boca Raton: CRC Press, 1995:27–30.

36. Prall J. Instrumental evaluation of the effects of cosmetic products on skin surfaces with particular reference to smoothness. J Soc Cosmet Chem 1973; 24:693–707.

37. Farinelli N, Berardesca E. The skin integument: variation relative to sex, age, race and body region. In: Serup J, Jemec G, eds. Handbook of Non-Invasive Methods and the Skin. Boca Raton: CRC Press, 1995:22–26.

38. Barlow T. Measuring skin hydration. Cosmet Toil 1999; 114(12):47–53.

39. Salter D. Study design. In: Loden M, Maibach H, eds. Dry Skin and Moisturizers: Chemistry and Function. Boca Raton: CRC Press, 2000:373–378.

40. Serup J. Prescription for a Bioengineering study: strategy, standards and definitions. In: Serup J, Jemec G, eds. Handbook of Non-Invasive Methods and the Skin. Boca Raton: CRC Press, 1995:17–21.

41. Spilker B. Guide to Clinical Trials. Philadelphia: Lippincott-Raven, 1996.
42. Serup J. EEMCO guidance for the assessment of dry skin (xerosis) and ichthyosis: clinical scoring systems. Skin Res Technol 1995; 1:109–114.
43. Seitz JC, Rizer RL, Spencer TS. Photographic standardization of dry skin. J Soc Cosmet Chem 1984; 35:423–437.
44. U.S. Food and Drug Administration. Sunscreen drug products for over-the-counter human use. Tentative Final Monograph; Proposed rule. 21 CFR 352.

23

Noninvasive Instrumental Methods for Assessing Moisturizers

**Gary L. Grove, Charles Zerweck,
and Elizabeth Pierce**
KGL Skin Study Center, Broomall, Pennsylvania

1   INTRODUCTION

Although the term *moisturizer* is in widespread use by both lay people and medical professionals, it is a neologism of the cosmetics industry and lacks a precise definition. It was conveniently coined by Madison Avenue to describe a treatment for dry skin, which remains one of the most frequent everyday skin problems. Unfortunately despite the fact that dry skin is a troublesome, disquieting problem for many millions of people, surprisingly little is known about its pathogenesis. We do know that dry skin is not a single entity, but rather a family of disorders that can originate in a variety of ways [1–4].

One type is the temporary dry skin condition which is the inevitable result of any kind of skin damage whether physical or chemical. This is a stereotypical response to injury and reflects a repair process in which new skin surface cells are formed at a greatly accelerated rate. This accelerated epidermopoiesis, which typically occurs after sunburn, chemical irritation, abrasion, or detergent damage, causes the skin to be dry and scaly, for example. As pointed out by Marenus [5] modern moisturizers often contain soothing agents to reduce chronic low level irritation.

We also know that some of the more severe dry skin conditions are genetically determined. Indeed, the biochemical defect in X-linked ichthyosis has been precisely identified as a lack of a specific enzyme, steroid sulfatase, which is essential for proper utilization of cholesterol in the keratinization process [6]. Other forms of dry skin are associated with an underlying disease such as psoriasis, atopic dermatitis, and diabetes or with nutritional problems.

By far the most general form of dry skin is that which is the primary concern of the typical moisturizer user and the focus of this chapter. For a thorough consideration of such common dry skin problems, one should read the excellent review by Chernosky [7].

Although it is certainly a gross oversimplification, historically, a reduced water content of the stratum corneum has been thought to be the key causative factor in skin dryness. There are two reasons for suggesting this. First, consider that dry skin problems are heavily influenced by weather conditions. Dry skin is far worse in the winter months when low relative humidity is often accompanied by low temperatures, strong icy winds, and dry overheated homes. The dry, hot climate of the desert is also apt to provoke dry skin. The critical factor, as shown by the thoughtful analysis provided by Gaul and Underwood [8], is the absolute moisture content of the air. Since the exposed stratum corneum will establish a hydration gradient in equilibrium with the surrounding air, any drop in the relative humidity of the environment will lead to a corresponding decrease in skin surface moisture levels. As shown by Middleton and Allen [9] the suppleness of the stratum corneum is closely related to its temperature and its water content. This means that such dry skin is relatively inflexible and inelastic under the previously mentioned adverse conditions. As a result, it will crack and fissure in order to accommodate body movements, producing one of the more characteristic signs of dry skin.

The second reason for believing that water content is a key factor in dry skin is a series of classic experiments performed by Blank [10,11]. He demonstrated very convincingly in the early 1950s that skin softening was most effectively achieved with water. Even long-term soaking of cadaver skin samples in various oils failed to produce a comparable degree of softening as a brief exposure to just water alone. Since that time, dermatologists and cosmetic chemists have emphasized that water is the principal plasticizer of the skin and critical in relieving the signs and symptoms of dry skin. Even if the therapy is based on anhydrous lipids, their effect on water content of the stratum corneum is still believed to be the keystone for an effective moisturizer.

Thus, it is not surprising that traditional moisturizers are formulated to increase the moisture content of the stratum corneum in two ways:

1. *Occlusion.* Coating the skin with oils such as petrolatum will retard the loss of surface water, thus increasing the moisture content of the underlying stratum corneum.

2. *By humectants.* Agents such as glycerin, sodium lactate, and PCA, which draw and strongly bind water, are added to a formulation and thus help trap water in the skin surface.

Of course, one should recognize that water alone can effectively eliminate all visual signs of dryness, although only temporarily. In this context, there are no ineffective cosmetic moisturizers, and the major difficulty facing investigators in this area is not to be unduly influenced by these transient effects. We must also heed the views of Prall et al. [12] as well as Wehr and Krochmal [13], who have found very little conclusive evidence to support a causative role of reduced water content with skin flakiness. They feel, and we concur, that the majority of moisturizers work by merely "sticking" loosened squames back onto the surface, thereby altering light scatter, causing the skin surface to appear more transparent, and hence less dry for a short period of time. We agree with Kligman [1,2] that such products should be classified as being "cosmetic" moisturizers in contrast to "therapeutic" moisturizers, which in fact modify the dry skin process rather than simply conceal it.

With these points in mind, let us review some of the clinical and instrumental methods that have developed to quantify skin dryness and thus allow us to evaluate moisturizers. Although Marenus [5] has provided some justification for extending the claims being made for modern moisturizers to include anti-aging, in this chapter we are going to limit ourselves to the more traditional claims of relieving the sings and symptoms of common dry skin.

2 EXPERIMENTAL DESIGNS FOR CLINICAL STUDIES

2.1 The Regression Method

By far the most widely used clinical method for assessing the efficacy of moisturizers is the regression method first proposed by Kligman [1,2] and later refined by Boisits, Nole, and Cheyney [14]. Such an approach can be used to identify products that are therapeutic moisturizers, which really modify the dry skin process, as opposed to cosmetic moisturizers, which merely conceal it temporarily. The most noteworthy change is our preference for middle-aged suburban housewives over young college co-eds as panelists. Although dry skin occurs across all age groups, we have found the housewives to have more consistent levels of dryness and, most importantly, to be far more reliable in complying with the requirements of the protocol, which include refraining from the use of any products except those provided during the study. We have also found that more mature volunteers are quite capable of self-administering the treatments whether using a controlled dosage or ad libitum application of the products. Nevertheless, we still prefer to have panelists report to our research center on a daily basis for at least their morning applications.

In recruiting volunteers for these types of clinical studies we screen for those individuals who have a history of dry skin problems of sufficient severity to require routine use of moisturizers during the dry skin season. We have found it best to enroll approximately twice as many subjects as needed and require them to refrain from the use of all products on the test sites for a 2-week pretrial period. Since many of our studies are run on the lateral aspects of the leg, we also impose restrictions on the scheduling and manner in which leg hair is removed. Restrictions are also placed on the use of such products as Buf-Pufs® (3M, St. Paul) loofa sponges, and bath oil beads.

At the end of this 2-week pretrial period, we select from these candidates the best subjects who have appreciable signs of dryness of equivalent magnitude on the paired test sites. This pretrial period also gives us a chance to determine the reliability of the panelists and their willingness to fully comply with the requirements of the experimental design, especially the restrictions.

Once a panel of 20 suitable subjects is selected, they are treated twice daily with the appropriate test products on each weekday for the next 2 weeks. In controlled dosing experiments, both applications are made by a technician, who applies liberal amounts of product with moderate hand pressure for a period of 30 s per leg. Disposable gloves are worn to prevent cross contamination of test products. Of course, at-home studies with ad libitum applications by the panelists themselves could also be conducted provided that the panelists are reliable and properly instructed.

The test sites are evaluated on the first two Mondays (days 7 and 14), and the study is terminated if improvement is negligible on the second Monday. Otherwise, follow-up observations are made on a daily basis every weekday for the next 2 weeks, or until the original level of dryness appears. During this regression period, the application of test products is discontinued, but all restrictions as to how the test sites are to be treated are maintained. Typical results based on the classic 6-week Kligman leg regression study schedule, which illustrates the behavior of a "cosmetic" moisturizer and a very effective "therapeutic" moisturizer, are shown in Fig. 1.

This basic design can be followed regardless of whether the test sites are the legs, arms, elbows, face, or other sites. The clinical expression of dry skin does vary from site to site, and the grading scale should be adjusted accordingly to reflect these differences. One effective way to do this is to utilize a comparative rating scheme in which the grader is forced to choose which of the paired sites is better and indicate by how much better using the terms slight, moderate, or dramatic to describe the degree of difference. Another equally valid approach is to use a well-characterized scoring scheme that has a sufficient number of grades (6 or more) to allow good resolution between products. We are very much in favor of the creation of standardized grading schemes which are accepted industry-wide such as EEMCO (European Expert Group on Efficacy Measurements of

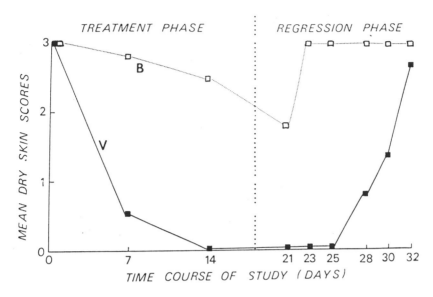

FIGURE 1 Comparative behavior of a "cosmetic" (B) and a "therapeutic" (V) moisturizer as revealed by the modified Kligman leg regression test. (From Refs. 1 and 2.)

Cosmetics and Other Topical Products) scoring system for evaluating dry skin in clinical studies [15]. This includes having the expert grader use a scoring scale which combines all of the major and minor signs of dry skin as well as individual grades of specific symptoms of scaling, roughness, redness, and cracks/fissures.

We also like the approach developed by Spencer's group [16] in which a reference set of standardized photos is used to visually define the grading scheme for the various attributes of dry skin being evaluated. Not only do such photographs serve as references for the expert graders to utilize during their actual assessments, but they can also serve in training and rating their proficiency through an external review process. Moreover, with such a photographic reference system, a much clearer understanding of the inclusion/exclusion criteria can be established. This is especially important in multicenter studies which involve different expert graders at different study sites.

It is also important to note that the relative merits of the test formulations as perceived by the panelists should also be ascertained. This can be done by a forced choice procedure, comparative visual analog scales, or written questionnaires. Also, as will be shown in the sections that follow, there are a number of instrumental methods that can be used to noninvasively measure various signs and symptoms of dry skin in a highly objective manner. Thus we have what is now known as the three-pronged approach to claims substantiation, which is based on ratings by an expert grader, instrumental measurements, and self-assessments by the panelist themselves [17,18].

2.2 The Mini-Regression Method

As a result of our considerable clinical experience with a wide variety of moisturizers and the classic Kligman regression test, we gained the impression that we could reliably detect meaningful differences on the Monday morning after the first treatment-free weekend. Prall's group [12] had reported similar experiences. This led to the development of the mini-regression method [19] in which the treatment and regression phases were compressed into a single week.

As can be seen from Fig. 2, the three-pronged approach also works quite well in these types of studies. Indeed, if a moisturizer is to be truly successful in

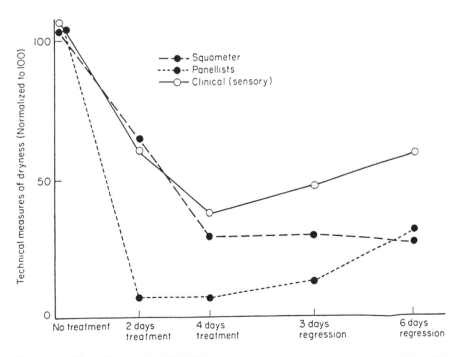

FIGURE 2 The effects of a 6% AHA-containing moisturizer as revealed by different evaluation methods employed during a mini-regression test. (Based on data presented in Ref. 12.)

the marketplace, then all three evaluations should be in good general agreement with regard to how effective a formulation is.

2.3 Short-Term Hydration Studies

In short-term testing, the effects are usually determined within a few hours after the initial application of a defined dose of test product to the dry skin site [20–24]. This type of testing is extremely useful during the product development process since it allows one to determine rapidly which of many possible prototypes might be the most desirable. The caveat here, and it is a big one, is that this approach clearly does not allow sufficient time for a therapeutic moisturizer to exert its effects. Nevertheless, variations on this approach enjoy widespread use. Since just water alone can provide a dramatic short-term effect, at least 3 hr should elapse before measurements are taken to eliminate this effect.

3 INSTRUMENTAL METHODS

Because of the increased demand for scientific documentation of advertising claims made for skin care products such as moisturizers, there has been considerable interest in developing instrumental methods for quantifying product efficacy in vivo [25–28]. The use of instrumental testing techniques by a number of premier companies has provided them with a significant marketing edge by providing functional claims and supportive research data to consumers. As a result, we have seen a large number of reports extolling the virtues of a wide variety of techniques which purportedly can be used to evaluate skin care product performance.

In the following sections we briefly review the most promising of the methods for their utility in documenting the efficacy of moisturizers. Although Marenus [5] has provided some justification for extending the claims made for modern moisturizers to include anti-aging, in this chapter we limit ourselves to the more traditional claims of relieving the signs and symptoms of common dry skin. The emphasis is on brevity, and the reader will be referred to appropriate reviews and research papers for details.

To provide a framework for these discussions we have arbitrarily grouped the instrumental methods into four broad areas based on some of the classic features of dry skin. First, we will deal with the appearance of the skin surface with its characteristic flaking and scaling. Next, we will examine a number of electrical and spectroscopic methods for determining the water content of the stratum corneum. Third, discussed will be various mechanical measurements of skin softness, extensibility, etc., that are an indication of the hydration state of the stratum corneum. Finally, we will discuss evaporative water loss measurements that can be used to show the effects of occlusive moisturizers. Of course these features are all interrelated to some degree and there can be considerable overlap in what is being measured by the various instruments.

3.1 Assessment of Skin Surface Appearance

3.1.1 Profilometry of Skin Surface Replicas

There are a number of different ways by which the skin surface topographic features can be noninvasively analyzed for degree of roughness. The reader is referred to a comprehensive review [29] for details of the present state of the art.

One of the most widely used methods has been to cast a replica of the skin surface by using one of the many excellent silicone rubber impression materials such as Silflo. A plastic positive can then be cast and measured with a computerized stylus instrument that provides a contour tracing of the surface. A number of different data formats are possible with such instruments, ranging from a simple plot of contour along a single axis to a three-dimensional stereograph of the skin surface topography. Provided that the movement of the stylus is sufficiently accurate, the problem becomes which of the many parameters that can be derived from such specimens are the best measure of skin surface roughness. As pointed out by both Cook [30,31] and Makki [32], certain roughness parameters appear to be more utilizable than others, and they can vary with scanning orientation and body area tested.

Despite its popularity [33], we do not advocate the use of replica profilometry to evaluate moisturizers, especially if the panelists have flakes and scales. There are many reasons for this. Among them is the fact that the application of the silicone rubber material most surely flattens and disturbs the uplifted scales, which is the primary feature of interest when evaluating a moisturizer.

3.1.2 Scanning Microdensitometry of Macrophotographs

Many investigators have shown that the visual benefits provided by a moisturizing cream can be photodocumented. Several attempts have been made by Marshall's group [34,35] to provide a more quantitative assessment of skin surface texture from such low magnification photographs. This includes using a scanning microdensitometer to detect the shadows and highlights of the skin surface captured in the photographic negative taken under standardized lighting conditions. The resulting contour line is quite similar to those obtained in replica profilometry, and calculation of roughness parameters can be done in much the same way. Although scanning densitometry has apparently been effective in following the clinical progression of patients with scaling disorders, such as psoriasis or ichthyosis, it seems less able to discriminate the degree of surface roughness in normal volunteers before and after application of various occlusive emollient agents. Thus, it seems that additional improvements must be made if this technique is to acquire the resolution needed to deal with more typical dry skin problems.

3.1.3 Squametry of Tape Strippings/D-Squame Adhesive Discs

The use of adhesive tape strippings to facilitate observations of the skin surface was first reported by Wolf [36]. When tape is pressed against the skin, the outermost, loosely adherent portion of the stratum corneum will stick to the tacky adhesive. Thus, upon removal the tape provides a specimen, which retains the topographical relationships of the skin surface and its pattern of desquamation (Fig. 3). This technique has been called squametry by Prall [12,37] and has been used extensively by both his group and ours [38] to provide an index of skin surface scaliness. More recently, D-Squame discs (CuDerm; Dallas, TX) have become a very popular way to sample the skin surface and objectively determine the degree of dryness [39–42]. Although there are a few subtle differences in the various approaches taken by different groups, the basic strategy is still the same, i.e., to use

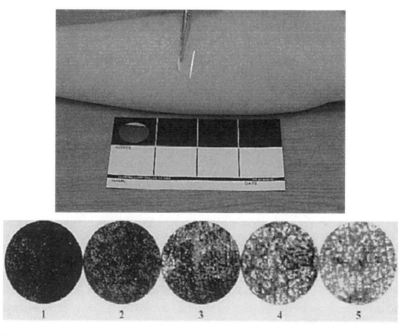

FIGURE 3 (Top) The use of D-Squame skin surface sampling disks for evaluating skin surface scaliness. (Bottom) Reference photos showing increasing scaliness levels. (Provided by CuDerm Corporation, Dallas, TX.)

an image-processing procedure to enhance and segment out the uplifted scales captured in such specimens. These objects of interest can be sized and counted to give a measure of the degree of skin surface scaliness.

3.1.4 In Vivo Image Analysis

Since an image-processing system has a video camera input, it is possible to directly record skin surface features. Indeed, we have been able to do a near real-time analysis of skin surface roughness with our Magiscan system [38]. To do so in a reliable fashion requires extreme attention to standardized lighting and critical camera angles. The use of special filters, such as those suggested by Dent [43], can also be used to enhance surface detail. Unfortunately, this all takes time, and we have found it more productive to take an intermediate photograph with a conventional 35-mm SLR camera system, similar to that described by Prall's group [12]. This means that this approach is converging on the macrophotographic technique described previously. Recently developed optical instruments (Scopeman, Microwatcher, Nikon) can collect and store electronic images directly from the skin surface. High-quality images can be evaluated by expert graders and/or quantified by image analysis techniques (Fig. 4).

3.2 Assessment of Stratum Corneum Hydration State

3.2.1 Electrical Properties

As pointed out in the excellent review by Leveque and de Rigal [44], the flow of electrical current through the skin surface is related to the water content of the stratum corneum, and thus offers a noninvasive method for assessing moisturization. They go on to describe that there are three distinct ways in which the application of an electrical field to the stratum corneum results in current flow. They are

1. Orientation of dipole moments of various constituents such as keratin
2. Ionic movement within the stratum corneum
3. Water mobility and proton exchange within the stratum corneum

It is obvious that water directly influences only the third mechanism, but it also indirectly facilitates current flow by enhancing dipole motion and ion mobility owing to decreased viscosity in hydrated stratum corneum. Unfortunately, agents other than water can lower skin impedance or resistance to flow. For example, urea, a common component in moisturizers, can induce changes in keratin dipole orientation by virtue of its protein denaturant properties. In addition, salts, whether as components of moisturizers or derived from perspiration, are intrinsically mobile and will cause a dramatic decrease in stratum corneum impedance. A

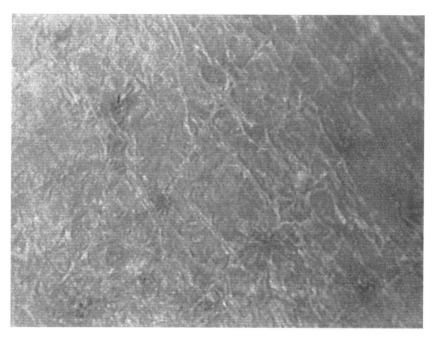

FIGURE 4 Image of scaling obtained by directly photographing skin surface using macrophotography.

concern for electrical measurements in some cases is that a product film on the skin surface can influence instrumental responses. The measurement of skin electrical impedance at different frequencies may help to exclude the effects of product residue on skin; however, no commercial instrument currently implements this technique [45].

Despite these problems, a number of investigators have found electrical measurements to be useful in assessing skin moisturization. Among the early workers was Clar [46], who worked at low frequencies where the net impedance of the stratum corneum is quite high. Unfortunately, her device required liquid junction electrodes to assure adequate current flow. Not only do these wet electrodes directly affect the hydration state of the underlying skin, they are also occlusive and must remain in place for approximately 20 min for each determination.

More recently, investigators have employed higher frequency impedance measurements that allow the use of dry electrodes. The most notable of these devices is the unit developed by Tagami and coworkers [47,48] that is now commercially available as the Skicon-200. This instrument operates at 3.5 MHz and uses an electrode of two concentric brass cylinders separated by a phenolic insulator. Their results from both in vitro and in vivo experiments show that impedance drops with increasing hydration. Furthermore, this method has been used by Tagami's group [48] and ours [49] to evaluate moisturizers as to their relative efficacy and duration of effect such as is shown in Fig. 5.

Other devices based on electrical measurements such as the Nova Dermal Phase Meter [50–52] and the laboratory-constructed wire mesh electrode instrument of Serban's group [53] have also been used to assess skin dryness and the effects of chronic treatments with such agents as creams, lotions, and raw materials. One of the more promising of the commercially available units is the DermaLab Moisture Meter with Pin Probe recently introduced by Cortex Technology (Hadsund, Denmark). As shown in Fig. 6 the probe configuration is not the typical flat electrode design but rather consists of a series of small pins. This arrangement offers two advantages over the conventional flat electrode design. For one, it is far less occlusive, especially when used with a stand-off device, and the problem of moisture accumulation under the probe with time is negligible. The other advantage is that it can be used on irregular and scaly surfaces such as the elbows or knuckles. With a flat electrode, the observed values are greatly influenced by how much skin surface is actually in intimate contact with the electrode surface [54].

Although it is assumed that these measurements are of the most superficial layers of the skin surface, the depth of the stratum corneum being probed with

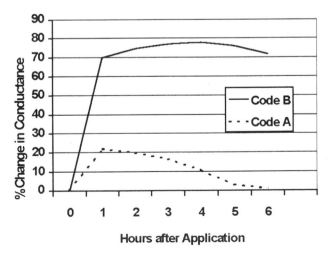

FIGURE 5 Impedance and stratum corneum hydration changes with time following the initial application of moisturizers of varying efficacies.

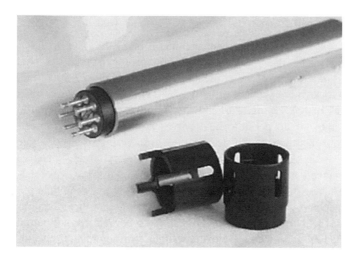

FIGURE 6 Close-up view of the pin probe used with the DermaLab Moisture Meter. This configuration is especially suited for making reliable measurements on rough scaly skin such as the hands and knuckles. (Photo courtesy of Cortex Technology, Hadsund, Denmark.)

any of these electrical devices has not been well established. Jacques and his coworkers [55–57] attempted to address this problem by utilizing a very high-frequency microwave device to measure the dielectric properties of the skin. They were operating in the region where the electrical fields will cause the water molecules to oscillate; and the amount of energy required to do so is dependent upon their number and hence their concentration. Clearly, microwaves can deeply penetrate within tissue; indeed, this is the basis for microwave ovens. To confine the microwave field to within a shallow depth of just a few microns, a focused microwave probe based upon fringe fields between closely spaced electrodes was created. The ability of the microwave probe to measure differences in skin surface water content was documented in vitro by following the water uptake of samples of human stratum corneum. In good agreement with other findings, these data showed biphasic behavior in which water was tightly bound at hydration levels of less than 30% (w/w), whereas it behaved like bulk liquid at higher levels. Jacques's focused microwave probe was also employed to measure the water concentration profile of human skin in vivo. This stratagraphic analysis was achieved by spacing the probe away from the skin surface with sections of inert Teflon film of varying thickness. As anticipated, and consistent with Fick's law, a nonlinear water concentration gradient across the stratum corneum was revealed in this manner.

3.2.2 Spectroscopic Methods

Photoacoustic Spectroscopy. Another technique that offers the potential for quantitatively measuring the water concentration profile is photoacoustic spectroscopy (PAS). For a review of the clinical applications of this PAS method, the reader is referred to several excellent reviews [58–61]. Briefly, PAS measures the thermal properties of the stratum corneum by modulating optical radiation with a beam chopper to create periodic heat waves within this compartment. These heat waves propagate through the stratum corneum, giving rise to periodic pressure waves that can be detected at the skin surface by an extremely sensitive microphone. The distance a heat wave can travel before being dissipated is related directly to the thermal diffusivity of the tissue and inversely to the modulation frequency. This means that by altering the modulation frequency of the optical radiation, one can probe the thermal properties of the stratum corneum as a function of depth. Although such measurements are experimentally difficult and time consuming, the effects of hydration-induced changes in the human stratum corneum water gradient have been evaluated both in vitro [62] and in vivo [63,64]. The results revealed that the stratum corneum is nonhomogeneous, and that the outermost surface layers dehydrate more rapidly than underlying tissue. The biggest problem with the PAS technique is that the probe is occlusive and water can build up during the consuming experiments leading to questionable results.

Infrared Spectroscopy. Attenuated total reflection infrared spectroscopy has been used by a number of investigators [65–68] to noninvasively examine the physicochemical interactions of skin and topically applied products. The basic premise of this approach is that the infrared (IR) absorbance spectrum of water can be, at least in principle, uniquely identified and effectively separated from the IR absorbance spectrum of everything else in the skin plus topical product system. Once this is achieved, the water content can be quantitatively determined from the intensity of IR absorbance in that particular region.

In early applications of this technique, the O-H stretching band from 3200 to 3600 cm was utilized to assess skin hydration [69]. More recent workers [70–72] have used the ratio of the amide I band at 1645 cm to the amide II band at 1545 cm to evaluate moisturizer efficacy. The idea here is that the amide I band is due to both protein and water absorbencies, whereas the amide II band is due to protein alone. Unfortunately, as pointed out by Potts [73], it seems that both the amide I and II bands of keratin, the major protein component of the stratum corneum (SC), change with hydration, thus removing the possibility of an absolute determination. Moreover, many moisturizers contain absorbencies which overlap with and therefore influence the intensity of the amide I band. Thus there are a number of difficulties inherent in quantitative evaluation of stratum corneum water content from amide I/II intensity ratios. Potts [74] is a strong advocate of the use of spectroscopy and feels that these problems can be overcome by using a ZWS crystal that has a low refractive index which closely approximates that of skin and enhances sensitivity. His Fourier Transform IR (FTIR) spectrophotometer allows rapid data collection and analysis. Moreover, he has chosen to use an incidence angle close to the critical angle to enhance the depth of penetration of the iodination into the skin and an optical path enclosed in a dry nitrogen purge to eliminate absorbencies due to atmospheric water vapor. With this arrangement, a minor absorbance band of water centered at 2100 cm has been found most useful in determining a quantity relative to the hydration of the stratum corneum.

Near-Infrared Spectroscopy. de Rigal et al. [75] have reported on a method for measuring skin surface hydration levels using near-infrared spectroscopy. By comparing the difference at 1100 nm, which is the wavelength at which the absorption of water is minimal, to that at 1940 nm, where it is strong, they were able to obtain a measurement that was well correlated to clinical scores of dryness (Fig. 7). In fact in their hands this measure proved to be far better correlated to the degree of skin dryness than did skin surface conductance.

Nuclear Magnetic Resonance. Most of the reports on the measurement of skin hydration using nuclear magnetic resonance (NMR) have been of the total skin including the dermis. However, Salter [76] has reported visualizing the hydration-dehydration process using MRI with a resolution of 0.06 mm. After 1 hr of occlusion with Vaseline, two layers could be observed in the stratum corneum of the finger pad. These differed in brightness with the degree of hydration, and over time the outer band disappeared as the surface "dried out." Unfortunately the

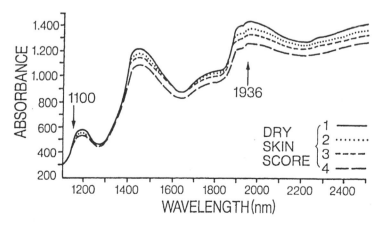

Figure 7 NIR absorption spectra of skin showing different levels of dryness. (From Ref. 75.)

resolution is still poor, and this observation has only been made in the finger pad which has a thick stratum corneum. Nevertheless, Szayna and Kuhn [77] have shown that the hydration effects of beauty care products on the stratum corneum could be demonstrated both in vivo and in vitro using high-field MRI and NMR microscopy.

3.3 Assessments of the Mechanical Properties of the Skin Surface

3.3.1 Gas-Bearing Electrodynamometer

The gas-bearing electrodynamometer (GBE) developed by Hargens [78] has proven to be quite useful in determining the viscoelastic properties of skin. The key element of this device is a highly compliant, virtually frictionless bearing of pressurized gas. Suspended upon this "gas bearing" is an armature, which mounts both the force coil and the core of a linear displacement transducer. The arrangement is such that the GBE measures the displacement of a small tab attached to the skin in response to a rapidly oscillating force placed parallel to its surface. The resulting dynamic stress–strain diagram (hystersis loop), which instantaneously appears on an oscilloscope, can be analyzed to reveal several characteristics such as stiffness, softness, and compliance. It is important to note that the GBE does not measure a fundamental property of the stratum corneum because there is a dermal component to these measured properties. Nevertheless, both Christensen et al. [79] and Cooper et al. [80] have observed a dramatic decrease in the elastic modulus immediately after the application of water to the skin. Such a rapid response could not result from the action of the applied water on the dermis and clearly indicates that the mechanical properties of the stratum corneum contribute significantly to the elastic modulus. Indeed, additional studies by both groups [79,80] as well as Maes et al. [81] have shown there to be a high degree of correlation of elastic modulus measurements with visual assessments of skin condition by a trained grader. In vitro studies [82] have also shown that dry skin is generally stiffer than normal skin, and effective treatments such as with glycerin can indeed soften the skin.

3.3.2 Twistometre and Dermal Torque Meter

The group of Leveque and de Rigal [83] have made extensive use of the Twistometre® (L'Oreal, Paris) to measure in vivo the influence of stratum corneum hydration on its extensibility. The Dermal Torque Meter is a commercially available variant of their device (Fig. 8). Both apply a weak torque to a rotating disk that is attached to the skin with a nonslip, tacky adhesive. The torque is held constant and the movement of the disk is monitored by a rotational sensor that is linked to a microprocessor that computes the main parameters. The area subjected to this twisting load is well delineated by a fixed guard ring that is con-

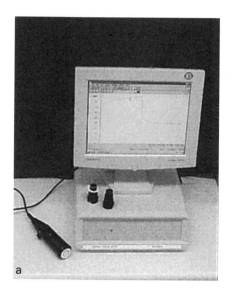 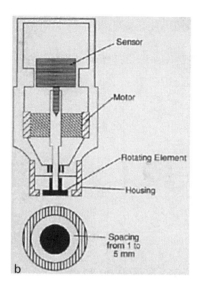

FIGURE 8 (a) The Dermal Torque Meter for measuring the torsional elasticity of the skin. (b) Schematic diagram of the Dermal Torque Meter. (Figure courtesy of Dia-Stron, Ltd., Andover, UK.)

centric to the inner rotating disk. When the distance between the disk and surrounding guard ring is less than 1 mm, the extensibility measurement (Ue) primarily reflects the resistance of the stratum corneum to stretching. Both short- and long-term studies with a variety of moisturizers and humectants have shown that this is a sensitive measure for rating such products as to their hydrating efficacy [83]. Indeed, it has been very nicely shown by Wiechers [84] that measurements of skin elasticity with the Diastron Dermal Torque Meter in combination with skin hydration levels by electrical conductance provides an excellent approach for the formulator to assess performance claims for skin care product ingredients. It has also been very clearly shown that there is a striking decrease in stratum corneum extensibility as the severity of dryness increases [85]. By far the most advanced application of this technology has been the creation of a "skin condition chart" based on the torsional mechanical properties of the skin as measured with the Dia-Stron DTM by Salter's group [86], as shown in Fig. 9.

3.3.3 Coefficient of Friction Devices

Skin friction plays an important role in both subjective and objective evaluations of many skin surface attributes including roughness and texture [87]. Devices which have been employed for this purpose include a rotating wheel [88,89], a re-

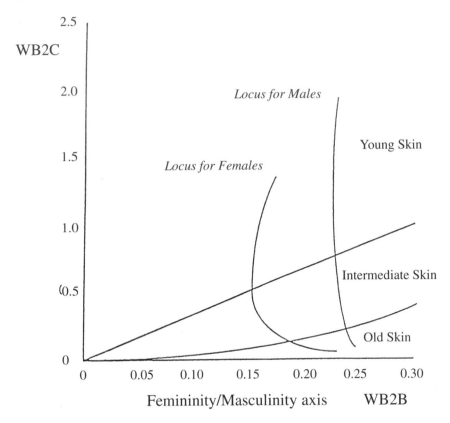

FIGURE 9 A "skin condition chart" based on the mechanical properties of the skin in vivo using the Dia-Stron Dermal Torque Meter. Any person can be located at a point indicating their overall skin condition in mechanical terms, and changes can be shown by movement across the plot. (From Ref. 85.)

volving ground glass disk [90,91], a sliding sled [92], and a modified viscometer [93–95]. In all cases, the underlying principle is that frictional properties of human skin in vivo can be assessed by determining how much force is required to drag an object across the skin surface. Although Weinstein [92] states rather matter of factly that "smoother skin requires less force," in actual practice the interpretation of differences in frictional properties induced by product application is very complicated. For example, moisturizers, which smooth and hydrate the skin, can actually increase friction as a result of increased contact area with the moving surface of the measuring device [88,90,92,95,96]. Nacht and coworkers [97] have suggested that these changes might also reflect an increased adhesiveness of the stratum corneum in a hydrated state. On the other hand, materials which act as surface lubricants do indeed lower the coefficient of friction, making the skin feel more slippery [88,96,98,99]. In the case of a greasy occlusive material such as petrolatum, a biphasic response can be observed in which initially the coefficient of friction decreases owing to its lubricant properties, then later it increases over baseline as a consequence of the increased hydration induced by occlusion [96].

Thus, it is not surprising that coefficient of friction measurements by themselves sometimes correlate very poorly with sensory scores of smoothness, as shown by Prall's group [90]. While additional studies in this area may correct this situation, at the present time such measurements do not seem to be useful in providing a precise and objective measure of skin roughness per se. Nevertheless, the use of this approach to screen topicals for their after-feel attributes of greasiness and their moisturizing properties as outlined by Nacht and coworkers [97] should prove worthwhile.

3.3.4 Scratch Resistance Test

Prall [90] has demonstrated that one of the physical properties of the skin that contributes to the overall perception of smoothness by the customer is hardness, as measured by the lowest pressure load which causes a stylus to just visibly scratch the skin surface. Although not widely employed, many individuals who suffer from dry skin problems will do an analogous procedure by scraping the skin surface with their fingernail to reveal underlying defects that might not be so obvious at first glance.

3.3.5 Sonic Wave Propagation

Experimental results from a number of laboratories have indicated that the mechanical properties of the skin vary dramatically with the stratum corneum hydration. These are often associated with subjective assessments of moisturization, especially with regard to the ability of the product to make the skin feel soft. For example, Torgalkar [100] utilized a vibrational device operating in the audible frequency range (approximately 700 Hz) to impart small amplitude oscillations normal to the skin surface. By scanning the frequency range, he was able to measure the resonant frequency of these "ripple waves" and from the known vibrational characteristics of the oscillator device calculate the energy loss of the viscous component of the skin. His results revealed that a continuous and rapid decline in energy loss occurred immediately after removal of an occlusive wrap that remained in place on the volar forearm of a subject for 14 hr. Indeed, a constant value was reached within 10 min after the wrap was removed, suggesting that the outer epidermal layers were primarily responsible for these changes in "softness."

More recently, Potts and his coworkers [101,102] have extended these studies of the effects of moisturizers on the viscoelastic properties of the stratum corneum. Their device consists of a vibrational stylus that lightly rests on the skin surface. The amplitude of the vibrations propagated on the skin surface is constant over the broad range of frequencies (20–1000 Hz) utilized in this method. A second pick-up stylus is positioned on the skin surface a few millimeters from the first. By using a spectrum analyzer, it was possible to determine the time required for these shear waves to travel through the skin surface and the degree of amplitude dampening as a function of frequency. As demonstrated in Fig. 10, the propagation velocity of hydrated skin was dramatically reduced, especially at the lower frequencies where the properties of the stratum corneum are primarily measured. This group has also shown [103] there to be seasonal and age-related changes that are consistent with the notion that this approach is indeed an indirect measure of the hydration state of the outer layers of the stratum corneum, although the exact relationship between frequency and depth needs to be established.

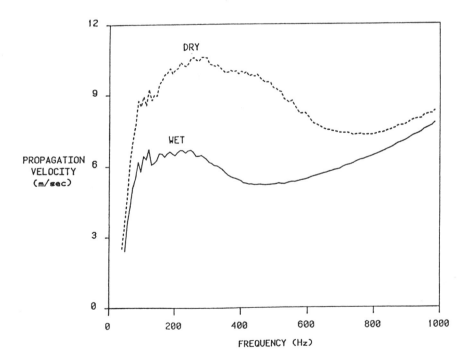

FIGURE 10 The propagation velocity versus frequency for shear waves in the skin of the dorsal hand for one individual. Data were obtained under ambient conditions (DRY) and after soaking the hand in water for 5 min followed by brief towelling (WET). (From Ref. 101.)

Dahlgren and Elsnau [104] have utilized a similar sonic velocity technique to assess the relative efficacy of moisturizers. Their results have shown that topically applied moisturizers do indeed decrease the sonic propagation velocity in skin and that this decrease is highly correlated with subjective assessments of moisturization. More importantly, the instrumental changes were noted after only a few days of use, whereas the subjective assessments took several weeks, indicating that sonic velocity can be a predictive measure.

3.4 Measurement of Stratum Corneum Barrier Function

The development of various methods for measuring trans-epidermal water loss (TEWL) have been comprehensively reviewed [105–108]. Leveque et al. [109] have shown that there is at least a trend toward higher than normal water loss values with dry skin. In more severe cases, where the skin is cracked and fissured, water loss rates are clearly elevated. One would expect that the greater the occlusivity of a product, the greater the reduction in TEWL upon its application, and this is certainly the case as shown by several studies [110–114]. With the commercially available instruments such as the computerized DermaLab TEWL Probe (Fig. 11) these types of assessments are straightforward and easy to accomplish [115,116]. Some care should be taken to ensure that the amount of product applied is relevant to the intended use conditions, as a thick film can give an unrealistically high value [117], and that the ambient temperatures are low so that sweating is not a factor [118]. In short-term experiments, it is important that suf-

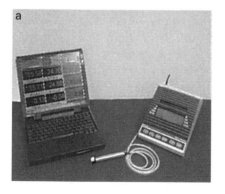
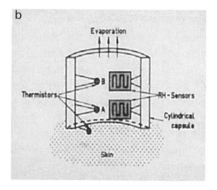

FIGURE 11 (a) The DermaLab TEWL Probe for measuring evaporative water loss from the skin surface. (b) Schematic diagram of the probe showing the paired RH and temperature sensors at fixed distance above the skin surface housed in an open chamber. (Figure courtesy of cyberDERM, Inc., Media, PA.)

ficient time be given for the volatiles to escape from the newly applied formulation as some of these can harm the sensors of the TEWL probe [119].

In dealing with moisturizers that are based on humectants, the situation is much more complex. Very early studies by Powers and Fox [120] demonstrated that trans-epidermal water loss was increased, not decreased, when treated with effective moisturizers. Rietschel [121,122] has confirmed these findings, especially with regard to the behavior of products containing glycerin. It is known that the diffusion coefficient increases with increased hydration of the stratum corneum [123–125], and thus water vapor will move through more readily. This means that more water is available to the outermost layers of the stratum corneum, thus leading to relief of the signs and symptoms of dry skin. Unfortunately, damaging products such as detergents will disrupt the barrier properties of the stratum corneum and also lead to increased flux and elevations in trans-epidermal water loss values. Of course, this is an undesirable consequence of product usage.

This means that there is a complex relationship between water content and flux in the stratum corneum that depends upon skin condition, which has been beautifully graphically summarized by Loden and Lindberg [20,21] as shown in Fig. 12.

4 SUMMARY

The methods for assessing the moisturizing efficacy of skin care products range from relying on the subjective assessments made by the panelists of their own skin to highly objective computer-assisted instrumental methods. No matter how accurate and precise an objective measurement may be, the question of relevance must always be considered. The measurement must ultimately correlate with the clinical perception of dry skin. At the moment, no one instrumental method can replace the experienced grader in rating dry skin. Devices invariably measure a single attribute, whereas the human brain integrates multiple inputs secured from vision and touch. By employing a battery of instrumental methods we can hope to gain a much fuller understanding of what defects are responsible for the dry skin problem, but this should be done in conjunction with, not instead of, the more classic clinical studies. Indeed, we strongly advocate that a three-pronged approach based on panelist self-appraisal, expert grader evaluations, and relevant instrumental measurements be utilized for adequately substantiating product performance.

Each of these methods has its own advantages, disadvantages, and idiosyncrasies. We recommend the use of multiple instruments in measuring the effects of moisturizing products on skin to characterize the broad spectrum of their effects. We would also encourage the adoption of standard operating procedures appropriate for the study design. Key methodological considerations include sever-

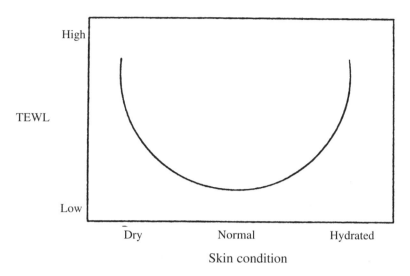

FIGURE 12 A simplified description of the relationship between TEWL and the degree of hydration of stratum corneum. (From Ref. 20.)

ity of dry skin being studied, product application procedures, time interval after application before measurement, study duration, and types of instruments used. We have found that the quality of instrumental measurements depends upon the use of a controlled environment (temperature and humidity) and the proper acclimation of the panelists to that environment.

We cannot stress enough that the operator must have a clear understanding of their instrument and how to consistently take correct measurements with it. Many of the modern instruments available today have been made extremely user friendly by their manufacturers. As a result anyone can plug in an instrument and within a few minutes begin to acquire readings without needing to understand anything else. If the readings show that their favorite product is the best, then they are very pleased with how the instrument performs. If on the other hand their favorite product doesn't fare so well, then most likely the new instrument will be blamed as performing poorly, not the product. Seldom is any consideration given by the investigator to undertake a proper validation study to learn the true limitations of the instrument and/or product.

Fortunately several groups have begun to address this problem of operator competency. Chief among them is the International Society of Bioengineering and the Skin as well as the American-based Dermal Clinical Evaluation Society, who have from time to time sponsored excellent workshops on how to use some of the more popular instruments properly. At least one firm, cyberDERM, Inc., has established a formal training program including educational course materials and proficiency exams that lead to certification of the operator according to factory authorized standards.

REFERENCES

1. Kligman AM. Regression method for assessing the efficacy of moisturizers. Cosmet Toil 1978; 93:27–35.
2. Kligman AM, Lavker RM, Grove GL, Stoudemayer T. Some aspects of dry skin and its treatment. In: Kligman AM, Leyden JJ, eds. Safety and Efficacy of Topical Drugs and Cosmetics. New York: Grune and Stratton, 1982:221–238.
3. Pierard GE. What does "dry skin" mean? Int J Dermatol 1987; 26:167–168.
4. Rieger MM. Skin, water and moisturization. Cosmet Toil 1989; 104:41–50.
5. Marenus KD. Skin conditioning benefits of moisturizing products. In: Aust LB, ed. Cosmetic Claims Substantiation. Melville, NY: Estee Lauder Research Laboratories, 1998:97–113.
6. Shapiro IJ, Weiss R, Webster D. X-linked ichthyoses due to sterol sulfatase deficiency. Lancet 1970; 1:70–72.
7. Chernosky ME. Clinical aspects of dry skin. J Soc Cosmet Chem 1976; 27:365–376.
8. Gaul LE, Underwood GB. Relation of dew point and barometric pressure to chapping of skin. J Invest Dermatol 1951; 18:9–12.
9. Middleton JD, Allen BM. The influence of temperature and humidity on stratum corneum and its relation to skin chapping. J Soc Cosmet Chem 1973; 24:239–243.
10. Blank IH. Factors which influence the water content of the stratum corneum. J Invest Dermatol 1952; 18:433–440.
11. Blank IH. Further observations on factors which influence the water content of the stratum corneum. J Invest Dermatol 1953; 21:259–271.
12. Prall JK, Theiler RF, Bowser PA, Walsh M. The effectiveness of cosmetic products in alleviating a range of skin dryness conditions as determined by clinical and instrumental techniques. Int J Cosmet Sci 1986; 8:159–174.
13. Wehr RF, Krochmal L. Considerations in selecting a moisturizer on the water distribution in human stratum corneum. Cutis 1987; 39(VI):512–515.
14. Boisits EK, Nole GE, Cheyney MC. The refined regression method. J Cutan Aging Cosmet Dermatol 1989; 1(III):155–163.
15. Serup J. EEMCO guidance for the assessment of dry skin (xerosis) and ichthyosis: clinical scoring systems. Skin Res Technol 1995; 1:109–114.
16. Seitz J, Rizer R, Spencer T. Photographic standardization of dry skin. J Soc Cosmet Chem 1984; 35:423.
17. Grove GL. Techniques for substantiating skin care product claims. In: Kligman AM, Leyden JJ, eds. Safety and Efficacy of Topical Drugs and Cosmetics. New York: Grune and Stratton, 1982:157–176.
18. Grove GL. Design of studies to measure skin care product performance. Bioeng Skin 1987; 3:359–373.
19. Grove GL. Skin surface hydration changes during a mini leg regression test as measured in vivo by electrical conductivity. Curr Ther Res 1992; 52 40:1–6.

20. Loden M, Lindberg M. Product testing—testing of moisturizers. In: Elsner P, Wilhelm K-P, Maibach HI, eds. Bioengineering of the Skin: Water and the Stratum Corneum. Boca Raton: CRC Press, 1994:275–289.

21. Loden M, Lindberg M. The influence of a single application of different moisturizers on the skin capacitance. Acta Derm Venerol (Stockholm) 1991; 71:79.

22. Serup J. A three-hour test for rapid comparison of the effects of moisturizers and active constituents (urea). Measurements of hydration, scaling and skin surface lipidization by non-invasive techniques. Acta Derm Venereol (Stockholm) 1992; (Suppl 177):29.

23. Blichmann CW, Serup J, Winther A. Effects of a single application of a moisturizer: evaporation of emulsion water, skin surface temperature, electrical conductance, electrical capacitance and skin surface (emulsion) lipids. Acta Derm Venerol (Stockholm) 1989; 70:400.

24. Grove GL. The effects of moisturizers on skin surface hydration as measured in vivo by electrical conductivity. Curr Ther Res 1991; 50 5:712–719.

25. Leveque JL. Physical methods for skin investigation. Int J Dermatol 1983; 22:368–375.

26. Kajs TM, Gartstein V. Review of the instrumental assessment of skin: effects of cleansing products. J Soc Cosmet Chem 1991; 42:249–271.

27. Takahaski M. Recent progress in skin bioengineering and its application to evaluation of cosmetics. SÖFW J 2000; 126:6–18.

28. Grove GL. Non-invasive methods for assessing moisturizers. In: Waggoner WC, ed. Clinical Safety and Efficacy Testing of Cosmetics. New York: Marcel Dekker, 1990:121–148.

29. Grove GL, Grove MJ. Objective methods for assessing skin surface topography noninvasively. In: Leveque JL, ed. Cutaneous Investigation in Health and Disease. New York: Marcel Dekker, 1988:1–32.

30. Cook TH. Profilometry of skin: a useful tool for the substantiation of cosmetic efficacy. J Soc Cosmet Chem 1980; 31:339–359.

31. Cook TH, Craft TJ, Brunelle RL, Norris F, Griffin WA. Quantification of the skin's topography by skin profilometry. Int J Cosmet Sci 1982; 4:195–205.

32. Makki S, Agache P, Mignot J, Zahouani H. Statistical analysis and three dimensional representation of the human skin surface. J Soc Cosmet Chem 1984; 35:311–325.

33. Dorogi PL, Zielinski M. Assessment of skin conditions using profilometry. Cosmet Toil 1989; 104(3):39–44.

34. Marshall R, Marks R. Assessment of skin surface by scanning densitometry of macrophotography. Clin Exp Dermatol 1983; 8:121–127.

35. Marshall R, Marks R. Quantification of skin surface texture of macrophotography and computer aided scanning densitometry. J Audiov Media Med 1983; 6:98–103.

36. Wolf J. Das oberflachen relief der menschlichen Haut. Z Mikrosk Anat Forsch 1940; 47:351.

37. Prall JK. Scaliness of human skin. Arch Biochem Cosmetol 1966; 9:27–43.

38. Grove GL. Dermatological applications of the Magiscan image analyzing computer. In: Marks R, Payne PA, eds. Bioengineering and the Skin. Lancaster, England: MTP Press, 1981:173–182.

39. Pierard GE, Pierard-Franchimont C, Saint Leger D, Kligman AM. Squamometry:

the assessment of xerosis by cyanoacrylate surface biopsies and colorimetry of D-Squame adhesive disks. J Soc Cosmet Chem 1992; 43:292–305.

40. Miller DL. D-Squame adhesive disks. In: Wilhelm K-P, Elsner P, Berardesca E, Maibach HI, eds. Bioengineering of the skin: skin surface imaging and analysis. Boca Raton: CRC Press, 1997:39–46.

41. Schatz H, Altmeyer PJ, Kligman AM. Dry skin and scaling evaluated by D-squames and image analyses. In: Serup J, Jemec GBE, eds. Handbook of non-invasive methods and the skin. Boca Raton: CRC Press, 1995:153–157.

42. Serup J, Winther A, Blichmann C. A simple method for the study of scale pattern and effect of a moisturizer—qualitative and quantitative evaluation by D-Squame tape in comparison with parameters of epidermal hydration. Clin Exp Dermatol 1989; 14:227–282.

43. Dent RV. The photographic aspects. J Lab Clin Med 1983; 26:1852–1862.

44. Leveque JL, de Rigal J. Impedance methods for studying skin moisturization. J Soc Cosmet Chem 1983; 34:419–428.

45. Salter DC. Examination of stratum corneum hydration state by electrical methods. Curr Probl Dermatol 1998; 26:38–47.

46. Clar EJ, Her CP, Sturelle CG. Skin impedance and moisturization. J Soc Cosmet Chem 1975; 26:337–353.

47. Tagami H, Ohi M, Iwatsuki K, Kanamaru Y, Ichijo B. Evaluation of the skin surface hydration in vivo by electrical measurement. J Invest Dermatol 1980; 75:500–507.

48. Tagami H. Impedance measurement for evaluation of the hydration state of the skin surface. In: Leveque JL, ed. Cutaneous Investigation in Health and Disease: Noninvasive Methods and Instrumentation. New York: Marcel Dekker, 1989:79–111.

49. Wortzman M, Grove GL. Assessment of long-lasting moisturizers by skin surface electrical hydrometry. Proceedings of 7th International Symposium of Bioengineering and the Skin, Milwaukee, WI, June 16–18, 1988.

50. Kohli R. Impedance measurements for the noninvasive monitoring of skin hydration-A reassessment. Int J Pharm 1985; 26:275–287.

51. Spencer TS, Anderson PJ, Seitz JC. Use of a phase angle meter to measure product effects on the skin surface. Bioeng Skin 1986; 2:153.

52. Gabard B, Treffel P. Hardware and measuring principle: the NOVA DPM 9003. In: Elsner P, Berardesca E, Maibach HI, eds. Bioengineering of the Skin: Water and the Stratum Corneum. Boca Raton: CRC Press, 1994:177–195.

53. Serban GP, Henry SM, Cotty VF, Cohen GL, Riveley JA. Electronic technique for the in vivo assessment of skin dryness and the effect of chronic treatment with a lotion on the water barrier function of dry skin. J Soc Cosmet Chem 1983; 34:383–389.

54. Berardesca E. EEMCO guidance for the assessment of stratum corneum hydration: electrical methods. Skin Res Technol 1997; 3:126–132.

55. Jacques SL. A linear measurement of the water content of the stratum corneum of human skin using a microwave probe. IEEE Eng Med Biol Soc Conf 1979; 180–182.

56. Jacques SL, Maibach HI, Susskind C. Water content in stratum corneum measured by focused microwave probe: normal and psoriatic. Bioeng Skin Newsletter 1981; 3:118.

57. Murahara RI, Hing SAO, Maibach HI, Roheim JR. The use of a microwave probe to evaluate the hydration of human stratum corneum in vivo. Bioeng Skin 1986; 2:235–247.
58. Rosencwaig A. Photoacoustic spectroscopy of biological materials. Science 1973; 181:657–658.
59. Rosencwaig A. Potential clinical applications of photoacoustics. Clin Chem 1982; 28:1878–1881.
60. Cahen D, Bults G, Garty H, Malkin S. Photoacoustics in life sciences. J Biochem Biophys Methods 1980; 3:293–310.
61. Campbell SD, Yee SS, Afromwitz MA. Applications of photoacoustic spectroscopy to problems in dermatological research. IEEE Transactions in Biomedical Engineering 1979; BME-28 26:220–227.
62. Pines E, Cunningham T. Dermatological photoacoustic spectroscopy. In: Marks R, Payne PA, eds. Bioengineering and the Skin. Lancaster, England: MTP Press, 1981:283–290.
63. Simon I, Emslie AG, Apt CM, Blank IH, Anderson RR. Determination of in vivo water concentration profile in human stratum corneum by a photoacoustic method. In: Marks R, Payne PA, eds. Bioengineering and the Skin. Lancaster, England: MTP Press, 1981:187–195.
64. Rosencwaig A, Pines E. A photoacoustic study of newborn rat stratum corneum. Biochim Biophys Acta 1977; 493:10–23.
65. Scheuplein RJ. A survey of some fundamental aspects of the absorption and reflection of light by tissue. J Soc Cosmet Chem 1964; 11:111–112.
66. Puttnam NA, Baxter BH. Spectroscopic studies of skin in situ by attenuated total reflectance. J Soc Cosmet Chem 1967; 18:469–472.
67. Puttnam NA. Attenuated total reflectance studies of the skin. J Soc Cosmet Chem 1978; 23:209–226.
68. Comaish S. Infrared studies of human skin in vivo by multiple internal reflection. Br J Dermatol 1968; 80:552–528.
69. Baier RE. Noninvasive, rapid characterization of human skin chemistry in situ. J Soc Cosmet Chem 1978; 29:283–306.
70. Osberghaus R, Gloxhuber H, Braig S. Hydagen-F, ein neuer Hautfeuchitigkeitsregulator Methoden und Ergebnisse des Wirkungsnachweises. J Soc Cosmet Chem 1979; 29:133–146.
71. Triebskorn A, Gloor M, Greiner F. Comparative investigation of the water content of the stratum corneum, using different methods of measurement. Dermatologica 1983; 167:64–69.
72. Stanfield JW, Kyriakopolour A. Substantivity of alpha keri bath oil® (Westwood Pharmaceuticals Inc., Buffalo, NY). Proceedings of 4th International Symposium in Bioengineering and the Skin, Bescanson, France, 1983.
73. Potts RO, Guzek DB, Harris RH, McKie JE. A noninvasive, in vivo technique to quantitatively measure the water concentration of the stratum corneum using attenuated total reflection infrared spectroscopy. Arch Dermatol Res 1985; 277:489–495.
74. Potts RO. Stratum corneum hydration: experimental techniques and interpretations of results. J Soc Cosmet Chem 1986; 37:9–33.

75. de Rigal J, Losch MT, Bazin R, Camus C, Sturelle C, Descamps V. Near infrared spectroscopy: a new approach to the characterization of dry skin. Proceedings of IFSCC International Congress, Yokohama, Japan 1992, pp. 1131–1146.
76. Ablett S, Burdett NG, Carpenter TA, Hall LD, Salter DC. Short echo time MRI enables visualization of the natural state of human stratum corneum water in vivo. Magn Reson Imaging 1996; 14(4):357–360.
77. Szayna M, Kuhn W. In vivo and in vitro investigations of hydration effects of beauty care products by high-filed MRI and NMR microscopy. J Eur Acad Dermatol Venereol 1998; 11(2):112–128.
78. Hargens CW. The gas-bearing electrodynamometer (GBE) applied to measuring mechanical changes in skin and other tissues. In: Marks R, Payne P, eds. Bioengineering and the Skin. Lancaster, England: MTP Press, 1981:113–122.
79. Christensen MS, Hargens CW, Nacht S, Gans EH. Viscoelastic properties of intact human skin: instrumentation, hydration effects, and the contribution of the stratum corneum. J Invest Dermatol 1977; 69:282–286.
80. Cooper ER, Missel PJ, Hannon DP, Albright GB. Mechanical properties of dry, normal, and glycerol-treated skin as measured by the gas-bearing electrodynamometer. J Soc Cosmet Chem 1985; 36:335–348.
81. Maes D, Short J, Turek BA, Reinstein JA. In vivo measuring of skin softness using the gas bearing electrodynamometer. Int J Cosmet Sci 1983; 5:189–200.
82. Missel PJ, Bowman WD, Benzinger MJ, Albright GB. An in vitro method for skin preservation to study the influences of relative humidity and treatment on stratum corneum elasticity. Bioeng Skin 1986; 2:203–214.
83. Leveque JL, de Rigal J. In vivo measurements of the stratum corneum elasticity. Bioeng Skin 1985; 1:13–23.
84. Wiechers JW. A supplier's contribution to performance testing of personal care ingredients. Proceedings of In Cosmetics, Kongresszentrum Süd, Düsseldorf, 1997, pp. 206–228.
85. Leveque JL, Grove G, de Rigal J, Corcuff P, Kligman AM, Saint Leger D. Biophysical characterization of dry facial skin. J Soc Cosmet Chem 1987; 82:171–177.
86. Salter DC, McArthur HC, Crosse JE, Dickens AD. Skin mechanics measured in vivo using torsion: a new and accurate model more sensitive to age, sex, and moisturizing treatment. Int J Cosmet Sci 1993; 15:200–218.
87. Wolfram LJ. Friction of skin. J Soc Cosmet Chem 1983; 34:465–476.
88. Comaish S, Bottoms E. The skin and friction: deviation from Amonton's laws, and the effects of hydration and lubrication. Br J Dermatol 1971; 84:37.
89. Comaish S, Harborow PRH, Hofman DA. A hand-held friction meter. Br J Dermatol 1973; 89:33.
90. Prall JK. Instrumental evaluation of the effects of cosmetic products on skin surfaces with particular reference to smoothness. J Soc Cosmet Chem 1973; 24:693–707.
91. Highley DR, Coomey M, DenBeste M, Wolfram LJ. Frictional properties of skin. J Invest Dermatol 1977; 69:303.
92. Weinstein S. New methods for the in-vivo assessment of skin smoothness and skin softness. J Soc Cosmet Chem 1978; 29:99–115.

93. Gerrad ED, Stimpson IM. A versatile friction meter based on a viscometer. Lab Pract 1984; 33:82–83.
94. Gerrard ED, Stimpson IM. The effect of treatment on skin friction coefficient in vivo. Bioeng Skin 1985; 1:229.
95. Naylor PFD. The skin surface and friction. Br J Dermatol 1955; 67:239.
96. El-Shimi AF. In vivo skin friction measurements. J Soc Cosmet Chem 1977; 28:37.
97. Nacht S, Close J, Yeung D, Gans EH. Skin friction coefficient: changes induced by skin hydration and emollient application and correlation with perceived skin feel. J Soc Cosmet Chem 1981; 32:55.
98. Cussler EL, Zlotnick SJ, Shaw MC. Texture perceived with fingers. Percept Psychophys 1977; 21:504.
99. Appeldoorn JK, Barnett G. Frictional aspects of emollience. Proc Sci Sect Toil Goods Assoc 1963; 40:28.
100. Torgalkar AM. A resonance frequency technique to determine the energy absorbed in stratum corneum, in vivo. In: Marks R, Payne PA, eds. Bioengineering and the Skin. Lancaster, England: MTP Press, 1981:55–65.
101. Potts RO. In vivo measurement of water content of the stratum corneum using infrared spectroscopy: a review. Cosmet Toil 1985; 100(10):27–31.
102. Potts RO. Stratum corneum hydration: experimental techniques and interpretations of results. J Soc Cosmet Chem 1988; 37:9–33.
103. Potts RO, Buras EM, Chrisman DA. Changes with age in the moisture content. J Invest Dermatol 1984; 82:97–100.
104. Dahlgren RM, Elsnau WH. Measurement of skin condition by sonic velocity. J Soc Cosmet Chem 1984; 35:1–20.
105. Idson B. In vivo measurement of transdermal water loss. J Soc Cosmet Chem 1976; 29:573–580.
106. Nilsson GE, Oberg PA. Measurement of evaporative water loss: methods and clinical applications. In: Rolfe P, ed. Non-Invasive Physiological Measurements. New York: Academic Press, 1979:279–311.
107. Grice KA. Transepidermal water loss and transepidermal water loss in pathological skin. In: Jarrett A, ed. The Physiology and Pathophysiology of the Skin. London: Academic Press, 1980:2115–2146, 2147–2155.
108. Miller DL, Brown AM, Artz EJ. Indirect measures of epidermal water loss. In: Marks R, Payne PA, eds. Bioengineering and the Skin. Lancaster, England: MTP Press, 1980:161–171.
109. Leveque JL, Garson JC, de Rigal J. Transepidermal water loss from dry and normal skin. J Soc Cosmet Chem 1979; 30:333–343.
110. Weldon AE, Monteith JL. Performance of a skin Evaporimeter. Med Biol Eng Comput 1980; 18:201.
111. Spruit D. Interference of some substances with water vapor loss from human skin. Am Perfumer Cosmet 1971; 86:27–32.
112. Baker H. Experimental studies on the influence of vehicles on percutaneous absorption. J Soc Cosmet Chem 1969; 20:239–252.
113. Weil I, Princen HM. Diffusion therapy analysis of transepidermal water loss through occlusive films. J Soc Cosmet Chem 1977; 28:481–484.
114. Seitz JC, Spencer TS. The use of capacitative evaporimetry to measure the effects

of topical ingredients on transepidermal water loss (TEWL). J Invest Dermatol 1982; 78:351.

115. Grove GL, Grove MJ, Zerweck C, Pierce E. Computerized evaporimetry using the DermaLab TEWL probe. Skin Res Technol 1999; 5:9–13.

116. Grove GL, Grove MJ, Zerweck C, Pierce E. Comparative metrology of the evaporimeter and the DermaLab TEWL probe. Skin Res Technol 1999; 5:1–8.

117. Berube GR, Berick M. Transepidermal moisture loss. II. The significance of the use thickness of topical substances. J Soc Cosmet Chem 1974; 25:397–406.

118. Thiele FAJ, Hemels HGWM, Malten KE. Skin temperature and water loss by skin. Trans St John's Hosp Dermatol Soc 1972; 58:218–223.

119. Morrison BM. ServoMed Evaporimeter: precautions when evaluating the effect of skin care products on barrier function. J Soc Cosmet Chem 1986; 37:351.

120. Powers DH, Fox CA. A study of the effect of cosmetic ingredients, creams and lotions on the rate of moisture loss from the skin. Proc Sci Sect Toil Goods Assoc 1957; 28:21–26.

121. Rietschel RL. A method to evaluate skin moisturizers in vivo. J Invest Dermatol 1978; 70:152–155.

122. Rietschel RL. A skin moisturization essay. J Soc Cosmet Chem 1979; 30:360–373.

123. Buettner KJ. The moisture of human skin as affected by water transfer. J Soc Cosmet Chem 1965; 16:133–143.

124. Blank IH, Moloney J, Emslie AG, Simon I, Apt C. The diffusion of water across the stratum corneum as a function of its water content. J Invest Dermatol 1984; 82:188–194.

125. Wu M, Yee DJ, Sullivan ME. Effect of a skin moisturizer on the water distribution on human stratum corneum. J Invest Dermatol 1983; 81:446–448.

24

Laboratory-Based Ex Vivo Assessment of Stratum Corneum Function

Claudine Piérard-Franchimont,
Veroniqué Goffin, and Gérald E. Piérard
University Medical Center Sart Tilman, Liège, Belgium

Marc Paye
Colgate-Palmolive, Milmort, Belgium

1   INTRODUCTION

The normal stratum corneum (SC) is composed of orderly interdigitating stacks of corneocytes coated by layers of intercellular lipids. The protein-enriched corneocytes are filled with a dense array of disulfide cross-linked keratin filaments bound to filaggrin. Permeating through this matrix are low molecular weight water-soluble molecules forming the natural moisturizing factor (NMF), which largely derives from the enzymatic degradation of filaggrin. The NMF avidly and effectively binds water. The resulting osmotic pressure inside the cells does not lead to their disintegration because corneocytes are made of so strong a cross-linked protein matrix surrounded by a thick cornified envelope, formed itself from highly cross-linked isopeptide bonded proteins. The lipid-enriched intercellular matrix provides a rate-limiting barrier to water evaporation from the skin surface and to the transport of other chemicals across the skin. With failure of the barrier, xerosis develops and may evolve to flaky and scaly presentations (Fig. 1). This represents an abnormal process of desquamation. In fact, the SC is not sim-

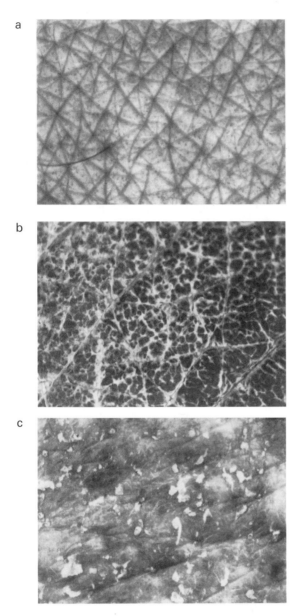

Figure 1 Aspect of the skin surface under ultraviolet illumination (Visioscan®). (a) Normal microrelief of a forearm; (b) xerosis (dry skin) of the limb, (c) kerosis (follicular xerosis) of the face.

ply a collection of dead cells, but rather represents a dynamic and metabolically active tissue interacting with subjacent cell layers that reacts to various environmental threats [1,2].

The integrity of the SC depends upon the intercellular cohesion provided by the corneodesmosomes, also called corneosomes [3]. There is ample evidence that regional differences are present on the body with respect of the structure, cohesion, thickness, and functions of the SC. Overall a critical level of hydration is required to allow the SC to maintain its flexibility and orderly desquamation [3]. Enzymatic degradation of corneodesmosomes by proteases along with glycosidases is inhibited at low environmental humidities [4–6]. Filaggrin hydrolysis giving rise to the intracellular NMF pool is similarly critically influenced by water activity in the SC. However, water is not the single modulator of SC functions. The nature and amount in intercellular lipids are also important. The renewal rate and thickness of the SC and the presence of parakeratotic cells are also key features. Laboratory-based in vitro methods may help in studying these parameters.

2 METHODS FOR SC HARVESTING

Half a century ago, the ex vivo usage of SC was pioneered to investigate its functions outside of the body influences. Stratum corneum was removed from foot callus and further dehydrated to demonstrate the effect of water upon flexibility of the samples [7]. This model proved to be useful and innovative. However, callus is not representative of SC from other body sites in terms of structure, thickness, and functions.

Powdered human SC is also a product made from foot callus which is cut into small pieces and ground with dry ice to form a powder. Sieving brings uniformity in particle size. The material retains some physical and chemical characteristics of human stratum corneum [8].

Other techniques of SC collection have been described from other body sites. They are described hereafter.

2.1 Separation of SC from Excised Skin Samples

Skin samples can be collected from cadaver, on surgery and from slaughterhouse animals. Different methods have been used to isolate the SC from the underlying tissues. The mechanical method involved repetitive stretching of the skin [9]. This procedure has only a historical value because it is nowadays rarely applied due to significant alteration of the SC.

Heat treatment of the skin samples is another approach [10]. Placing the sample for 1 min in a water bath at 60°C allows easy subsequent removal of the SC with a grip. Minor variants in temperature and incubation time have been described [11]. This treatment is likely to alter the SC structure and functions. However, permeability properties of the membrane appear unaffected by the procedure [11]. Thickness was found to range between 10–15 μm. Due to the absence of chemical treatment, this method is still used by some research groups.

Exposure of skin for 1 to 3 hr to ammonia vapor in a dessicator jar followed by water immersion allows the epidermis to be separated from the dermis [12]. Epidermal cells are then gently scraped off to leave the SC with a thickness around 25 μm.

Enzymatic treatment using trypsin digestion of the living tissues is still another approach [13]. The skin sample is incubated several hours at 37°C or overnight at 4°C in a buffered 0.5 or 1% trypsin solution, after which the SC can be easily peeled off. Trypsin is then inhibited using soybean trypsin inhibitor, and the SC is abundantly rinsed in water. Other enzymes like dispase can be used similarly. However, an enzymatic technique should be reserved for some specific aims when it has been demonstrated that the treatment is unlikely to interfere with the SC function under investigation.

2.2 SC Harvesting from Human Volunteers

An SC sheet can be collected from the forearm using a surgical knife and a tweezer. This method preserves the SC from any chemical or mechanical alteration and is often preferred to trypsin treatment for hydration studies [14]. Suction blisters under negative pressure (2 atmospheres) is applied on a small area of the volar forearm of the volunteers using a vacuum pump for about 1 to 2 hr [15]. When the blister is formed, its roof is cut off and the living epidermis rubbed away with a cotton swab moistened in saline solution. The SC may be full thickness, composed of 14 to 17 layers.

Cyanoacrylate skin surface stripping is an ancillary method used to collect a few layers of the outer portion of the SC [16–19]. Corneocytes are tightly bound to the plastic or glass support used for the harvesting process. Horny casts within the upper part of the hair follicles are also ripped off [20,21].

The stripping of corneocytes from the skin surface using casual adhesive tapes [22] is nowadays often replaced by calibrated strippings with adhesive-coated discs (SACD). This method removes fragments of the upmost outer layer of corneocytes with better reproducibility. Cells collected represent those whose bond with the underlying SC layers is weaker than with the bond of the adhesive present on the collecting disc [18,19,23–25]. The pressure applied to the disc should be carefully controlled [18,19,25]. The contact time between the disc and the skin affects the data [19,25,26]. There may be some seasonal influence on the amount of SC collected [27].

The detergent scrub method removes individual corneocytes from the stratum disjunctum [28]. A buffered solution of 0.05% Triton X-100 is placed in a glass cylinder held firmly on the skin. The skin surface is rubbed or scrubbed for 30–60 s. The wash fluid contains individual corneocytes.

Forced desquamation using a motorized scrub apparatus with controlled application force onto the SC represents a significant improvement of the method [29]. Still another device generates an air current by a turbine, and a woollen pad serves as a friction element to remove corneocytes [30].

In many experiments, the amount of SC harvested is critical for the interpretation of data. In fact, it may represent the primary parameter to be evaluated after an in vivo intervention. It may also affect significantly other outcomes in purely ex vivo experiments. Weighing samples is difficult to perform accurately due to the variability in the SC dessication according to the ambient temperature, relative humidity (RH), and air movement. Other methods include chemical quantification [31], optical spectroscopy [32], and squamometry [18,19,25]. The latter method consists of a colorimetric assessment (Chroma C*) after staining the SC with a solution of toluidine blue and basic fuschin at pH 3.4.

3 SC AND XENOBIOTICS

Many xenobiotics are absorbed to, stored in, and/or transported across the SC. The SC binding/partitioning of chemicals correlates well with percutaneous absorption. These biological features can be studied ex vivo on harvested human SC. Water represents a particular example of such interactions.

3.1 Chemical Partitioning Inside the SC

Many experiments have been conducted to predict chemical partitioning into the SC in vitro. Most were based on quantitative structure–activity relationships (QSARs) or on related chemicals to determine the partitioning process.

Human SC has been used as an in vitro model to explore percutaneous absorption and risk of dermal exposure [33,34]. The traditional method of preparation uses physicochemical and enzymatic processes to separate the SC from whole skin. However, it is time consuming and, in some cases, difficult to control the size and thickness of a sheet of SC.

Powdered human SC can be used to study the partitioning process of diverse compounds and to determine which decontaminant might be able to remove hazardous chemicals from human skin [35,36].

3.2 In Vitro Adsorption on SC

Isolated SC can be used in vitro to investigate the adsorption of various chemicals [37–41]. This is especially important in the case of products which have to be rinsed off like body cleansing products. During the development of cosmetics and toiletries with skin moisturizing claims, or at least aiming to respect the skin surface moisture, the SC adsorption tests can be used to optimize the formulation in two ways, namely, by minimizing the adsorption of anionic surfactants and/or by maximizing the adsorption of emollients or humectants.

The residual anionic surfactants bound to the skin surface induce a perception of rough and dry skin to the consumer, independently of a loss of moisture [42]. Understanding and controlling surfactant adsorption to the SC is thus a key step toward consumer acceptance of cleansing products claiming skin surface hydration. In such a study, SC isolated by trypsin from hairless guinea pig and human cadaver skin can be used for testing different radiolabeled anionic surfactants [41]. After a defined incubation period, the amount of surfactant bound to the SC is determined by scintillation counting and corrected for the weight of SC. The adsorption of several surfactants to SC can be compared, and the effect of concentration, temperature, and pH of the solutions is conveniently assessed.

Humectants are ingredients which adsorb onto the SC and hold water in it like a sponge. Examples are sodium lactate, urea, glycerol, amino acids, pyrollidone carboxylic acid, and peptides. Emollients participate in increasing the SC hydration by forming an occlusive coating between the SC and the environment to avoid the evaporation of moisture from the SC. In both cases, the delivery of molecules to the SC is a key step which can be investigated in vitro using isolated SC and revelation techniques depending on the ingredient to be detected and on the level of quantification which is required [38–40].

3.3 Skin Permeation

The absorption of chemicals through skin can be assessed in vivo and in vitro. With the current efforts to suppress tests on animals, in vitro tests on excised skin have become more and more popular for percutaneous absorption studies [43]. For water-soluble compounds the absorption rate-limiting barrier is the SC, while for lipophilic compounds, the living epidermis is the major barrier to absorption.

Depending on the compounds to be tested, skin permeation studies can be performed on full or split skin thickness. When the interest is mainly in investigating the passive barrier function of the SC to substances applied to its external side, the split thickness model is preferred. The skin piece, checked for integrity, is placed between two compartments. The chamber beneath the skin serves as a container for a receptor fluid, while the compartment above the skin serves to receive the topical preparation. Many parameters need to be carefully controlled, including the temperature of the receptor fluid, the hydration level of the skin, the vehicle of the test compound and its application mode, and an adequate mixing of the receptor fluid. Other models using dynamic flux also exist. However, these skin permeation tests are essentially used in toxicological studies, rather than for SC hydration investigations, and the reader is referred to specific literature for a more detailed description [43,44].

3.4 Predicting Surfactant-Induced Skin Irritation with the SC Swelling Test

In the original swelling test, square (2 × 2 cm) pieces of guinea pig SC were weighed and incubated in the appropriate test solutions and reweighed after the incubation to estimate the extent of swelling of the sample [45]. A revised method used SC collected by heat or trypsin treatment of cadaver skin samples [46]. Similar results were obtained by both procedures. After isolation and drying, the SC is cut crosswise to the longitudinal axis of the cadaver into strips 0.5 cm wide and 4 cm long. At each end of the strips, plastic tabs are glued resulting in final exposed dimensions of 0.5 × 2.5 cm, and the membranes are hung by one end. The membranes are then soaked into the solutions of surfactant to be tested and remain overnight in a refrigerator. Usually five to six strips are used as replicates. Swelling of the SC is estimated by measuring the change in length of the long axis of the strips and the weight.

The more irritant the test solution, the more the swelling of the SC (Table 1). Variants to the technique were described with SC from isolated pig skin [47] and different incubation conditions (30 min at 40°C). Swelling is evaluated by gravimetry. Nowadays, the SC sheets are often replaced by commercially available dried collagen membranes [48,49]. This procedure is faster, does not suffer from the lack of reproducibility due to the SC preparation, and provides results similar to the original SC swelling test.

Using these methods, a large series of anionic surfactants were tested and showed excellent predictability of their skin irritation potential [43,46,48,49]. Nonionic surfactants do not induce SC swelling. Relative to anionic surfactants, they are usually very mild and this could be considered as an acceptable prediction of their skin irritation, with however a degree of uncertainty. In contrast, amphoteric and cationic surfactants show no swelling or even swelling inhibition, although several of them are clearly irritants for the skin. The SC swelling test is thus not appropriate for those classes of surfactants in single solutions. In more complex systems including surfactants from different classes, the presence of nonionic, amphoteric, or cationic surfactant is able to improve the skin compatibility of anionic surfactants; such an effect can be easily predicted through SC or collagen swelling tests, which have proved their usefulness in those circumstances [50].

As a predictor of the skin mildness/irritation potential of surfactant-based compositions, the SC swelling test should be considered when developing a prod-

TABLE 1 Factors Affecting SC Swelling

Temperature	Swelling increases with temperature up to a plateau.
Incubation time	Swelling increases with incubation time up to a plateau.
Concentration	Maximum swelling at 2–5% of surfactant and then decreases.
Divalent cations	Magnesium inhibits swelling, not skin irritation.
pH	pH rise increases the swelling due to anionic surfactants.
Carbon chain length	Maximum swelling around C10–C12 chain length.

uct with skin surface hydration claims. Indeed, an aspect of improvement of skin surface hydration properties relies on a gentle cleansing system. Any irritant hygiene product will tend to dehydrate the SC.

3.5 Corneosurfametry and Corneoxenometry

Cyanoacrylate skin surface strippings are the substrate used ex vivo to test the reactivity and binding of surfactants and other xenobiotics on human SC. Samples are sprayed onto or immersed inside the test solutions under controlled temperature and for a defined period of time [18,24,51]. Microwave activation can also be used [52,53]. Samples are stained by a toluidine blue/basic fuschin solution. Colorimetric assessments are used in a reproducible way. Corneosurfametry and corneoxenometry can predict some aspects of skin irritation when the product interacts with the SC [54]. Alternatively, data are interpreted as the expression of the product binding to the corneocytes.

Both bioassays are influenced by regional variations in the SC structure. They are also affected by the previous biological history and cumulative environmental threats at the site of SC harvesting. Repeated contacts with dishwashing liquids significantly increase the corneosurfametry reactivity to a subsequent standard challenge with a surfactant. Such a negative preconditioning is less prominent when a moisturizer is regularly applied before harvesting the stratum corneum for the bioassay (Fig. 2). Indeed, the moisturizer helps to eliminate the altered corneocytes in vivo, somewhat cleaning the skin surface from partly adherent and altered corneocytes. These latter cells strongly bind the corneosurfametry dyes.

3.6 Effect of Surfactants on Corneocyte Aspect

The damaging effects of soaps and surfactants on human SC can be assessed using small SC discs collected from suction blisters [15]. Samples are incubated for

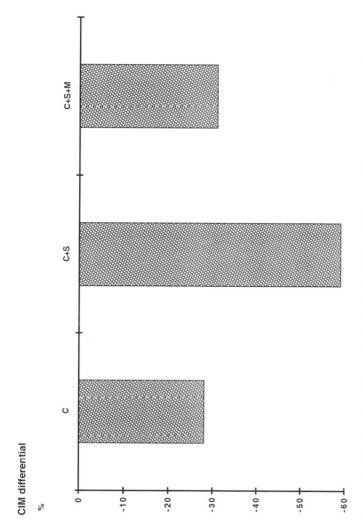

CIM differential

%

Figure 2 Reduction in the colorimetric index in mildness (CIM) at the corneosurfametry test following an in vivo challenge (C) after repeated forearm immersion in a regular dishwashing liquid. A cumulative deteriation is observed when the stratum corneum is further placed in contact with the surfactant SLS (S) in vitro. The effect is less severe when a moisturizer (M) is applied in vivo at the test site. Data are expressed as percentages of variation in CIM compared to unchallenged intact skin.

6 hr at 60°C in solutions of surfactants or soaps. Cytological alternations of corneocytes can be evaluated through different parameters: the number of corneocytes released from the SC with time, their size (swelling), and their changes in shape. This method allows a classification of the tested soaps according to their irritancy potential. Nonionic and cationic surfactants do not appear significantly different from water, although some cationic surfactants are skin irritants. Anionic surfactants release more corneocytes, but induce less swelling and changes. This test is a useful screening tool to determine the irritation potential of soaps. It also provides insights in the understanding of the interaction of surfactants with the SC.

Stratum corneum harvested by SACD can also be used to assess the corneocyte integrity after an in vivo challenge. The method is called squamometry S [25]. Samples are stained by a toluidine blue/basic fuschin solution at a pH about 3.4. The color (Chroma C*) is measured by reflectance colorimetry. In addition, the microscopic assessment brings information about the shape and intercellular cohesion of corneocytes [18,25,55].

4 SC AND WATER

4.1 Prediction of Water Uptake by SC

Several groups have run ex vivo studies to investigate water uptake by SC. The moisture content of the SC is essentially determined by gravimetry [7] and spectrometric techniques [56]. In the first case, samples of SC were prepared by trypsin treatment from human cadavers, dried, cut into small pieces, and weighed. The SC pieces were placed at equilibrium at constant temperature, but variable RH, when the samples were reweighed [9]. The gain of weight, relative to the water uptake from the environment, was calculated. Up to 50–60% RH, water uptake is moderate, while further increase in RH up to 90–95% leads to exponential water uptake. Ambient temperature seemed to affect the uptake of water in the low humidity range, while not above 50–60% RH, suggesting two different mechanisms. Gravimetric techniques were also used to determine the effect of formulations on SC hydration [57].

Spectrometric methods used to measure skin hydration of SC include infrared [58], Raman [59,60], and nuclear magnetic resonance (NMR) [61] assessments. Such methods not only provide a quantification of the water content in the SC, but also bring information on the interaction and mobility between the water molecules with SC proteins. Among these assessment methods, only NMR is able to quantitate the hydration profile of the various SC layers and to provide information on the concentration gradient of water within the SC [62]. Proton NMR can determine in the same samples both the total amount and the bound nonfreezing water by recording the spectra below 0°C [61].

Altogether, the data collected in vitro from the gravimetric and spectrometric technique demonstrate that at low RH water molecules quickly adsord to the SC and are tightly bound to the SC proteins. Increasing the ambient RH leads to a slowdown the uptake of water by the SC and make it less temperature dependent. Water also becomes less tightly bound. At very high RH, part of water is in a liquidlike state [54].

4.2 SACD and SC Hydration

In some instances xerosis, flakiness, and scaliness are related to desiccation of the superficial part of the SC [2,6]. Assessments of SACD samples can be used to quantify such a physiological ailment [18,49,63–65]. Several methods of quantification have been proposed. Measuring light transmission through the samples [63] and weighing them are either not validated or difficult to handle properly. In particular, data are significantly affected by RH after SACD has been harvested. Image analysis appears more reliable although technically difficult to handle because a sophisticated softwave program is mandatory to cope with both area and thickness of scales [64,65]. Squamometry X (for xerosis) entails staining SACD using a toluidine blue/basic fuschin solution and subsequently measuring the color (Chroma C*) using reflectance colorimetry [18,19,25]. The effect of moisturizers can be elegantly assessed by this method (Fig. 3). In fact, moisturizers exhibit an indirect corneodesmolytic effect. As a result the amount of corneocytes harvested by SACD is abated. Time to recurrence after stopping the moisturizing treatment evaluates the lingering effect of the product.

4.3 Water Diffusion Through SC

When water evaporation through SC is studied on human volunteers, some environmental variables and the volunteer physiology need to be rigorously controlled [66]. Temperature, humidity, air flux, psychologic status, sweating, food consumption, and water hygiene procedure can affect the so-called trans-epidermal water loss (TEWL). Measurements often yield high interindividual variability.

Using isolated SC in vitro allows one to better standardize the variability factors linked to the individuals. Furthermore, due to the small size of the samples, they can be placed in test chambers with well-controlled ambient conditions [67]. In those studies the SC membrane is mounted, external face side up, above a water-containing reservoir. Water is maintained at a constant and defined temperature and separated from the SC by a small vapor space. Water diffusion through the SC membrane can be evaluated by measuring the weight loss from the water reservoir [7], the water uptake in the environment [68], the flux of radiolabeled water through the SC [69,70], or the water vapor gradient at the external side of the SC [67]. Also in the in vitro tests, several parameters need to be

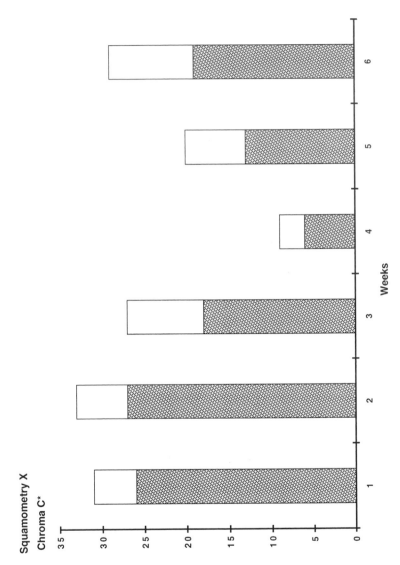

FIGURE 3 Evaluation of the effect of a moisturizer using Squamometry X. Data (mean ± SD) show baseline values (weeks 1 and 2), the improvement during a 2-week treatment (weeks 3 and 4), and the regression phase after stopping the applications of the moisturizer (weeks 5 and 6).

well controlled. Changes in RH affect the SC water content and hence the water diffusion rate through the SC [71]. The thickness of the SC also affects the water diffusion [72]. Studies using SC from different body sites showed huge differences in water flux, with up to 20-fold differences between abdominal and scrotal SC [73]. Any treatment of the skin before isolating the SC can also have significant consequences on water diffusion, mainly if those treatments cause SC lipid extraction or disorganization [73] or if they cause any mechanical damage to the SC.

Well-controlled in vitro studies using a computer-based Evaporimeter® system yield a threefold higher precision in TEWL in vitro measurement compared to human studies [67]. With such a precision, the role of the corneocyte envelope and intercellular lipids were shown on the skin barrier function. In addition, the effect of treatment with anionic surfactants, skin permeation enhancers, and high $CaCl_2$ concentrations were demonstrated.

5 EFFECT OF TREATMENTS ON SC LIPIDS USING IN VITRO TESTS

Lipids play a prominent role in the water-holding capacity of the SC. Such a function has been demonstrated in vitro on isolated SC by differential scanning calorimetry (DSC) [74,75] and ultrastructural studies [14,76]. Briefly, the piece of SC is dried and then hydrated in excess. The total amount of water in the SC is determined by the gain of weight after rehydration. For DSC measurements, the SC samples are first frozen to –40°C and then progressively heated at a constant, slow rate up to 20°C. The melting behavior of the water contained within the SC is recorded. Unbound water in the SC causes an endothermic peak between –17 to –6°C. When the SC is hydrated to less than 33.3%, no peak can be observed in this area. This is the approximate amount of bound water in intact SC which never freezes, even at –40°C, and thus has no endothermic peak when reheating. The depletion in SC lipids by acetone/ether treatment causes the SC bound-water content to markedly decrease. Electron microscopic observations reveal the removal or alteration of intercellular lamellae. In contrast, application of a mixture of SC lipids to the acetone/ether treated SC is able to re-increase the bound water content in the SC and to refill the intercellular spaces induced by the treatment with multiple lamellae [14]. These studies demonstrate the usefulness of in vitro investigations on isolated SC to understand and control the moisture of the SC. Using an in vitro model of SC lipids, glycerol helped to maintain the SC lipids under a liquid crystalline state, even at low relative humidity [77]. Such an effect participates in keeping SC well moisturized. The same model was used to investigate the effect of several cosmetic additives in preventing lipid phase transition in vitro [78].

In vitro studies have also been performed to determine how much and which lipids could be extracted from the SC by surfactants. The effects of sodium lauryl sulfate (SLS) and linear alkyl benzene sulfonate (LAS) were studied on isolated SC [79]. The extracted lipids were analyzed by high performance thin layer chromatography (HPTCL) after elimination of the surfactants. Both surfactants at various concentrations removed lipids only above the critical micelle concentration (CMC). Even at high concentrations, only very small amounts of SC lipids were extracted. Such in vitro extractions of lipids from SC can also be used for rapid screening of lipid biochemical abnormalities of scaling skin disorders [80]. Extraction and analysis of lipids by HPTLC can also be performed on cyanoacrylate skin surface. However, this method may look more tedious as it is necessary to completely remove glue residues from the extracted lipids before the chromatographic analysis can be performed.

6 SC AND MOISTURIZER DEVELOPMENT

As described, many methods are available to harvest human SC and to study its interaction with xenobiotics in vitro. Some of these approaches can be used for moisturizer development. The study design may involve a spontaneously developed xerosis or scaly skin. A similar aspect can also be induced by different means including barrier disruption by organic solvents, occlusive surfactant dressing, and decreased environmental dew point. The effect of a moisturizer can be performed in a second step in vitro. In these instances, squamometry is one of the cheapest, most rapid, and most reliable objective in vitro tests.

REFERENCES

1. Elias PM. Stratum corneum architecture, metabolic activity and interactivity with subjacent cell layers. Ext Dermatol 1996; 5:191–201.
2. Piérard GE, Goffin V, Hermanns-Lê T, Piérard-Franchimont C. Corneocyte desquamation. Int J Mol Med 2000; 6:217–221.
3. Chapman SJ, Walsh A. Desmosomes, corneosomes and desquamation. An ultrastructural study of adult pig epidermis. Arch Dermatol Res 1990; 282:304–310.
4. Bernard D, Camus C, Nguyen QL, Serre G. Proteolysis of corneodesmosomal proteins in winter xerosis. J Invest Dermatol 1995; 105:176.
5. Rawlings AV, Harding CR, Watkinson A, Banks J, Ackerman C, Sabin R. The effect of glycerol and humidity on desmosome degradation in stratum corneum. Arch Dermatol Res 1995; 287:457–464.
6. Harding CR, Watkinson AW, Rawlings AV, Scott IR. Dry skin, moisturization and corneodesmolysis. Int J Cosmet Sci 2000; 22:21–52.
7. Blank IH. Factors which influence the water content of the stratum corneum. J Invest Dermatol 1952; 18:433–440.
8. Wester RC, Mobayen M, Maibach HI. In vivo and in vitro absorption and binding to powdered stratum corneum as methods to evaluate skin absorption of environmental

chemical contaminants from ground and surface water. J Toxicol Environ Health 1987; 21:367.

9. Anderson RL, Cassidy JM, Hansen JR, Yellin W. Hydration of the stratum corneum. Biopolymers 1973; 12:2789–2802.

10. Kligman AM, Christophers E. Preparation of isolated sheets of human stratum corneum. Arch Dermatol 1963; 88:70–73.

11. Scheuplein RJ. Mechanism of percutaneous adsorption. I. Routes of penetration and the influence of solubility. J Invest Dermatol 1965; 45:334–346.

12. Faucher JA, Goddard ED. Sorption of a cationic polymer by stratum corneum. J Soc Cosmet Chem 1976; 27:543–553.

13. Lampe MA, Burlingame AL, Whitney JA, Williams ML, Brown BE, Roitman E, Elias PM. Human stratum corneum lipids: characterization and regional variations. J Lipid Res 1983; 24:120–130.

14. Imokawa G, Kuno H, Kawai M. Stratum corneum lipids serve as a bound-water modulator. J Invest Dermatol 1991; 96:845–851.

15. Shukuwa T, Kligman AM, Stoudemayer TJ. A new model for assessing the damaging effects of soaps and surfactants on human stratum corneum. Acta Derm Venereol 1997; 77:29–34.

16. Marks R, Dawber RPR. Skin surface biopsy: an improved technique for the examination of the horny layer. Br J Dermatol 1971; 84:117–123.

17. Piérard-Franchimont C, Piérard GE. Skin surface stripping in diagnosing and monitoring inflammatory, xerotic and neoplastic diseases. Ped Dermatol 1985; 2:180–184.

18. Piérard GE, Piérard-Franchimont C. Drug and cosmetics evaluation with skin strippings. In: Maibach H, ed. Dermatologic Research Techniques. Boca Raton: CRC Press, 1996:133–148.

19. Piérard GE, Masson P, Rodrigues I, Berardesca E, Lévêque JL, Loden M, Rogiers V, Sauermann G, Serup J. EEMCO guidance for the assessment of dry skin (xerosis) and ichthyosis: evaluation by stratum corneum strippings. Skin Res Technol 1996; 2:3–11.

20. Piérard GE, Piérard-Franchimont C, Goffin V. Digital image analysis of microcomedones. Dermatology 1995; 190:99–103.

21. Piérard-Franchimont C, Piérard GE. Comedogenicity. In: Elsner P, Merk HF, Maibach HI, eds. Cosmetics: Controlled Efficacy Studies and Regulations. Berlin: Springer, 1999:268–274.

22. Haidl G, Plewig G. Exfoliative cytology of stratum corneum and the effects of topical retinoids on the physical properties of corneocytes. J Soc Cosmet Chem 1988; 39:53.

23. Piérard GE, Piérard-Franchimont C, Saint Léger D, Kligman AM. Squamometry: the assessment of xerosis by colorimetry of D-Squame adhesive discs. J Soc Cosmet Chem 1992; 47:297–305.

24. Piérard GE, Goffin V, Piérard-Franchimont C. Squamometry and corneosurfametry in rating interactions of cleansing products with stratum corneum. J Soc Cosmet Chem 1994; 45:269–277.

25. Piérared-Franchimont C, Henry F, Piérard GE. The SACD method and the XLRS squamometry tests revisited. Int J Cosmet Sci 2000; 22:437–446.

26. Tokumara F, Ohyama K, Fujisana H, Suzuki M, Nukatsuka H. Time-dependent changes in dermal peeling force of adhesive tapes. Skin Res Technol 1999; 5:33–36.

27. Tokumara F, Ohyama K, Fujisawa H, Nukatsuka H. Seasonal variation in adhesive tape stripping of the skin. Skin Res Technol 1999; 5:208–212.

28. McGinley KJ, Marples RR, Plewig G. A method for visualizing and quantitating the desquamating portion of the human stratum corneum. J Invest Dermatol 1969; 53:107.

29. Roberts D, Marks R. The determination of regional and age variations in the rate of desquamation: a comparison of four techniques. J Invest Dermatol 1980; 74:13.

30. Corcuff P, Chatenay F, Saint Léger D. Hair–skin relationships: a new approach to desquamation, Bioeng Skin 1985; 1:133.

31. Dreher F, Arens A, Hostynek JJ, Mudumba S, Ademola J, Maibach HI. Colorimetric method for quantifying human stratum corneum removed by adhesive tape-stripping. Acta Derm Venereol 1998; 78:186–189.

32. Weigmann HJ, Lademann J, Meffert H, Schaefer H, Sterry W. Determination of the horny layer profile by tape stripping in combination with optical spectroscopy in the visible range as a prerequisite to quantify percutaneous absorption. Skin Pharmacol Appl Skin Physiol 1999; 12:34–45.

33. Surber C, Wilhelm KP, Hori M, Maibach HI, Guy RH. Optimization of topical therapy: partitioning of drugs into stratum corneum. Pharmceut Res 1990; 12:1320.

34. Potts PO, Guy RH. Predicting skin permeability. Pharmaceut Res 1992; 9:663.

35. Wester RC, Maibach HI, Sedik L, Melendres J, Wade M. In vivo and in vitro percutaneous absorption and skin decontamination of arsenic from water and soil. Fundam Appl Toxicol 1993; 20:336–340.

36. Hui X, Wester RC, Magee PS, Maibach HI. Partitionng of chemicals from water into powdered human stratum corneum (callus)—a model study. In Vitro Toxicol 1995; 8:159–163.

37. Faucher JA, Goddard ED. Interaction of keratinous substrates with sodium lauryl sulfate. I. Sorption. J Soc Cosmet Chem 1978; 29:323–337.

38. Goddard ED, Leung PS. Protection of skin by cationic cellulosics: in-vitro testing methods. Cosmet Toil 1982; 97:55–69.

39. Turowski A, Adelmann-Grill BC. Substantivity to hair and skin of ^{125}I-labelled collagen hydrolysates undeer application simulating conditions. Int J Cosmet Sci 1985; 7:71–84.

40. Goddard ED, Harris WC. Adsorption of polymers and lipids on stratum corneum membranes as measured by ESCA. J Soc Cosmet Chem 1987; 38:295–306.

41. Ananthapadmanabhan KP, Yu KK, Meyers CL, Aronson MP. Binding of surfactants to stratum corneum. J Soc Cosmet Chem 1996; 47:185–200.

42. Kawai M, Imokawa G. The induction of skin tightness by surfactants. J Soc Cosmet Chem 1984; 35:147–156.

43. Bronaugh RL, Collier SW. In vitro methods for measuring skin permeation. Cosmet Toil 1990; 105:86–93.

44. Diembeck W, Beck H, Benech-Kieffer F, Courtellemont P, Dupuis J, Lovell W, Paye M, Spengler J, Steiling W. Test guidelines for in vitro assessment of dermal absorption and percutaneous penetration of cosmetic products. Food Chem Toxicol 1999; 37:191–205.

45. Putterman GJ, Wolfram NF, Laden K. The effect of detergents on swelling of stratum corneum. J Soc Cosmet Chem 1977; 28:521–532.
46. Robbins CR, Fernee KM. Some observations on the swelling of human epidermal membrane. J Soc Cosmet Chem 1983; 34:21–34.
47. Zeidler U. Physico-chemical in vitro methods for the determination of the skin compatibility of surfactants. J Soc Cosmet Chem (Japan) 1986; 20:17–26.
48. Blake-Haskins JC, Scala D, Rhein LD. Predicting surfactant irritation from the swelling response of a collagen film. J Soc Cosmet Chem 1986; 37:199–210.
49. Goffin V, Paye M, Piérard GE. Comparison of in vitro predictive tests for irritation induced by anionic surfactant. Contact Dermatitis 1995; 33:38–41.
50. Rhein LD, Simion FA. Surfactant interactions with skin. In: Bender M, ed. Interfacial Phenomena in Biological Systems. New York: Marcel Dekker, 1991:33–49.
51. Henry F, Goffin V, Maibach H, Piérard GE. Regional differences in stratum corneum reactivity to surfactants: quantitative assessment using the corneosurfametry bioassay. Contact Dermatitis 1997; 37:271–275.
52. Goffin V, Piérard-Franchimont C, Piérard GE. Microwave corneosurfametry. A minute assessment of the mildness of surfactant-containing products. Skin Res Technol 1997; 3:242–244.
53. Goffin V, Piérard GE. Microwave corneosurfametry and the short-duration dansyl chloride extraction test for rating concentrated irritant surfactants. Dermatology 2001; 202:46–48.
54. Goffin V, Henry F, Piérard-Franchimont C, Piérard GE. Penetration enhancers assessed by corneoxenometry. Skin Pharmacol Appl Skin Physiol 2000; 13:280–284.
55. Paye M, Cartiaux Y. Squamometry: a tool to move from exaggerated to more and more realistic application conditions for comparing the skin compatibility of surfactant-based products. Int J Cosmet Sci 1999; 21:59–68.
56. Potts RO. Stratum corneum hydration: experimental techniques and interpretations of results. J Soc Cosmet Chem 1986; 37:9–33.
57. Gehring W, Fluhr J, Gloor M. Influence of vitamin E acetate on stratum corneum hydration. Arzneimittel-Forschung 1998; 48:772–775.
58. Potts RO, Guzek DB, Harriss RR, McKie JE. A non invasive, in vivo, technique to quantitatively measure water concentration of the stratum corneum using attenuated total-reflectance infrared spectroscopy. Arch Dermatol Res 1985; 277:489–495.
59. Williams AC, Lawson EE, Edwards HGM, Barry BW. In vitro–in vivo correlation of FT-Raman spectra of human stratum corneum. Pharm Res 1997; 14:S454.
60. Caspers PJ, Lucassen GW, Wolthuis R, Bruining HA, Puppels GJ. In vitro and in vivo Raman spectroscopy of human skin. Biospectroscopy 1998; 4:S31–S39.
61. Gilard V, Malet-Martino M, Riviere M, Gournay A, Navarro R. Measurement of total water and bound water contents in human stratum corneum by in vitro proton nuclear magnetic resonance spectroscopy. Int J Cosmet Sci 1998; 20:117–125.
62. Querleux B, Richard S, Bittoun J, Jolivet O, Idy-Peretti I, Bazin R, Lévêque JL. In vivo hydration profile in skin layers by high-resolution magnetic resonance imaging. Skin Pharmacol 1994; 7:210–216.
63. Serup J, Winther A, Blichmann C. A simple method for the study of scale pattern and effects of a moisturizer—qualitative and quantitative evaluation by D-squame tape compared with parameters of hydration. Clin Exp Dermatol 1989; 14:277–282.

64. el Gammal C, Pagnoni A, Kligman AM, el Gammal S. A model to assess the efficacy of moisturizers—the quantification of soap-induced xerosis by image analysis of adhesive-coated discs (D-squames®). Clin Exp Dermatol 1996; 21:338–343.

65. Lagarde JM, Black D, Gall Y, Del Pozo A. Image analysis of scaly skin using Dsquame samples: technical and physiological validation. Int J Cosmet Sci 2000; 22:53–65.

66. Rogiers V, EEMCO group. EEMCO guidance for the assessment of the transepidermal water loss (TEWL) in cosmetic sciences. Skin Pharmacol Appl Skin Physiol 2001; 14:117–128.

67. Norlen L, Engblom J, Andersson M, Forslin B. A new computer-based evaporimeter system for rapid and precise measurements of water diffusion through stratum corneum in vitro. J Invest Dermatol 1999; 113:533–540.

68. Smith G, Fischer RW, Blank IH. The epidermal barrier. A comparison between scrotal and abdominal skin. J Invest Dermatol 1961; 36:337–342.

69. Blank IH, Moloney J, Emslie AG, Simon I, Apt C. The diffusion of water across the stratum corneum as a function of its water content. J Invest Dermatol 1984; 82:188–194.

70. Potts RO, Francoeur ML. The influence of stratum corneum morphology on water permeability. J Invest Dermatol 1991; 96:495–499.

71. El-Shimi AF, Princen HM. Water vapor sorption and desorption behavior of some keratins. Colloid Polym Sci 1978; 256:105–114.

72. Blank IH. Further observations on factors which influence the water content of the stratum corneum. J Invest Dermatol 1953; 21:259–271.

73. Smith WP, Christensen MS, Nacht S, Gans EH. Effect of lipids on the aggregation and permeability of human stratum corneum. J Invest Dermatol 1982; 78:7–11.

74. Golden GM, Guzek DB, Harris RR, McKie JE, Potts RO. Lipid thermotropic transitions in human stratum corneum. J Invest Dermatol 1986; 86:255–259.

75. Golden GM, Guzek DB, Kennedy AH, McKie JE, Potts RO. Stratum corneum lipid phase transitions and water barrier properties. Biochemistry 1987; 26:2382–2388.

76. Imokawa G. In vitro and in vivo models. In: Elsner P, Berardesca E, Maibach HI, eds. Bioengineering of the Skin: Water and the Stratum Corneum. New York: Marcel dekker, 1994:23–47.

77. Froebe CL, Simion FA, Olmeyer H, Rhein LD, Mattai J, Cagan RH, Friberg SE. Prevention of stratum corneum lipid phase transition in vitro by glycerol—an alternative mechanism for skin moisturization. J Soc Cosmet Chem 1990; 41:51–65.

78. Mattai J, Froebe CL, Rhein LD, Simion FA, Ohlmeyer H, Su DT, Friberg SE. Prevention of model stratum corneum lipid phase transitions in vitro by cosmetic additives—differential scanning calorimetry, optical microscopy, and water evaporation studies. J Soc Cosmet Chem 1993; 44:89–100.

79. Froebe CL, Simion FA, Rhein LD, Cagan RH, Kligman A. Stratum corneum lipid removal by surfactants: relation to in vivo irritation. Dermatologica 1990; 181:277–283.

80. Melnik BC, Hollman J, Erler E, Verhoeven B, Plewig G. Microanalytical screening of all major stratum corneum lipids by sequential high-performance thin-layer chromatography. J Invest Dermatol 1989; 92:231–234.

25

Formulation of Skin Moisturizers

Steve Barton
The Boots Company, Nottingham, United Kingdom

1 INTRODUCTION

Earlier chapters in this treatise on skin moisturizers have provided detailed analysis of skin physiology and function or described conditions resulting from perturbations in these. Other chapters have discussed some common moisturizer ingredients and means of assessing their efficacy. This chapter attempts to bring all this into perspective for those wishing to understand how the knowledge may be used to develop and manufacture a skin moisturizer.

This cannot hope to be a comprehensive directory on the art of formulating a moisturizer; the range of raw materials alone is prohibitive. For formularies and details of raw material nomenclature and function the reader can access specific texts [1–3]. Here I will identify the major issues to be considered in this process of moisturizer product development.

Some assumptions are required. The first of these is recognition that the challenge is both technologically and commercially driven. This chapter will focus on the technology but always with a view to commercial factors, the principal of which is consumer need. This gives rise to the second assumption; no attempt will be made to artificially separate "cosmetic skin care" from "therapeutic skin care" since these can be seen to derive from slightly different consumer needs, but with often very different regulatory constraints. The third, related, assumption is recognition of the fact that any topical product will have a *physiological* action.

It is therefore clear that all raw materials contained within the final product have a potential contribution toward efficacy, safety, stability, and consumer acceptability.

Recognition of these potentially conflicting interdependencies—technical/commercial, pharmacological/physiological, single material/whole product—is an essential first step to understanding what drives decisionmaking on the final constituents of a moisturizer.

Figure 1 shows some of these interrelated factors to be discussed in the following pages; others will have been covered in other chapters. The objective of this chapter is to outline the challenge presented by attempting to create products that are stable, safe, and in a form acceptable to the user. Consumers have in-

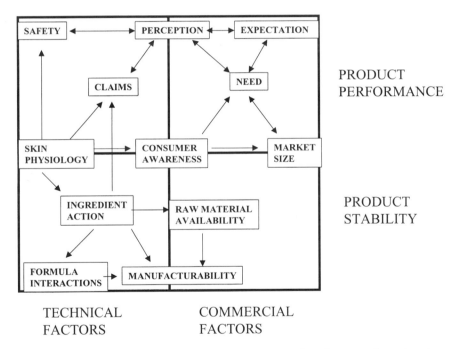

FIGURE 1 Some of the factors that influence moisturizer product development can derive from technical or commercial considerations. Their impact may be greater on product stability or product performance. Understanding the elements of these interactions helps to define key product development criteria. Some relationships are predominantly one-way (e.g., skin physiology defines safety, ingredient action, and claims). Others are iterative (e.g., consumer awareness of skin physiology will determine the market, but as this grows it will reinforce greater consumer awareness).

creasingly high expectations of these performance criteria with the consequence that "acceptable" is being replaced by "esthetically pleasing and efficacious."

2 BACKGROUND

The term *skin moisturizer* is a misleading anachronism from a technical or scientific viewpoint, since the means of achieving "moisturized" skin may have little to do with adding water. The benefit perceived by the person using the moisturizer will depend on several factors, including skin type, product type, and expected benefit, and again may not necessarily relate to moisture. Alongside this there has been constant growth in the added benefits delivered by a moisturizer. This has had the effect of changing the meaning of moisturizer to become a class of skin care products in their own right. Whilst this may seem to create an initial difficulty in deciding how to formulate a moisturizer, it can help focus on the key attributes the target consumer requires (see Table 1).

This is the first stage of developing a product, to be assessed alongside many other factors including total market size, anticipated market share, price, competitor products/benchmarks, and any promotional or advertizing requirements. Consideration of these factors will help a product developer to focus on the technical options and cost constraints required to deliver the targeted benefits.

Table 1 also introduces specific considerations, worthy of more detailed analysis, which may help to provide a comprehensive background to developing a moisturizer. These can be loosely termed demographics—skin type, age, gender, ethnicity, and intention to purchase (see this volume, chapter by Johnson, for more detail). Such information will help describe the target user and required product function of a given moisturizer—conventional moisturizer, specialist moisturizer, or a product with a secondary moisturizing action. These insights will help define the technical delivery options. Table 1 summarizes some of these factors and Fig. 2 shows one way of defining where a product is positioned, thus helping to identify the technological options available to satisfy consumer expectations.

2.1 Technological Influences

The earlier chapters within this book explore more fully the many biological factors that undoubtedly drive the development of moisturizers. Not only do these factors suggest options for achieving improved skin condition, they also influence how this improvement can be assessed.

Understanding the role of the skin's own moisturizing components also presents options, e.g., should we directly address the "deficiency" by replacement or allow the skin to replenish its own integrity by use of a protective product?

TABLE 1 Anticipated Importance of Performance Attributes for Different Moisturizer Product Types and Users

Change to skin attribute	Product Type			
	Therapeutic dry skin product	Baby lotion	Anti-aging face cream	Antenatal body cream
Reduce dryness	Expected	Expected	Expected	Desirable
Reduce flakiness	Expected	Nonessential	Nonessential	Nonessential
Reduce scaling	Expected	Nonessential	Nonessential	Nonessential
Improve dull appearance	Desirable	Desirable	Expected	Desirable
Improve smoothness	Expected	Expected	Expected	Desirable
Improve softness	Desirable	Expected	Expected	Desirable
Improve suppleness	Desirable	Expected	Expected	Expected
Improve flexibility	Expected	Specific product[a]	Desirable	Expected
Reduce wrinkled appearance	Specific product[a]	Nonessential	Desirable	Nonessential
Reduce appearance of fine lines	Specific product[a]	Nonessential	Expected	Nonessential
Reduce leathery appearance	Nonessential	Nonessential	Desirable	Nonessential

[a]Specific product indicates where the performance attribute would not normally be expected but may be delivered by products designed specifically with this attribute in mind.

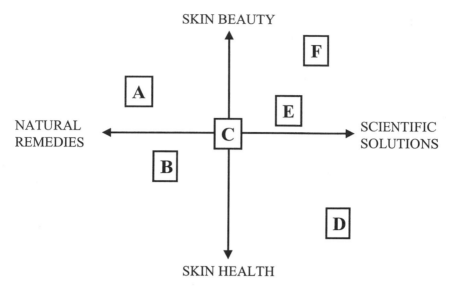

FIGURE 2 Consumers may be driven by different needs (health or beauty) and may have different values which influence their preferred solution. This figure shows one way of treating such choices. Hypothetical solutions are described to help illustrate this using product or ingredient considerations. (A) Botanical extracts to improve normal skin condition; (B) lanolin or beeswax to improve skin health; (C) basic moisturizer; (D) single entity (e.g. retinoic acid for acne-prone skin); (E) hyaluronic acid to plump skin; (F) vitamin A to improve fine lines and wrinkles.

The transfer of technology from skin physiology through therapeutic product to cosmetic product is clear from examples such as α-hydroxyacids and vitamin A, but it may skip directly to mass market product as evidenced by the early incorporation of natural moisturizing factor and ceramides into consumer products. What may not be clear from the previous parts in this book are the other technological aspects that enable this technology transfer.

2.1.1 Raw Material Availability and Performance

Most mass market moisturizers are multicomponent systems, with each material contributing more than one property to the final product. It is therefore rare to attribute unique properties to an individual component. Consumer-defined product attributes may impose limitations on choice of raw materials, requirements such as oil-free, nongreasy, or hypoallergenic may automatically exclude certain classes or species.

Specific comments on useful raw materials are given later in this chapter. However, some general comments on raw materials are worthwhile.

Identification of a useful raw material (e.g., ceramide) is only the first stage in providing a means of modifying stratum corneum. Producing a material in commercial quantities, to an acceptably reproducible standard, in a form that may be easily and safely used in the manufacture of moisturizers represents a major challenge. Commercial and regulatory considerations will influence whether a material is suitable for a therapeutic or mass market product.

The essential fatty acid linoleic acid has been shown to improve dry skin in essential fatty acid deficiency, and the natural source (sunflower seed oil) was also shown to be beneficial [4].

Other sources such as evening primrose oil have also been shown to provide skin benefits, but cost, esthetic, and stability considerations dictate that mass market products use limited proportions of these materials.

Natural raw materials or blends of raw materials are thus an important and attractive source of moisturizing ingredients. Natural sources present other challenges, some of which are dealt with elsewhere (see this volume, chapters by Flower, Young). The key technical factors include stability (including resistance to microbial degradation), variability in identifiable "active" constituents, consistency of supply, and removal of unwanted components.

In the case of plant extracts where skin benefits are attributable to particular components (e.g., chamomile extract) the method of extraction, species, cultivar, time, and place of harvest may also be considerations a product developer wishes to take into account. Where the desirable element within the plant is not readily available, the extraction process may help to provide a more usable form without compromising benefit. The saponification of plant structures is an example where this occurs. Insoluble components can be made available as modified waxes or oils. Alternatively, useful materials can be left in the unsaponifiable fraction. This may have the added advantage of reducing the bulk of the material, hence making it easier to handle and formulate into products. An alternative approach to using natural materials is to use synthetic processes to provide "nature identical" molecules (e.g., lactic acid/panthenol). In such cases the proportion of different isomers may or may not be an important consideration. The purity and reproducible quality of synthetic sources may outweigh any cost disadvantage.

Many of the basic raw materials for moisturizers originate from the petroleum industry. Cost, bulk availability, and reproducible quality were influential in their introduction, though undoubtedly the coincidental growth in affluence and the petrochemical and cosmetics industries also played a part. Materials such as white soft paraffin and light liquid paraffin (mineral oil) remain relatively cheap, standard components for many moisturizing products.

Other important petrochemical byproducts are emulsifiers. These are not only important in themselves, in allowing stable oil and water emulsions to be formulated, but also form the major tool for modifying other raw materials such as vegetable oils or waxes to allow their easy incorporation into the moisturizer. Such modification of raw materials may have several purposes. Changing the solubility, fluidity, or sensory properties are important, but a secondary aim may be to improve the bulk handling properties.

Where novel raw materials have been identified there are additional considerations of safety and registration or patenting. Whilst the latter may not seem a technical issue it may place constraints on the timing of testing. Placing the invention in the public domain before the patent application is accepted may constitute "prior art."

2.1.2 Manufacturability

Raw material bulk handling has already been recognized as an important factor in the previous section. The level of human exposure to a raw material in a manufacturing environment will be different to that anticipated in a product, thus assessment of safe levels under both conditions is important.

Such raw material factors will be considered alongside the processes used to manufacture the bulk. Size of batch, heating/cooling requirements, energy required for dispersion, water content, transfer to pack, pack material and size, will all be considerations in the choice of final formulation. It is also clear that processing itself is an important component of the final formula since viscosity, clarity, and appearance are all dependent on achieving reproducible processing. These factors are considered in more detail later in this chapter.

2.1.3 Performance Testing

The practicalities of performance testing have been discussed elsewhere (see this volume, chapters by Jarret, Grove, Pierard). In formulating a moisturizing product the claims, regulatory requirements, and performance expectations will influence which raw materials and testing methods are to be used and will thus affect the total time and cost of new product development.

2.2 "Extraneous" Constraints

In starting out to develop a new moisturizer there are several other nontechnical issues which will play a part. These are dealt with in detail elsewhere (see this volume, chapters by Flower, Young). For a given raw material, different markets will impose various conditions upon what may or may not be used from the point of view of safety and claims. Additionally, its use in the various product categories and limitations on level of incorporation into a product will impose constraints on the product developer. Patent searching is also an important early step in the product development process—what is freely used in one market may be protected in another.

Various guidelines will exist for good manufacturing practice and good clinical practice for testing efficacy. There are also existing guidelines for claims substantiation testing, e.g., COLIPA guidelines [5]. Thought will need to be given to the promotional activity supporting the postlaunch marketing. Various geographic regions will have their own advertizing standards guidelines which need to be borne in mind in order to help decide, at an early stage, how the product benefits are to be communicated. Outside of these formal systems there will also exist an awareness of attitudes, concerns, and product performance requirements within the healthcare professionals community, particularly dermatologists.

3 DESIGNING MOISTURIZERS: BASIC PRINCIPLES

Moisturizing products are to be applied to the skin and left there to replace lost moisture to improve hydration, protect from drying, and improve the various outward signs of dryness such as scaling or flaking and generally smooth the skin (see Table 1). Bringing together all the materials to achieve the desired result(s) requires an understanding of their benefits to the skin and physicochemical behavior if the three key criteria of safety, stability, and esthetics are to be achieved.

3.1 Cosmetic Emulsions

The delivery options open to a product developer may seem straightforward, but given that most mass market moisturizing products are emulsions, one could be forgiven for asking why this is the case. Table 2 summarizes some of the reasons for choosing an emulsion. In most cases the emulsion will comprise oil and water.

Emulsions are multiphase systems where one phase (the continuous phase) contains droplets of the other (dispersed) phase(s). Commonly skin care emulsions are two-phase systems where the relative volume of the continuous phase is usually, but not necessarily, greater than the dispersed phase. Droplet size is usually, but not necessarily, large enough to interfere with the path of light and thus emulsions will be at least opalescent and usually white. Special cases exist where the particle size is so small that the liquid is clear (microemulsions) or where the emulsion structure becomes a liquid crystalline matrix (ringing gels). Three-phase systems can also exist, but all these systems tend to follow the basic principles described herein.

The theoretical approach to emulsions is helpful in formulating personal care products, but the underlying principles are often based on highly simplified systems. Experience and intelligent use of these principles rather than exact science underlies much of the skill of the formulator. To formulate cost-effective moisturizers the basic challenge is to overcome the problem that oil and water are immiscible. It is thermodynamically preferable for the two phases to exist in discrete layers, minimizing the interfacial tension.

TABLE 2 Why Use an Emulsion?

Benefit	Example
Esthetics	Elegant, pleasant to use; water content improves skin feel and cooling effect better than oil alone.
Range of physical forms	Cream, lotion, milk, paste.
Vast range of properties	From light through to heavy. From lubricious through to "draggy". From quickly absorbed through to maintained film on skin.
Inclusion of actives	Simultaneous delivery of incompatible materials, e.g., oil soluble with water-soluble actives in the same base. Allows use of these materials at levels appropriate to their benefit.
Cost	Water content reduces overall cost.

Agitating mixtures of oil and water, in whatever proportion, will increase the surface area between the phases, thereby increasing the surface energy of the system. Thus any oil/water system, in the absence of external energy input, will ultimately configure itself in the lowest possible energy state—in this case by minimizing the amount of contact between two phases and reorganizing itself into two separate layers. The solution is to reduce the interfacial tension between the two layers and thereby reduce the surface energy of the system.

Generally we use a combination of chemical and mechanical energy to achieve an emulsion that will retain its stability for an acceptable period of time (equivalent to what is often referred to as the shelf-life). The main source of chemical energy is from emulsifiers or surfactants (the terminology can become confusing and the term *emulsifier* will be used throughout this chapter). These change interfacial tension and, depending on various factors, will produce either oil-in-water (o/w) or water-in-oil (w/o) emulsions.

Mechanical energy input into the emulsification process is an underrated consideration. High shear, applied to the phases under continuous agitation, will reduce the size of emulsified particles. Generally, the smaller the particle size, the greater the stability, so mechanical energy can contribute greatly to the overall emulsion stability and esthetics. The usual means of achieving this is to force the agitated mixture through a small orifice under pressure. The design and geometry of the tools to achieve this will vary, but a turbine drawing up the mixture and forcing it back through mesh is a common format. The size and shape of the mixing vessel, the speed of mixing, and the rate of heating and cooling will also play a role since heat energy is conventionally another means of facilitating emulsification.

Alternatives to simple emulsions have been prepared and used in personal care products: multiple phase emulsions (e.g., oil-in-water-in-oil), liquid crystal emulsions, etc. Silicone oils can also form part or all of one of the phases of an emulsion. Space does not permit a full description of the differences, but energy requirements, particle size, and different manufacturing conditions required are amongst the considerations a product developer would consider when choosing one of these special types of emulsion. The principal considerations to be described will be similar for these specialized cases.

The process of emulsification also finds use in cleansers (see this volume, chapter by Simion) where oil droplets are suspended in an aqueous environment thereby removing oil-bound dirt. Emulsifiers are amphipathic molecules that act by partitioning themselves at the boundary between the oil and water phases. Since conventional emulsions comprise water and oil it is their relative preference for, or solubility in, water and oil that dictates the characteristics of an emulsifier. The partitioning between the phases will also be influenced by the physicochemical characteristics of the two phases—for example, the melting point of the combined oil phase and the salt concentration of the water phase, each of which, separately but indirectly, may contribute to the effectiveness of emulsification.

The factors responsible for determining the physical format of the emulsion (lotion, cream, etc.) include emulsifier selection, physicochemical nature of oil phase components, relative phase volume, and droplet particle size. The mechanical energy applied to the system can also influence greatly the droplet size and therefore the whole outcome.

One clear source is energy during manufacture, however secondary sources worthy of consideration from a stability and esthetics standpoint are pumping from manufacturing vessel into pack and dispensing from pack during use.

3.1.1 Emulsifier Types

There are various types of emulsifier described by their chemical nature. The earliest used chemical emulsifiers were probably soaps. These have a charged, hence hydrophilic, group and a fatty, hence hydrophobic, portion. These early anionic emulsifiers—named on the basis of the nature of the ion providing the polar or hydrophilic region—demonstrate some of the problems of turning emulsification into an exact science.

Soaps from tallow and coconut have very different proportions of fatty acid species. Even within coconut soaps the proportion of particular carbon chain lengths will vary between batches and the source of coconut oil starting materials. This variation will affect the physicochemical behavior at the oil–water interface, since the oil partitioning will depend upon fatty chain length, and thus there will be a range of emulsifying performance resulting from the chemical heterogeneity of the starting raw material. Refinement of the starting material can produce more reliable performance but at a higher cost. Crude material, e.g., hydrogenated vegetable oils can be "cut" to produce mixed fatty alcohols, e.g., cetearyl alcohol, and further refined to produce purer materials, e.g., polyglyceryl-3 oleate. This principle applies as much to emulsifiers as it does to other oil phase ingredients commonly used in formulating moisturizers.

Many original skin care emulsions were produced by in situ neutralization of stearic acid with sodium hydroxide. The resulting soap acts as an emulsifier. There are problems with such systems, particularly their pH and susceptibility to heavy metal salts. In particular their aggressiveness on skin has tended to rule them out of favor moreso in leave-on moisturizers than wash-off cleansers (see this volume chapter by Simion). More sophisticated anionic systems do however still find use in emulsions. Modified coconut oils still form the basis of the sulfate and ether sulfate anionic emulsifiers (such as sodium lauryl sulfate and sodium lauryl ether sulfate). The substitution of the fatty chain using an ether group reduces the hydrophobic nature of the fatty chain, hence the emulsifier, and produces an emulsion system less aggressive to the skin [6].

Nonionic emulsifiers are commonly used in personal care moisturizers, and as the name implies they have no charge. Instead their amphipathic nature derives from their long carbon chains imparting hydrophobic nature (e.g., fatty acids) or hydrophilic nature (e.g., alcohols). Unsaturated carbon chains are easily substituted with ethylene oxide. This process of ethoxylation can be carried out to varying degrees on the same starting material to give a range of different amphipathic behaviors. When combined with varying lengths and branching of the carbon chain, this has produced a vast array of different molecules; many of which have become the workhorses for skin care formulators.

Cationic emulsifiers also exist and do have some use in skin care formulations. Many of those used also demonstrate some antimicrobial activity; this may be considered of benefit. Cationic emulsifiers do not have the same problem as anionics with metal salts, but may be prone to instability at high pH and negative ion concentration. They also have a property that can be either detrimental or beneficial. The skin surface has a net negative charge, and cationic emulsifiers may thus bind to the substrate.

Polymeric emulsifiers are also common in moisturizer formulations. Examples include those based on silicone or polyacrylic acids. These polymers distribute themselves along the oil/water interface with side groups of lipophilic and hydrophilic nature inserted into their respectively preferred phase.

It is not uncommon to find mixed types of emulsifier in a given emulsion. Indeed many raw material suppliers combine anionic and nonionic emulsifiers as a blend for commercial purposes. The skill of the formulator will be to recognize where one of the particular properties mentioned is required, understand the consequences and compromises this confers on the emulsion, and act accordingly.

3.1.2 Emulsifier Choice

This is not straightforward but has been simplified by the introduction, around 50 years ago, of the HLB system. The system accompanied the increased use of nonionic emulsifiers where it finds greatest use. The HLB number (hydrophile/lipophile balance) represents the balance of the size and strength of the hydrophilic (or polar) and lipophilic (or nonpolar) groups within the emulsifier molecules. This can be visualized in terms of how the emulsifier molecule will position itself at the oil–water interface (Fig. 3).

The more polar one part of the molecule is (often referred to as the headgroup), the more it will insert itself into the water domain of an emulsion. Conversely, the more nonpolar the other part (or the tailgroup), the more it will be part of the oil phase. The relative polarity will not only affect the final position of the emulsifier within the interface, but also the stability and fluidity of this boundary.

The HLB system uses this relative preference on a scale from 1 to 20 and provides most emulsifiers, particularly nonionic emulsifiers, with such a number. The usefulness of the HLB system is that it is additive. Thus combining equal proportions of emulsifier of different HLB (e.g., 5 and 15) will produce a system of average HLB (i.e., 10). This property of the HLB system can be used to calculate the most appropriate emulsifier for an oil phase of unknown requirements. Simple experimental determinations can be carried out, using a range of emulsifier mixtures with a known range of HLB, to show the HLB value(s) that result in good emulsification. An appropriate emulsifier, or blend of emulsifiers, can then be chosen having the equivalent HLB number. In practice the task is not always that simple, however the HLB system provides a useful guide. The HLB values are normally published in suppliers' literature and are therefore often readily available.

The factors that influence HLB include the chemistry, stereochemistry, and purity for each emulsifier and their miscibility with other oil and water phase components (rarely do we wish to produce an emulsion of a single oil with pure water). These factors can usefully be taken into account alongside the HLB. It is also necessary to point out that HLB determinations will produce two conclusions, one for oil-in-water the other for water-in-oil systems.

The usefulness of the HLB system, the range of physical forms, and relative mildness (compared to anionics and cationics) have made nonionic emulsifiers the commonest choice.

Milder anionics have become more available and more appropriate for leave-on products and blends of nonionics and anionics are useful starting points for emulsions, combining the advantages of both emulsifier types. However non-

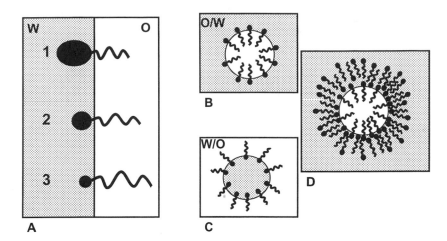

FIGURE 3 Emulsifiers cross the oil–water interface as shown in this diagrammatic representation.
(A) Emulsifier 1 has greater affinity for water than oil (e.g., HLB 12–15). The stereochemistry of the polar headgroup may contribute to its performance. As spherical droplets of oil form in water this stereochemistry will limit the number of emulsifier molecules that are used per unit surface area of oil droplet. Emulsifier 2 has a more even affinity for oil and water (HLB 5–12) and may be able to contribute more molecules per unit area provided that the lipophilic domains do not sterically hinder this. Emulsifier 3 will readily form water in oil emulsions (HLB 1–5). It can be seen that combinations of more than one emulsifier will enable greater numbers of emulsifier molecules per unit surface area of droplets.
(B) Alignment of emulsifiers in oil-in-water emulsions. (C) Alignment of emulsifiers in water-in-oil emulsions. (D) The concept of using a secondary emulsifier with higher HLB to stabilize the emulsion. A bilayer effect is produced around the oil droplet as the polar heads and nonpolar tails orient themselves in alternating fashion. The outer portion of the spherical droplet is therefore hydrophilic, and the hydrophilic heads of primary and secondary emulsifiers align themselves at the oil–water interface. It is also likely that secondary emulsifiers insert lipophilic tails into the oil droplet. The overall result is greater emulsion stability.

ionics have other advantages. They are more stable to pH changes and less influenced by salt concentration, and they are more easily combined as emulsifier blends. By using the same carbon chain length backbone and different degrees of ethoxylation an emulsifier blend can be created which, though it has an equivalent HLB as a single emulsifier of similar chain length, produces a better quality emulsion. The rationale for this lies in the packing of the individual emulsifier molecules into the oil–water interface; single species will compete for space, whereas mixed species will take up complementary spatial distribution (see Fig. 3).

3.1.3 Stability

Stability is a term used in the cosmetics and toiletries industry to describe how the product may be expected to respond to storage and use after manufacture, packing, and temporary storage in warehouse or point of sale. As with many of the issues discussed in this particular chapter there are no absolutes; much will be determined by assessing risk on the basis of experience and laboratory simulation. Cosmetic emulsions are in thermodynamic equilibrium and changes in this status quo can destabilize the emulsion structure in a number of ways.

To help understand why we use some ingredients in a moisturizer it can be useful to look at what might go wrong. A formulator, having understood the compromises mentioned, will think ahead to some of these possibilities and modify the formula appropriately. Table 3 is a brief and incomplete summary of some of the factors. It is designed to show how the factors affecting emulsion stability are interlinked. We can rarely pinpoint a single variable and change it to effect a desired end. For example, increasing the viscosity (actually the rheology, since the system is in equilibrium) of the continuous phase using a thickener will reduce the effects of dispersed phase Brownian motion.

However, the use of such additives (e.g., waxes for continuous oil phase or polymers for a continuous water phase) will also increase the specific gravity of the continuous phase, change the interfacial behavior at the water–oil interface and thus affect the fluidity of this layer.

The overall effects on the emulsion may be beneficial, but simultaneously changing other emulsion components or processing parameters will render it difficult to know which emulsion characteristic has been changed and how, hence the inexact science!

Coalescence resulting from fusion of two droplets of the dispersed phase may be minimized by the changes mentioned (through limiting the effects of Brownian motion), but the void space (between the dispersed phase particles) and the particle size are important contributory factors. Changing the relative volume and/or the emulsifier can effect changes to these emulsion attributes. Concentration of emulsifier is also important in maintaining the phase separation at the interface, and minimizing the possible confluence of droplets if they do come into contact. Increasing the concentration of a nonionic emulsifier in this way to overcome the risk of coalescence may however create other problems—flocculation, for example. Options for overcoming this eventuality may include substituting some anionic for nonionic emulsifier. Here again the concept of emulsifier blends helps to achieve the desired end (see Fig. 3).

Where dispersed phase droplets become extremely tightly packed, phase inversion can occur, e.g., oil-in-water emulsion changes to water-in-oil. There

TABLE 3　Emulsion Stability Factors and Their Implications for Formulation Development

Symptom	Causes	Some formulation implications
Coalescence of disperse phase droplets	Proximity of droplets. Instability at oil–water interface. Brownian motion.	Improve strength of interface—emulsifier blend choice effect on stability. Change relative volume of phases. Continuous phase thickeners.
Flocculation of disperse phase droplets	Attraction of droplets via van der Waal's forces results in effectively larger droplets.	Change charge of droplet surface. Change relative volume of phases. Continuous phase thickeners.
Sedimentation or floating of dispersed phase droplets	Large differences in specific gravity of phases.	Change specific gravity of phases. Change viscosity of continuous phase. Reduce dispersed phase particle size.
Phase inversion	High relative volume of dispersed phase. Instability at oil–water interface	Change relative volume of phases. Change emulsifier blend. Change processing—increased shear reduces particle size.
Ostwald ripening	Large dispersed phase droplets formed at expense of small ones. Instability at oil–water interface.	Change solubility characteristics of dispersed phase components to prevent migration into continuous phase.

will be a critical volume fraction for the dispersed phase beyond which the thermodynamics will favor the dispersed phase becoming continuous. The risk of phase inversion can be a particular problem in water-in-oil emulsions where high relative volumes of water are favored to reduce the oily feel. The choice of emulsifier influences whether a system favors a water-in-oil or oil-in-water emulsion, but the rate of addition of the dispersed phase or the degree of mixing can influence whether or not an emulsion phase inverts. This potential problem has been exploited in manufacturing some sophisticated emulsion types.

Many of the potential problems may also be modified by use of "co-emulsifiers." These too have amphipathic nature and can be thought of as outer coatings around the individual droplets. Using as an example cetyl alcohol in oil-in-water systems, the hydrophilic domain (alcohol group) will co-locate with the primary emulsifier hydrophile. The hydrophobic tail (fatty chain) will not be physicochemically compatible with the aqueous phase, but more easily associated with other hydrophobes. As a result some hydrophilic heads project back toward the aqueous phase, their hydrophobic tails aligning together forming a bilayer (see Fig. 3). As an extension of this principle a network of structured lamellae can form a matrix throughout the continuous phase—the so-called liquid crystalline emulsions being the result.

The advantage here is that the structure adds stability to the system and may even add skin care benefits of longer-term moisturization and improved esthetics. The intercorneocyte lipid arrangement in skin is an analogous system that not only helps explain how this structure works, but also shows how it may help in "selling" an emulsion of this type into a skin care product or the skin care market.

The enhanced stability provided by liquid crystalline structures is a specific example of how polymeric systems can stabilize the emulsion. A variety of polymeric systems can be used in the water phase of o/w systems (celluloses, alginates, etc.). Another commonly used polymer matrix used to stabilize emulsions can be seen with polyacrylic acid copolymer systems (carbopols). In extreme cases these can act as the sole emulsifier and modified carbopols can make useful "emulsifier-free" emulsions.

Other symptoms of instability such as "creaming" (oil droplets floating to surface in oil-in-water system) or "sedimentation" (water droplets sinking in water-in-oil systems) can also be addressed by altering the viscosity with polymers. Balancing the differences in the specific gravity of the dispersed and continuous phases will also minimize this effect. Again processing to achieve small particle size in the dispersed phase is also a key factor.

In systems where dispersed phase components are partially soluble in the continuous phase—cetyl alcohol can exist in both the oil and water phase—Ostwald ripening may occur. Larger droplets are formed at the expense of smaller ones, another manifestation of the dynamic status that emulsions exhibit.

The formulator has a number of tools available to assist in assessing the behavior of the emulsion and the likely stability implications (Table 4).

As can be seen from the foregoing, the type and number of raw materials in the formulation required for producing a stable emulsion already appears large. This has stability implications, but controlling the symptoms of instability may also change the esthetics of the product. Many of the materials used are chosen for their esthetic properties, so the process of understanding this interdependency between stability and esthetics can be convoluted.

Once other materials are added the potential interactions increase logarithmically. The skill of the formulator will be to understand the physicochemical

TABLE 4 Some Tools to Assist in Determining Emulsion Characteristics in Short-Term and Long-Term Stability

Tool	Principle	Comments
Microscopy	Visualization of phase differences	Very useful qualitative tool Dark field; phase contrast, polarized light and Nomarski optics very useful modes of visualization Can require emulsion to be disturbed (squashed) in the process
Laser particle sizer	Droplet disturbs the laser beam in proportion to its size	Usually requires diluted samples
Tensiometer	Measures force required to pull a ring or plate through the interface between two layers	Gives basic information on interfacial tension but can only be carried out where a large surface area interface can be achieved
Rheometer	Measures the changes in viscoelastic properties of the emulsion under known stress	Stress conditions and parameters of interest can be specific to particular emulsion types
Turbidometry	Examines bulk light scattering properties	Gross stability rapidly assessed if used with accelerated testing

properties of the raw material used and, by combining this with experience of previous products, predict what may be a suitable solution for the consumer need.

It has already been pointed out that a "simple moisturizer" may also have other required functions. Example formulations are presented in Sec. 4 detailing examples of these classes to help demystify the ingredient labeling nomenclature.

3.1.4 Stability Testing

Why conduct stability tests? This question, if thought through, should provide all the necessary parameters with which to assess the risk of failing to deliver consumer expectation. The consumer wants a safe, effective product. What may make it unsafe or ineffective? The consumer wants a product that will be pleasurable to use. What may detract from this pleasurable experience? The consumer wants to be able to use it in the course of their daily routine. What is that likely to be and how will the product respond? Many of these questions are common to the general principles underlying formulation of a successful product.

The formulator will test the initial batch(es) of the product to assess fit with consumer expectation; what happens once the product is opened or stored for long periods?

Physicochemical and Organoleptic Stability. As detailed in Table 4 there are a number of physicochemical characteristics that can help determine stability. Viscosity and microscopic appearance are commonly used as laboratory tools in this way. Rapid change in viscosity over time will suggest a change in the emulsion structure. Both increased and decreased viscosity can have implications for stability and each may affect the delivery from the pack.

Microscopy can be helpful in understanding the reasons underlying the change in stability. Emulsion structure and homogeneity of droplet in terms of size and structure can be visualized. Emulsification of complex lipid mixtures can result in droplets containing different lipid phases; their stability can be assessed from how well defined and how consistent these phases are within and between individual lipid droplets. Crystallization of water-soluble or oil-soluble components can be seen using polarizing light microscopy, and the special case of liquid crystalline emulsions can be assessed for consistency and appearance.

Many of the other criteria for stability assessment focus on the sensory aspects—odor, color, and viscosity, in particular. Changes in these are likely to be noticed by the customer and have an effect on the perceived as well as the real performance. Objective characteristics such as pH and viscosity are easy to record; sensory properties often require reference to a standard sample, usually the one stored at room temperature.

Amongst other factors that may change, the pH of the product will be the most often tested, and changes here may have safety implications. This can only be assessed in an oil-in-water emulsion, and pH changes in a water-in-oil formulation could affect the overall product stability.

One of the requirements during the initial formulation work will be to rapidly assess potential stability problems. Exposure to elevated temperatures (60°C) is often used as an indicator, since many of the potential problems are a consequence of the thermodynamics of emulsification. Temperature cycling can also be used in a similar way to stress the potential formulation, but the method finds use in longer-term testing for anticipated changes that may result from warehouse storage, travel, and export to other countries.

Many of the stability characteristics will be dictated by the pack. Whilst glass is fairly inert, many of the other commonly used plastics can impose constraints on formulation raw materials. Some esters used in formulations can solubilize certain pack types. The resulting effect varies from softening and deformation of the pack to reduction of permeability of the pack material. The latter change will reduce the physical barrier allowing gaseous exchange to occur and even result in microbial spoilage. Testing in the appropriate pack is therefore essential.

Clear packs also impose some constraints. Colored products can fade in a clear pack and inclusion of a sunscreen in the product or pack required may resolve the problem. Testing to mimic the exposure to light in the shop window or bathroom window is therefore another means of ensuring that the esthetics of the product do not change on storage.

Microbial Stability. The most important of the potential risks in the safety category is microbial contamination. Sources of contamination occur throughout the supply chain—raw material, raw material storage and processing, packaging, final product storage, and product use and storage by the consumer. There may be particular considerations that influence the risk analysis. For instance baby moisturizer products for the diaper area will be exposed to fecal contamination. Eczema sufferers have increased risk of skin staphylococcal contamination. Botanical extracts for incorporation in skin moisturizers may contain microbial contamination at source.

Particular parts of the machinery used to process the product may have reservoirs susceptible to contamination or prove difficult to clean in between manufacturing batches, pumps in particular. The pack in which the product is presented also plays an important part. Whilst pump packs and squeeze bottles prevent the introduction of contamination from the fingers or outside world, the "suck-back" from a squeeze bottle could siphon contamination back in and provide a false sense of security. Once the product has been used a number of times, there is a large air space and condensation on the side of pack can create an environment for microbial growth.

The response to all of these risks is to incorporate a degree of preservation. Incorporating preservatives or using barrier methods (e.g., pump pack; single-dose format) are two common strategies but these should be as protection against accidental contamination postmanufacture. Primary risk reduction should always come from good manufacturing practice—avoidance of contamination in the first place. The implication for the product developer is that no raw material or process used should increase the risk of microbial contamination. Use of freeze-dried or alcoholic or glycolic rather than aqueous plant extracts is one level of risk limitation.

The processes used for testing microbial stability are termed challenge testing. Here inoculation of the product with known organisms is carried out and their subsequent survival monitored. The protocols used and the criteria for passing and failing may be laid down in prescribed monographs [7]. Such testing will be conducted on samples from first laboratory or small-scale batches as well as on these samples after storage for a given period. Full microbial counting after manufacture and before release for sale may also be used to assess the quality of the factory batch prior to delivery.

3.2 Processing and Packaging

Whilst the focus of this chapter is the formulation aspects of moisturizers, processing and packaging cannot be excluded as they impose limitations and create opportunities for the formulator.

Skin care moisturizers are produced in large quantities worldwide. Many different batch sizes, processes, and plant specifications exist, and economics often dictate the role played by human operator or automated machine. Small-scale production runs up to 1000 L can be managed by small enterprises without much sophistication. Where large-scale volumes permit, continuous processing can be achieved, but this is probably the exception. Similarly, dispensing lotions into 30-mL narrow-necked bottles will impose different economic constraints than filling 500-g tubs with a thick cream. Whichever the case, raw material handling, water purity, and plant hygiene are of prime concern.

The technical and formulation constraints imposed by different manufacturing conditions are a key part of formulation development and can command considerable resource. The key issues that require control will be speed of heating and cooling, speed of addition of one phase to another, shear, duration, and energy input during mixing. Some of the other constraints imposed will be addition of volatiles (e.g., fragrance) or heat-sensitive raw materials (e.g., vitamins, botanical extracts).

Where oils are added to water there is the likelihood of crystallization of some high–melting point components if the water temperature differs too greatly from the oil. Water phase thickeners also pose potential problems since thorough dispersion is required to prevent the formation of gelatinous lumps; hydration of the external layer can occur, preventing adequate hydration of the central mass. Overagitation can introduce air into the mixture and with some emulsifier levels and types, this aeration can be retained all the way through into the pack.

Another area of potential risk is incorporation of mineral particulates such as talc, zinc oxide, or titanium dioxide. These create a high surface area and require adequate "wetting" if incorporated in water phase or dispersion into oil phase. The effect on the overall emulsification requirements will not be simply assessed via HLB calculations.

In some cases processing conditions can be the vital element in producing the desired product and here, or where other factors dictate, small-scale trial or pilot batches may be desirable.

4 FORMULATION EXAMPLES

A number of example formulations are presented and ingredients discussed to illustrate the issues highlighted earlier in the chapter. The formulations will also be referred to later in the chapter when discussing performance aspects.

4.1 Basic Moisture Lotion

Formula I (Table 5) is a basic moisturizing lotion, which requires that some of the oil phase will remain fluid at room temperature. Shorter chain esters are more fluid contributing to this property in this formulation. Mineral oils are also useful here but with added benefits of stability (lower risk of rancidity than esters) and lower bulk cost. However the esthetics of a solely mineral oil formula would not be very good and incorporating esters improves the skin-feel without reducing lubricity. Cetyl alcohol helps stabilize the emulsion and provides some viscosity. Its higher molecular weight fatty chain length and relative hydrophobicity contribute to this action. The ratio of oil to water will be around 1:3 and this will influence the overall viscosity. Silicone oils usually count toward the oil phase, and the type and concentration of silicone oil will depend on the intended product use. Higher levels of barrier can be achieved with higher molecular weight silicones.

Water phase thickeners not only provide added stability, but also increase the bulk or body of the lotion. Such viscosity modifiers are also important when considering how the product is dispensed. Pumping through nozzles creates high shear forces. Some rheology modifiers tolerate these better than others and the formulator must choose the correct combinations for this and "rub-in" properties. In the case of alginates or carbomers the effects of salts also require consideration.

Salts present on the skin have a thinning effect on these systems and this can be put to use to achieve "quick break" effects on application. Glycerin is an all-purpose moisturizing ingredient that is cost effective and widely available from a variety of sources. The level of incorporation and claims associated with glycerin depend on the target market. In some markets urea might be another expected moisturizing ingredient though its mode of action would be different. Urea also introduces stability constraints—pH and preservative and thickener compatibility being examples.

Since pump delivery has the added benefit of reducing the risk of spoilage via microbial contamination, this can be a popular pack choice for baby lotions.

TABLE 5 Formula I: Basic Moisture Lotion—Oil-in-Water Emulsion, Lotion Consistency

Ingredient name	Function	Comment
Aqua	Solubilize and deliver aqueous phase ingredients; provide cooling effect	Continuous phase.
Paraffinum Liquidum	Provide occlusive layer for emollience, protection, and smooth skin-feel	Disperse phase; low cost; low risk of oxidation; low miscibility with water phase.
Glycerin	Humectant	Polar nature enhances water binding.
Caprylic/capric Triglyceride	As mineral oil but with better esthetics as a result of its esterified structure	Relatively short chain length to maintain lotion characteristic of this formulation.
Dimethicone	Adds some slip to the skin-feel on application and adds to barrier produced by the oil phase components	Different grades of silicone oils (chain length, viscosity) give different benefits to the barrier and feel characteristics.
Glyceryl stearate	Nonionic emulsifier	Lipophilic>lipophobic HLB 4.
PEG 100 stearate	Nonionic emulsifier	Lipophilic<lipophobic HLB 18.
Cetyl alcohol	Co-emulsifier/wax	Stabilizes disperse phase droplet interface and acts as viscosity builder.
Carbomer	Aqueous phase thickener	Improves stability; adds body to lotion; breaks quickly as product is rubbed in to enhance esthetics.
Potassium hydroxide	Neutralize acidic groups on carbomer	
Tetrasodium EDTA	Sequestrant to prevent metal ions being bound to cationic groups on aqueous phase thickeners	Also enhances microbial stability by removing metal ions.
Parfum[a]		
Preservative[b]		

[a]Fragrance may or may not require special consideration during formulation.
[b]Choice of preservative will depend on local market regulations and preservation needs.

4.2 Water-in-Oil Cream

Whilst water-in-oil creams (Formula II, Table 6) may be expected to have high proportions of oil, this is not axiomatic. Use of a combination of low HLB non-ionic and silicone emulsifier systems to obtain highly stable small droplet size water phase can contribute to an increased water content. The rich feel can come from the high oil loading, and the emulsifier combination enhances this by providing a shear-thickening effect in use. This is counteracted by silicone fluid helping provide final rub-in characteristic. In the case of this formulation the C12–C15 ester makes up the bulk of the oil phase. This material has good solubilizing properties for other oil phase components and has lower cost and greater predictability and quality compared with other oil phase components. The lanolin and bees wax add structure. The ratio of these structuring waxes and the fluid ester will help define the final viscosity. The glycerin in the water phase is "trapped" within the lipid matrix and when applied to skin may be released more slowly.

4.3 Anhydrous Emollient Cream

Where cost and efficacy permit, such anhydrous systems as Formula III (Table 7) can deliver moisturized skin via emollience and occlusion. Lanolin performs this dual role well but in the case of this formulation the cost is reduced by blending petroleum based oils and waxes, silicones and carnauba wax (also a common structural wax ingredient for lipsticks). Dispersion is aided by stearic acid. Microbial spoilage is unlikely in the absence of water but rancidity of lanolin and other oils can be prevented by the inclusion of anti-oxidants such as butylated hydroxy toluene.

4.4 Basic Dry Skin Cream

A basic dry skin cream is described by Formula IV (Table 8). Where products for therapeutic use are required, there are limitations imposed by regulatory bodies on permitted raw materials.

Here the bulk of the oil phase is from mineral oil/wax to achieve a suitable consistency occlusive film that rubs in well without being too greasy. Lanolin is added for its emollient properties.

The combination of PEG-20 stearate and cetearyl alcohol is an example of a commercially available mixed emulsifier system. This one known as Polawax™ is commonly used in therapeutic skin care products. It provides very thick but not particularly elegant emulsions. Oil phase components have well-documented tolerance and pharmacopoeia specifications. Other ingredients may be included for therapeutic purposes—urea, lactic acid introduced into the water phase; additional oil phase components rich in linoleic acid (borage oil, evening primrose oil, etc.). Anti-oxidant may be included for formulation stability rather than skin benefit.

TABLE 6 Formula II: Cold Cream—Water-in-Oil Emulsion, High Viscosity

Ingredient name	Function	Comment
Aqua	Solubilize aqueous phase ingredients	Disperse phase; effect more prolonged since it is trapped in oil phase.
C12–15 alkyl benzoate	Provide emollience, protection, smooth skin-feel	Mixed chain length ester provides better combination of occlusion without waxiness (e.g., compared to paraffin). Allows incorporation of other waxes.
Cetyl stearate	Emollient	
Polyglyceryl-3-oleate	Nonioinic emulsifier/thickener	HLB 5.
Cetyl dimethicone Copolyol	Silicone emulsifier	
Lanolin alcohols	Provide emulsifying and emollient properties, protection, smooth skin-feel	Branched nature provides a balance between occlusion and protection. Also has HLB 4
Cyclomethicone	Slip on application, subsequent evaporation means that it does not add to occlusion	To balance against shear thickening of cream during rub-in.
Cera alba	Provides emollience, protection, smooth skin-feel	Waxy nature also provides structure to the formulation to give high viscosity.
Glycerin	Humectant	In disperse phase, slower release possible.
Preservative		

4.5 Upper-Mass Cosmetic Moisturizer

More sophisticated products inevitably comprise more ingredients. This may seem self-serving in terms of ensuring the customer appears to get more for their money. However such complex mixtures are required to create the desired textural properties. Formula V describes an upper-mass cosmetic moisturizer formulation (Table 9).

TABLE 7 Formula III: Anhydrous Emollient Cream—Ointment Consistency, High Viscosity Cream

Ingredient name	Function	Comment
Lanolin	Emollient; protective; occlusive; smooth skin-feel	Lanolin is a complex material and its many components provide a variety of advantages to the skin.
Paraffinum liquidum	Occlusive; protective	Allows the bulk volume of the product to be substituted by this cheaper and more stable raw material.
Paraffin	Occlusive	Blend of liquid and this solid matches overall lanolin consistency to achieve above.
Stearic acid	Dispersing agent (anionic emulsifier)	In this case there is no water to create an emulsion, but the material aids the dispersion of all the components.
Carnauba	Structuring agent	Together with the paraffins, this wax creates a lanolinlike consistency.
Cyclomethicone	Skin slip on application	
BHT	Butylated hydoxytoluene; anti-oxidant	Prevents the lanolin from oxidizing (going rancid) on storage.

In the case of this cream the backbone is a nonionic emulsion system using the common C18 carbon chain backbone. Stearyl alcohol with 2 and 21 moles ethoxylation respectively together with cetearyl alcohol co-emulsifier produce a structuring effect that has liquid crystalline properties. This enhances stability and mimics the structure of the stratum corneum lipids. Other oil phase components are emollient esters; some, such as dioctyl maleate, have secondary action, in this case as a solubilizer for the UV filters added to provide a level of UV protection. Petrolatum, caprylic/capric triglycerides, isopropyl lanolate, and Theobroma oil provide a balance of solid/liquid oils. Theobroma oil has a melting point close to skin temperature and thus excellent skin-feel properties.

TABLE 8 Formula IV: Basic Dry Skin Cream—Oil-in-Water Emulsion, Thick Cream Consistency

Ingredient name	Function	Comment
Aqua	Provide cooling, moisturizing effect, consistent with expectation	Continuous phase; allows some reduction in cost.
Paraffinum liquidum	Protective; occlusive	Bulk of oil phase.
Paraffin	Protective; occlusive	Combination of liquid and solid paraffin allows thick consistency to be formed.
Lanolin alcohols	Emollient	
PEG-20 stearate	Nonionic emulsifier	HLB 1.4.
Cetearyl alcohol	Co-emulsifier; structuring agent	HLB 1.3.
Preservative		

Humectant properties of glycerin and butylene glycol ensure a mixed, prolonged moisturization, which can be measured instrumentally.

Dimethicone adds "slip" during application to the skin. The water phase is thickened using polyacrylamide and modified cellulose providing increased stability for this complex oil phase. The former gels but is more watery and cooling, and "breaks" on application; the cellulose persists longer.

The skin benefits provided by the combination of vitamins A, E, and C are common amongst modern anti-aging skin creams.

4.6 Moisturising Gel

The gel formula (Formula VI, Table 10) provides a rapid, cooling watery feel to the skin and would be common for after-sun or body massage products. In order to deliver more than transient moisture, the formula comprises humectants seen in other formulae, but also amino acids to mimic the role played by natural moisturising factor. Aloe barbadensis is reputed for soothing properties and would fit well within an after-sun product. The source and quality would dictate what strength of claim could be made for the product.

Alcohol adds additional cooling as well as augmenting the resistance to microbial challenge. The level of alcohol chosen needs to balance these properties with the potentially drying effects on the skin that alcohol may have.

The bulk of the gel is carbomer cost effective and highly stable in these product types, particularly in the presence of alcohol. The only emulsification required is to solubilize fragrance.

TABLE 9 Formula V: Upper Mass Cosmetic Moisturizer—Oil-in-Water
Emulsion, Cream Consistency but Light with Good Break Properties

Ingredient name	Function	Comment
Aqua	Solubilize and deliver aqueous phase ingredients; provide cooling effect	Continuous phase.
Butylene Glycol	Humectant	More expensive than glycerin, but better efficacy.
Paraffinum liquidum	Emollient; protective	
Dicaprylyl maleate	Emollient ester; good skin-feel and solubilising properties for UV filters	
Petrolatum	Emollient; protective	
Glycerin	Humectant	
Caprylic/capric triglyceride	Emollient ester	Relatively short chain length to add to sophisticated skin-feel
Octyl methoxycinnamate	UV filter	Peak absorbance around erythemal (UVB) part of spectrum.
Steareth-2	Nonionic emulsifier	HLB 8.
Cetearyl alcohol	Co-emulsifier; structuring and stabilizing agent	
Butyl methoxy-dibenzoyl-methane	UV filter	Absorbance in UVB and UVA regions of spectrum.
Steareth-21	Nonionic emulsifier	HLB 15.5 Combined with steareth-2, cetearyl alcohols give liquid crystalline structure to emulsion.
Isopropyl lanolate	Conditioner; emollient	Lanolin derivative adds lubricity.
Theobroma cacao	Structuring agent; good skin-feel on application and on skin	Solid with melting point at skin temperature.
Dimethicone	Added slip during application	
Polyacrylamide	Aqueous phase thickener; stabilizer; viscosity enhancer	Breaks quickly as product is rubbed in to enhance esthetics.

TABLE 9 Continued

Ingredient name	Function	Comment
Hydroxyethyl cellulose	Aqueous phase thickener; stabilizer; viscosity enhancer	Adds body to lotion; slower break to encourage rub-in characteristics.
Tocopheryl acetate	Anti-oxidant	
Ascorbic acid	Anti-oxidant	Combination of vitamins E and C improves anti-oxidant action.
Retinyl palmitate	Vitamin effect	Effective in rebuilding epidermal lipids.
Tetrasodium EDTA	Sequestrant	Prevents metal ions interfering with water phase thickener.
Parfum		
Preservative		

5 PERFORMANCE CRITERIA

The performance of moisturizers has been continually referred to throughout the chapter. Some of the important aspects of this are discussed here alongside the regulatory and safety considerations, which the formulator will need to assimilate.

5.1 Esthetics

Earlier in this chapter, and elsewhere in this book (Chapter 1), reference has been made to the need for moisturization and the benefits conferred by various types of product. When the question Why are there so many to choose from? is asked, part of the answer lies in esthetic considerations. This property (including the packaging and branding) drives much of the purchasing behavior. There is a spectrum of needs from a moisturizer but the pleasurable experience that moisturizers convey is important. I want to touch upon the esthetic considerations affecting choice of raw material. The relationship between esthetics and stability referred to earlier in this chapter will again become evident.

The role of fragrance is of undoubted importance in choice of most mass market moisturizers. I shall not deal with this particular aspect since, though fragrance stability in the formulation is vital, limitations imposed by fragrance on raw material choice are few and often idiosyncratic. Fragrance can be a means of masking unpleasant odors from some of the raw materials.

TABLE 10 Formula VI: Moisturizing Gel—Aqueous Gel, Pumpable Thick Viscosity

Ingredient name	Function	Comment
Aqua	Bulk of product	
Alcohol denat	Provides cooling effect on application	Also provides solubilization and ehancement to preservation.
Butlyene glycol	Humectant	Prolongs moisturization effect beyond initial application.
Glycerin	Humectant	Prolongs moisturization effect beyond initial application.
Polysorbate-20	Fragrance solubilizer	HLB 16.7
Triticum vulgare	Source of amino acids	Mimics NMF in skin.
Glycine soya	Source of amino acids	Mimics NMF in skin.
Carbomer	Structuring agent	The only source of structure in the product, this is chosen for its stability to alcohol and pumping. Pump packs reduce the risk of introducing microbial agents and (like alcohol) enhance preservation.
Aloe barbadensis	Moisturizing ingredient	Quality and quantity of aloe extract will dictate what benefits can be conferred on the product.
Potassium hydroxide	Neutralizing ingredient	
Tetrasodium EDTA	Sequestrant	
Parfum		
Preservative		

5.1.1 Sensory Properties

The key characteristics will differ between consumer groups but some will be universal. Definitions of these properties vary from person to person and the industry has long had an interest in using sensory panels to help them understand exactly what the criteria are and how they can be influenced by product formulation—raw material *and* processing.

In comparing emulsions one of the most obvious characteristics is its visual impact. Bright, white, shiny emulsions are achieved with good processing and small particle size. Earlier in the chapter the role of emulsifiers has been discussed. Some stabilizers, such as higher molecular weight waxes, can induce some graininess and crystallike appearance, especially if heating and cooling has not been well controlled. Use of water phase thickeners and stabilizers can induce a watery whiteness. A high degree of order, as exhibited in liquid crystalline emulsions, can confer a translucent appearance.

In order to understand these properties expert panels can be used. These comprise persons with a high degree of sensory perception. By recognizing the skill and developing it by suitable training the panel can detect and reproducibly describe in a quantitative manner many of the attributes that consumers demand of the product. In doing so they are acting in a similar way to instrumental analysis, providing numeric information with which to compare many different properties from a given set of products. Ultimately the measures are comparative, and the use of benchmarks is essential to make any comparison between sets of data.

Sensory testing can only be a test under ideal conditions, and relating this to in-use conditions is another essential part of understanding product esthetics. Factors that must be borne in mind include the variations in skin site (e.g., face versus body). Even on the face the underlying bone and musculature will vary within individuals and with other factors such as age. Thus formulations targeted at older facial skin types will first need to consider the sensory properties preferred by the target group prior to testing these using expert sensory panels. The final stage will be to confirm the result in a large number of the target population.

Results from product comparisons using sensory analysis will provide an understanding of the qualitative differences between products (see Fig. 4). Converting these findings into quantitative changes in the raw material components of the formulation will require skill and experience from the formulator. Like many other factors in formulation technology, changing one component rarely results in a single change in one product characteristic. As an example of this I shall briefly touch on some of the sensory properties that may be exhibited in a product and show how they may be altered.

> *Rub-in.* This property can be described as the ease with which a product disappears on application. It will be a function of several things including initial viscosity, viscosity change under shear, compatibility of oil phase with the skin, the amount of water, and whether the water is the continuous or dispersed phase. Improving rub-in of Formula I (Table 5) could be achieved in several ways. Increasing the aqueous phase thickener concentration whilst reducing the cetyl alcohol will maintain the viscosity and decrease the rub-in. Increasing the ratio of caprylic/capric triglyceride to liquid paraffin in Formula I, or increasing the ratio of C12–15 alkyl benzoate to cetyl stearate and or lanolin alcohols in For-

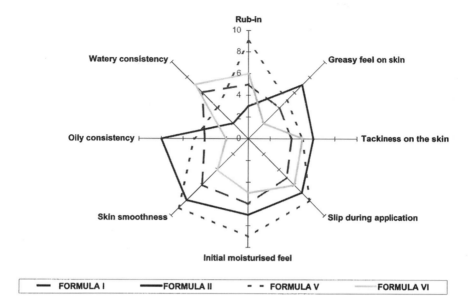

Figure 4 Predicted sensory properties of four formulations referred to in the text. This shows how the different performance attributes can be analyzed using this technique. Customer expectation of particular attributes will help to define final formulation performance, usually against a benchmark.

mula II (Table 6) would similarly reduce rub-in. Increasing the water phase in either of these formulae will reduce rub-in, but with very different consequences for stability since the water-in-oil emulsion may already be close to its maximum water content. However this option is not possible in Formula III (Table 7), where altering of the ratio of liquid to soft paraffin or the introduction of lower viscosity oil may be required to improve rub-in. The structure of the emulsion also plays a major part in sensory properties. Liquid crystal structures tend to smooth the rub-in characteristics (Formula V, Table 9).

Greasiness. Greasiness on the skin can be determined by visual and tactile signals. The changes in oil phase components suggested to improve rub-in may increase the greasiness, whilst increasing the water phase may reduce greasiness. Improving the compatibility of oil phase components with the skin by reducing the reliance on mineral oils and waxes or changing to natural esters may also improve the relative greasiness of Formula III. Whilst the possible change in *degree* of greasiness for this formula may appear to be small in comparison to the lotion in Formula I, sensory analysis (comparing like with like) may show where improvements have been achieved. Smaller particle size o/w emulsions will also have reduced perception of greasiness.

Tackiness. Although self-explanatory, this property can manifest itself during or after application to the skin and can stem from oil or water phase components. Tacky oils include lanolins, cetyl and cetearyl alcohols, and high viscosity modified silicones. Water phase components such as proteins, panthenol, and some aqueous phase thickeners will produce a tacky feeling if used in too high a concentration. Thus the ranges in which these can be used to improve stability are limited by their adverse effects on sensory properties. Anhydrous systems such as Formula III will have an inherent tackiness during application; this could be reduced by changing the ratios of higher and lower melting point components or increasing the level of silicone. However "oil-free" moisturizers are not without tackiness. Polyols and proteins added to provide substantive moisturization (beyond the transient addition of water to stratum corneum) can confer some tacky after-feel to the skin if used at inappropriate levels.

Slip. This expresses how the product glides across the skin. In some ways this is related to "break" (see following). The lubricity of a product can be highly pleasurable and an indicator of the "premium" position of a product. Likewise a moisturizer for compromised skin will require a degree of slip in order to prevent putting a dry or friable skin under undue stress during application. Esters are among the best sources of slip in a formulation, but mineral oils and silicones are also important. Where massage is an important attribute of the product in-use (e.g., ante-natal body creams), slip might need to be balanced against provision of some resistance to encourage more rub-in (e.g., shear thickening properties of Formula II, Table 6).

Break. This can be seen as the initial slip and is more a descriptor of the formulation than its action on the skin. A thick, gel-like cream may actually contain relatively low oil phase and very quickly break down under the stress of rubbing in. Such systems need to be stable to other forms of stress (e.g., pumping), and the presence of salts on the skin helps to de-structure the polymer matrix and achieve the break. Such products when placed on the skin without any rubbing can sometimes be seen to melt and flow across the skin as the gel structure breaks down. Certain emulsifiers can also impart this property.

Moisturized after-feel. This is obviously a highly important factor for a moisturizer. However there are other sensory characteristics contributing to this, e.g., softness, smoothness, suppleness. To understand their relative importance, further breakdown of the sensory properties may be required if the consumer group targeted actually wants a specific moisturizing effect. However for basic moisturizers satisfying moisturized after-feel may be sufficient. The formulation choices will depend in part on which of these different needs are to be fulfilled.

It is important to point out that these sensory descriptors and any others that may be generated for a particular product are of no inherent value without an understanding of their contribution to consumer expectation or demand. Thus a high level of tackiness may be a negative influence in formulating a premium moisturizer, but neutral or of no importance for a therapeutic dry skin cream. It is also important to understand the role of fragrance and minimize its impact in comparing products by using unfragranced samples or masking the sensory panel's sense of smell in some way. Understanding the relationship between sensory characteristics and consumer expectation can be difficult for innovative products, but for existing product types the use of a benchmark will help define the key parameters that will drive choice of formulation.

It is also clear that there are an enormous number of raw material combinations that will achieve a required sensory profile. Thus different combinations may provide sensory properties so similar that they are beyond perception.

5.1.2 Rheology

The process of rubbing a product into the skin involves placing the product under shear, and the sensory performance of products under these conditions are key to our understanding of the consumer acceptability. For this reason product rheology is studied in an attempt to produce objective instrumental data on product behavior during shear. This has the added benefit of assisting understanding of product performance during processing, packing, and delivery.

Under increased shear, a proportional linear increase in the induced stress (Newtonian flow) is rarely seen in emulsions. Usually the response will exhibit some form of curve describing viscoelastic behavior. Where increasing shear rate causes an initially steep but then plateau response in stress, the flow is pseudoplastic. This would be typical for a rich cream that resisted initial massage but then flowed into the skin. When increasing shear rate produces an initially low shear stress response which then rises exponentially, the flow is dilatant. This would be typical for a lotion which flowed but then thickened as the water disappeared into the skin and the mixture became thicker in texture.

5.1.3 Ensuring Continued Product Use

From a therapeutic or commercial standpoint this is an important factor since a product will be best used if it is pleasant, easily absorbed, and well tolerated in use. For therapeutic moisturizers the skin-feel during application may be less important than the skin texture after application, and skin comfort will probably override both. Skin texture will be important for users of cosmetic products but less important than elegance on application and skin residue. The role of raw materials in providing these sensory properties is vital, as is to a lesser extent how the product is processed prior to sale.

In assessing the compliance factors and the trade-offs a consumer may make in approving a product, the formulator will need to use a number of methods. The sophistication of the method will vary depending on the cost of getting it wrong. Large-scale consumer testing using identified target consumers will bring better information but is not a useful screening method for candidate formulations. There exists an array of methods that can help the formulator refine and/or select the final product. In many of the cases it is the qualities of the formulation that are under test rather than the total product (pack, design, claims, etc.).

5.2   Regulatory Influence

These issues are covered elsewhere in this book, but it is worth noting their importance in driving choice in formulation components, testing, and delivery. The product must fulfill consumer expectation not only from a legal standpoint, but also from commercial necessity. Understanding the formulation constraints of (say) α-hydroxyacids is as important from a technical standpoint as a legal one if safety and efficacy are to be delivered.

5.2.1   Interaction of Product with the Skin

It is clear that combining the complexity of skin biochemistry, in particular that of the stratum corneum, with the complex chemistry of moisturizer formulation, in particular emulsification, produces a system with little in the way of predictive behavior. Deleterious effects of raw materials can be detected in simple systems, but once formulated the picture becomes less clear. The product developer has the task of assessing raw material performance (including safety) from a number of sources, including previous experience. In light of this, limitations on new raw material introduction and product innovation need to be balanced against issues of ethics and safety.

The formulator must design for safety (and efficacy a close second!) from the bottom up. Some authors have suggested that long-term use of emulsions will adversely affect the skin [8], and routine testing of skin tolerance should ideally be achieved using more than a single use. It has also been suggested that emulsifier choice contributes to the skin intolerance often attributed to other formulation components such as fragrance or preservative [9].

Whilst the relative risk here is probably low, future developments in technology and consumer expectation of moisturizer formulations will undoubtedly involve continued tailoring of the emulsifiers to the skin.

Elsewhere in this chapter the need for preservatives is discussed. There is increasing interest in the prevalence of skin hypersensitivity to particular preservatives. This is also the case for sunscreens and fragrances. The product developer will be aware of these issues and prior to inclusion in a formulation will assess the rationale for incorporating any raw material with a likely sensitization risk. Consideration will be given to target customer (e.g., infants, people with sensitive skin), conditions of use (where on skin, how often, etc.), use rate (daily, weekly), and geographical market (European, global). Product testing will also help to inform a final assessment of the risk.

5.2.2 Interaction with the Skin and Ensuring Claims Substantiation

In the context of regulatory influence it is also true that the cosmetics industry has other challenges. The increasing desire to control products appears to be driven from several angles. One suggests that since cosmetic products are "trivial," the risk/benefit analysis should err toward greater control of safety. More recently the increased understanding of skin physiology has led to the belief that cosmetics can have beneficial effects on skin physiology and products should reflect these benefits in claims on the packaging. This has again resulted in a belief that control along the lines of drug status or "cosmeceuticals" is desirable (see Chapters 16 and 28).

The challenge for the product developer is to ensure that the claims remain within the legal definition of a cosmetic. Ensuring that the product actually delivers a claim is also vital, since claims are increasingly seen as the means of product differentiation. This is especially important where ingredients referred to on the label are used to justify or help deliver claims. Whilst this is a legislative issue the formulator (and marketer) should consider this high on the list of product specification, since *not* delivering a claim can be commercially disastrous. Industry guidelines on claims do exist but since the market moves very quickly it is impossible to define a particular test to support a given claim. The European Guidelines propose an approach to claims substantiation rather than prescribed methods [5].

It is important to return to the fact that skin moisturizers now encompass many products that do more than moisturize (see Chapter 1). Skin lightening, anti-aging, sun protection, and cell renewal are all claimed to be delivered from a daily moisturizer. Much of the rest of this book is dedicated to understanding the underlying skin physiology and some of the means of influencing this. Here I will briefly touch on issues that exercise the formulator's thoughts in designing moisturizers with "actives."

The formulator is often first confronted by data from suppliers of candidate raw materials. In previous times such data may have been from animal studies, which were sometimes performed irrespective of ethical factors and were of limited value in scientific interpretation. Today data from in vitro tests is frequently provided.

The formulator needs to understand the limitations of the test(s), the influence of formulations used in these tests, particularly where cells grown in aqueous media are used, and the relevance to human in vivo exposure. The development of three-dimensional, fully differentiated human epidermal skin models of reproducible quality has gone some way to assisting the formulation scientist in this task [10].

With these factors taken into account, there is often a residual question to be answered. How much of raw material X do I need to achieve the desired effect? The response is to work through the available data in order to choose a level of ingredient that is both safe and efficacious prior to testing the final product in human volunteers to assess if a claim is measurable and perceivable. (See this volume Chapters by Jaret; Grove; Pierard).

5.2.3 Fitting Performance to Skin Physiology

This aim would appear to be sensible in order to maintain the safety and performance expectations of the consumer. However, even where a case appears straightforward, there can be complex issues that influence the formulator's final decision. The case of UV protection in daily moisturizers is an example.

The influence of ultraviolet light exposure from the sun on premature skin aging (photoaging) is well accepted though compounded by other factors [11]. The role of short wavelength ultraviolet light (UVB) in burning the skin is also accepted, but the relationship between frequency and intensity of burning and premature skin aging has not been defined. What is clear is that those who have outdoor occupations show higher degrees of photoaging than those with indoor occupations.

The role of longer wavelength ultraviolet light (UVA) in burning is approximately 1000 times less than UVB, but there is still damage caused by increased exposure to UVA alone. This has been termed aging damage, though both UVB and UVA are involved.

Sun protection factors (SPF) can be derived for products using accepted and standardized human test methods to deliver protection against burning. However the protection is not complete; even SPF 60 products allow 1.7% of the burning UV rays to get through to the skin. The raw materials used as UV filters in the formulation rarely act like a neutral density filter. Therefore the burning UVB wavelengths may be absorbed, protecting against burning without absorbing the longer wavelengths to the same efficiency. Therefore there may be a risk of overexposing the skin to the longer wavelengths by use of these products. This has led to the use of other measures of assessing sun protection against longer wavelength ultraviolet (UVA) penetration.

The consumer need for SPF numbers is protection against burning, and the product is usually applied when deliberate, recreational exposure is anticipated, e.g., whilst at the beach. Daily moisturizers are not used globally as protection against burning, and only in markets where the occasional, accidental exposure to UV constitutes a threat of burning is the SPF number really relevant.

Where the consumer need is protection against premature aging the role of the SPF number has become the consumer short-hand. In the absence of anything better, the message has become "sun protection is important therefore SPF numbers are important."

This message has been given great support by dermatologists and the beauty press, and as a consequence we find ourselves using SPF numbers (possibly inappropriately) to help deliver a consumer need. We cannot guarantee what level of SPF is appropriate since we do not have the direct supporting evidence, but SPF 15 has become the recommendation for protection against UV in daily skin care based on the opinion of a number of experts. Discussion of the value of this number and the basis for this recommendation has been overtaken by events.

Perhaps more importantly there are other considerations for the formulator. A once-per-day application of a moisturizer claiming SPF 15 would require that it deliver this level of protection throughout the day. Beach use products normally include advice on pack to reapply ever hour or two. In terms of consumer expectation, the package wording needs consideration. Neither is it easy to formulate an SPF 15 moisturizer with high quality esthetics; the UV filter loading required produces heavy and greasy skin-feel. From a safety standpoint, there is also the issue of exposure to UV filters. The risk of contact sensitization has been raised though not quantified. The safety assessments made on UV filters used exposures based on infrequent holiday use rather than daily exposure via a moisturizer. Thus even with an active with a known action, physiological endpoint, and standard test methods, there are difficulties for the formulator to overcome.

6 SUMMARY

Formulation of a moisturizer requires an understanding of technical and commercial factors and the restrictions that they can impose. As discussed in Chapter 1, many new moisturizers launched on the market do not survive. The overall success can depend on such factors as promotion and professional support, which though they are outside the developer's control should be part of the early planning. Understanding how the various factors interact is as important as understanding the physicochemical interactions within the formulation. Delivering a stable, safe, and esthetically pleasing product that meets consumer expectation is the aim of all product developers. This chapter has identified some of the technical elements that go toward supporting successful product development.

ACKNOWLEDGMENTS

The author would like to thank Ed Owen, Claire Wilson, Patrick Love, and Nicki Lenton for their help in preparing this manuscript.

REFERENCES

1. Hunting ALL. A Formulary of Cosmetic Preparations. Vol. 2: Creams, Lotions and Milks. Micelle Press, 1993.
2. Cosmetic Bench Reference. Cosmet Toil 2001; 115(13).
3. Wenninger JA, Canterberry RC, McEwen GN, eds. International Cosmetic Ingredient Dictionary and Handbook. 8th ed. The Cosmetic, Toiletries and Fragrance Association, 2000.
4. Prottey C, Hastop PJ, Press M. Correction of the cutaneous manifestations of essential fatty acid deficiency in man by application of sunflower seed oil to the skin. J Invest Dermatol 1975; 64:228–234.
5. Guidelines for the Evaluation of the Efficacy of Cosmetic Products. 2nd ed. The European Cosmetic, Toiletry and Perfumery Association, 2001.
6. Hubbard AW, Moore LJ, Clothier RH, Sulley H, Rollin KA. Use of in-vitro methodology to predict the irritancy potential of surfactants. Toxic *In-Vitro* 1994; 8(4):689–691.
7. Efficacy of anti-microbial preservation. Sec. 5.1.3. In: European Pharmacopoeia. 3rd ed. Supplement 2001. European Directorate for Quality of Medicines Within Council of Europe, Strasbourg.
8. Held E, Sveinsdottir S, Agner T. Effect of long term use of moisturisation on skin hydration, barrier function and susceptibility to irritants. Acta Derm Venereol 1999; 79(1):49–51.
9. Maes D, Declercq L, Muizzuddin N, Fthenakis C, McKeever MA, Collins D, Mammone T, Dicanio D, Marenus K. Optimisation of safety testing for better product development. Proceedings of 21st IFSCC Congress, Berlin, 2000, pp. 321–327.
10. Rognet R, Tessoneaud E, Gagne C, Teissler MH, Cohen C, Leclaire J. Use of standardised reconstructed epidermis kit to assess in-vitro the tolerance and efficacy of cosmetics. Int J Cosmet Sci 2000; 22(6):409–419.
11. Malvy DJM, Guinot C, Preziosi P, Valliant L, Tenenhans M, Galan P, Hercberg S, Tschachler E. Epidemiologic determinants of skin photo ageing: baseline data of the SU.VI.MAX cohort. J Am Acad Dermatol 2000; 42(1):47–55.

26

Formulation and Assessment of Moisturizing Cleansers

David C. Story and
Frederick Anthony Simion
The Andrew Jergens Company, Cincinnati, Ohio

1 INTRODUCTION

Very few types of cleansing products have the ability to truly moisturize the skin, either by enhancing the residual moisture content of the stratum corneum, removing dry skin flakes, or increasing skin elasticity. Many cleansing products claim to be, or are trademarked as, moisturizing cleansers but during typical use they do not deliver these benefits. The objectives of this chapter are to provide an explanation of what constitutes a moisturizing cleanser in today's market and outline methods of measuring the benefits.

The most common and economical form for cleansing is bar soap. Soap is the comparative standard for all personal cleansers. If a product is milder, more moisturizing, less drying, etc., it is always milder than soap, more moisturizing than soap, and less drying than soap.

Simplistically, soap is the sodium and/or potassium salt of a fatty acid. When sodium potassium soaps are used with conventional water, the divalent and trivalent metallic ions will exchange with the Na^+ or K^+ ion to form multivalent salts that are insoluble. The multivalent metal soaps readily precipitate on the skin and any other available surface. These insoluble soaps are referred to as lime soaps or soap scum. This phenomenon is important since it affects the sensory properties of cleansing products. The scum deposition is not observed with the synthetic detergents used in moisturizing cleansers.

The pH of toilet soaps is approximately 10 [1]. This high pH and its cleansing properties promote the loss of water and water-binding materials from the stratum corneum. These characteristics establish the basic precepts for moisturizing cleansers. By substituting different surfactants for all or part of the soap and lowering the product pH closer to physiologic values, the product becomes less disruptive to the skin barrier, and therefore less residual water is lost. The first products to apply these precepts were combination bars that used a mixture of sodium soap and synthetic detergents. These products were shown to be less drying than conventional soap bars and subsequently became thought of as moisturizing cleansers. The most common synthetic detergent added to bars is isethionate.

2 FORMULATION

Isethionates were one of the first surfactants used in the moisturizing category. This class of surfactants is a monovalent metallic salt of an alkyl carboxyethane sulfonate. Their properties make them ideal for solid cleansers. They possess a high melting point and are stable when added to soap bars. Isethionates are effective dispersants for lime soaps and thus decrease the surface deposition of soap scum. Soap bars containing isethionate are stable at a pH of 7.

The solid cleansing products have now given way to the liquid cleansers, which are less drying than the combination bars and allow for a high degree of flexibility in formulation and the delivery of new benefits. The liquid cleansers are essentially the same formulations as today's hair shampoos. The approach for formulating moisturizing cleansers will be detailed in the following sections.

2.1 Ingredients

2.1.1 Surfactants

The surfactants are classified usually by the inherent charge associated with the surface-active moiety of the molecule. The surfactant classes are anionic (negative charge), cationic (positive charge), zwitterionic (both positive and negative charges), and nonionic (no charge).

Primary. The products are usually assembled with a mixture of detergent types. The primary detergents are almost always anionic. The alkyl sulfates may be included as the primary detergent for their lather characteristics and durability in the presence of soil loads. They are inexpensive but are much too irritating to the skin to be the only surfactant in a cleansing product. The linear alkylbenzene sulfonates have also been used as the primary detergents. Although as a class they are milder than the alkyl sulfates, they are considered skin irritants. The most prevalent anionic surfactant used in moisturizing products today is the alkyl ether sulfates. This class of detergents usually has a C12 alkyl group (lauryl) and 2 to 3 moles of ethylene oxide (ethoxylation) to form the ether linkage of the molecule. If lower degrees of ethoxylation are used, the surfactant will produce better foaming characteristics and have lower water solubility, higher propensity for irritating or drying skin, and higher Krafft temperatures. The 2–3 moles of ethoxylation seem to be the best balance at cleansing, foaming, and mildness. Longer carbon chains will produce some lather but at a much lower volumes and more dense when compared to the C12 alkyl chain.

Other anionic surfactants have been used as the primary cleanser but usually have some disadvantage when compared to sodium laureth sulfates, e.g., monoalkylphosphates, ammonium isethionates, and lauryl or cocoyl sarcosinates. Primary surfactants can be combined to achieve the ideal balance between mildness and lather characteristics (volume and durability). The primary surfactants are commercially available with various counterions. The counterion can affect the solubility, formula compatibility, and overall mildness. Na^+, K^+, and Mg^{2+} are the more common counterions seen in today's moisturizing liquid cleansing products. The active concentration for the primary surfactants is typically in a range of 8–20 w/w%.

Co-Surfactants. The co-surfactants are added to moisturizing liquid cleansers for a multitude of reasons. If co-surfactants were used as the primary detergent, they would be inferior by consumer standards for lather volume and density. Consumers typically would rate the products as diluted, weak, and inefficient. When the co-surfactant is combined with the primary anionic detergent, the formulation will produce results that increase consumer acceptance and are less destructive to the stratum corneum barrier.

The usual co-surfactants are anionic or zwitterionic. In some specialized products, nonionics will be used to decrease the harshness of the cleanser to skin and eyes. The nonionic co-surfactants are generally found in products marketed for children or babies. Adding nonionics to liquid moisturizing cleansers is a challenge since they suppress lather volume and durability. In many moisturizing liquid cleansing compositions, two or three co-surfactants will be used. The zwitterionics are more prevalent due to their various properties. Zwitterionics diminish the harshness of the primary surfactants and have a propensity to adsorb to the skin, thus providing some conditioning benefit. The most common zwitterionics are imidazoline, amino acid, and betaine derivatives. The inherent charge of the zwitterion surfactant molecule is pH dependent. Adjusting the pH to an acidic or basic range can control the character of the composition. The amphoteric (or zwitterionic) detergents will as a rule produce a better quality of lather at basic pH since they assume a negative charge (anionic). When the pH of the formula is acidic, the amphoteric surfactant becomes cationic (positively charged) and produces a conditioning effect since it is now substantitive to skin or hair. It is well documented that irritation and eye stinging can be significantly reduced by the addition of amphoterics to conventional cleansing systems [2].

The newest class of co-surfactants is the polyglucosides. This group of detergents is formed from the reaction of glucose and fatty alcohols. The polyglucosides are mild and have a low potential for irritation. They are nonionic in character and possess better foam properties than the amphoteric class of detergents. They are not well adsorbed by skin and therefore have no conditioning effect. The application of polyglucosides is detailed in the referenced patent [3].

One of the mildest anionic co-surfactant classes is the sodium alkyl sulfosuccinates or alkyl ether sulfosuccinates. Sulfosuccinates are restricted to a narrow formula pH of 4 to 6 because they are prone to base catalyzed hydrolysis.

The amino acid–derived co-surfactants include the sarcosinates, propionates, glutamates, and taurates. The mildness and conditioning effects of these detergents are well documented. They are often included in specialized hair shampoos and moisturizing body cleansers.

The co-surfactants have the significant ability to influence the consumer sensory properties of moisturizing cleansers. In general applications, the total active concentration for co-surfactants can range from as low as 2 w/w% and as high as 15 w/w%. The use concentration in moisturizing formulas is frequently limited by product economics.

2.1.2   Conditioning/Moisturizing Agents

This diverse group of materials provides the distinctive features of marketed moisturizing cleansers. The discussion in this section has been limited to the more common ingredients. These agents are used for their effects on skin, whether they would be physiological, sensory, or a combination of the two.

The deposition of these ingredients on skin is a true dichotomy since the intent of cleansing is to remove foreign material from the target surface. Promoting the deposition of the conditioning or moisturizing agent while selectively removing dirt is a significant challenge for the product formulator. The deposition of the selected materials must be highly efficient since only 5 to 15 g of product are used during the cleansing treatment. Considering, on average, an adult has 2 m^2 of skin, this calculates to be 0.75 mg cleansing product per square centimeter. Since the conditioning or moisturizing ingredient is usually less than 10% of the cleansing composition, and if 20% of this material would be adsorbed, the amount of material remaining on the skin is less than 15 $\mu g/cm^2$. Another factor which can, and usually does, interfere with the deposition of these beneficial materials is the use of an accessory, e.g., a washcloth, a polyethylene puff or pouf, or even a sponge. Often the target material deposits or adsorbs to the accessory and very little is delivered to the skin. Finally, the most significant obstacle to skin deposition is the constant elution of the adsorbed agent by the rinse water. It becomes more apparent that delivering an effective amount of the conditioner or moisturizer to the skin is not a simple task and presents a true challenge to the technical formulator.

Lipids and Oils. If moisturizing or conditioning the skin were simply adding a lipid or oil to the cleansing product, then this discussion would be brief. Simply adding these materials to a cleansing formula usually results in a product failure. The lipophilic ingredients suppress the lathering characteristics and often lead to phase separation of the cleansing product. There must be a balance between the detergent and conditioning ingredients in the formula. Ethoxylation of the oil or lipid will facilitate its incorporation into the formula, but if the material is too soluble or too dispersible in water, it can easily be rinsed from the skin. Another concern about the inclusion of an oil or lipid in the cleansing formula is that the lipophilic material may enhance the solubility of the skin lipids and facilitate their removal during treatment. There are commercial hard-surface cleaning products that have successfully applied the synergy of oil and detergents. Obviously, skin is not a hardsurface and this is not a desired outcome for a moisturizing cleansing product.

Another technology that is used to incorporate the lipid in the cleansing composition is structured surfactants. Albright and Wilson developed this technology in the 1980s. A simple analogy of the technology is an onion [4]. The onion is composed of multiple layers, in this case surfactant layers, and sandwiched between the surfactants is the lipid ingredient. When this material is applied during cleansing, the structure collapses when diluted (rinsing) and the lipid is deposited on the skin. The technology provides a significant lipid payload to skin.

The cleansing accessory must also be included in this discussion. With the rapid commercialization of the polyethylene body pouf or sponge, cleansing formulas no longer needed high levels of surfactants. The open weave of the accessory provided a high number of nucleation sites for bubble or lather generation, in other words the device mechanically compensates for low lather volumes and slow lather-building systems. This allowed formulators to use higher percentages of lipophilic ingredients and maintain consumer acceptability of the product when used with the accessory.

There are many examples of oils and lipids used in marketed moisturizing cleansers. Glycerides from vegetable oils, e.g., capric, cacprylic, and soybean, which are usually unsaturated or short carbon chains, are often added as the moisturizing ingredient. Giret discloses the utility of some of these oils [5]. The unsaturated or branched carbon chains have lower melting points and tend be liquid or semisolid at room temperature, which is desirable for ease of incorporation into the formula and product stability. Hydrocarbons, such as petrolatum or paraffin, have been used successfully in key moisturizing cleansing brands. The usual use level of these materials is 3–5 w/w%, but some products may contain as much as 8–10 w/w%.

Polymers. This discussion will include synthetic and natural polymers since both are used as conditioners in moisturizing cleansers. The majority of the polymers has a cationic net charge and is substantive to skin. The molecular charge is usually from a quaternized structure in which N^+ is the cationic moiety. These large chains attach to the negative sites on the skin and create the sensory effect of smoothness and softness. Many of the polymers have a cellulosic or repeating sugar backbone. The polymers must be hydrated, to facilitate their electrostatic attachment to the skin. The conditioning effect is transient since the polymers eventually will dehydrate and be sloughed from the skin's surface. After the polymers are fully hydrated, they are tolerant to the anionic detergents without flocculation or precipitation. This phenomenon will be discussed in more detail later in the chapter. A few examples of these polymers are polyquaternium-10, polyquaternium-7, polyquaternium-11, and chitosan. The active polymer concentration normally found in cleansing products is 0.1–1.0 w/w%.

Proteins. The original use of proteins in moisturizing cleansing products was found in marketed hair shampoos. The proteins, which can be animal or plant derived, are usually hydrolyzed or chemically modified to improve their physical properties, such as odor, color, and their affinity for skin or hair. This discussion of proteins also includes polypeptides since these ingredients all have similar characteristics. They are somewhat substantive to areas of the skin where some protein denaturation has occurred. These ingredients may also be cationic and attracted to the skin via the electrostatic forces. Proteins exhibit a sensory effect similar to the polymers, i.e., skin smoothness and softness. Their effect is also transient since these materials will also wear from the skin. The concern of using proteins, especially animal derived, is the potential for developing sensitivity to the material. The use level of proteins is relatively small due to material cost and the adverse influence they can impart to the quality of the marketed cleanser. The active protein concentration is usually restricted to less than 1 w/w%.

Silicones. Silicones have been used as a conditioning or moisturizing agent in cleansing products for over a decade. One of the first applications of silicones in a cleansing product was reported by Bolich et al. [6]. He disclosed how to suspend the silicone gums in a detergent system (shampoo). Upon rinsing (dilution) the silicone suspension is destabilized and the gum is uniformly deposited on the hair or skin. One of the inherent properties of silicones is to efficiently spread and form single layers on a surface. The expectation would be the same for skin. The silicone spreads evenly on the skin surface providing a sensory effect and possibly forming a barrier to reduce water loss. The sensory effect is a smooth, powdery feeling on the skin. The challenge with using silicones is the fact they are known to be one of the most efficient antifoam materials available. In a personal cleansing product the lack of lather will make the product's performance completely unacceptable. The most common approach for adding silicones to cleansing compositions is to suspend the material separately and then incorporate this suspension into the detergent phase. The mixing of the two phases uses minimal shear, which allows them to form a uniform macrosuspension, without physical interaction. The preferred range of silicone in a moisturizing cleansing product is 1–5 w/w% active.

2.1.3 Preservatives and Fragrances

These two classes of ingredients are not necessary for cleansing or moisturization, but are required to prevent spoilage and to drive consumer acceptance of the product. A variety of preservatives are available that have different types of action retarding spoilage of the formula. Microbial spoilage is usually controlled with a formaldehyde donor, such as DMDM hydantoin, imidazolidinyl urea, diazolidinyl urea, methylchloroisothiazolinone and methylisothiazolinone. Other types of microbicides that are common to toiletries include iodopropynyl butylcarbamate, methylparaben, propylparaben phenoxyethanol, benzyl alcohol, and ethanol. Often times chelating agents and anti-oxidants are added to prevent oxidation and color change of the product or to enhance the effectiveness of the microbicides. These materials are highly effective at low levels in cleansing products. The phenoxyethanol is usually 1 w/w% or lower and ethanol is usually more than 10 w/w%. The other preservatives are usually no more than 0.2 w/w%. It is always desirable to use the minimum effective level of these ingredients since some consumers may react to the preservatives (hypersensitivity).

Fragrances are an essential component to most cleansing products. The obvious benefit of a fragrance is to impart a pleasant odor to the product so that during use it creates a positive emotional experience. Fragrances can be designed to be retentive to the skin, which will maintain the pleasant odor character for an extended period of time. Even though fragrances do not usually have a physical or chemical effect on the moisturizing cleanser, they can be the single most important point of differentiation for the product. The formulator carefully selects the fragrance based on several factors:

> The inherent odor of the formulation
> The product concept and emotional message
> Consumer satisfaction and approval of the product's aroma (in the package and during use)

Oftentimes the fragrance will determine whether the product is a market success or failure, regardless of other formula benefits.

2.1.4 Viscosity Modifiers

A broad definition for the viscosity modifiers would be a single ingredient (or group of ingredients) that will increase or decrease the apparent viscosity when added to a liquid cleanser. Since these cleansers are complex mixtures of surfactants, electrolytes, and conditioning or moisturizing ingredients, the effects of viscosity modifiers are highly unpredictable. These materials almost always have significant interaction with the available water in the formulation. They often have the ability to increase or reduce the water solubility of the other ingredients in the composition. If the viscosity modifier increases the water solubility (hydrotrope) of other formula ingredients, frequently the viscosity will decrease. If the modifier decreases the water solubility of materials in the composition, the viscosity of the formula increases. If the modifying material has impact on the surfactant dynamics (structure), it also will affect the apparent viscosity of the product. As a generality, if more organization occurs in the detergent network, then characteristically the viscosity will increase; and if the network is disrupted, the viscosity decreases.

Polyols are well known for their hydrotropic actions in detergent mixtures and are one of the most effective materials for reducing the viscosity of liquid cleansers. Short chain alcohols, e.g., methanol, ethanol, propanol, etc., will also act as a hydrotrope and effectively decrease viscosity. Electrolytes that are polyvalent often will reduce viscosity since they can disrupt the dynamics of the surfactant network. From the formulator's perspective reducing the viscosity is not difficult and usually is a minor modification to the composition.

Thickening liquid cleansers is more challenging than reducing the product viscosity. The simple approach is to modify the electrical properties of surfactant network by adding NaCl to the formula. The formulator can construct a curve of added salt versus apparent viscosity of the formula. Typically, by adding a small percentage of NaCl to the composition, the viscosity will increase. The electrolyte influences the surfactant network by encouraging the multilamellar units to build upon themselves [7] and have less interaction with external ingredients. The NaCl may also reduce the water solubility of other ingredients in the composition and, as explained previously, lead to higher viscosity in the formulation. Since NaCl is easily added to the liquid cleansers and is very economical, it typically is the formulator's first choice for increasing the product viscosity.

The next major class of viscosity-building agents is the polymers. Acrylates and cellulosics are the most common polymers used to increase viscosity. The acrylates require a basic pH for maximum efficiency and impact on the product viscosity. The acrylates are somewhat sensitive to the inherent electrolyte in the formula. This may prevent the polymer chain from unfolding, and subsequently the polymer does not create its typical network. This phenomenon precludes any significant increase in viscosity. The combination acrylates are less sensitive to the electrolyte contaminants. These copolymers, such as acrylates/steareth-20 itaconate copolymer, tend to increase viscosity regardless of the electrolyte present. The cellulosics are equally efficient as the acrylate copolymers. Cellulosics such as methylcellulose, hydroxyethylcellulose, and hyrdoxypropyl methylcellulose, are not excessively sensitive to electrolyte after hydration and usually will build the product viscosity. The advantage of the cellulosics is that they are neutral (have no charge) and therefore are more compatible with multiple classes of surfactants and conditioners. The cationic polymers may add to the product viscosity, but this is a secondary benefit to their conditioning properties.

The alkanolamides are one of the most common classes of viscosity building agents. They are easily incorporated into liquid cleansing compositions and enhance the lather properties of the composition. They synergistically build the product viscosity with small amounts of electrolyte. The alkanolamides, which includes the monoethanolamides and diethanolamides, are insoluble in water but dispersible. This property allows them to build within the surfactant network, which leads to higher viscosity. This alkanolamide–surfactant network increases the compatibility with the air interface, which leads to more stable and denser foams or lather. Although the alkanolamides are highly effective, there are some concerns associated with their purity and the free amine present in the material. Free diethanolamine is considered to be a precursor to nitrosoamines, which are known carcinogens. Industry has responded to this concern by manufacturing superamides, which have less than 1% free amine. This has not eliminated all concern and the issue remains unsettled. The monoethanolamides are of less concern since the free monoethanolamine does not form the precursor that is required to generate the nitrosoamines. In spite of the apprehension associated with alkanolamides, their use has not declined in liquid cleansing products.

Another type of thickener that acts as the alkanolamides do is the high molecular weight, ethoxylated fatty acid esters. Several examples are the PEG-150 pentaerythrityl tetrastearate, PEG-120 methyl glucose dioleate, and PEG-18 glyceryl oleate/cocoate. These large molecules are water dispersible, with some small degree of solubility and contribute to the product viscosity by promoting the surfactant network structure.

There are numerous materials that may not be included in a classical discussion of thickeners but are used by formulators to increase product viscosity. Many times these viscosity-building materials are formula specific, and their effects are due exclusively to their interaction with that formula. The one such group of materials is the amine oxides. These ingredients significantly enhance lather formation and density and often contribute to the product viscosity. There are several concerns with using amine oxides in personal care products. Since amine oxides have a propensity to form the nitrosoamines precursor, these materials must be extremely pure and be stabilized to prevent conversion to the nitrosoamines. The first commercial materials were known to have free amine contaminants, which caused human reactions. The materials no longer have these high levels of impurities but the concerns associated with nitrosoamine formation still exist. It is unfortunate, since the amine oxides are amphoteric or cationic (pH dependent) and condition as well as enhance product lather and viscosity.

2.1.5 Opacifying/Pearling Agents

The natural appearance of many liquid cleansing products is clear or slightly turbid. When products are pearled or opaque, additional ingredients were added to create this effect. These specific materials have very limited water solubility and usually have a particle size greater than 15 μm. Materials that have these properties and are commonly used in personal care products for their opaque characteristics include fatty alcohols (C16 to C18), glycol monostearates and distearates, propylene glycol or glycerol monostearates, latex emulsions, and titanium dioxide. Some of these materials have a tendency to form large reflective crystals (especially the glycol diesters). The reflective properties impart a pearled appearance to the product, or pearlescence. These ingredients normally have no functional benefit in the formulation other than to embellish the product appearance. The use percentage is usually 1–3% except for the latex emulsions and titanium dioxide, which are used at less than 1%.

Example formulations of liquid moisturizing cleansers are shown in Tables 1 and 2.

TABLE 1 Moisturizing Cleanser 1

Part	Ingredient	Percent of active (ww)	Function
A	Polyquaternium-10	0.20	Conditioning agent/moisturizer
	Deionized water	QS	
B	Glycerin	1.00	
C	Cocamidopropylbetaine	5.25	Secondary Surfactant
	Sodium myreth sulfate	4.80	Primary Surfactant
	Decyl glucoside	2.00	
	PEG-150 Pentaerythrityl tetrastearate	0.30	Viscosity Building Agent
	Sodium chloride	QS	
D	Preservative	QS	
	Fragrance	QS	
	Citric acid	QS	

Procedure: Disperse the polyquaternium-10 into the water with adequate mixing. Add Part B to A. Heat Part C to 50°C to dissolve the PEG-150 pentaerythrityl tetrastearate. Add Part AB to C. Cool to room temperature (35°C) and add Part D. Bring to total weight.

TABLE 2 Moisturizing Cleanser 2

Part	Ingredient	Percent of Active (w/w)	Function
A	Quaternium-61	3.00	Conditioning agent moisturizer
B	Deionized water	QS	
C	Cocamidopropylbetaine	3.00	Secondary surfactant
	Sodium laureth sulfate	8.00	Primary surfactant
	Dioctyl sodium sulfosuccinate	10.50	Secondary surfactant
	Acetamide MEA	3.00	Conditioning agent/moisturizer
	Glycerin	1.50	
	Di-isostearyl dimer dilinoleate	1.00	Refatting agent/emollient
D	Preservative	QS	
	Citric acid	QS	
	Fragrance	QS	

Procedure: Add Part A to B and mix until dissolved. Add Part C ingredients individually to Part AB and mix. Add Part D to Part ABC and mix until uniform.

3 SOLUTION/SUSPENSION STRUCTURE

The liquid cleansing products can assume various physical forms, from a classical solution to a multiphase suspension. In this section the more common product forms will be discussed, i.e., those represented in today's market. Most commercial liquid cleansers will not be limited to one type but take multiple physical forms, e.g., liquid crystals within a suspension.

3.1 Suspensions

The common definition of a suspension is an insoluble particle dispersed in a uniform concentration throughout a continuous vehicle. Many of the moisturizing liquid cleansing products are suspensions, since the lipid or silicone is insoluble in the aqueous-based detergent vehicle. The typical approach is to formulate these suspensions with rather large lipophilic particles so that they have less interaction with the surfactant and subsequently less suppression of the lather. All suspensions are formulated so that the insoluble particles remain dispersed throughout the vehicle. Liquid cleansers are no exception. The vehicle separates the macrolipophilic particles from each other, and the inherent viscosity of the vehicle prevents the settling or coalescence (fusing) of these particles. The shelf-life of the composition is a primary concern for the formulator, since suspensions are thermodynamically unstable. The intent is to have the product remain stable throughout its life cycle. Most of the suspensions are unstable by design. The suspension while in a concentrated state is stable. During use, the consumer applies the product to their skin and then rinses. The dilution associated with rinsing destabilizes the suspension and the moisturizing ingredient is delivered to the skin (or hair). Suspensions allow the formulator to target and control the delivery of the moisturizing ingredient. Although this is somewhat simplistic, it is a cost-effective delivery system for liquid moisturizing products.

3.2 Solutions

Very few moisturizing liquid products would conform to the ideal definition of a solution. The ideal solution is one in which there is no change in the properties of the components, other than dilution, when they are mixed to form the solution [8]. The less complicated product forms would fall into this class. These are usually simple mixtures of detergents with an ethoxylated refatting ingredient. The ethoxylation allows the moisturizing ingredient to be solubilized in the aqueous detergents. When the product is used for cleansing, a small amount of the refatting ingredient will deposit on the skin and remain throughout the rinse (theoretically). Those formulators experienced in the art usually find this product form to be inefficient for any significant delivery of a moisturizing or conditioning material. A great majority of the refatting agent is lost during rinsing.

3.3 Coacervates/Colloids

Coacervates refers to the polymer-rich phase that occurs when dilute solutions separate into a solvent phase practically free of polymer and a viscous liquid phase that contains almost all of the polymer still with a significant amount of solvent. How is this phenomenon relevant to moisturizing cleansers? Coacervation is another method for delivery of conditioning ingredients to the skin during the dynamics of cleansing and rinsing. When more than one polymer is in solution and then incorporated into the detergent phase of the formulation coacervates can form which build the product viscosity and temporarily stabilize the mixture [9]. When this mixture is applied to the skin during cleansing, the product is diluted. As it undergoes infinite dilution during rinsing the coacervate structure is eliminated allowing the polymer to readily deposit on the skin. Often during the mixing of polymer phases coacervation is undetectable, except for a slight increase in the formulation viscosity.

Colloidal solutions are another common form for moisturizing liquid cleansers. These are not true solutions and often exhibit a Faraday–Tyndall effect [10]. This is the effect when a strong light beam passing through a colloidal solution causes the colloidal particles to scatter the light to form a cone, usually blue in color. Although the mixture appears to be clear, it is a dispersion with particles of size less than 5μm. Since many of the conditioning polymers are cationic and have a limited, if any, compatibility with the anionic detergents, it is likely they form colloidal solutions. The presence of colloidal solution can be confirmed by testing for the Faraday–Tyndall effect. The colloidal solution upon dilution will exhibit characteristics of a true solution. The cationic polymers will have a higher affinity for the skin than the anionic solution. The product then delivers its conditioning effect during rinsing.

It is very difficult to determine which phenomenon is responsible for the moisturizer/conditioner delivery but from the formulator's perspective, it is not necessary, since the consumer benefit is still realized.

3.4 Liquid Crystals

There are three types of liquid crystal phases relevant to detergents. They are one-dimensional periodicity, which is lamellar; two-dimensional periodicity, hexagonal; and three-dimensional periodicity, cubic. These liquid crystal phases are important since they have very different rheological properties. The hexagonal phase is the most viscous and is often preferred by the formulator [11]. The hexagonal liquid crystal structure allows the suspension of noncompatible materials into the aqueous vehicle. The liquid crystalline structure is very stable until the concentration of the surfactant is altered. The surfactant concentration is changed when the product is used in the cleansing and rinsing process. When the cleansing composition is applied, the suspending properties are lost and the non-compatible polymer or lipophile is readily available for deposition on the skin.

The knowledge of liquid crystals and their stability has been extensively applied to emulsion products for many years. The liquid crystal formation from surfactants is now being applied in a similar manner to temporarily stabilize oils that would be commonly used in emulsions. The delivery dynamics are different but the end result is similar.

4 STRATEGIES FOR FORMULATING MOISTURIZING CLEANSERS

There are two approaches to enhancing skin condition. First is not to damage the skin. The second is to deliver moisturizing agents that improve its condition. These approaches are not mutually exclusive and can be used simultaneously.

4.1   Reducing Skin Damage

Skin irritation can take many forms. This includes primary irritation (erythema and edema), skin dryness and roughness, as well as sensory irritation. It is likely that these phenomena are caused by different mechanisms—different interactions between the skin and surfactants. Therefore it is important to develop formulations that minimize the different interactions thereby reducing all forms of irritation.

4.1.1   Primary Irritation

Prolonged and repeated surfactant exposure to the skin can produce erythema (redness) and edema (swelling). The relative ability of the surfactants to cause primary irritation has been well documented especially for anionic and cationic surfactants. For anionic surfactants, primary irritation potential reaches its maximum for C12 surfactants [12]. Either reducing or increasing the alkyl chain length reduces primary irritation. Other factors that can reduce irritation of the surfactant molecule are

> Increasing the degree of ethoxylation
> Increasing the size of the hydrophilic headgroup
> Reducing the charge density of the hydrophilic headgroup

4.1.2   Mechanisms Inducing Primary Irritation by Anionic Surfactants

The key step by which anionic surfactants start the irritation process is the interaction with the skin surface. The two main factors in this process are (1) the number of surfactant monomers available and (2) their ability to bind to the skin's surface. In examining the dose response of surfactants to swell the stratum corneum, it is apparent that both parameters increase it until the critical micelle concentration (CMC) is reached [13,14]. Further increases in surfactant concentration do not cause additional swelling. As the concentration of surfactant monomer also ceases to increase at the CMC, it has been hypothesized that the surfactant monomers are key contributors to irritation. This hypothesis is supported by the alkyl ether sulfates. Increasing the degree of ethoxylation reduces both their CMC and their primary irritation potential [14].

There are alternative models that account for many of all these effects. For instance, the ability of surfactants to bind to the stratum corneum surface and to cause the denaturation of the skin, are important steps.

4.1.3   Surfactant Binding to Skin Causes Primary Irritation and Skin Dryness

Imokawa and his colleagues have proposed that surfactant binding to the stratum corneum surface has an important effect on its potential to cause dryness and roughness [15]. It may also play an important role in primary irritation. They modeled normal use of surfactant solutions by exposing the skin to a surfactant solution for 10 min, once a day, for four consecutive days. A trained evaluator assessed the extent of skin roughness. A rank order for the surfactants' ability to induce roughness in vivo was determined:

$$SLS > LAS > AOS > SLES\text{-}3EO > C_{12}(EO)_7$$

There were two in vitro parameters that correlated with this in vivo order:

The ability of the surfactants to bind to the stratum corneum
The ability of the surfactants to denature bovine serum albumin

Its is known that the first step of the denaturing interaction of surfactants with the bovine serum albumin is ionic absorption onto the protein [16]. This initial denaturation appears to have two important effects. First, it is the basis of superhydration, the ability of surfactants to cause rapid swelling of the stratum corneum. Wilhelm et al. demonstrated that even a short, 10-min exposure to a surfactant solution will cause a significantly greater uptake of water than exposure to a buffer solution [12]. Although this swelling is temporary and reverses when the solution is removed, the stratum corneum does not go back to its original condition. The small hydrophilic molecules in the stratum corneum, known as natural moisturizing factors, are probably leached out. Conversely, the damaging surfactants that bind to the stratum corneum proteins probably remain in place to further damage the skin. Wilhelm's data also showed a correlation between the superhydration caused by alkyl sulfates of different chain lengths and their primary irritation potential. This observation is probably the basis of using the in vitro stratum corneum and protein film swelling assays to predict irritation potential of anionic surfactants and cleansers.

Further support for the binding models of irritation comes from the work of Warren et al. [17]. They were able to show that increasing water hardness, especially in the rinse, increased soap binding and soap-induced skin irritation. This is probably caused by the formation of insoluble calcium soaps, scum, on the skin's surface. Irritation caused by anionic surfactant based bars was less influenced by water hardness. The calcium salts of these surfactants are more soluble than that of soap.

This mechanism of irritation is probably more relevant for cationic surfactants. Dodecyl trimethyl ammonium chloride (DTAC) does not swell the stratum corneum or protein film, yet in occlusive patching it can be as irritating as SLS [18,19].

4.1.4 Percutaneous Penetration of Surfactants Has Little Effect on Irritation Potential

Ironically, the ability of surfactants to penetrate the stratum corneum barrier does not appear to have much effect on their irritation potential. Sodium lauryl sulfate penetrates more slowly than its ethoxylated analog [SLES-3EO], which in turn penetrates more slowly down its unsulfated analog laureth-3EO [C_{12}–$(EO)_3$] [20,21]. The primary irritation potential is in the reverse order.

However it is known that SLS will significantly increase in the percutaneous penetration of other molecules such as water and hydrocortisone. This probably relates to its ability to damage the stratum corneum [22].

4.1.5 Strategies for Enhancing Formulation Mildness

There are three approaches to enhance formulation mildness:

Use of mild surfactants
Use of interactive surfactants
Addition of polymers

Use of Mild Surfactants.   The substitution of a harsh surfactant by a milder one will reduce the overall irritation potential of the product. However, mildness is not the only parameter that needs to be optimized; the ability to produce lather/foam is also critical for consumer acceptability. Unfortunately, many mild surfactants do not lather as well as their harsher analogs.

Use of Interactive Surfactants.   The irritation of harsh anionic surfactants can be reduced by the addition of a secondary milder surfactant, even though the level of the more irritating ingredient remains unchanged. This was demonstrated by Rhein et al., who added increasing levels of SLES-7EO to a fixed concentration of SLS [23]. As a result, the primary irritation potential was reduced. There are two explanations for this behavior. First, the formation of mixed micelles (SLS + SLES-7EO). This mixture has a lower CMC than SLS alone, so the concentration of free SLS monomers available to induce irritation is reduced. A second explanation is the competitive binding between the two molecules. Adding additional SLES reduces the amount of SLS bound to the stratum corneum surface and therefore the amount of irritation. There are insufficient data to determine which model is correct.

Similar interactions have been observed in vitro and in vivo using other surfactants. Each of the models are supported by different systems. Faucher and Goddard showed that the nonionic surfactant (Tergitol 15-S-9) reduces SLS binding to hair by modifying its solution properties [24]. Adding increasing levels of Tergitol to the SLS reduces the CMC, meaning that there is less SLS monomer available for binding. As little Tergitol binds to hair, this argues that this is the solution properties, rather than competitive binding that has the primary effect on SLS binding.

Conversely Dominguez et al. showed that betaine and SLS compete for binding sites on skin callus [25]. This competition is affected by the pH and the alkyl chain length of the betaine. Such interactions can reduce irritation in vivo.

A second paper by Dominguez et al. showed that mixtures of betaine and SLS caused less ocular irritation than either surfactant alone [26]. However it is often suggested that the interaction between SLS and betaine is a charge neutralization, especially at pH 6 and below, where betaine will carry a positive charge. This observation is similar to that of Rhein et al., who showed that amine oxides, which carry a partial positive charge, can also reduce the irritation potential of SLS [13].

Recently McFadden et al. demonstrated that the cationic surfactant dodecyl trimethyl ammonium chloride (DTAC) can reduce SLS-induced irritation even when it is added after the SLS application [27]. This suggests that the formation of a "pseudononionic" complex via charge neutralization can reduce irritation potential.

Addition of Cationic Polymers. Another example of charge neutralization is the interaction of anionic surfactants with cationic polymers. Cationic polymers are frequently used in body washes and hair shampoos as conditioning agents and are readily deposited on keratinous surfaces. They have been demonstrated to reduce irritation and dryness caused by anionic surfactants. Certainly, in solution they will complex with anionic surfactants and may carry them to the skin. However as they are in the form of pseudononionic complexes, the surfactants will be relatively mild.

4.1.6 Deposition of Moisturizing Ingredients on the Skin

It has long been recognized that cleansing systems can be used to deliver useful amounts of ingredients to the skin. These include antidandruff shampoos, antibacterial agents from bar and liquid soaps, and silicone and hydrocarbon hair conditioners from two-in-one shampoos. There is no reason why a skin conditioner cannot be delivered to the skin in an analogous way. One of the challenges of delivering a moisturizer to the skin from a cleanser is the detergency of the cleansing base. Indeed, much of the conditioning agents will be rinsed away. Parkhani showed that this was a function of the surfactant's structure as well as its concentration [28].

An approach to increasing retention of the moisturizing agent on the skin during washing and rinsing is to increase the affinity between the two. For zinc pyrithione, an antidandruff agent, this means reducing the pH to 5 so the molecules bears a positive charge. This enables the pyrithione ion to bind to the negatively charged sites on the skin and hair.

The linkage does not have to be direct. Story et al. showed that the cationic polymer polyquaterium 6 can be used as a bridge between the anionic conditioner sulfated castor oil and the skin [29]. This significantly increases the conditioner's substantivity.

5 ASSESSMENT OF MOISTURIZING POTENTIAL OF CLEANSERS

5.1 Consumer Testing

Moisturizing cleansers are consumer personal care products, and ultimately their benefits should be recognizable to consumers. If they do not deliver against their promise, that is, to leave the skin feeling and looking moisturized, or at least less dry, they will not be successful in the marketplace. Therefore it is important to assess whether potential consumers recognize the product's benefits in normal use conditions. Such data from a properly designed test can be used for claims support as well as to assure the scientists developing the product that it successfully delivers the benefits promised. The review of how to design and implement such consumer studies is beyond the scope of this chapter.

5.2 Clinical Testing Overview

Previously, most evaluations of cleanser effects have been to assess primary irritation or drying potential. Such studies start with the skin in good condition, and the extent by which parameters such as erythema and dryness worsen is evaluated. However, moisturization potential carries the implication that it is improving skin condition. Therefore a different experimental design is required. Such studies should incorporate aspects of moisturizer efficacy testing especially with regard to (1) starting with dry skin, to enable improvement to be observed and (2) the use of moisturizer end points such as assessments of skin dryness and skin hydration, together with (3) an application method that reflects how cleansing products are used.

Ideally the application method should not greatly affect, especially decrease, the degree of dry skin. Thus the method initially described by Lukakovic et al. in 1988 is probably more appropriate than methods that involve rubbing for longer periods, e.g., the flex wash or the volar forearm wash test [30]. For the latter studies, the prolonged rubbing has the potential to remove skin flakes, and as a result the methods will lose sensitivity [31,32].

5.2.1 Experimental Design

In order to demonstrate that the cleanser delivers a benefit to the skin, the skin must start out in poor condition. As with moisturizer efficacy studies, the skin should be dry at baseline (dryness score of 2 or more on a 0–4 scale). The test should be run on a body site that readily shows skin dryness. This includes the lower legs or the dorsal aspect of the forearms. The lower leg, in particular, has sufficient area to enable multiple products (and a no-product control) to be tested simultaneously. Using a within-subject design enables potentially large person-to-person variations to be eliminated. There are three main ways to produce dry skin:

Cold weather frequently, occurring during the winter, can often produce dryness.

As people age they exhibit more dry skin, especially at the extremities.

Washing the test area with a drying cleanser will induce dryness.

Combining the first and second methods is probably the best approach. Relying on the weather alone can be risky, as a few warm humid days will significantly reduce the level of dryness observed. Giving the panelists a drying soap bar for regular cleansing has two great disadvantages. First, the soap bar may interfere with the effects of the moisturizing cleanser. Then, consumers usually do not use two cleansing products on the same body sites. Second, Ertel et al. suggested that artificially drying out the skin with a cleanser reduces subsequent responses compared with naturally dry skin [33]. The basis of this is unclear, but it contrasts with the increased irritation response observed when subclinically or mildly irritated skin is re-exposed to an irritant. There are several hypotheses for the different behavior of dry skin, but all reflect that we have studied dryness much less than irritation.

5.2.2 Measuring the Clinical Effects of Products on the Skin

Based on the approaches used to assess moisturizer efficacy, the two main parameters to assess the moisturizing potential of cleansing products are skin dryness and skin hydration. It is always advisable to use multiple methods for assessing efficacy, as each individual method has potential shortcomings. The use of a basket of methods will yield a fuller assessment of skin condition.

Skin Dryness. Traditionally skin dryness has been evaluated by a trained observer using an ordinal scale. However, this approach has two major problems. It is very dependent on the evaluator, and great care must be taken to ensure reproducibility between evaluators, studies, and different testing laboratories. For this, a standardized photographic scale is very helpful. Second, there are many factors that can reduce the appearance of dryness without there being any benefit to the skin. These include short-term humidity and occlusive lotions that matte the dry skin flakes down without removing them. These problems can be overcome by using a sticky tape to sample the skin's surface, e.g., DeSquame® tape (CuDerm Inc., Dallas, TX). The tape is pressed onto the skin's surface and then removed. The greater the scaling, the more skin flakes are removed by the tape. These can be quantified by using an analog scale or by image analysis. The tape will remove the flakes even if they are matted down or obscured by warm, humid weather. This was demonstrated in a single-wash study (see Fig. 1). After a baseline assessment, dry skin on the dorsal forearm was washed once by the method of Lukakovic et at. [30]. The skin condition was reassessed three hours later. Re-

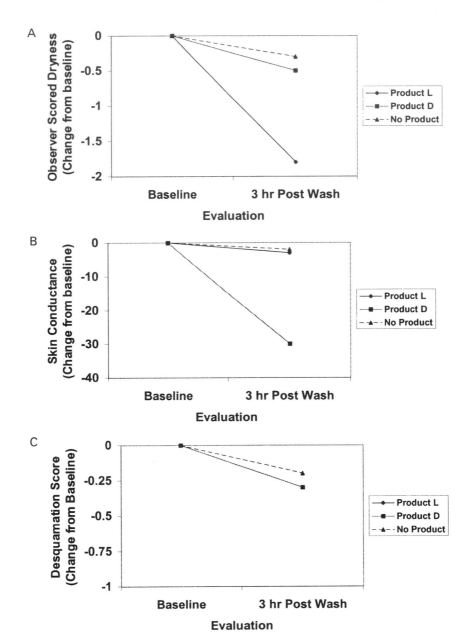

Figure 1 The effect of liquid cleansers on (A) observable dryness, (B) skin conductance, and (C) desquamation 3 hr after a single wash wash. The method used was that of Lukacovic et al. [31].

sults show that Product L reduces observable dryness more than product D or no product. However the DeSquame tape indicates that flakes are still present, just masked. This conclusion is supported by the conductance readings, which had not increased.

Conductance and Capacitance. Conductance and/or capacitance are frequently used to measure skin hydration. This approach has been supported empirically by Morrison and Scala, who showed a strong correlation between observable dryness and reduction in skin conductance (measured by a Skicon 200) and capacitance (measured by a dermal phase meter) [34]. There are two reasons that explain how skin conductance may measure dryness. First, as the skin becomes drier, the concentration of water in the stratum corneum is reduced. Since water is a good conductor compared with the more hydrophobic stratum corneum, a reduction in water activity will reduce conductance. Another possible mechanism by which dryness reduces conductance is that as scales develop, air pockets are formed in the damaged stratum corneum. Since air is a poor conductor, this scaling also results in reduced conductance. Clearly these two mechanisms are not mutually exclusive and may occur simultaneously.

It should be stressed that residues left on the skin's surface may modify conductance in the absence of dryness. For instance, petrolatum, silicones, and mineral oil are good insulators and can reduce conductance even as they moisturize the skin. Conductance data should be evaluated based on the product's composition and with an understanding of which ingredients may remain on the skin after rinsing.

Stained DeSquames. Staining skin flakes on the DeSquame tape with hydrophilic dyes can give a measure of the integrity or degree of damage. From irritation testing, Pierard and his colleagues demonstrated that even mild insults will damage the stratum corneum surface and cause an increase in dye uptake [35]. This is readily quantified using a color meter such as a Minolta Chromameter. Damage that is not readily observable to the naked eye can be detected by this method. This approach has been extended to moisturizer efficacy testing. Simion has shown that glycerin-based moisturizers are good at removing dry damaged skin from the surface, revealing undamaged corneocytes below [36]. As yet, this method has not been used to assess the efficacy of moisturizing cleansers.

5.3 Irritation Testing

Skin dryness and primary irritation are frequently separate phenomena and can be induced by different mechanisms. It has been demonstrated that dryness from repeated hand washing can be induced in the absence of erythema [37]. However, dryness is frequently produced as a sequala to primary irritation as the skin begins to repair itself [38]. Therefore it is important to assess irritation potential of

Table 3 Effect of Cleansers on Skin After a Single 24-hr Occlusive Patch Soap Chamber Test

	Erythema[a]	Stratum corneum barrier damage[b]
Soap	1.67	10.35
Detergent bar	0.69	7.27
Liquid cleanser L	0.29	5.62
Liquid cleanser E	0.44	4.76

Notes: Method used is that of Simion et al. [39]. n = 26 responsive skin volunteers.
[a]Erythema scored on a 0–4 scale; baseline value of erythema = 0.
[b]Stratum corneum barrier damage assessed by trans-epidermal water loss; data shown are change from baseline in g water/m^2/hr.

cleansers, especially to prevent a low-level irritation from causing dryness that the product is supposed to reverse. Table 3 shows the irritation potential of bar and liquid cleansers after 24 hr occlusive patching on the skin of responsive panelists using the soap chamber test [39].

5.3.1 Methods for Assessing Primary Irritation

Closed (occlusive) patch testing is used to assess the dermal primary irritation potential of chemicals including detergents and cleansing products. Frequently panels of 50 volunteers from a general population are occlusively patched for 24 to 48 hr. This will give an overall assessment of irritation potential. There are two ways to increase the method's sensitivity—either patch for longer periods of time or recruit a sensitive skin population. The former approach is the basis of the cumulative irritation test. This is frequently used to assess very mild products. Occlusive patching for 14 to 21 days will significantly weaken the stratum corneum barrier and result in more irritation. Care must be taken to ensure that the correct concentration of cleanser is used. Too high will produce overwhelming irritation; if the concentration is too low, then nothing will be seen.

Frosch and Kligman developed the soap chamber test, which utilizes "sensitive" skin panelists to increase the response [40]. Panelists are patched with 5 to 8% soap solutions for 24 hr, then for 6 hr on the next 4 days. Three days later both erythema and skin dryness are assessed. This method is especially effective at differentiating the irritation potential of different surfactants. Simion et al. were able to shorten the patching duration to two consecutive days [39]. In this case, erythema and trans-epidermal water loss are measured.

The responsiveness of the skin can be increased artificially. The chamber scarification test relies on mechanical trauma to damage the barrier [41]. Frosch and Kligman showed that the responsiveness to hydrophilic material was greatly increased. For instance, the threshold for SLS to produce irritation was reduced fiftyfold.

6 SUMMARY

For centuries, soap has been the primary product used for personal cleansing. Although it is an effective cleanser, it can also leave the skin dry and irritated. The development of synthetic surfactants in the 20th century has enabled the formulation of milder cleansers that do not damage the skin as much as soap. This results in consumers experiencing less dryness and irritation. However, these cleansers can go beyond reducing skin damage and deliver benefits to the skin. This can be done from soap bars, e.g., through delivery of triclocarban from antibacterial soap, but is more effective from liquid cleansers. Unlike a bar such as soap, which is mainly detergents, or cocoyl isethionate, liquid cleansers have a much lower surfactant load. Thus their ability to wash away beneficial ingredients is reduced. However, they still are able to adequately cleanse most consumers that can afford their higher price, as these individuals usually do not need all the cleansing potential that a bar car deliver.

This chapter described the use of the different components required for a liquid cleanser, whose formulation is more complex than that of a bar of soap. Constituents include primary and secondary surfactants for cleansing and lathering. A foam booster is frequently added as well. Thickeners, opacifiers, color, and fragrance are needed to optimize the esthetic acceptability of the product to consumers. Finally, preservatives are required to prevent microbial growth in the aqueous base.

Beyond having a milder product, beneficial ingredients can be delivered to the skin. These include antibacterial ingredients such as triclosan, triclocarban, and antidandruff agents such as zinc pyrithione. Cationic polymeric skin conditioners will bind to anionic sites on the skin and be retained after rinsing. These polymers can leave the skin feeling softer and smoother. However, it must be stressed that the vast proportion of any beneficial agent is rinsed away due to the detergency of the surfactant system. To effectively deliver greater benefits, especially when using effective but expensive ingredients, requires new methods of delivering the agents and preventing them from washing away during rinsing. However, for the foreseeable future, this approach will remain less effective at delivering beneficial agents than leave-on products such as lotions. For example, an anti-aging cleanser may not dry and roughen the skin as much as soap, so the fine lines associated with dryness are less evident. However, delivery of sunscreens, retinol, or other materials that prevent damage boost the skin's moisture content or stimulate the skin's self-repair mechanism is still done more effectively with a lotion.

There are two approaches to measuring the clinical effects of moisturizing cleansers on the skin. The first is to ensure that the cleansing system causes minimal damage to the skin, for which traditional irritation testing is used. Second is to measure moisturizing efficacy, which requires a paradigm shift toward the techniques used for assessing lotion efficacy. Irritation assessments such as closed patch tests and exaggerated arm washes are used to assess a product's ability to increase irritation from a negligible starting point. In contrast, to measure the product's ability to deliver a benefit such as moisturization, the skin must start with a deficiency, i.e., it must be dry. Then the methods used to assess leave-on moisturizers, such as conductance and DeSquame tape, can be used to assess the moisturizing cleanser.

REFERENCES

1. Gloxhuber C, Künstler K. Anionic Surfactants: Biochemistry, Toxicology, Dermatology. 2nd ed. Vol. 43, Surfactant Science Series. New York: Marcel Dekker, 1992:212.
2. Bluestein BR, Hilton CL. Amphoteric Surfactants. Vol. 12, Surfactant Science Series. New York: Marcel Dekker, 1982:145–150.
3. Ramon LA. U.S. patent 4,663,069.
4. Phillips BM, Akred BJ. U.S. patent 5,039,451.
5. Giret MJ, Langlois A, Duke RP. U.S. patent 5,409,640.
6. Bolich RE Jr., Williams TB. U.S. patent 4,788,006.
7. Ogino K, Abe M. Mixed Surfactant Systems. Vol. 46, Surfactant Science Series. New York: Marcel Dekker, 1993:235–247.
8. Martin AN, Swarbrick J, Cammarata A. Physical Pharmacy. 2d ed. Philadelphia: Lea & Febiger, 1969:149.
9. Gennaro AR. Remington's Pharmaceutical Sciences. 18th ed. Easton, PA: Mack Publishing, 1990:292.
10. Martin AN, Swarbrick J, Cammarata A. Physical Pharmacy. 2d ed. Philadelphia: Lea & Febiger, 1969:449.
11. Ogino K, Abe M. Mixed Surfactant Systems. Vol. 46, Surfactant Science Series. New York: Marcel Dekker, 1993:248–251.
12. Wilhelm KP, Cua AB, Wolff HH, Maibach HI. Surfactant-induced stratum corneum hydration in vivo: prediction of the irritation potential of anionic surfactants. J Invest Dermitol 1993; 101:310–315.
13. Rhein LD, Robbins CR, Fernee K, Cantore R. Surfactant structure effects on swelling of isolated stratum corneum. J Soc Cosmet Chem 1986; 37:125–139.
14. Blake-Haskins JC, Scala DD, Rhein LD, Robbins CR. Predicting surfactant irritation from the swelling response of a collagen film. J Soc Cosmet Chem 1986; 37:199–210.
15. Imokawa G, Sumura K, Katsumi M. A correlation between adsorption of surfactant onto callus and skin roughness caused by the surfactant. J Jpn Oil Chem Soc 1974; 23:17–23.

16. Cooper ER, Berner B. Vol. 16, Surfactant Science Series. Rieger MM, ed. New York: Marcel Dekker, 1985:195–208.

17. Warren R, Ertel KD, Bartolo RG, Levine MJ, Bryant PB, Wong LF. The influence of hard water (calcium) and surfactants on irritant contact dermatitis. Contact Dermatitis. 1996; 36:337–343.

18. Imokawa G, Takeuchi T. Surfactants and skin roughness. Cosmet Toil 1976; 91:32–46.

19. Cutler RA, Droebek HP. Toxicology of Cationic Surfactants in Cationic Surfactants. Jungerman E, ed. New York: Marcel Dekker, 1970:527–616.

20. Howes D. The percutaneous absorption of some anionic surfactants. J Soc Cosmet Chem 1975; 26:47–63.

21. Prottey C, Ferguson T. Factors which determine the skin irritation potential of soap and detergents. J Soc Cosmet Chem 1975; 26:29–46.

22. Wilhelm KP, Surber C, Maibach HI. Effect of sodium lauryl sulfate–induced skin irritation on in vivo percutaneous penetration of four drug. J Invest Dermatol 1991; 97:927–932.

23. Rhein LD, Simion FA, Hill RL, Cagan RH. Matti J, Maibach HI. Human cutaneous response to a mixed surfactant system: role of solution phenomena in controlling surfactant irritation. Dermatologica 1990; 180:18–23.

24. Faucher JA, Goddard ED. Interaction of keratinous substrates with sodium lauryl sulfate. I. Sorption. J Soc Cosmet Chem 1978; 29:323–337.

25. Dominguez JG, Balaguer F, Parra JL, Pelejero CM. The inhibitory effects of some amphoteric surfactants on the irritation potential of alkylsulfates. Int J Cosmet Sci 1981; 3:57–68.

26. Dominguez JG, Parra JL, Infante MR, Pelejero CM, Balaguer F, Sautre T. A new approach to the theory of adsorption and permeability of surfactants on keratinic proteins: the specific behavior of certain hydrophobic chains. J Soc Cosmet Chem 1977; 28:165–182.

27. McFadden JP, Holloway DB, Whittle EG, Basketter DA. Benzalkonium chloride neutralizes the irritant effects of sodium dodecyl sulfate. Contact Dermatitis 2000; 43:264–266.

28. Parkhani N. The effect of surfactants on lipid deposition from liquid cleansers to the skin. Master's Thesis, University of Cincinnati, 1995.

29. Story DC, Gott RE, Asbury MT, Phifer K, Simion FA. U.S. patent 6,024,952.

30. Lukacovic MF, Dunlap FE, Michails SF, Visscher MO, Watson DD. Forearm wash test to evaluate the clinical mildness of cleansing products. J Soc Cosmet Chem 1988; 39:355–366.

31. Strube DD, Koontz SW, Murahata RI, Theiler RF. The flex wash test: a method for evaluating the mildness of personal washing products. J Soc Cosmet Chem 1989; 40:297–306.

32. Sharko PT, Murahata RI, Leyden JJ, Grove GL. Arm wash with instrumental evaluation—a sensitive technique for differentiating irritation potential of personal washing products. J Derm Clin Eval Soc 1991; 2:19–27.

33. Ertel KD, Neumann PB, Hartwig PM, Rains GY, Keswick BH. Leg wash protocol to assess the skin moisturization potential of personal cleansing products. Int J Cosmet Sci 1999; 21:383–387.

34. Morrison BM, Scala DD. Comparison of instrumental measurements of skin hydration. J Toxicol Cut Ocular Toxicol 1999; 15:305–314.

35. Pierard GE, Goffin V, Pierard-Franchimont C. Corneosurfametry: a predictive assessment of the interaction of personal care products with human stratum corneum. Dermatology 1994; 189:152–156.

36. Simion FA. Use of stained sticky tape to enhance assessment of the moisturization efficacy of lotions. 59th American Academy of Dermatology Annual Meeting, Washington, D.C., 2001.

37 Simion FA, Babulak SW, Morrison BM, Rhein LD, Scala DD. Experimental method soap induced dryness in the absence of erythema. 50th American Academy of Dermatology Annual Meeting, Dallas, TX, 1991.

38. Wilhelm KP, Freitag G, Wolff HH. Surfactant-induced skin irritation and skin repair: evaluation of a cumulative human irritation model by non-invasive techniques. J Am Acad Dermatol 1994; 31:981–987.

39. Simion FA, Rhein LD, Grove GL, Wojtowski J, Cagan RH, Scala DD. Sequential order of skin responses to surfactants in a soap chamber test. Contact Dermatitis 1991; 25:242–249.

40. Frosch PJ, Kligman AM. The soap chamber test: a new method for assessing irritancy of soaps. J Am Acad Dermatol 1979; 1:35–41.

41. Frosch PJ, Kligman AM. The chamber scarification test for irritancy. Contact Dermatitis 1976; 2:314–324.

27

Safety Assessment of Cosmetic Products

Christopher Flower
The Cosmetic, Toiletry, and Perfumery Association,
London, United Kingdom

1 INTRODUCTION

It is clearly not possible in a short chapter such as this to cover in detail safety assessment programs to comply with the legislative environment surrounding cosmetic products in each of the major markets of the world. Neither is it possible to provide in-depth instruction on toxicological testing methods and interpretation of data. Such a program would, and indeed should, become outdated as scientific methods evolve. In fact, during the writing of this chapter, the Organisation for Economic Co-operation and Development (OECD) agreed to delete the LD_{50} test from its list of official protocols [1]. The shortcomings of this test have been known to toxicologists for a long time, but getting agreement for it to be delisted has also taken a long time. Instead, therefore, the intention of this chapter will be to provide something of the philosophy of cosmetic product safety to guide rather than train from scratch the safety assessor and to help colleagues understand the needs of the safety assessor.

Although the European Community Cosmetics Directive (76/768/EEC) is seen as a model for legislation by an increasing number of countries in the world, significant markets operate under quite different regimes. The nonalignment of different definitions of what constitutes a cosmetic complicates the situation, with some borderline products being regulated quite differently in different markets around the world depending on their final classification in each country. Underlying each regime, though, is the basic demand that cosmetic products, however defined, should be safe for their intended purpose and not cause harm to the consumer. The regimes run from those which, like the United States, restrict very few ingredients to those, like Japan until recently, where only permitted ingredients may be used in cosmetic products. The EU regime is somewhat midway between the two. There are lists of prohibited and restricted substances and several positive lists too. Any other substance may be used as an ingredient subject to an overriding safety requirement. It is this basic safety requirement and how a cosmetic is assessed for compliance that is the subject of this chapter.

The successful cosmetic product will be used by large numbers of people, repeatedly and for a considerable time. Its mode of use will be governed partly by custom or past experience and partly by the manufacturer's instructions. Rarely will use be under professional supervision although that may be the case sometimes. Yet experience shows this situation is satisfactory; by and large, cosmetic products do not lead to personal injury or worse [2], and today they are amongst the safest products in the major markets of the world to which general consumers are exposed.

This has not always been the case. The historical use of substances such as white lead, arsenic, and belladonna for cosmetic purposes is well documented and even today some traditional cosmetics are still available which might not pass the assessment process being described here.

That is not to say cosmetic products are not subject to controls or regulations. On the contrary, in all member states of the European Union, cosmetic products are closely regulated by their own specific directive, the Cosmetics Directive [or, to give it its full title, Council Directive of 27 July 1976 on the approximation of the laws of the Member States relating to cosmetic products (76/768/EEC)]. The Cosmetics Directive is a safety directive. This is made clear in the recitals where it is stated, "Whereas the main objective of these laws is the safeguarding of public health." To this end, the Cosmetics Directive first defines what is a cosmetic product (Article 1) and then immediately requires of them that they should be safe (Article 2). Both the degree of safety required and the circumstances to be considered are indicated in this article. Furthermore, the directive requires that each cosmetic product should be subject to a safety assessment to ensure compliance with Article 2.

Thus, cosmetic products are defined in European Community law, and each cosmetic has to undergo a safety assessment prior to marketing to ensure compliance with the safety requirement. Guidelines have been written elsewhere to help in this regard [3,4].

2 THE SAFETY REQUIREMENT

Article 2 of the Cosmetics Directive states, "A cosmetic product put on the market within the Community must not cause damage to human health when applied under normal or reasonably foreseeable conditions of use, taking account, in particular, of the product's presentation, its labelling, any instructions for use and disposal as well as any other indication or information provided by the manufacturer or his authorised agent or by any person responsible for placing the product on the Community market. The provision of such warnings shall not, in any event, exempt any person from compliance with the other requirements laid down in this Directive."

The wording of Article 2 is very important. It requires that a cosmetic product must not cause damage to human health, but does not require that a cosmetic must not provoke any adverse reaction. Thus, absolute safety is not required—indeed could not be achieved—but a degree of safety is required, and the appropriate degree is defined as a freedom from damage to human health.

Compliance with the safety requirement is a matter of professional judgement and will be considered in greater depth later, but it will involve the evaluation of factors such as severity of possible adverse reactions, their duration and reversibility, and their prevalence or likelihood in the normal population. Reactions judged to be mild, readily reversible, or rare tend to support the safety of a product, whereas responses judged to be severe, long-lasting, or common would not.

Article 2 also requires that the product be "safe" under normal or reasonably foreseeable conditions of use. There is no requirement for a product to be safe under all circumstances; misuse and deliberate abuse, therefore, need not be considered. However, particular care needs to be given as to what is reasonably foreseeable and to the value warning labels might have.

For example, a shampoo might cause some discomfort should it get into the eyes. A warning advising against allowing that to happen and what action to take in the event is quite reasonable. However, because shampoo getting in to the eyes in normal use is reasonably foreseeable, any adverse reactions that occur should not be so severe as to constitute damage to human health.

Finally, the safety requirement is not qualified but is absolute. In other words, it is not possible to weigh the risks against the benefits, as one may do with a pharmaceutical for example. No matter what benefits may be provided by a cosmetic, the cosmetic product must not cause damage to human health. This is, therefore, a very stringent requirement.

Compliance with the safety requirement of Article 2 is through the conduct of an "assessment of the safety of human health of the finished product. To that end the manufacturer shall take into consideration the general toxicological profile of the ingredient, its chemical structure and its level of exposure" [Article

7a(d)]. Although the foregoing relates specifically to the situation in the member states of the European Community, the principles expounded will also apply to safety assessments conducted under other regulatory regimes.

The process of safety assessment is a multistep one which comprises a number of stages:

Hazard identification. This step essentially collects all the adverse data pertaining to the product and its constituent ingredients to identify the hazards.

Risk characterisation. This step compares the hazard data with the anticipated exposure conditions to determine which hazards could constitute risks to human health. In essence, this step identifies the relevant hazards for further consideration.

Risk evaluation. This step is a further refinement of risk characterisation in which the potential risks are quantified and gauged against known risks. This step requires detailed information regarding actual exposure.

Safety assessment. In the final step, the safety assessor must judge whether the potential risks are deemed acceptable and therefore whether the product is safe to market.

Before going through each of these steps in detail, it is appropriate to consider practical aspects of importance to the safety assessment process. This is information that is essential if the safety assessor is to be in a position to perform an adequate assessment.

2.1 Assess the Right Product

Companies often have complex development programs and many alternative formulations may be under simultaneous evaluation prior to deciding which candidate is to be selected for the market. Product brand or variant names may change during the course of development and a means of tracking these changes must be in place. If each formula is assigned a unique reference number, then a clear and unambiguous link can be established between the marketed product and its safety assessment regardless of other changes to its name.

Then, if each adjustment to a formula, no matter how slight, generates a new unique formula reference number, a new review or safety assessment is automatically triggered. Without this trigger, there is a risk that formulae may be repeatedly modified until the original assessment becomes remote from the marketed product. It is not acceptable that a product formula should be changed without reference to the safety assessor. Manufacturers should be aware that the safety assessor cannot be held responsible for the safety of a formula changed without his or her knowledge, and manufacturers should be aware that it is they and not the safety assessor who runs the risk of prosecution under the Cosmetic Directive.

2.2 Know the Formula

The complete formula must be available to the safety assessor, including the chemical name, INCI name, and any in-house name by which each ingredient is known.

Since most cosmetic ingredients are available in various grades or qualities, the specification for each as actually used must be available. Some raw materials are presented as mixtures, sometimes with additives to enhance stability or for preservation. The specifications for these ingredients should show such additives.

Where necessary, the safety assessor may determine which grades are to be used by defining appropriate quality criteria. The manufacturer should ensure substitution is not possible without the approval of the safety assessor. Product made from ingredients that do not comply with a defined quality would not necessarily be covered by the safety assessment.

2.3 Exact Level of Ingredients

The final level of each specific ingredient must be known when they are added from different sources. Some ingredients will be added in variable amounts, q.s., or *quantum satis;* pH and viscosity adjusters are typical. The likely ranges and maximum limits for these must be specified. Some ingredients may react during manufacture and reaction products must be identified; others are added as pre-mixes and their constituents must be known.

Safety assessors must be given details of the method of manufacture and a description and the specification of the final product. They must also understand what changes take place during manufacture to know to what the consumer will be exposed when using the product.

2.4 Product Stability

The product must be stable and an assurance of this is required by the safety assessor; written assurance of stability or actual reports of stability tests should be provided. In addition, the safety assessor may wish to see analytical data on a typical product, particularly regarding levels of "active" ingredients or undesirable degradation products or contamination substances both before, during, and after storage testing. It is important to take account of storage conditions likely in use and consider whether that may affect product stability and safety.

2.5 Microbiological Quality

The finished product must have an acceptable microbiological specification. The safety assessor needs to know this and must be sure that the product meets its specification. Again, reports of microbiological testing or written assurance of microbiological quality may be required by the safety assessor.

Stability testing and microbiology are specialist fields in their own right. Although large companies will probably have expertise in house, smaller concerns may have to employ contractors. In either case, the safety assessor needs to be satisfied that the product is microbiologically and chemically stable throughout the anticipated shelf-life of the product, bearing in mind normal storage conditions in the anticipated market. Consideration must be given to the capacity of the preservative system to cope with normal contamination once the product has been opened and in use.

2.6 Packaging, Instructions, and Labeling

Safety assessors should see the proposed packaging to consider what impact that might have on safety. For example, child-resistant closures may be appropriate in some cases or the maximum pack size might need to be limited in other situations. They should also see instructions for use and any warning labels to be included, and must be able to influence these where safety is affected. In particular, compliance with any mandatory warnings needs to be checked, a task that may be handled by the safety assessor.

A copy of the INCI ingredient declaration should be supplied and linked to the formula as a check to ensure no ingredients are omitted.

2.7 Efficacy

Although efficacy and claims support are not generally the province of the safety assessor, in certain circumstances (suncare products are good examples) efficacy does become a safety issue. Copies of efficacy study reports should be available to the safety assessor where there may be a safety aspect, but the safety assessor is not required to determine efficacy per se nor to endorse product claims.

If human trials have been carried out, any adverse effects must be reported to the safety assessor as this constitutes relevant information. Copies of trial reports must be made available.

2.8 Adverse Effects Reports

The safety assessor must have access to reports of adverse effects notified to the company on this or similar products; ideally, the number of such events should be related to the number of product units sold. Such reports can be tabulated periodically to provide a continuous record, but a system of highlighting severe or particularly unusual events should be considered.

2.9 Toxicity Data

The safety assessor must have access to toxicity and safety data on each of the ingredients, on the final product or similar products where available and should have knowledge of possible ingredient interactions. These data would include material safety data sheets from ingredient suppliers and letters of safety assurance from fragrance suppliers confirming the fragrance conforms to the code of practice of the fragrance industry [5] as well as conventional toxicological data, in vitro as well as in vivo, and human volunteer studies. In addition, authoritative sources, such as the Cosmetic Ingredient Review in the United States, should be consulted [6].

2.10 Exposure Estimation

Before commencing a safety assessment proper, it is essential to know the category of cosmetic product that is to be assessed and how, in general terms, it is to be used: e.g., whether it is for hair care or skin care, whether it is to be left in situ or rinsed off, whether ingestion or inhalation are likely, whether it is diluted before or during use, and so on. Later, it will be necessary to refine this general understanding to gain an accurate exposure assessment and to consider also how the product may be misused, perhaps accidentally, and whether there is potential for deliberate abuse.

Specifically, therefore, the following information is required:

Type of cosmetic product
Intended mode of use
Quantity used each time
Frequency of application
Duration of contact
Site of contact
Area of contact
Unintentional contact
Nature of consumers and numbers
Other factors (e.g., exposure to sunlight, potential for abuse, interaction with other products)

2.11 Hazard Identification

The first step in the safety assessment of cosmetics, as with any other consumer product, has to be that of hazard identification. First and foremost, you have to know what hazards might be associated with each of the ingredients in the product, and not just the ingredients but also any contaminants and possible degradation products. Later, the safety assessor must also consider possible reaction products and ingredient interactions, either with one another or with the packaging.

Hazard identification is primarily achieved through conventional toxicological testing both in vivo and, to an increasing extent, in vitro. Much data will be obtained from the literature and from toxicology databases as well as from ingredient suppliers. The quality of the data needs to be considered, not just the apparent quantity [7]; it is the interpretation of the significance of the data in terms of its applicability to the use of the ingredient in a cosmetic product that is the primary role of the toxicologist/safety assessor. For this reason, original reports and publications should be consulted whenever possible rather than relying solely on reported data. Particular attention should be given to the actual substance tested and its description to gauge whether the data are relevant to the ingredient in question.

Toxicity tests are frequently defined in terms of their endpoints and, for convenience, that is how they are considered here. Thus, for each ingredient, one needs to consider

Acute toxicity
Irritancy to skin, eyes, and mucous membranes
Sensitization and photosensitization
Subchronic or repeated exposure toxicity
Mutagenicity and genotoxicity
Long-term toxicity and carcinogenicity
Photomutagenicity, photogenotoxicity, and photocarcinogenicity
Toxicokinetics (absorption, distribution, metabolism, and excretion)
Human data

2.11.1   Acute Toxicity

Some estimate of the acute toxicity of a substance to be used as an ingredient in a cosmetic product must be available. This does not automatically mean an LD_{50} test, although historically the LD_{50} was often used for such a purpose. What is required is evidence that the ingredient will not be acutely toxic at a relevant exposure level and by an appropriate route of exposure. With the imminent deletion of the LD_{50} test from the OECD guidelines, more information and less severe studies should become the norm in the absence of in vitro alternatives.

Normally, pre-existing data are often limited to gavage studies in rodents up to a dose limit (typically 2 g/kg or a dose volume of 10 mL/kg). Oral dosing may be appropriate for an ingredient likely to be ingested, but such studies require careful interpretation before extrapolating the results to dermal exposure scenarios. Consideration must be given to the effects of dermal absorption [8,9], metabolism by the skin, and to differences in body compartment distribution resulting from dermal exposure, as opposed to absorption from the gastrointestinal tract with its potential for first-pass hepatic metabolism and other differences likely in distribution and excretion. The all-important target tissue concentration of the active toxic principle may be very different depending on the route of exposure.

2.11.2   Local Tolerance—Skin, Eye, and Mucous Membrane Irritancy

Estimation of the irritancy of the substance to both skin and eyes may be appropriate depending on the type of end product use envisaged and the concentration to be used. Without care, because of use of excessively high doses or concentrations or the use of a sensitive or reactive model (such as the rabbit eye), data from local tolerance studies may prove misleading by suggesting the existence of a hazard which is unlikely to be encountered in practice. This, however, will be reconsidered in the next sections, those of risk characterization and risk evaluation, when such hazards will be identified as unlikely or irrelevant risks.

Ingredients to be used in specialized cosmetic products, such as those for oral care, intimate hygiene, or on infants, may require data on their mucous membrane compatibility. Whilst conjunctival reactions seen from ocular test results can be useful, they can only serve as a guide in the absence of clear benchmarks.

Again, frequently such local tolerance data are pre-existing, having been generated on the basic substance as required under chemicals legislation. Problems arise when the data are only generated for high doses or high concentrations and there has been no attempt to characterize the dose–response relationship.

2.11.3   Sensitization and Photosensitization

Sensitization and, increasingly, photosensitization data are required if the sensitizing potential of a product is to be estimated. Various in vitro tests have been developed over the years to model aspects of the sensitization process, but they are not yet able to replace in vivo studies completely at the present time. Nevertheless, there have been reductions in the severity of the in vivo procedures [10], with the murine local lymph node test [11] now being accepted as a fully validated alternative to the more stressful guinea pig maximization methods.

One crucial factor for skin sensitization is that exposure be considered in terms of dose of substance per unit area of skin, rather than as simple concentration in the vehicle. It is important to remember this when considering the final product safety assessment. For example, a spray-on cologne based on a volatile solvent such as alcohol contains a given concentration of any ingredient; as the solvent evaporates from the skin, the concentration of ingredient in the remaining product rises, but the dose of the ingredient per unit area of skin remains unchanged.

Photosensitization (and phototoxicity) data are becoming ever more important when considering ingredients which will be used in products such as sunscreens [12,13]. Evidence that a substance is capable of absorbing UV light should be taken as a trigger for considering the need for phototoxicity and photosensitization data.

2.11.4   Repeat Dose or Subchronic Toxicity

These studies provide valuable information on any toxic effects which occur following repeated exposure to a substance. Investigations normally involve post mortem examination of all major organ systems as well as numerous in vivo investigations. As with acute studies, both the dose levels used and the routes of exposure must be taken into account when extrapolating the findings to a cosmetic product safety assessment.

Ideally, the results of a repeated exposure study would allow the identification of doses which could be termed the no effect level (NEL), no adverse effect level (NAEL), no observed effect level (NOEL), or no observed adverse effect level (NOAEL). The differences in meaning of these terms needs to be understood and their accurate use checked.

Strictly, since one cannot guarantee that all possible effects which might have occurred in a study were actually detectable, any reference to effects should be qualified as relating to observed effects only. The NOEL would be the highest dose at which no effects due to treatment could be detected; such animals would, to all intents and purposes, be identical to animals sham-treated with vehicle as controls. Where effects were noticed, there is then a judgement as to whether the effects were adverse or not. Thus, the NOAEL is the highest dose level at which any changes observed are judged not to be adverse ones. The NOAEL may be the same dose level as the NOEL, or may be higher.

In either case, these estimates of doses which appear not to cause harm are used as markers when attempting to establish safety margins for human exposures. Safety margins are introduced in toxicology to make allowance for uncertainty; just because a given dose was without toxic effect in one study on one species does not mean to say that same dose would always be equally benign. Individuals within a species vary in many ways, including in their susceptibility to a putative toxin. Similarly, whole species may differ from one another in susceptibility. Because it is rare for the most susceptible and the most resistant members within a species to differ by more than tenfold, a safety factor of 10 is applied to take account of this. In the same way, the difference between the most and the least susceptible species is rarely greater than tenfold, so an additional factor of 10 is applied here too.

Thus, if, by chance, a measure of toxicity had been established in a resistance species the application of a 100-fold safety factor would take account of the most sensitive member of the most sensitive species (as man is assumed to be). For example, if a dose of 100 mg/kg was "safe" in an animal study (i.e., produced no observed adverse effects), applying a 100-fold safety factor means that 1 mg/kg should be "safe" in man.

2.11.5 Mutagenicity and Genotoxcity

Mutagenicity is the capacity to induce mutation, which is a permanent change in the amount or structure of the genetic material of an organism that may result in a heritable change in the characteristics, or phenotype, of the organism. Mutations may involve single genes, blocks of genes, or whole chromosomes, and the processes include point mutations (changes to a single base or the addition or deletion of a base), clastogenicity, or chromosome aberrations (gaps, breaks, or translocations) as well as aneuploidy (changes in chromosome numbers).

Genotoxicity is the specific adverse effect upon the genome of living cells that may be expressed as a mutagenic or carcinogenic effect. Interaction by a chemical or its metabolites may be with the DNA directly or to the apparatus which regulates the fidelity of the genome. Interference with the process of chromosome segregation during meiotic or mitotic cell division can lead to aneuploidy without there necessarily being mutation of the DNA itself.

In vitro tests exist to detect all three mutation endpoints, namely, gene mutation, clastogenicity, and aneuploidy, but there is currently no single, validated test that can provide information on them all. A range of tests will be required and these may involve a variety of organisms, from bacteria and yeasts through cultured mammalian cells to whole mammal studies. In general, testing strategy follows a hierarchical approach whereby absence of activity in an in vitro study is taken as encouraging, but a positive effect is not proof of a potential human hazard, only that further investigation is warranted. The underlying principle is to see whether activity seen in vitro can be expressed in vivo. If it cannot, that is taken as an indication that in vitro result may be given less emphasis.

Considerable expertise in conducting the tests themselves and in understanding the underlying mechanisms is essential if the results are to be interpreted correctly.

2.11.6 Long-Term Toxicity and Carcinogenicity

Increasingly, questions are asked about the potential adverse effects of long-term exposure to substances and whether those effects may include carcinogenicity. Where pre-existing data are available, again the quality of those data and their relevance to the proposed use of the substance must be taken into account. However, the need for studies to generate such data should be carefully weighed against the value of the information they could usefully provide. It is here that information on the likely exposure to and fate of the substance is most valuable.

Many examples exist of substances that are toxic or carcinogenic at very high doses and for which clear thresholds can be demonstrated below which toxicity or carcinogenicity are not manifest, or which exert their toxicity through mechanisms known not to be relevant for man. Nevertheless, since exposure to cosmetic ingredients is generally of the long-term and low level kind, a consideration needs to be given to the potential for subtle, long-term changes in fields such as immunotoxicity and hormonal toxicology. Identification of thresholds is likely to become more relevant.

2.11.7 Photomutagenicity, Photogenotoxicity, and Photocarcinogenicity

Information relating to these endpoints is needed when the proposed conditions of use would include prolonged exposure to sunlight, as would be the case with the UV filters present in sun protection cosmetics. Since the absorbed energy of the filtered UV is not destroyed, some consideration is required as to how this energy is handled by the filter.

The absorbed energy could, theoretically, be re-emitted as visible light or sound, but in practice it is more likely to be emitted as heat or as an energetic particle, such as a free radical. The skin protective benefit comes from the re-emission taking place near the external surfaces of the skin where the nearby tissues which form the primary target (stratum corneum and upper epidermis) are subject to constant renewal, so avoiding the accumulation of subcritical toxic insults which could otherwise develop into overt toxicity. Without a sun protection product, UV rays penetrate deeper into the skin and are able to interact directly with viable cells.

2.11.8 Toxicokinetics

Toxicokinetics is the effect the body has on the substance and refers to the absorption, distribution, metabolism, and excretion of the substance in question. Knowledge of the mathematics of toxicokinetics allows an estimate to be made of the concentration and duration profile of the substance, or its metabolites, at the tissue site of interest, and thereby a better assessment of the likelihood of a hazard is gained.

For example, a substance which is either very poorly absorbed through the skin or is extensively and rapidly metabolized there is most unlikely to have the same effects following topical application as it would have after ingestion or following gavage dosing.

2.11.9 Human Data

Human data are extremely valuable to the safety assessor of cosmetic products since they are obtained from the intended target species. Ethical considerations relating to the use of human volunteers must be evaluated carefully [14], but human data may come from a variety of sources:

> *Market experience.* A history of safe use of the substance in similar products for a substantial period of time is a valuable benchmark against which to judge the proposed product.
>
> *Human volunteer studies.* A variety of studies in which volunteers are deliberately exposed to the substance in question or to a formulated product again provides good background data. These may be in-use or preference trials of the market research kind, efficacy trials under clinical conditions, or clinical tests to determine kinetic data [15,16].
>
> *Accidents and industrial exposures.* The literature may record incidents in which humans have been exposed to the substance and provide descriptions of the consequences. The details surrounding such incidents are of vital importance if their relevance to cosmetic use is to be assessed accurately.
>
> *Epidemiology studies.* Epidemiology studies require particular care in their interpretation. By their very nature they are inherently subject to bias and the influence of confounding variables. Although epidemiology studies may indicate an association or link between two factors, by itself such a link, even if statistically significant, is not necessarily of biological significance and should not be taken as indicative of a causal relationship. Even if the results of one study are replicated in others, each may have suffered from the same bias or failed to have controlled the same confounding factors.
>
> When reviewing epidemiology studies as part of a safety assessment program, the original reports should certainly be evaluated by an expert in this field if the risk of being misled is to be avoided.
>
> In spite of this, epidemiology data have a very real part to play in the safety assessment of cosmetic products both prospectively, when a review of the consequences of past exposure aids future safety predictions, and retrospectively, in establishing that past exposures have not led to damage to human health. Since most human exposure to cosmetic ingredients outside the industrial setting is to low doses but for prolonged periods, epidemiological methods are likely to become ever more pertinent.

At this stage, data will have been accumulated on each of the ingredients and, to some extent, on the finished product itself or on comparable products. These data will be incomplete; that is inevitable. Even so, the safety assessor must now consider whether there is enough data to proceed or whether vital information is missing and must be made available first.

Moving on at this time does not preclude a return to this point in the future to obtain further data to clarify issues or questions as they arise. Figure 1 provides

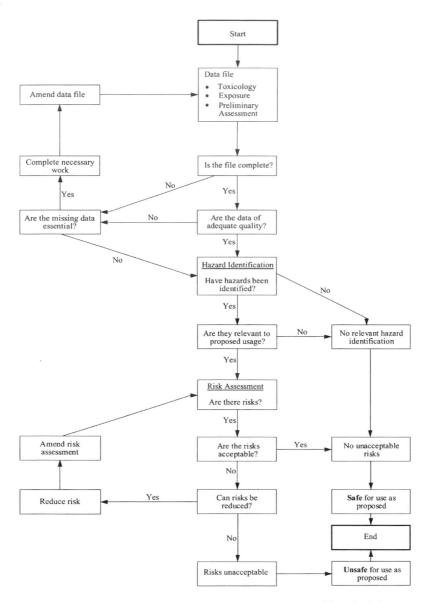

Figure 1 General safety assessment decision tree. The decision tree provides a structured approach to the safety assessment of an individual ingredient. By starting with the accumulated data relating to that ingredient and working through the tree one eventually reaches the end via the conclusion that the ingredient is either safe or unsafe for use as proposed. The same tree can also be used when making the final safety assessment of the proposed cosmetic product.

a decision tree applicable to evaluating individual substances and, by analogy, completed products by guiding the safety assessor through the sequence of questions in a logical manner.

If vital information on potential hazards are not available, effort to uncover them must be made. Previous literature searches could be extended and additional suppliers questioned. Should vital data not exist, then no further progress on establishing the safety of a product is possible until those data are generated. The viability of the project as a whole will need to be reassessed, taking account of the time and cost involved in any proposed testing and the risk that the data generated will not actually support the safety of the product. The possibility of generating adverse data must be faced in a realistic manner.

In addition, if the data can only be obtained by animal testing, the client or company policy on that issue must be fully understood and followed, as must the legislation applicable in the territory concerned. This chapter is not the appropriate place for a discussion of the question of animal testing [17,18]. Instead, if an animal study is the only way of obtaining vital data which are not available by any other means and if company policy (and legal issues) allow such studies, they must be carried out to the highest scientific standards and with full regard to the three Rs of reduction, refinement, and replacement. Guidelines on the testing of substances specifically for use as cosmetic ingredients are available [19,20].

> *Reduction,* of course, means using the fewest animals consistent with the scientific objective being pursued, but an adequate number is still required. If too few are used such that a poor study is carried out, in effect all those animals will have been wasted. Therefore, experimental design and statistical interpretation are vital factors to be considered and should be fully evaluated before any study is commissioned.
>
> *Refinement* means that the procedure adopted should produce the least stress, discomfort, or interference with the animals' normal functioning, physiology, and well being as possible, consistent with aims and purpose of the study. Remember that a stressed animal will rarely respond normally and abnormal responses can compromise the integrity of the study. In any study, good science must be the goal, for good science is compatible with the three Rs; bad science is not.
>
> *Replacement* can mean more than simply replacing an animal study with an alternative not involving animals. By extension, it can also mean replacing the particular ingredient with another for which testing is not required or it may mean replacing animal test data with analogy, interpretation, or calculation to see whether the data are, in fact, needed. Replacement presents an opportunity to recheck the need for an animal study before it commences. However, the absence of animal test data has been used to criticize the use of some ingredients and as an opportunity to challenge industry in the past.

2.12 Risk Characterization

This is the second main step of the safety assessment process and it is the one where all the hazard data on each of the ingredients are given a review with the aim of categorizing them in the light of information relating to likely exposure. In essence, this is the first step in converting hazard identification into risk assessment. At this stage the safety assessor needs to be familiar with the mode of use of the cosmetic product.

Hazards that are only manifest under conditions quite unrelated to the anticipated usage can be put to one side. For example, lung damage following inhalation is a hazard that presents an unlikely risk if that ingredient cannot be inhaled, such as when used in a skin lotion. Similarly, liver enzyme induction following prolonged ingestion is a hazard that would be unlikely to present a risk from most topical cosmetics. In each case, the rationale for categorizing each hazard from each ingredient as an unlikely risk should be recorded.

Conversely, hazards that might related to actual usage conditions need to be identified for priority consideration. For example, severe irritation or corrosivity associated with an ingredient for a leave-on cosmetic needs to be noted, as does inhalation toxicity with an ingredient of an aerosol. At this time, there should be no attempt to quantify the risk; the purpose of risk characterization is to identify for further assessment hazards that may pose risks.

There will be a number of ingredients which present hazards whose significance is not clear at this stage and need to be assigned to a third, intermediate category for further consideration, for example, toxicity following ingestion of a substance destined for use in an oral care product or lip product.

Risk characterization therefore results in a list of potential high risks where an evaluation of the actual risk should begin, a list of moderate or unknown risks that need to be evaluated next, and a third category or low of unlikely risks that can be double-checked last. Taken together, they begin to build up a picture of where any risks to human health may lie with the product and, inevitably, allow a degree of assessment as to the final level of confidence in the product safety. This then leads into the third step, risk evaluation.

2.13 Risk Evaluation

Although the distinction between risk characterization and risk evaluation is, in some respects, artificial, nevertheless it does represent a shift of emphasis from deciding whether the identified hazards present risks in general terms (and in what priority should they be handled) to a more specific quantification of the individual risks as they apply to the product in question.

In this step, each high priority hazard is considered in the context of the use of that substance in the product. The chance or likelihood that any particular hazard would manifest itself as harmful needs to be weighed in terms of likely severity of adverse effect and in the frequency or likely prevalence of adverse effect. In turn, these will depend on exposure (concentration of the substance in the product, quantity of product used at each application, and frequency of use) and numbers of people exposed.

It is at the risk evaluation stage that the safety assessor needs to know likely consumer exposure, in terms of quantity of product used and concentration of substance in the product. Also to be considered at this stage is whether the cosmetic product is intended for any special category of consumers (e.g., products for infants or products intended for people with sensitive skin) as this may affect likely exposure patterns or possible susceptibility of the consumer to adverse reactions.

2.14　Safety Assessment

This is the final step in the process of determining whether a particular cosmetic product is likely to be safe for release to the market. The final decision is rarely easy and rarely straightforward.

Of course, there may be occasions when the product being assessed is but a minor variation on a well-known product with a long history of safety in use. Approval is readily granted and the certainty factor is high.

Alternatively, the product under investigation may be judged to present clear and unacceptable risks to human health and, again, a decision is readily taken with a high certainty factor, but this time it is a decision not to market.

However, in the majority of cases, the decision will only be made after a reappraisal of the data to hand and a reassessment of the risks involved. The objective is to reduce the uncertainty involved in making the decision and to increase personal confidence. Remember, the underlying basis of the decision is a positive approval saying the product is safe to market and it is that decision that must be justifiable.

What then are the actual steps that need to be completed to justify the marketing decision? First, the hazards from each ingredient will have been listed, the relevant ones identified and those of little or no relevance placed to one side, with a note of justification. Second, the likelihood of each hazard being manifest will have been judged based on the human exposure, in turn based on the concentration of the ingredient, the quantity and frequency of use, the mode of use, and the particular characteristics of the intended consumers and their numbers.

By this time, only those risks judged likely to be of relevance to the consumer remain to be assessed. This judgment cannot be performed in isolation; it must be gauged against established criteria, yardsticks, or benchmarks. The experienced safety assessor working within an established product field will have ready access to such benchmarks from historical records which will justify the acceptance of certain levels of risk. For example, the acceptability of a new shampoo can be judged quite accurately by comparison of its formula with that of established products.

If no such benchmark is apparent, then other ways are needed to achieve a resolution. For example, if an ingredient is found to contain variable amounts of an impurity shown to be a genotoxic carcinogen and no substitute is available, can that ingredient be used and, if so, what impurity limits should be set?

In such a circumstance, one would look to quantifying the risk over a lifetime of exposure and working back from a value deemed acceptable (the benchmark, in this case, is therefore the acceptable lifetime risk figure) to set a limit for the level of that impurity in the final product. If the impurity level can be maintained below the limit, the product would have an acceptable safety assessment, but if the impurity level exceeds the limit, the product must be rejected.

Such calculations are relatively common in the assessment of exposure to toxic substances in an industrial setting or in assessing the consequences of exposure to toxic substances present in the environment. Therefore, the safety assessor of cosmetic products must have an awareness of toxicology in its broadest sense if support is to be sought from related fields.

Having established that neither the ingredients nor their impurities constitute an unacceptable risk to human health in the proposed product, there needs to be a final re-evaluation of the finished product. The safety assessor needs to check that the combination of impurities from different sources does not become excessive or that exposure to two or more substances in combination might not compromise safety. Finally, there should be a simple logic check in which the safety assessor reflects upon the decision made and the level of confidence. Are there doubts? Can they be expressed and dealt with? Is the labeling adequate or excessive? Only when all these voices have been answered can the safety assessor say the assessment stage has been completed.

Having decided that the proposed cosmetic is safe for marketing to the public, the safety assessor must communicate this information to colleagues and must also ensure any caveats are understood. The simplest way is to issue a signed document stating exactly which formula has been assessed, when, and by whom; the outcome of that assessment; and most importantly any restrictions that are to be applied.

For example, the safety assessor may approve the product only if the level of a certain impurity is controlled either in one of the raw materials or in the finished product itself, or only if a specific warning phrase is present on the pack (in addition to any mandatory warnings), or only if the pack has a child-resistant closure, etc.

The safety assessor may, if necessary, issue a provisional approval for limited release to the market, with full approval only being granted following an evaluation of the feedback from the market. Postmarketing surveillance is discussed later.

An outline of a suitable document is provided as Fig. 2. The safety assessor should include a copy of such a document with a full report of the safety assessment. Whilst the report need not include copies of all scientific papers and study reports consulted, these should be referenced and stored in a library or archive. The report should be a logical argument of the process by which the assessor reached the conclusion that the cosmetic product was safe to market. In particular, it should refer to the ingredients and their toxicological profile and to any interactions or combined effects likely from the finished product.

3 POSTMARKETING SURVEILLANCE

The EU Cosmetics Directive requires a manufacturer to maintain a record of adverse reactions to a cosmetic product. Such records, whether or not they are required by law, can provide essential data for the safety assessor. In essence, they provide evidence indicating whether the decision to market was correct.

Adverse reactions are generally held to be those that

Involve an identified individual
Are directly related to a specific product
Are verified by an appropriate professional (doctor, dentist, nurse, etc.)

Unless all three conditions are met, it is not possible to be sure that an adverse reaction actually occurred or that the cause was the product in question.

The background level of adverse reactions to cosmetic products is low, with there being typically only one reaction for every several hundred thousand or even million units sold. Should the frequency of adverse reactions rise, the safety assessor should be informed of this fact and of the nature of those reactions. Such figures could be indicative of a previously unsuspected problem arising or they could mean nothing more than a chance cluster of events.

The rarity of adverse reactions to cosmetics is both testimony to the safety of this class of consumer product and an indicator of the problem facing the safety assessor; even an unacceptable level of adverse events of, say, 1 in 10,000 is still a very rare event. Animal studies, in vitro studies, and even human volunteer studies are statistically quite incapable of detecting so low an incidence, much less determining the difference between two similar products, unless exposure conditions are exaggerated to the point of being provocative. That is the reason any studies are carried out under exaggerated conditions, so that a comparison can be made between the proposed product and a benchmark control. Postmarketing surveillance provides the evidence to justify the decision made to proceed to market.

STATEMENT OF OPINION

Statement number:
Version number:
Date of issue:
Supersedes statement number:

I, (name of safety assessor), am a (registered medical practitioner/registered pharmacist/chartered biologist/chartered chemist) duly authorized according to The Cosmetic Products (Safety) Regulations 1996, as amended, to conduct and take responsibility for the safety assessment of cosmetic products. The following statement has been prepared in accordance with those Regulations and, in particular, Regulation 3, 8(1)(d), 8(1)(e), 8(2) and 8(3).

Product name (brand and variant):
Formula reference number:

Taking into consideration the general toxicological profile of each ingredient used, its chemical structure and its level of exposure, the presentation of the product, its labeling and instructions for use and disposal and any other information provided, it is my opinion that the cosmetic product identified above is not liable to cause damage to human health when it is applied under normal or reasonably foreseeable conditions of use.

This statement of opinion is valid only for the product that complies with the following specific, additional requirements:

(List here those restrictions, if any, deemed to be applicable or state NONE.)

This statement is valid until (specify expiry date, if applicable.)

Signature of safety assessor: _____

Date of signing: _____

Name and qualifications:

Address:

Figure 2 Safety assessment statement of opinion. This general format may be adapted to suit the specific regulations applicable in a territory. It provides formal documentary evidence that a specific product and formula has been assessed by a named person and is an unambiguous presentation of the opinion of the safety assessor.

Although the frequency of true or verifiable adverse reactions to cosmetic products is low, most manufacturers receive a number of customer complaints. Those that allege adverse reactions, particularly if the allegations are of severe or potentially long-lasting effects, need to be handled sympathetically by a specialist from within the company. Although many of these allegations may turn out to be groundless, some may become verified as true reactions. In any event, the pattern of complaints must be monitored and the data made available to the safety assessor. How they are handled will also reflect the public image projected by the company.

A higher level of customer complaints does not of itself indicate a safety issue, but it could be indicative of poor consumer acceptance. This is clearly of importance to the manufacturer. A transient rise in complaints frequently follows the launch of a new product or relaunch of a previous one. However, if the increase fails to fall back to the level expected from past experience, the nature of the complaints should be investigated. Remedial action may be warranted.

4 CRISIS MANAGEMENT

In the worst circumstances, a sudden rise in the number or severity of complaints could indicate a serious fault in a batch of product, with possible implications for human health. Alternatively, a new hazard may become apparent and require remedial action. Manufacturers should have a plan prepared to manage such a crisis, and the safety assessor should be part of the crisis management team. His knowledge and expertise will be vital in helping to decide whether the problem might even require product recall and stock uplift.

5 SUMMARY

This chapter has tried to show not only what is involved is the safety assessment of cosmetic products and how to go about the process itself, but also to indicate the central role a safety assessor can play in a cosmetic company. That role can extend far beyond a simple "pass or fail" statement on the safety of a proposed new product.

Safety assessors should be involved in project development planning and in ensuring that adequate time is allowed for the safety assessment. They should be involved in product formula development to advise of possible ingredient safety issues throughout the development. They should be involved with marketing and advertizing and with product packaging and labeling, etc. Finally, they should be involved with customer relations and with crisis management. All of these supplement their primary role of actually assessing product safety prior to launch. If utilized fully, the safety assessor can avert many problems early in product development and so directly contribute to effective use of time and resources.

It has been said that anyone can become a toxicologist in two easy lessons, each of which takes ten years. To that I would add that the safety assessment of cosmetic products also requires experience.

REFERENCES

1. Organisation for Economic Co-operation and Development. OECD Guidelines for Testing of Chemicals. Section 4, Health Effects. Paris: OECD.
2. de Groot AC. Adverse Reactions to Cosmetics. Groningen, The Netherlands: State University of Gronongen, 1988.
3. Colipa. Guidelines for the safety assessment of a cosmetic product. Brussels: Colipa, 1997.
4. SCCNFP. Opinion concerning the revision of annex 7 of the notes for guidance for the safety assessment of the finished cosmetic product. Brussels: European Commission, 24 October 2000. http://europa.eu.int/comm/food/fs/sc/sccp/out 129_en.html
5. International Fragrance Association. Code of Practice. 33rd amendment. Geneva: IFRA, 1999.
6. Cosmetic Ingredient Review. 2000 CIR Compendium. Washington, D.C.: CIR, 2000.
7. SCCNFP. Opinion of the SCCNFP concerning basic requirements for toxicological dossiers to be evaluated by the SCCNFP. Brussels: European Commission, 17 February 2000. http://europa.eu.int/comm/food/fs/sc/sccp/out111_en.html
8. SCCNFP. Opinion on in vitro methods to assess percutaneous absorption of cosmetic ingredients. Brussels: European Commission, 20 January 1999. http://europa.eu.int/comm/food/fs/sc/sccp/out48_en.html
9. SCCNFP. Opinion concerning basic criteria for the in vitro assessment of percutaneous absorption of cosmetic ingredients. Brussels: European Commission, 23 June 1999. http://europa.eu.int/comm/food/fs/sc/sccp/out86_en.html
10. SCCNFP. Opinion concerning the predictive testing of potentially cutaneous sensitising mixtures of ingredients. Brussels: European Commission, 17 February, 2000. http://europa.eu.int/comm/food/fs/sc/sccp/out102_en.html
11. National Institute of Environmental Health Sciences. The murine local lymph node assay: a test method for assessing the allergic contact dermatitis potential of chemicals/compounds. NIH publication No. 99-4494. Bethesda: NIEHS, 1999.
12. European Commission. Commission Directive 2000/33/EC of 25 April 2000 adapting to technical progress for the 27th time Council Directive 67/548/EEC on the approximation of laws, regulations and administrative provisions relating to the classification, packaging and labelling of dangerous substances. In vitro tests for: B40—skin corrosion and for B41—phototoxicity, in vitro 3T3 NRU phototoxicity test. Official Journal of the European Communities, 2000; L136:90–107.
13. SCCNFP. Opinion on the in vitro methods to assess phototoxicity in the safety evaluation of cosmetic ingredients or mixtures of ingredients. Brussels: European Commission, 25 November 1998. http://europa.eu.int/comm/food/fs/sc/sccp/out46_en.html

14. SCCNFP. Opinion—guidelines on the use of human volunteers in the testing of potentially cutaneous irritant cosmetic ingredients or mixtures of ingredients. Brussels: European Commission, 25 November 1998. http://europa.eu.int/comm/food/fs/sc/sccp/out45_en.html

15. SCCNFP. Opinion concerning guidelines on the use of human volunteers in compatibility testing of finished cosmetic products. Brussels: European Commission, 23 June 1999. http://europa.eu.int/comm/food/fs/sc/sccp/out87_en.html

16. SCCNFP. Opinion concerning basic criteria of the protocols for the skin compatibility testing of potentially cutaneous irritant ingredients or mixtures of ingredients on human volunteers. Brussels: European Commission, 18 December 1999, SCCNFP/0245/99/final. http://europa.eu.int/comm/food/fs/sc/sccp/out101_en.pdf

17. SCCNFP. Opinion concerning the present development and validation of adequate alternative methodologies to the use of animals in safety testing of cosmetics. Brussels: European Commission, 23 June 1999. http://europa.eu.int/comm/food/fs/sc/sccp/out84_en.html

18. SCCNFP. Opinion on the use of alternative methods to animal testing in the safety evaluation of cosmetic ingredients (with three annexes) and the updating of notes of guidance for testing of cosmetic ingredients for their safety evaluation (with two annexes). Brussels: European Commission, 20 January 1999. http://europa.eu.int/comm/food/fs/sc/sccp/out49_en.html

19. SCCNFP. Notes of guidance for testing of cosmetic ingredients for their safety evaluation. 3d revision. Brussels: European Commission, 23 June 1999. SCCNFP/0119/99/final. http://europa.eu.int/comm/food/fs/sc/sccp/out12_en.pdf

20. SCCNFP. Notes of guidance for testing of cosmetic ingredients for their safety evaluation. Brussels: European Commission, 24 October 2000, SCCNFP/0321/00.

28

Regulatory Assessment of Cosmetic Products

Simon Young

Unilever Research, Port Sunlight Laboratory,
Bebington, Wirral, United Kingdom

1 INTRODUCTION

This chapter is not intended to offer the reader an extended view of the history or theory of the regulation of skin moisturization products. It is intended to focus on the regulations which affect the development and marketing of such products in Europe, offer a practical guide to ensuring that products comply with these regulations, and give a very brief overview of cosmetic regulations in the United States and Japan.

2 CONTROL OF COSMETIC PRODUCTS IN THE EUROPEAN COMMUNITY

The Cosmetic Products Directive (76/768/EC [1] as amended) has two main aims, first, to ensure consumer safety and, second, to create a single European market for cosmetic products to enable free trade. The requirement for product safety is enshrined in Article 2 of the directive and is dealt with extensively by another chapter of this book. Free trade is enabled by common rules on what constitutes a cosmetic product, ingredients, labeling and data requirements which have been enacted in member state legislation in response to the directive.

2.1 Definition of a Cosmetic Product in the EU

Article 1 of the Cosmetic Products Directive gives the following definition of a cosmetic

> A cosmetic product shall mean any substance or preparation intended to be placed in contact with the various external parts of the human body (epidermis, hair system, nails, lips and external genital organs) or with the teeth and the mucous membranes of the oral cavity with a view exclusively or mainly to cleaning them, perfuming them, changing their appearance and/or correcting body odours and/or protecting them or keeping them in good condition.

Further clarification of what constitutes a cosmetic product is given in Annex I of the Directive. This is an "illustrative list" and is not exhaustive. It was put in place when the directive was first produced to give clarity as to what kinds of products should be considered to be included within the scope of cosmetic products. This list includes product types, such as antiperspirants and anti-dandruff shampoos that are regulated in other markets either as medicines or in a class (or classes) between cosmetics and medicines. Examples of these systems are over-the-counter (OTC) drugs in the United States, quasi-drugs (Japan), specially-controlled cosmetics (Thailand) and Risk Category 2 cosmetics (Brazil). Products fall into these categories either by virtue of making specific functional claims or by containing nominated functional ingredients. The level of safety and efficacy support required for these intermediate classes is generally between that of a cosmetic and that of a drug.

2.1.2 Borderline Products in the European Union

There is an overlap between the definitions of cosmetic products and medicinal products within European regulations. Current EC regulations that cover the borderline area are the Cosmetics Directive (76/768/EC as amended) and the Medicines Directive (65/65/EC [2] as amended). These provide definitions of cosmetic and medicine as follows:

> A cosmetic is

> Any substance or preparation intended to be placed in contact with the external parts of the human body . . . or with the teeth and the mucous membranes of the oral cavity with a view exclusively or mainly for cleaning them, perfuming them, changing their appearance and/or correcting body odours and/or protecting or keeping them in good condition.

> A medicinal product is

> Any substance or combination of substances presented for treating or preventing disease in human beings or animals *or* Any substance or

combination of substances which may be administered to human beings or animals with a view to making a medical diagnosis or to restoring, correcting or modifying physiological functions in human beings or animals.

When the Cosmetics Directive was enacted in 1976, the Council of Europe was aware of the possibility of an overlap between the definition of a cosmetic and a medicine and that some products could fall under both regimes. In an attempt to avoid this, the Council made it clear in the preamble to the Cosmetics Directive that it intended to draw a dividing line between medicines and cosmetics. The recital reads

Whereas this Directive relates only to cosmetic products and not to pharmaceutical specialities and medicinal products; whereas for this purpose it is necessary to define the scope of the Directive by delimiting the field of cosmetics from that of pharmaceuticals; whereas this delimitation follows in particular from the detailed definition of cosmetic products which refers both to their areas of application and to the purposes of use; whereas this Directive is not applicable to products that fall under the definition of cosmetic products but are exclusively intended to protect from disease.

In order to understand the thought processes behind the words it does help to look at the way that the original 1976 definition was modified in 1993 [3].
Original:

Any substance or preparation intended for placing in contact with the external parts of the human body . . . or with the teeth and the mucous membranes of the oral cavity with a view exclusively or principally to cleaning them,[1] perfuming them[2] or protecting them[3] in order to keep them in good condition,[4] change their appearance[5] or correct body odour.[6]

Current

Any substance or preparation intended to be placed in contact with the external parts of the human body . . . or with the teeth and the mucous membranes of the oral cavity with a view exclusively or mainly for cleaning them,[7] perfuming them,[8] changing their appearance[9] and/or correcting body odours[10] and/or protecting[11] or keeping them in good condition.[12]

By removing the words "in order to" and replacing the three functions [1–3] and three objectives [4–6] by six individual purposes [7–12], the 1993 definition removes several legal anomalies including the one that effectively excluded all decorative products from being cosmetics.

It should be noted that the phrase "exclusively or principally" has been changed to "exclusively or mainly" reinforcing the fact that the regulators recognize that cosmetic products may have functions other than those six individually listed.

While the Medicinal Products Directive defines a products presented for treating or preventing a disease as a medicine, the Cosmetics Directive implies that a product intended for external application with a view exclusively or mainly for one of the six cosmetic purposes could remain a cosmetic provided that it is not exclusively or mainly intended to protect from disease. This has been interpreted in most member states of Europe as meaning that a cosmetic product could have a secondary, minor therapeutic function provided that its prime purpose was a cosmetic one. An example of this is the marketing of sensitive teeth toothpastes as cosmetic products in all EC member states with the exception of the United Kingdom. Here there is clearly some overlap between the two definitions. Cosmetics sometimes claim to prevent disease, e.g., use of a fluoride toothpaste reduces the incidence of caries and use of a sensitive teeth toothpaste reduces the perception of dentinal sensitivity. The cosmetics directive states that cosmetic products must deliver "exclusively or mainly" the types of cosmetic benefits listed in the definition. However, the word "mainly" means that a cosmetic product can make a therapeutic claim as long as this is secondary to the cosmetic claim. This is supported by the preamble in the Cosmetics Directive that "This directive is not applicable to cosmetic products . . . exclusively intended to protect from disease." In the case of a toothpaste the primary cosmetic function is to clean and keep the teeth in good condition, the secondary function is to reduce the incidence of caries. If the product contains fluoride at a cosmetically acceptable level (<1500 ppm), it is classified as a cosmetic. If a similar product had no cleaning function or contained fluoride at >1500 ppm, it would be classified as a medicine.

It can also be argued that cosmetics often "restore, correct or modify physiological function." Indeed it would be difficult to identify any product applied to the skin that had no effect at all on physiological function. Again this is an area of overlap between the definitions of a cosmetic and a drug. The decision as to whether the product should be regulated as a cosmetic or not is made by each national authority in the light of a number of factors. For example, will the averagely well-informed consumer think that they are buying a medicine? This will be largely driven by the claims made in the context of the product and its presentation as a whole. Does the product claim to treat or prevent a disease or to interfere with the normal operation of a physiological function of the human body. Other factors that will be taken into account by the competent authorities in making this decision will include

Medicinal implications of the product name, e.g., UlcerOut.
Medicinal presentation of the product, e.g., as a tablet, or in a package typ-

ically used for medicines, or sold in pharmacies next to medicinal products.

Medicinal implications of data made available to the public by the marketing company which reports a therapeutic effect. This is true whether it is given directly through advertisements and helplines or indirectly via a third party, e.g., in a newspaper article to which the marketer has contributed.

Medicinal implications of specifically marketing the product at particular sections of the population with, or vulnerable to, a specific adverse condition.

Each country in Europe independently controls what claims are permitted for cosmetic products in their own market. There is no central EU list of permitted and banned claims for cosmetics and there is no central EU organization responsible for deciding whether a claim is cosmetic or medicinal for the following reasons:

Culture, historical treatment of products, habits, and attitudes vary from country to country. The acceptability of claims in each country must be assessed by local nationals for local nationals.

Claims are made up of words which communicate a subtle message to consumers in the context of their own language and culture. Translation of a common list into all of the languages of the EU would lead to differences in meaning.

Any list of claims would require constant revision and agreement at technical, bureaucratic, and political levels between all 15 countries to cover new, innovative product types and claims. This would create an enormous workload and lead to long delays to new product/claim introduction.

Industry can be very creative in developing new products and wording new claims to avoid rigid positive and negative lists.

The current approach allows for rapid classification of completely new product types and claims using the rationale and tools laid down by the EU as interpreted by local regulators.

Confirmation of this of this national approach was given by the European Court of Justice (ECJ) in 1988. The Medicines Directive defines a medicinal product partly by its action on disease. However, it does not actually define what constitutes a disease. When this was examined by the ECJ they decided that

It is for the national authorities to determine, subject to judicial review, whether or not, having regard to its composition, the risk which its prolonged consumption may entail or its side-effects and, more generally, all of its characteristics, a product presented as counteracting certain conditions or sensations, such as hunger, heaviness in the legs, tiredness or itching constitutes a medicinal product.

The case of Delattre was referred to the European Court of Justice for consideration and decision on what constituted a medicinal product (Case C-369/88[1991] ECR 1487). The Court ruled that

> A product may be regarded as being presented as a medicine if its form and the manner in which it is packaged render it sufficiently similar to a medicinal product and, in particular, if on its packaging and in the information provided with it reference is made to research by pharmaceutical laboratories, to methods or substances developed by medical practitioners or even to certain testimonials from medical practitioners commending the qualities of the product. A statement that the product is not medical is persuasive evidence which the national court may take into consideration but is not, in itself, conclusive.

One of the few borderline cases which has come to the European Court of Justice for resolution was that of *Upjohn vs. Farzoo* (Case C-112/89 [1991] ECR I-1703) in which Farzoo was marketing Upjohn's minoxidil-based hair growth product Regaine® in the Netherlands as a cosmetic product. Upjohn claimed that this was against EC law as the product was a medicine. In its judgement the ECJ decided for Upjohn, rejecting the claim of Farzoo that a medicine could only be defined in relation to the notion of illness. The ECJ also clarified that the definition of a medicine that Regaine fell under was the second definition, i.e., "restoring, correcting or modifying physiological functions . . . (65/65/EC)." The key sections of the judgement are as follows:

21. With regard to what must be understood by "to restore, correct or modify physiological function" . . . this expression must be understood in a manner which is sufficiently wide so as to include all substances which may have an effect on the function of the body.
22. However this criterion does not include substances which while having an influence on the human body, as for instance certain cosmetics, do not have a significant effect on the metabolism which therefore strictly speaking do not modify the condition of its function.
23. It is necessary for the national judge to proceed case by case on the necessary categorization taking account of the pharmacological properties of the product and the consideration of its methods of use, the extent of its distribution, and the knowledge of its customers.

2.2 The Sixth Amendment

In 1993 major modifications were made to the Cosmetics Directive by the sixth amendment Council Directive (93/35/EEC[4]), the most significant of which addressed

Ingredient labeling
Product information requirements
Implications of animal testing

2.2.1 Ingredient labeling

Article 6 of the Cosmetics Directive lists labeling requirements for cosmetic products. The sixth amendment introduced a requirement for a label on the outer package to carry a list of all ingredients. Prior to the sixth amendment, the only ingredients which had to be designated on the label were those mandated within the annexes of the directive.

Article 6(1)(g) of the amended directive requires that all ingredients are labeled by descending order of weight at the time that they were added. Once the list reaches those ingredients added at less than 1%, it does not need to be in weight order.

The nomenclature used should be the common names adopted by the European Commission. Article 5a of the Cosmetics Directive established an inventory of these names. Since the publication of the original inventory of cosmetic ingredients in June 1996 there have been approximately 1500 additions and 900 changes made. The Scientific Committee on Cosmetics and Non-Food Products (SCCNFP) published the first update of the inventory, adopted 28 June 2000, on the internet at http://europa.eu.int/comm/food/fs/sc/sccp/out123_en.pdf

International Nomenclature of Cosmetic Ingredients (INCI) names for novel ingredients can be easily obtained by submission of a package of chemicophysical data on the substance to the INCI Committee with a suggested INCI name. To address concerns of trade secrecy Commission Directive 95/17/EC established a provision that enables manufactures to request a code number instead of an INCI name for ingredient listing. Once granted, confidentiality codes may be used for up to 5 years and may be extended for a further 3 years.

Exceptions from these general ingredient labeling rules are as follows:

Ingredients added for the purposes of flavor or fragrance do not need to be named but can be covered by the terms "aroma" or "parfum."

Raw material impurities do not have to be listed, neither do subsidiary technical materials such as solvents or perfume carriers used in strictly necessary quantities.

For color cosmetics, the label can mention all of the colors in the product range.

2.2.2 Product Information

Probably the greatest change to the Cosmetics Directive introduced by the sixth amendment was the requirement for every party responsible for placing a cosmetic product on the market in the European Community to maintain certain data readily accessible to government authorities. These data must be kept readily available at an address specified on the product label. The information required is as follows:

> The qualitative and quantitative composition of the product (in the case of perfume compositions and perfumes, the name and code number of the composition and the identity of the supplier).
>
> The physicochemical and microbiological specifications of the raw materials and the finished product and the purity and microbiological content of the cosmetic product.
>
> The method of manufacture complying with good manufacturing practice laid down by Community law or, failing that, laid down by the law of the member state concerned. The person responsible for manufacture or first importation into the Community must possess an appropriate level of professional qualification or experience in accordance with the legislation and practice of the member state which is the place of manufacture or first importation.
>
> An assessment of the safety for human health of the finished product.
>
> The name and address of the qualified person/people responsible for the safety assessment. They must hold a diploma as defined in Article 1 of Directive 89/48/EC in the filed of pharmacy, toxicology, dermatology, medicine, or a similar discipline.
>
> Existing data on undesirable effects on human health resulting from use of the cosmetic product.
>
> Proof of the effect claimed for the cosmetic product, where justified by the nature of the effect or product.

This information is the property of the company but may be viewed by the competent authority designated by the government in each member state. The data package has to be readily accessible to the competent authority. It is generally accepted that 24–72 hours is considered an adequate response time.

2.2.3 Implications of Animal Testing

The use of animals for safety and efficacy testing is an emotive issue in Europe which has ethical, political, and technical aspects, and it is right that the use of animals in testing of cosmetic products and ingredients is subject to scrutiny. In regulatory terms, Article 2 of the Cosmetics Directive demands that a cosmetic product put on the market within the Community must not cause damage to human health when applied under normal or reasonably foreseeable conditions of use. Article 7 of the directive then states that ". . . the manufacturer shall take into consideration the general toxicological profile of the (cosmetic) ingredient, its chemical structure and its level of exposure."

Although there are no set methodologies imposed by the cosmetics directive to enable this safety assessment to be performed, there is some guidance from the Commission's Scientific Committee on Cosmetics and Non-Food Products. ("See Notes for Guidance on the Safety Assessment of Cosmetic Ingredients," SCCNFP, 1997). Some animal-based toxicological tests, used to ensure the safety of pharmaceuticals, agrochemicals, dangerous substances, etc., are recommended. These test methods are detailed in The Organisation of Economic Co-operation and Development (OECD) publications and have been incorporated into EU legislation as Annex V test methods for the Dangerous Substances Directive [5].

In 1993, the sixth amendment addressed concerns regarding the use of animal testing by the cosmetics and associated industries by including the clause "Member States . . . shall prohibit the marketing of cosmetic products containing ingredients or combinations of ingredients tested on animals after 1 January 1998 in order to meet the requirements of this Directive." This amendment also acknowledged that prohibition depended on the development of satisfactory, validated, nonanimal alternative tests, and made provision for a postponement for not less than 2 years if the alternative methods were not available. Following a review of progress toward validation of nonanimal methodologies carried out in 1997 the marketing ban was postponed until 30 June 2000, with provision for a further reassessment of progress by 1 January 2000.

2.3 Control of Ingredients

When assessing an ingredient for use in a cosmetic formulation to be marketed within the European Community there are two principal pieces of regulation to be considered. First, the Dangerous Substances Directive and, second, the Cosmetics Directive.

2.3.1 The Dangerous Substances Directive

The aim of the Dangerous Substances Directive (67/548/EC [5] as amended) is to protect people and the environment from the possible harmful effects of chemical substances and to create a single market in new substances across the EU. It aims to reinforce the latter by ensuring that chemical notification requirements are identical in all 15 member states and that there is mutual recognition of notifications, i.e., a notification accepted in one member state is valid for all of them.

This regulation was issued in the form of a European Directive and has been enacted into national legislation by member states. Each member state has designated its own competent authority which has the responsibility of running the system. In the United Kingdom the competent authority is the Health and Safety Executive and the Department of the Environment, acting jointly.

From the perspective of the Dangerous Substances Directive (DSD), potential ingredients for cosmetic products for the European market are considered to be one of the following:

Existing chemical substances
Notified chemical substances
New chemical substances

If the ingredient is either existing or notified, then no further action will be required with reference to the DPD by the cosmetic formulator. If the ingredient is new, then it has to be notified before use in a cosmetic product unless covered by one of the exemptions described here in Section 2.4.5.

In terms of structures, the DSD has three important components, a closed inventory [6], an open inventory [7], and a notification process.

The European Inventory of Existing Chemical Substances (EINECS). This is a list of over 100,000 substances which were on the European market between 1 January 1971 and 18 September 1981. Substances on this list are considered to be "existing" as opposed to "new." The list is "closed" in that no substances can be added to it. The EINECS was published in the *Official Journal* of the European Community on 15 June 1990 (Vol. C146A). Substances on this list carry a number of the format 2XX-XXX-X or 3XX-XXX-X.

The European List of Notified (New) Chemical Substances (ELINCS). Since 1981 any substance placed on the European market which was not included in EINECS has had to be notified to one of the member state competent authorities. The process is described briefly in the next subsection. The successful outcome being that the new substance is added to the ELINCS list and becomes a notified substance. These are given an ELINCS number in the format 4XX-XXX-X.

Notification Process. The notification process involves submission of a package of physicochemical characterization, toxicology, and ecotoxicology data to the competent authority. The nature and level of data required are proportional to the annual and cumulative tonnage of the material to be placed on the market in the EU and are defined in the regulations. Receipt of this data submission is formally acknowledged by the competent authority, and unless the notifier is contacted within 30 or 60 days (dependent upon the level of the notification) of this acknowledgement then the material may be placed on the market. It is strongly advised that discussions with the competent authorities on the scope of the data submission are held during the planning phase of a notification.

Practical Implications. From a practical point of view then, the first step is to determine whether the ingredient of interest already exists or has been notified. This can often be done by the supplier of the material. If this is not possible, there can be difficulties due to the differences in chemical nomenclature systems in use by chemical suppliers around the world. Identification of the chemical abstracts system (CAS) number of the material is extremely helpful as a common denominator which is used within the published EINECS/ELINCS documentation. When searching EINECS it should also be noted that not all of the entries in EINECS are for specific chemicals; many substances of plant and origin are described in more general terms.

Electronic versions of the EINECS, including annually updated copies of the ELINCS, are also available commercially and reduce search times considerably. If the ingredients of interest are already included in one of the inventories, then there is no need to notify them.

Exemptions from the Dangerous Substances Directive. In terms of the cosmetics industry in Europe there are two important exemptions from the notification requirements of the regulations.

COSMETIC PRODUCTS. New ingredients which are placed on the EU only as part of cosmetic products are exempt from notification. In practical terms this means that cosmetic products containing a new chemical substance may be imported from outside the EU without notification of that substance. This exemption does not cover new chemical substances which are manufactured by a chemical supplier within the EU for use only in cosmetic products, as the transfer between the separate legal entities of the supplier and the cosmetic company is covered by the definition of "placing the ingredient on the market."

SUBSTANCES NO LONGER POLYMERS. Polymers are treated differently from other materials by these regulations and are not subject to the same notification requirements. The definition of a polymer in the original regulation (67/548/EC) was modified in 1992 by the seventh amendment to the DSD (92/32/EC [8]), and some substances which were covered (and hence exempt from notification) by the 1967 definition of a polymer were outside the 1992 definition of a polymer given in the amending directive. Any of the materials that were inside the 1967 definition, outside the 1992 definition, and were placed on the EC market between 1 January 1971 and 1 November 1993 are considered to be exempt from notification.

SUBSTANCES TREATED AS HAVING ALREADY BEEN NOTIFIED. Three categories of notifiable chemical substances of importance to the cosmetics industry can be treated as having already been notified under the requirements of the DSD. These are technically complex and subject to interpretation by the competent authorities. It is strongly recommended that assistance and clarification are sought from the local competent authority when operating in these areas.

POLYMERS. Polymers (as defined by the directive) which meet the following conditions do not require notification:

Those which are produced by polymerization of EINECS-listed substances only.

Those which are produced by polymerization of EINECS-listed substances only, with postpolymerization reaction with another EINECS-listed substance.

Those which contain less than 2% (in bonded form) of a non–EINECS-listed substance. This includes incorporation of the non-EINECS listed substance in the initial polymerization or by postpolymerization reaction. In this case, notification may not be required if it is decided by the competent authority that the polymer is identical with an existing polymer produced with EINECS-listed substance(s) that is already available on the EU market.

NEW CHEMICAL SUBSTANCES FOR SCIENTIFIC RESEARCH AND DEVELOPMENT. Substances intended specifically for scientific research and development in quantities less than 100 kg per annum do not need to be notified to the competent authority. It should be noted that the interpretation of the scope of this exemption may vary between competent authorities, and certain information may have to be provided to the competent authority and/or maintained in-house.

NEW CHEMICAL SUBSTANCES FOR PROCESS-ORIENTATED RESEARCH AND DEVELOPMENT. Notification is not required for substances used for these purposes. However, certain information, up to that for a reduced notification at the 100 kg per annum level, does have to be provided to the competent authority. Again, it should be noted that the interpretation of the scope of this exemption may vary between competent authorities.

2.4 The Cosmetics Products Directive

Once a potential ingredient has been assessed against the Dangerous Substances Directive the next regulatory check is to ascertain whether it will be permitted for use in a cosmetic product to be placed on the market in the European Union. The Cosmetics Directive (76/768/EEC as amended) controls the use of ingredients permitted to be used in cosmetic products to be placed on the EC market by means of a negative list, a restricted list, and three positive lists. These lists are regularly updated by means of Adapting Directives which reflect advances in technical progress.

2.4.1 Annex II (The Negative List)

Annex II is a single list of over 400 substances which must not form part of the composition of cosmetic products to be placed on the EC market. It should be noted that cosmetic products may be placed on the EC market if they contain traces of these materials provided that their presence is technically unavoidable in good manufacturing practice and that they conform with the safety requirements for cosmetic products laid down in Article 2 of the Directive. Annex II includes both specific chemicals, e.g. spironolactone, and wider classes of substances, e.g., alkyne alcohols, their esters, ethers, and salts.

The remaining annexes are each divided into two parts. The first part of each annexe is a permanent list, the second a provisional list. Presence of an ingredient on a provisional list indicates that it is under review and is permitted for inclusion in cosmetic products subject to the restrictions indicated until the review date attached to the entry. After this date the material may be transferred to the permanent section of the annex, modified, deleted, or the period of review extended.

2.4.2 Annex III (The Restricted List)

Annex III lists substances which cosmetic products must not contain except subject to certain restrictions. Substances may be restricted to certain types of products, certain levels or both. The restriction may also include compulsory labeling text. An extract of an Annex III entry is shown in Table 28.1.

2.4.3 Annexes IV, VI, and VII (The Positive Lists)

These annexes mandate the ingredients that can be used as coloring agents (Annex IV), preservatives (Annex VI), and UV filters (Annex VII) in cosmetic products. If an ingredient is to be used for one of these three functions, then it must appear on the appropriate annexe. Ingredients within the annexes are subject to individual restrictions such as limitations in field of use, concentration limits, and warning statements.

TABLE 1 Sample Extract of an Annex III Entry

Substance	Field of application/use	Maximum authorized concentration in the finished product	Conditions of use and warnings which must be printed on the label
Hydrogen peroxide, and other compounds or mixtures that release hydrogen peroxide, including carbamide peroxide and zinc peroxide	Skin care preparations	4% of H_2O_2 present or released	Contains hydrogen peroxide Avoid contact with eyes Rinse eyes immediately if product comes into contact with them

2.4.4   Changes to the Annexes

There is a process in place within the European Commission for updating the ingredient annexes to reflect progress in technical knowledge. Scientific support to this process is given by a body of independent academic experts known as the Scientific Committee on Cosmetics and Non-Food Products intended for Consumers. Activity can be initiated by member state governments or by industry via the European Cosmetics Industry Trade Association (COLIPA).

2.5   Impact on Selection of Potential Ingredients

The logic flows used when assessing a potential ingredient against the annexes of the cosmetics directive are as follows:

> A substance may be used as an ingredient in a cosmetic product for purposes other than as a colorant, preservative, or UV filter provided that it is not banned by inclusion in annexe II or restricted for intended purpose by annexe III and that the product is safe.
>
> A substance may only be used as an ingredient in a cosmetic product as a colorant, preservative, or UV filter if it appears in the appropriate annexe and the product is safe.

3   OVERVIEW OF CONTROL OF COSMETIC PRODUCTS IN THE UNITED STATES

Cosmetics marketed in the United States are regulated under the federal Food, Drug and Cosmetic Act (FD&C Act) [9] and the Fair Packaging and Labeling Act (FPLA) [9].

The FD&C Act defines cosmetics as articles intended to be applied to the human body for cleansing, beautifying, promoting attractiveness, or altering the appearance without affecting the body's structure or functions. Included in this definition are moisturizing skin creams and lotions and any material intended for use as a component of a cosmetic product. As in the European Union there is no premarketing approval process for cosmetic products, and the person placing the product on the market carries responsibility for the safety of the product.

With the exception of color additives and a few prohibited ingredients, any raw material may be used as a cosmetic ingredient without prior approval. The law requires that color additives used in food, drugs, and cosmetics must be tested for safety and approved by the FDA for their intended uses. The color additives approved for use in cosmetics are listed at 21 CFR 73, 74, and 82 [9]. The use of the following ingredients is either restricted or prohibited in cosmetics: bithionol, mercury compounds, vinyl chloride, halogenated salicylanilides, zirconium complexes in aerosol cosmetics, chloroform, methylene chloride, chlorofluorocarbon propellants, and hexa-chlorophene.

4   OVERVIEW OF CONTROL OF COSMETIC PRODUCTS IN JAPAN

Products which are typically considered to be cosmetics in Europe are regulated under two separate systems in Japan. Product claims which the authorities consider to be more active are classified as "quasi-drugs". In terms of skin products these include those skin lotions making specific claims in areas such as chapping and roughness, prevention of razor burn, keeping the skin healthy, and supplying the skin with moisture. In order to make such a claim, the product must contain a quasi-drug active which has been approved for that specific class of product and must only make claims in the area defined within the quasi-drug regulations [12]. It should be noted that once preapproved by the authorities for marketing, quasi-drugs can be sold freely through retail outlets.

Control of general cosmetic products was deregulated in Japan from 1 April 2001, moving away from the previous system which imposed tight restrictions on which ingredients could be used for each type of product toward a system where internationally accepted ingredients can be used. Major changes to the regulatory system include abolition of the premarket approval system, the adoption of ingredient labeling, and the implementation of positive lists for UV filters, colors, and preservatives. Although implementation is still at an early stage, most cosmetic ingredients will be freely available for use in Japan. These new regulations cover ordinary skin lotions making general skin moisturization claims. Details of these new cosmetic regulations which contain ingredient lists, rules for prior approval of products containing ingredients not on the lists, and new labeling requirements have been published by the Japanese authorities [13].

5   SUMMARY

Products making simple skin moisturization claims only are generally classified as cosmetics around the world. Regulations controlling cosmetics are currently in a state of evolution across the world, moving generally in the direction of a harmonized system based upon the general principles of regulation in the European Union as follows:

A standard definition of cosmetic products which clearly delineates them from drugs and foods

An illustrative list of product types, e.g., creams, face masks, toilet soaps, perfumes, etc.

No borderline categories between cosmetics and other product types

Responsibility for product safety clearly with the manufacturer and/or marketer

Clear restriction of certain ingredients

Standardization of cosmetic Good Manufacturing Practice

Appropriate labeling to ensure safe use of products
Use of in-market control to verify fraud or negligence
Standardization of minimum labeling requirements
Ingredient labeling using INCI
Scientifically valid system for restricting and banning ingredients for use in
   cosmetic products
System for regular updating of restrictions

Good progress against these principles is already being made in many countries around the world and every step toward harmonization facilitates supply to the consumer of safer and more innovative cosmetic products. However, the challenge presented to industry by these rapid changes to industry is to stay abreast of the current situation, predict short-term changes, and work with regulators during regulatory transition to assure that products meet the regulations in all target markets.

REFERENCES

1. Council Directive 76/768/EEC of 27 July 1976 on the approximation of the laws of the Member States relating to cosmetic products. Official Journal L 262, 27/09/1976 P. 0169.
2. Council Directive 65/65/EEC of 26 January 1965 on the approximation of provisions laid down by law, regulation or administrative action relating to proprietary medicinal products. Official Journal B 022, 09/02/1965, pp. 0369–0373.
3. Council Directive 93/35/EEC of 14 June 1993 amending for the sixth time Directive 76/768/EEC on the approximation of the laws of the member states relating to cosmetic products. Official Journal L 151, 23/06/1993, pp. 0032–0037.
4. Council Directive 93/35/EEC of 14 June 1993 amending for the sixth time Directive 76/768/EEC on the approximation of the laws of the Member States relating to cosmetic products. Official Journal L 151, 23/06/1993, pp. 0032–0037.
5. Council Directive 67/548/EEC of 27 June 1967 on the approximation of laws, regulations and administrative provisions relating to the classification, packaging and labelling of dangerous substances. Official Journal B 196, 16/08/1967, pp. 0001–0005.
6. EINECS Volumes I and II. Notice number 90/C 146A/01. Official Journal C146A, Volume 33, 15 June 1990.
7. Third Publication of ELINGS. Notice numbers 93/C 130/01 and 93/C 130/02. Official Journal C130, Volume 36, 10 May 1993.
8. Council Directive 92/32/EEC of 30 April 1992 amending for the seventh time Directive 67/548/EEC on the approximation of the laws, regulations and administrative provisions relating to the classification, packaging and labelling of dangerous substances. Official Journal L 154, 05/06/1992, pp. 0001–0029.
9. Code of Federal Regulations, Title 21.
10. PAB Notification No. 44, February 8, 1961; No. 287, July 17, 1961; and No. 470, November 18, 1961.
11. Pharmaceutical Publication No. 990, MHW Ordinances 125, 330, and 331, Medical Safety Bureau of the Ministry of Health and Welfare, September 29, 2000

Index